Novel Biomarkers for Heart Disease

Novel Biomarkers for Heart Disease

Editor

Michael Lichtenauer

MDPI • Basel • Beijing • Wuhan • Barcelona • Belgrade • Manchester • Tokyo • Cluj • Tianjin

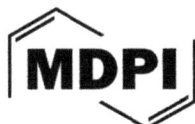

Editor
Michael Lichtenauer
Paracelsus Medical University Salzburg
Austria;
Department of Internal Medicine II,
University Clinic Salzburg
Austria

Editorial Office
MDPI
St. Alban-Anlage 66
4052 Basel, Switzerland

This is a reprint of articles from the Special Issue published online in the open access journal *Journal of Clinical Medicine* (ISSN 2077-0383) (available at: https://www.mdpi.com/journal/jcm/special_issues/Biomarker_Heart_Disease).

For citation purposes, cite each article independently as indicated on the article page online and as indicated below:

LastName, A.A.; LastName, B.B.; LastName, C.C. Article Title. *Journal Name* **Year**, *Volume Number*, Page Range.

ISBN 978-3-03943-883-9 (Hbk)
ISBN 978-3-03943-884-6 (PDF)

Cover image courtesy of Michael Lichtenauer.

© 2020 by the authors. Articles in this book are Open Access and distributed under the Creative Commons Attribution (CC BY) license, which allows users to download, copy and build upon published articles, as long as the author and publisher are properly credited, which ensures maximum dissemination and a wider impact of our publications.
The book as a whole is distributed by MDPI under the terms and conditions of the Creative Commons license CC BY-NC-ND.

Contents

About the Editor ix

Peter Jirak, Moritz Mirna, Bernhard Wernly, Vera Paar, Uta C. Hoppe and Michael Lichtenauer
Assessment of Cardiac Remodeling—A Chance for Novel Cardiac Biomarkers?
Reprinted from: *J. Clin. Med.* **2020**, *9*, 2087, doi:10.3390/jcm9072087 1

Peter Jirak, Rudin Pistulli, Michael Lichtenauer, Bernhard Wernly, Vera Paar, Lukas J. Motloch, Richard Rezar, Christian Jung, Uta C. Hoppe, P. Christian Schulze, Daniel Kretzschmar, Rüdiger C. Braun-Dullaeus and Tarek Bekfani
Expression of the Novel Cardiac Biomarkers sST2, GDF-15, suPAR, and H-FABP in HFpEF Patients Compared to ICM, DCM, and Controls
Reprinted from: *J. Clin. Med.* **2020**, *9*, 1130, doi:10.3390/jcm9041130 5

David Niederseer, Sarah Wernly, Sebastian Bachmayer, Bernhard Wernly, Adam Bakula, Ursula Huber-Schönauer, Georg Semmler, Christian Schmied, Elmar Aigner and Christian Datz
Diagnosis of Non-Alcoholic Fatty Liver Disease (NAFLD) Is Independently Associated with Cardiovascular Risk in a Large Austrian Screening Cohort
Reprinted from: *J. Clin. Med.* **2020**, *9*, 1065, doi:10.3390/jcm9041065 17

Isabel Galeano-Otero, Raquel Del Toro, Agustín Guisado, Ignacio Díaz, Isabel Mayoral-González, Francisco Guerrero-Márquez, Encarnación Gutiérrez-Carretero, Sara Casquero-Domínguez, Luis Díaz-de la Llera, Gonzalo Barón-Esquivias, Manuel Jiménez-Navarro, Tarik Smani and Antonio Ordóñez-Fernández
Circulating miR-320a as a Predictive Biomarker for Left Ventricular Remodelling in STEMI Patients Undergoing Primary Percutaneous Coronary Intervention
Reprinted from: *J. Clin. Med.* **2020**, *9*, 1051, doi:10.3390/jcm9041051 27

Moritz Mirna, Albert Topf, Bernhard Wernly, Richard Rezar, Vera Paar, Christian Jung, Hermann Salmhofer, Kristen Kopp, Uta C. Hoppe, P. Christian Schulze, Daniel Kretzschmar, Markus P. Schneider, Ulla T. Schultheiss, Claudia Sommerer, Katharina Paul, Gunter Wolf, Michael Lichtenauer and Martin Busch
Novel Biomarkers in Patients with Chronic Kidney Disease: An Analysis of Patients Enrolled in the GCKD-Study
Reprinted from: *J. Clin. Med.* **2020**, *9*, 886, doi:10.3390/jcm9030886 47

Anna Klimiuk, Anna Zalewska, Robert Sawicki, Małgorzata Knapp and Mateusz Maciejczyk
Salivary Oxidative Stress Increases with the Progression of Chronic Heart Failure
Reprinted from: *J. Clin. Med.* **2020**, *9*, 769, doi:10.3390/jcm9030769 65

Naufal Zagidullin, Lukas J. Motloch, Diana Gareeva, Aysilu Hamitova, Irina Lakman, Ilja Krioni, Denis Popov, Rustem Zulkarneev, Vera Paar, Kristen Kopp, Peter Jirak, Vladimir Ishmetov, Uta C. Hoppe, Eduard Tulbaev and Valentin Pavlov
Combining Novel Biomarkers for Risk Stratification of Two-Year Cardiovascular Mortality in Patients with ST-Elevation Myocardial Infarction
Reprinted from: *J. Clin. Med.* **2020**, *9*, 550, doi:10.3390/jcm9020550 87

Hiroyuki Naruse, Junnichi Ishii, Hiroshi Takahashi, Fumihiko Kitagawa, Hideto Nishimura, Hideki Kawai, Takashi Muramatsu, Masahide Harada, Akira Yamada, Wakaya Fujiwara, Mutsuharu Hayashi, Sadako Motoyama, Masayoshi Sarai, Eiichi Watanabe, Hideo Izawa and Yukio Ozaki
Urinary Liver-Type Fatty-Acid-Binding Protein Predicts Long-Term Adverse Outcomes in Medical Cardiac Intensive Care Units
Reprinted from: *J. Clin. Med.* **2020**, *9*, 482, doi:10.3390/jcm9020482 103

Erik Nilsson, Jens Kastrup, Ahmad Sajadieh, Gorm Boje Jensen, Erik Kjøller, Hans Jørn Kolmos, Jonas Wuopio, Christoph Nowak, Anders Larsson, Janus Christian Jakobsen, Per Winkel, Christian Gluud, Kasper K Iversen, Johan Ärnlöv and Axel C. Carlsson
Pregnancy Associated Plasma Protein-A as a Cardiovascular Risk Marker in Patients with Stable Coronary Heart Disease During 10 Years Follow-Up—A CLARICOR Trial Sub-Study
Reprinted from: *J. Clin. Med.* **2020**, *9*, 265, doi:10.3390/jcm9010265 115

Elke Bouwens, Victor J. van den Berg, K. Martijn Akkerhuis, Sara J. Baart, Kadir Caliskan, Jasper J. Brugts, Henk Mouthaan, Jan van Ramshorst, Tjeerd Germans, Victor A. W. M. Umans, Eric Boersma and Isabella Kardys
Circulating Biomarkers of Cell Adhesion Predict Clinical Outcome in Patients with Chronic Heart Failure
Reprinted from: *J. Clin. Med.* **2020**, *9*, 195, doi:10.3390/jcm9010195 127

Kuang-Fu Chang, Gigin Lin, Pei-Ching Huang, Yu-Hsiang Juan, Chao-Hung Wang, Shang-Yueh Tsai, Yu-Ching Lin, Ming-Ting Wu, Pen-An Liao, Lan-Yan Yang, Min-Hui Liu, Yu-Chun Lin, Jiun-Jie Wang, Koon-Kwan Ng and Shu-Hang Ng
Left Ventricular Function and Myocardial Triglyceride Content on 3T Cardiac MR Predict Major Cardiovascular Adverse Events and Readmission in Patients Hospitalized with Acute Heart Failure
Reprinted from: *J. Clin. Med.* **2020**, *9*, 169, doi:10.3390/jcm9010169 143

Ewa Romuk, Wojciech Jacheć, Ewa Zbrojkiewicz, Alina Mroczek, Jacek Niedziela, Mariusz Gąsior, Piotr Rozentryt and Celina Wojciechowska
Ceruloplasmin, NT-proBNP, and Clinical Data as Risk Factors of Death or Heart Transplantation in a 1-Year Follow-Up of Heart Failure Patients
Reprinted from: *J. Clin. Med.* **2020**, *9*, 137, doi:10.3390/jcm9010137 159

Alexandre Meloux, Luc Rochette, Maud Maza, Florence Bichat, Laura Tribouillard, Yves Cottin, Marianne Zeller and Catherine Vergely
Growth Differentiation Factor-8 (GDF8)/Myostatin Is a Predictor of Troponin I Peak and a Marker of Clinical Severity after Acute Myocardial Infarction
Reprinted from: *J. Clin. Med.* **2020**, *9*, 116, doi:10.3390/jcm9010116 175

Radka Kočková, Hana Línková, Zuzana Hlubocká, Alena Pravečková, Andrea Polednová, Lucie Súkupová, Martin Bláha, Jiří Malý, Eva Honsová, David Sedmera and Martin Pěnička
New Imaging Markers of Clinical Outcome in Asymptomatic Patients with Severe Aortic Regurgitation
Reprinted from: *J. Clin. Med.* **2019**, *8*, 1654, doi:10.3390/jcm8101654 185

Stasė Gasiulė, Vaidotas Stankevičius, Vaiva Patamsytė, Raimundas Ražanskas, Giedrius Žukovas, Žana Kapustina, Diana Žaliaduonytė, Rimantas Benetis, Vaiva Lesauskaitė and Giedrius Vilkaitis
Tissue-Specific miRNAs Regulate the Development of Thoracic Aortic Aneurysm: The Emerging Role of KLF4 Network
Reprinted from: *J. Clin. Med.* **2019**, *8*, 1609, doi:10.3390/jcm8101609 199

Toshiaki Nakajima, Ikuko Shibasaki, Tatsuya Sawaguchi, Akiko Haruyama, Hiroyuki Kaneda, Takafumi Nakajima, Takaaki Hasegawa, Takuo Arikawa, Syotaro Obi, Masashi Sakuma, Hironaga Ogawa, Shigeru Toyoda, Fumitaka Nakamura, Shichiro Abe, Hirotsugu Fukuda and Teruo Inoue
Growth Differentiation Factor-15 (GDF-15) Is a Biomarker of Muscle Wasting and Renal Dysfunction in Preoperative Cardiovascular Surgery Patients
Reprinted from: *J. Clin. Med.* **2019**, *8*, 1576, doi:10.3390/jcm8101576 215

Josip A. Borovac, Duska Glavas, Zora Susilovic Grabovac, Daniela Supe Domic, Domenico D'Amario and Josko Bozic
Catestatin in Acutely Decompensated Heart Failure Patients: Insights from the CATSTAT-HF Study
Reprinted from: *J. Clin. Med.* **2019**, *8*, 1132, doi:10.3390/jcm8081132 231

Daniel Dalos, Georg Spinka, Matthias Schneider, Bernhard Wernly, Vera Paar, Uta Hoppe, Brigitte Litschauer, Jeanette Strametz-Juranek and Michael Sponder
New Cardiovascular Biomarkers in Ischemic Heart Disease—GDF-15, A Probable Predictor for Ejection Fraction
Reprinted from: *J. Clin. Med.* **2019**, *8*, 924, doi:10.3390/jcm8070924 249

Yi-Lin Shiou, Hsin-Ting Lin, Liang-Yin Ke, Bin-Nan Wu, Shyi-Jang Shin, Chu-Huang Chen, Wei-Chung Tsai, Chih-Sheng Chu and Hsiang-Chun Lee
Very Low-Density Lipoproteins of Metabolic Syndrome Modulates STIM1, Suppresses Store-Operated Calcium Entry, and Deranges Myofilament Proteins in Atrial Myocytes
Reprinted from: *J. Clin. Med.* **2019**, *8*, 881, doi:10.3390/jcm8060881 261

Yi-Cheng Chang, Shih-Che Hua, Chia-Hsuin Chang, Wei-Yi Kao, Hsiao-Lin Lee, Lee-Ming Chuang, Yen-Tsung Huang and Mei-Shu Lai
High TSH Level within Normal Range Is Associated with Obesity, Dyslipidemia, Hypertension, Inflammation, Hypercoagulability, and the Metabolic Syndrome: A Novel Cardiometabolic Marker
Reprinted from: *J. Clin. Med.* **2019**, *8*, 817, doi:10.3390/jcm8060817 277

David de Gonzalo-Calvo, David Viladés, Pablo Martínez-Camblor, Àngela Vea, Andreu Ferrero-Gregori, Laura Nasarre, Olga Bornachea, Jesus Sanchez Vega, Rubén Leta, Núria Puig, Sonia Benítez, Jose Luis Sanchez-Quesada, Francesc Carreras and Vicenta Llorente-Cortés
Plasma microRNA Profiling Reveals Novel Biomarkers of Epicardial Adipose Tissue: A Multidetector Computed Tomography Study
Reprinted from: *J. Clin. Med.* **2019**, *8*, 780, doi:10.3390/jcm8060780 293

Weronika Bulska-Będkowska, Elżbieta Chełmecka, Aleksander J. Owczarek, Katarzyna Mizia-Stec, Andrzej Witek, Aleksandra Szybalska, Tomasz Grodzicki, Magdalena Olszanecka-Glinianowicz and Jerzy Chudek
CA125 as a Marker of Heart Failure in the Older Women: A Population-Based Analysis
Reprinted from: *J. Clin. Med.* **2019**, *8*, 607, doi:10.3390/jcm8050607 313

Margaret A. Drazba, Ida Holásková, Nadine R. Sahyoun and Melissa Ventura Marra
Associations of Adiposity and Diet Quality with Serum Ceramides in Middle-Aged Adults with Cardiovascular Risk Factors
Reprinted from: *J. Clin. Med.* **2019**, *8*, 527, doi:10.3390/jcm8040527 325

Zornitsa Shomanova, Bernhard Ohnewein, Christiane Schernthaner, Killian Höfer, Christian A. Pogoda, Gerrit Frommeyer, Bernhard Wernly, Mathias C. Brandt, Anna-Maria Dieplinger, Holger Reinecke, Uta C. Hoppe, Bernhard Strohmer, Rudin Pistulli and Lukas J. Motloch
Classic and Novel Biomarkers as Potential Predictors of Ventricular Arrhythmias and Sudden Cardiac Death
Reprinted from: *J. Clin. Med.* **2020**, *9*, 578, doi:10.3390/jcm9020578 339

Abrar Alfatni, Marianne Riou, Anne-Laure Charles, Alain Meyer, Cindy Barnig, Emmanuel Andres, Anne Lejay, Samy Talha and Bernard Geny
Peripheral Blood Mononuclear Cells and Platelets Mitochondrial Dysfunction, Oxidative Stress, and Circulating mtDNA in Cardiovascular Diseases
Reprinted from: *J. Clin. Med.* **2020**, *9*, 311, doi:10.3390/jcm9020311 371

Richard Rezar, Peter Jirak, Martha Gschwandtner, Rupert Derler, Thomas K. Felder, Michael Haslinger, Kristen Kopp, Clemens Seelmaier, Christina Granitz, Uta C. Hoppe and Michael Lichtenauer
Heart-Type Fatty Acid-Binding Protein (H-FABP) and Its Role as a Biomarker in Heart Failure: What Do We Know So Far?
Reprinted from: *J. Clin. Med.* **2020**, *9*, 164, doi:10.3390/jcm9010164 395

About the Editor

Michael Lichtenauer was born in Vienna, Austria. He attended primary and secondary school in Vienna's 19th district and finished his Matura exams in 2003 with distinction. After serving his civilian service in the years 2003 and 2004, he registered himself as a student in human medicine at the Medical University Vienna in autumn 2004. He started his career in biomedical sciences in 2006 when he joined a research group at the Department of Cardio-Thoracic Surgery at the Medical University Vienna. Shortly after, he was assigned a research project focusing on regenerative medicine that investigated the positive influence of apoptotic cells in an animal model of acute myocardial infarction. In a follow-up project, he analyzed the effects of apoptotic cells on cellular protective signaling mechanism leading to a reduction in the damage caused by myocardial infarction in a small and large animal model. In his PhD thesis, he described these protective effects which were primarily attributed to soluble ("paracrine") mediators release by apoptotic cell. After earning his degree in human medicine in 2010, he started his residency in Internal Medicine and Cardiology at the Friedrich Schiller University Jena, Germany (Head: Prof. Figulla). In 2010, he was awarded the First Prize in Basic Science for his research on cell protective mechanisms at the annual meeting of the Austrian Society of Cardiology in Salzburg. In 2012, he finished his PhD thesis and was nominated researcher of the month at the Medical University of Vienna. At the University of Jena, he joined the research group of Prof. Christian Jung and focused on biomarker research in cardiovascular diseases and prevention. In 2014, he returned to Austria and continued his residency in Internal Medicine and Cardiology at the University Hospital Salzburg (Head. Prof. Hoppe). A year later, he filed his application for the venia docendi (Habilitation) at the Paracelsus Medical University. In 2017, he finished his residency and is has been employed as consultant physician since then. In 2019, Dr. Lichtenauer was summoned as Associate Professor in Internal Medicine at the Paracelsus Medical University. He has been awarded national and internal prizes of the scientific community, is acting as a reviewer for international peer-reviewed journals, and is involved in the organization the curriculum of Human Medicine at the Paracelsus Medical University. Furthermore, he holds multiple memberships of national and international medical associations and societies.

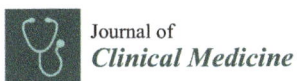 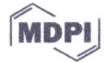

Editorial

Assessment of Cardiac Remodeling—A Chance for Novel Cardiac Biomarkers?

Peter Jirak, Moritz Mirna, Bernhard Wernly, Vera Paar, Uta C. Hoppe and Michael Lichtenauer *

Department of Internal Medicine II, Division of Cardiology, Paracelsus Medical University Salzburg, 5020 Salzburg, Austria; p.jirak@salk.at (P.J.); m.mirna@salk.at (M.M.); b.wernly@salk.at (B.W.); v.paar@salk.at (V.P.); u.hoppe@salk.at (U.C.H.)
* Correspondence: m.lichtenauer@salk.at; Tel.: +43-57855-57130

Received: 21 June 2020; Accepted: 29 June 2020; Published: 3 July 2020

1. Background

Biomarkers are defined as "cellular, biochemical or molecular alterations that are measurable in biological media such as human tissues, cells, or fluids", providing "biological characteristics that can be objectively measured and evaluated as an indicator of normal biological processes, pathogenic processes, or pharmacological responses to a therapeutic intervention "according to Hulka et al. as well as Naylor et al. [1,2]. Depending on their respective role in physiologic and pathophysiologic processes, biomarkers can be used for different purposes such as disease diagnosis, risk stratification, screening, as well as prognosis [2]. In recent decades, biomarkers have gained major clinical significance, especially in the cardiovascular field. Above all, the introduction of natriuretic peptides and highly sensitive troponin assays have led to significant facilitation and improvement in clinical practice.

However, while these markers represent indispensable diagnostic tools in clinical routines, their prognostic impact remains limited. Accordingly, the evaluation of prognosis remains a clinical challenge, even to date. In contrast to the aforementioned markers, novel biomarkers targeting the critical factors for prognosis and outcomes in cardiovascular disease, cardiac fibrosis, and remodeling could be of additional value on this account [3,4]. Cardiac remodeling: The term cardiac remodeling describes changes in the size; mass; geometry; and, consequently, function of the heart in response to acute and chronic myocardial damage [5]. While acute myocardial damage is usually induced by ischemic processes such as myocardial infarction, chronic damage comprises inflammatory processes, dysregulated metabolic pathways, toxic damage, as well as a chronic increase in cardiac strain [6–8].

Interestingly, in contrast to natriuretic peptides as well as troponin, most novel heart failure biomarkers do not provide a comparable amount of organ specificity [9,10]. However, due to their involvement in multiple pathophysiologic processes, novel cardiac biomarkers represent promising tools to refine the assessment of cardiac remodeling and fibrosis and thus also of prognosis [4,11].

2. sST2

The most promising marker on this regard represents soluble suppression of tumorigenicity 2 (sST2), which has also found entrance into current guidelines to some extent. sST2 represents a versatile marker, predominantly used in heart failure patients [12]. sST2 was shown to be elevated in acute and chronic heart failure as well as in acute coronary syndrome [13,14]. Besides, elevated levels have also been reported in pulmonary hypertension and peripheral artery disease, emphasizing its involvement in different disease entities [15,16].

Regarding its molecular background, two different isoforms have been identified, a soluble form (sST2) and a membrane-bound form (ST2L) [17]. Interleukin-33 (IL-33) represents the only known ligand for ST2 and is responsible for the induction of cardioprotective effects by binding to the ST2L receptor [17]. Besides, IL-33 is also involved in immunomodulation through the secretion and the interaction of T helper 2 (TH2) cells, mast cells, group 2 innate lymphoid cells, (ILC2s) regulatory T (Treg) cells, TH1 cells, CD8+ T cells, and natural killer (NK) cells, among others, further elucidating the involvement of sST2 and ST2L in inflammatory processes [18]. On the other hand, sST2 can counteract the cardioprotective effects by acting as a decoy receptor for IL-33 [17]. Hence, an increase in sST2 results in a decrease of cardioprotective IL-33, consequently leading to cardiac damage and increased cardiac strain [17].

In short, sST2 incorporates different pathophysiological processes involved in cardiac remodeling and fibrosis such as inflammation and increased cardiac strain. Accordingly, sST2 represents a promising new marker in the assessment of prognosis of heart failure patients. sST2 was shown to predict all-cause mortality as well as cardiovascular mortality in chronic heart failure patients [19]. Additionally, sST2 was reported to predict mortality in acute heart failure [11]. With regards to therapy monitoring, an sST2 cut-off below 35-ng/mL was proposed to significantly improve outcomes in heart failure patients (Pres-ageassay, Critical Diagnostics, SanDiego, California, USA) [19].

3. microRNAs

While sST2 has already found entrance into current guidelines, the field of microRNAs (miRNAs) is currently limited to investigative research, although previous trials have reported promising results regarding their diagnostic and therapeutic applicability in cardiovascular disease entities. MiRNAs comprise a group of small (19–24 nucleotides) ribonucleic acids (RNAs), which play a pivotal role in posttranslational gene silencing (PTGS) and hence regulation of protein synthesis [20,21]. In recent studies, several miRNAs were found to be involved in cardiac remodeling by promoting myocardial inflammation, as well as pro-fibrotic and -apoptotic pathways. Consequently, patients with acute and chronic heart failure show dysregulated plasma concentrations of various pathological miRNAs, which gives rise to novel diagnostic approaches in these patients. For example, Ovchinnikova et al. recently identified several significantly dysregulated miRNAs (miR-18a-5p, miR-26b-5p, miR-27a-3p, miR-30e-5p, miR-106a-5p, miR-199a-3p, and miR-652-3p) in acute heart failure (AHF), which were also associated with adverse outcomes in these patients [22]. Furthermore, another trial reported that a combination of miR-30c, miR-221, miR-328, and miR-375 could adequately discriminate heart failure with preserved ejection fraction (HFpEF) from heart failure with reduced ejection fraction (HFrEF) [23], which is to this extent not possible using conventional cardiovascular biomarkers [24]. Consequently, analysis of the miRNA expression pattern ("miRNome") could provide substantial additional information in the clinical management of patients with HF in the future.

Besides their application in diagnostics, miRNAs also constitute interesting targets for novel therapeutic approaches. Since myocardial inflammation and cardiac fibrosis are considered potentially reversible processes in the course of cardiac remodeling, miRNAs interacting with these pathways represent promising targets in the management of patients with HF. For example, miR-21 was found to enhance myocardial fibrosis by targeting the extracellular signal-regulated kinase (ERK)–mitogen-activated protein (MAP) kinase pathway, and silencing of miR-21 by synthetic antagonist significantly attenuated myocardial fibrosis in an animal model [25]. Since miR-21 was also found to be involved in myocardial inflammation by targeting T-cell development, it constitutes an interesting drug target in the management of HF and certainly warrants further investigation in future studies.

4. Conclusions

Despite the long time period since the establishment of natriuretic peptides and troponin in clinical practice, the evaluation of prognosis in cardiovascular disease remains challenging. The assessment of cardiac remodeling and fibrosis with the help of novel biomarkers represents a promising approach for a more sophisticated evaluation of prognosis and consequently also therapy guiding. In this regard, their versatility regarding their involvement in numerous different organ systems might be a considerable benefit over natriuretic peptides and troponin with regards to their prognostic value. As cardiac remodeling is strongly correlated with a worse prognosis in cardiovascular disease, the implementation of biomarkers addressing this issue holds great potential to improve outcomes further.

Funding: This research received no external funding.

Conflicts of Interest: The authors declare no conflict of interest.

References

1. Hulka, B.S.; Wilcosky, T.C.; Griffith, J.D.; Rynard, S.M. Biological markers in epidemiology. *Am. J. Hum. Biol.* **1990**, *3*.
2. Naylor, S. Biomarkers: Current perspectives and future prospects. *Expert Rev. Mol. Diagn.* **2003**, *3*, 525–529. [CrossRef]
3. Lichtenauer, M.; Jirak, P.; Wernly, B.; Paar, V.; Rohm, I.; Jung, C.; Schernthaner, C.; Kraus, J.; Motloch, L.J.; Yilmaz, A.; et al. A comparative analysis of novel cardiovascular biomarkers in patients with chronic heart failure. *Eur. J. Intern. Med.* **2017**, *44*, 31–38. [CrossRef]
4. Zagidullin, N.; Motloch, L.J.; Gareeva, D.; Hamitova, A.; Lakman, I.; Krioni, I.; Popov, D.; Zulkarneev, R.; Paar, V.; Kopp, K.; et al. Combining Novel Biomarkers for Risk Stratification of Two-Year Cardiovascular Mortality in Patients with ST-Elevation Myocardial Infarction. *J. Clin. Med.* **2020**, *9*, 550. [CrossRef] [PubMed]
5. Azevedo, P.S.; Polegato, B.F.; Minicucci, M.F.; Paiva, S.A.; Zornoff, L.A. Cardiac Remodeling: Concepts, Clinical Impact, Pathophysiological Mechanisms and Pharmacologic Treatment. *Arq. Bras. Cardiol.* **2016**, *106*, 62–69. [CrossRef]
6. Talman, V.; Ruskoaho, H. Cardiac fibrosis in myocardial infarction-from repair and remodeling to regeneration. *Cell Tissue Res.* **2016**, *365*, 563–581. [CrossRef] [PubMed]
7. Li, L.; Zhao, Q.; Kong, W. Extracellular matrix remodeling and cardiac fibrosis. *Matrix Biol.* **2018**, *69*, 490–506. [CrossRef]
8. Nakamura, M.; Sadoshima, J. Mechanisms of physiological and pathological cardiac hypertrophy. *Nat. Rev. Cardiol.* **2018**, *15*, 387–407. [CrossRef]
9. Savic-Radojevic, A.; Pljesa-Ercegovac, M.; Matic, M.; Simic, D.; Radovanovic, S.; Simic, T. Novel Biomarkers of Heart Failure. *Adv. Clin. Chem.* **2017**, *79*, 93–152.
10. Correale, M.; Monaco, I.; Brunetti, N.D.; Di Biase, M.; Metra, M.; Nodari, S.; Butler, J.; Gheorghiade, M. Redefining biomarkers in heart failure. *Heart Fail. Rev.* **2018**, *23*, 237–253. [CrossRef]
11. Aimo, A.; Januzzi, J.L., Jr.; Bayes-Genis, A.; Vergaro, G.; Sciarrone, P.; Passino, C.; Emdin, M. Clinical and Prognostic Significance of sST2 in Heart Failure: JACC Review Topic of the Week. *J. Am. Coll. Cardiol.* **2019**, *74*, 2193–2203. [CrossRef] [PubMed]
12. McCarthy, C.P.; Januzzi, J.L., Jr. Soluble ST2 in Heart Failure. *Heart Fail. Clin.* **2018**, *14*, 41–48. [CrossRef] [PubMed]
13. Jenkins, W.S.; Roger, V.L.; Jaffe, A.S.; Weston, S.A.; AbouEzzeddine, O.F.; Jiang, R.; Manemann, S.M.; Enriquez-Sarano, M. Prognostic Value of Soluble ST2 After Myocardial Infarction: A Community Perspective. *Am. J. Med.* **2017**, *130*, 23. [CrossRef]
14. Pascual-Figal, D.A.; Lax, A.; Perez-Martinez, M.T.; del Carmen Asensio-Lopez, M.; Sanchez-Mas, J. Clinical relevance of sST2 in cardiac diseases. *Clin. Chem. Lab. Med.* **2016**, *54*, 29–35. [CrossRef] [PubMed]
15. Jirak, P.; Mirna, M.; Wernly, B.; Paar, V.; Thieme, M.; Betge, S.; Franz, M.; Hoppe, U.; Lauten, A.; Kammler, J.; et al. Analysis of novel cardiovascular biomarkers in patients with peripheral artery disease (PAD). *Minerva Med.* **2018**, *109*, 443. [CrossRef]
16. Mirna, M.; Rohm, I.; Jirak, P.; Wernly, B.; Baz, L.; Paar, V.; Kretzschmar, D.; Hoppe, U.C.; Schulze, P.C.; Lichtenauer, M.; et al. Analysis of Novel Cardiovascular Biomarkers in Patients with Pulmonary Hypertension (PH). *Heart Lung Circ.* **2020**, *29*, 337–344. [CrossRef]
17. Kakkar, R.; Lee, R.T. The IL-33/ST2 pathway: Therapeutic target and novel biomarker. *Nat. Rev. Drug Discov.* **2008**, *7*, 827–840. [CrossRef]
18. Cayrol, C.; Girard, J.P. Interleukin-33 (IL-33): A nuclear cytokine from the IL-1 family. *Immunol. Rev.* **2018**, *281*, 154–168. [CrossRef]

19. Aimo, A.; Vergaro, G.; Passino, C.; Ripoli, A.; Ky, B.; Miller, W.L.; Bayes-Genis, A.; Anand, I.; Januzzi, J.L.; Emdin, M. Prognostic Value of Soluble Suppression of Tumorigenicity-2 in Chronic Heart Failure: A Meta-Analysis. *JACC Heart Fail.* **2017**, *5*, 280–286. [CrossRef]
20. Kim, S.; Song, M.L.; Min, H.; Hwang, I.; Baek, S.K.; Kwon, T.K.; Park, J.W. miRNA biogenesis-associated RNase III nucleases Drosha and Dicer are upregulated in colorectal adenocarcinoma. *Oncol. Lett.* **2017**, *14*, 4379–4383. [CrossRef]
21. Mohr, A.M.; Mott, J.L. Overview of microRNA biology. *Semin. Liver Dis.* **2015**, *35*, 3–11. [CrossRef] [PubMed]
22. Ovchinnikova, E.S.; Schmitter, D.; Vegter, E.L.; Ter Maaten, J.M.; Valente, M.A.; Liu, L.C.; van der Harst, P.; Pinto, Y.M.; de Boer, R.A.; Meyer, S.; et al. Signature of circulating microRNAs in patients with acute heart failure. *Eur. J. Heart Fail.* **2016**, *18*, 414–423. [CrossRef] [PubMed]
23. Watson, C.J.; Gupta, S.K.; O'Connell, E.; Thum, S.; Glezeva, N.; Fendrich, J.; Gallagher, J.; Ledwidge, M.; Grote-Levi, L.; McDonald, K.; et al. MicroRNA signatures differentiate preserved from reduced ejection fraction heart failure. *Eur. J. Heart Fail.* **2015**, *17*, 405–415. [CrossRef] [PubMed]
24. Jirak, P.; Pistulli, R.; Lichtenauer, M.; Wernly, B.; Paar, V.; Motloch, L.J.; Rezar, R.; Jung, C.; Hoppe, U.C.; Schulze, P.C.; et al. Expression of the Novel Cardiac Biomarkers sST2, GDF-15, suPAR, and H-FABP in HFpEF Patients Compared to ICM, DCM, and Controls. *J. Clin. Med.* **2020**, *9*, 1130. [CrossRef] [PubMed]
25. Thum, T.; Gross, C.; Fiedler, J.; Fischer, T.; Kissler, S.; Bussen, M.; Galuppo, P.; Just, S.; Rottbauer, W.; Frantz, S.; et al. MicroRNA-21 contributes to myocardial disease by stimulating MAP kinase signalling in fibroblasts. *Nature* **2008**, *456*, 980–984. [CrossRef] [PubMed]

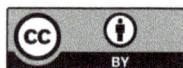

© 2020 by the authors. Licensee MDPI, Basel, Switzerland. This article is an open access article distributed under the terms and conditions of the Creative Commons Attribution (CC BY) license (http://creativecommons.org/licenses/by/4.0/).

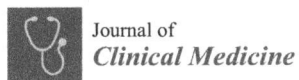 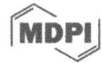

Article

Expression of the Novel Cardiac Biomarkers sST2, GDF-15, suPAR, and H-FABP in HFpEF Patients Compared to ICM, DCM, and Controls

Peter Jirak [1,*,†], Rudin Pistulli [2,†], Michael Lichtenauer [1], Bernhard Wernly [1], Vera Paar [1], Lukas J. Motloch [1], Richard Rezar [1], Christian Jung [3], Uta C. Hoppe [1], P. Christian Schulze [4], Daniel Kretzschmar [4], Rüdiger C. Braun-Dullaeus [5] and Tarek Bekfani [5]

[1] Clinic of Internal Medicine II, Department of Cardiology, Paracelsus Medical University of Salzburg, 5020 Salzburg, Austria; m.lichtenauer@salk.at (M.L.); b.wernly@salk.at (B.W.); v.paar@salk.at (V.P.); l.motloch@salk.at (L.J.M.); r.rezar@salk.at (R.R.); u.hoppe@salk.at (U.C.H.)
[2] Division of Vascular Medicine, Department of Cardiology and Angiology, University Hospital Muenster, Albert-Schweitzer-Campus 1, Munster, North Rhine-Westphalia, 48149 Münster, Germany; Rudin.Pistulli@ukmuenster.de
[3] Division of Cardiology, Pulmonology, and Vascular Medicine, Medical Faculty, University Duesseldorf, 40225 Duesseldorf, Germany; Christian.Jung@med.uni-duesseldorf.de
[4] Department of Internal Medicine I, Division of Cardiology, Angiology, Pneumology and Intensive Medical Care, University Hospital Jena, Friedrich Schiller University Jena, 07740 Jena, Germany; Christian.Schulze@med.uni-jena.de (P.C.S.); daniel.kretzschmar@med.uni-jena.de (D.K.)
[5] Department of Internal Medicine I, Division of Cardiology, Angiology and Intensive Medical Care, University Hospital Magdeburg, Otto von Gericke University, Magdeburg, 39120 Magdeburg, Germany; r.braun-dullaeus@med.ovgu.de (R.C.B.-D.); tarek.bekfani@med.ovgu.de (T.B.)
* Correspondence: p.jirak@salk.at
† These authors contributed equally to the paper.

Received: 27 February 2020; Accepted: 8 April 2020; Published: 15 April 2020

Abstract: Background: Heart failure with preserved ejection fraction (HFpEF) remains an ongoing therapeutic and diagnostic challenge to date. In this study we aimed for an analysis of the diagnostic potential of four novel cardiovascular biomarkers, GDF-15, H-FABP, sST2, and suPAR in HFpEF patients compared to controls as well as ICM, and DCM. Methods: In total, we included 252 stable outpatients and controls (77 DCM, 62 ICM, 18 HFpEF, and 95 controls) in the present study. All patients were in a non-decompensated state and on a stable treatment regimen. Serum samples were obtained and analyzed for GDF-15 (inflammation, remodeling), H-FABP (ischemia and subclinical ischemia), sST2 (inflammation, remodeling) and suPAR (inflammation, remodeling) by means of ELISA. Results: A significant elevation of GDF-15 was found for all heart failure entities compared to controls ($p < 0.005$). Similarly, H-FABP evidenced a significant elevation in all heart failure entities compared to the control group ($p < 0.0001$). Levels of sST2 were significantly elevated in ICM and DCM patients compared to the control group and HFpEF patients ($p < 0.0001$). Regarding suPAR, a significant elevation in ICM and DCM patients compared to the control group ($p < 0.0001$) and HFpEF patients ($p < 0.01$) was observed. An AUC analysis identified H-FABP (0.792, 95% CI 0.713–0.870) and GDF-15 (0.787, 95% CI 0.696–0.878) as paramount diagnostic biomarkers for HFpEF patients. Conclusion: Based on their differences in secretion patterns, novel cardiovascular biomarkers might represent a promising diagnostic tool for HFpEF in the future.

Keywords: HFpEF; heart failure; HFrEF; biomarker; sST2; suPAR; H-FABP; sST2

1. Introduction

With an overall prevalence of 2%, heart failure (HF) represents one of the leading causes of morbidity and mortality in the western world and thus also an important economic factor [1]. About 50% of all heart failure patients suffer from heart failure with preserved ejection fraction (HFpEF). HFpEF is characterized by a deterioration of cardiac relaxation resulting in an impaired diastolic filling of the left ventricle, mainly triggered by arterial hypertension along with obesity and metabolic disorders [2,3]. In contrast to heart failure with reduced ejection fraction (HFrEF), the left ventricular ejection fraction in HFpEF remains preserved [2,3].

The cellular processes involved in the development of HFpEF are heterogeneous. One of the most generally accepted hypotheses is that cellular hypertrophy combined with a reduction in cellular relaxation and an increase in tissue fibrosis could contribute strongly to the development of ventricular stiffening [4,5]. Furthermore, obesity, which is a very frequent co-morbidity of HF, leads to adipose tissue dysfunction along with elevated leptin levels and can trigger an upregulation of aldosterone, leading to sodium retention [6]. In consequence, higher levels of aldosterone trigger a volume expansion leading to increased filling pressures, thereby promoting cardiac remodeling, myocardial hypertrophy and fibrosis [6].

While numerous advancements have been made in the pharmacologic treatment of heart failure with reduced ejection fraction over the last decades (e.g., ARNIs), no evidence-based therapy for HFpEF patients exists to date [3,7]. Despite huge efforts, studies failed to show a significant prognostic benefit of pharmaceutical therapies in HFpEF, with the "PARAGON-Trial" as most prominent example [8]. Accordingly, the prognosis in HFpEF remains poor [9].

In addition to the lack of an evidence-based therapy, the actual diagnosis of HFpEF remains challenging and the precise diagnostic criteria are still matter of ongoing debates [9]. According to the current ESC guidelines, HFpEF is defined as a combination of: (I) Typical signs and symptoms of heart failure, (II) elevated levels of natriuretic peptides, (III) LVEF > 50%, (IV) evidence of diastolic dysfunction and/or structural heart disease (left ventricular hypertrophy or left atrial enlargement) [3]. Given the vague diagnostic criteria, the need for novel and additional diagnostic markers for HFpEF is evident.

In the last years, novel cardiac biomarkers have emerged as promising diagnostic tools for the assessment of different cardiovascular disease entities [10,11]. As a result to the complex pathophysiological background of most cardiovascular diseases, a multi-marker approach was reported as most effective for diagnosis, therapy monitoring and risk prediction due to the incorporation of different pathophysiologic processes covered by each respective marker [10,12].

Among the tested markers in previous studies, H-FABP (myocardial ischemia), sST-2 (myocardial strain and inflammation), GDF-15 (inflammation, remodeling), and suPAR (inflammation, remodeling) proved to be promising tools in achieving an improvement in the diagnosis and prognosis of cardiovascular diseases [13–16]. Accordingly, some of the listed markers are already included in the current guidelines and used in clinical routine [17].

Given the evident need for novel diagnostic tools in HFpEF we aimed for a head-to-head analysis of these four novel cardiovascular biomarkers in patients with heart failure with preserved ejection fraction compared to controls. Additionally, as the aforementioned markers are well studied in HFrEF patients, we aimed for a head-to-head analysis of HFpEF and HFrEF patients to put our findings into reference.

2. Experimental Section

The present study was conducted in accordance with the Universal Declaration of Helsinki and was approved by the local ethics committee at the University Hospital Jena, Germany. In total, we included 252 patients in this retrospective single-center study. Seventy-seven patients diagnosed with DCM, 62 patients with ICM, and 18 patients diagnosed with HFpEF were enrolled. Additionally, a control group of 95 patients was included. In these patients, coronary artery disease was excluded by coronary angiography. During visits in the outpatient ward, serum samples of all patients were obtained and analyzed for GDF-15, H-FABP, sST2, and suPAR.

The diagnosis of ICM, DCM and HFpEF was made according to the current guidelines of the European Society of Cardiology [3]. Clinical examination, assessment of medical history, laboratory analysis as well as transthoracic echocardiography was performed in all patients in the outpatient ward. Additionally, ICM and DCM patients underwent coronary angiography for diagnosis/exclusion of coronary artery disease. Controls also underwent coronary angiography because of suspected coronary artery disease and a relevant risk profile (hypertension, smoking etc.) and evidenced a rule out. All patients were in a stable, non-decompensated state at the timepoint of inclusion and clinical examination and were on a stable treatment regimen. Decompensated HF patients were not enrolled in this study. All examinations were performed by an experienced heart failure specialist. Laboratory analysis was conducted in all patients after informed consent. Serum samples were analyzed by means of ELISA and were stored at −80°C until measurements were conducted. Exclusion criteria were defined as: (I) Age under 18 years, (II) acute or chronic infections, (III) malignancies, (IV) advanced stages of renal failure (as indicated by a glomerular filtration rate less than 30 mL/min), (V) decompensated heart failure, (VI) hyperthyroidism, (VII) medication with immunosuppressive agents, and (VIII) recent acute coronary syndrome. For HFpEF patients a glomerular filtration rate under 60 ml/min was an exclusion criterion to rule out a potential cardiorenal confounder in this cohort.

2.1. Laboratory Analysis

Routine analysis of blood samples was performed at the Department of Clinical Chemistry (University Hospital Jena). The analyses comprised high-density lipoprotein (HDL; mmol/L), low density, lipoprotein (LDL; mmol/L), triglycerides (mmol/L), and C-reactive protein (CRP, mg/L) and hematological parameters. The glomerular filtration rate was calculated according to the CKD-EPI equation. Serum levels of sST2, GDF-15, suPAR, and H-FABP were measured using commercially available ELISA kits (DuoSet ELISA, DY523B, DY957, DY807, DY1678, and DFTA00, R&D Systems, Minneapolis, Minnesota, USA) in accordance with the instructions provided by R&D. ELISA analyses were performed at room temperature. In brief, 96-well plates were coated with the provided capture antibody according to the certificate of analysis and manufacturer's instructions. The multiwell plates were incubated overnight on a horizontal shaker. The next day, plates were washed using 0.5% Tween 20 (Carl Roth, Karlsruhe, Germany) in 1× phosphate buffered saline (PBS) and were then blocked with 1% bovine serum albumin (BSA; Carl Roth, Karlsruhe, Germany) in 1× PBS for one hour. After a further washing step, serum and the appropriate standard concentrations for sample quantification were added onto the wells and incubated for two hours. Again, the plate was washed and the provided biotin-labelled detection antibody was added to each well, followed by an incubation of another two hours. Thereafter, ELISA plates were washed again, before a provided streptavidin-horseradish-peroxidase (HRP) solution was added and incubated for 20 min. After a final washing step, the addition of the substrate tetramethylbenzidine (TMB; Sigma Aldrich, St. Louis, Missouri, USA) resulted in a blue color reaction which was stopped by adding 2 N sulfuric acid (H_2SO_4; Sigma Aldrich, St. Louis, Missouri, USA), changing the color to yellow. Optical density (OD) was measured at 450 nm on an ELISA microplate reader (iMark Microplate Absorbance Reader, Bio-Rad Laboratories, Wien Austria).

2.2. Statistical Analysis

Statistical analysis was performed using GraphPad-Prism software (GraphPad-Software, La Jolla, CA, USA), SPSS (22.0, SPSS Inc., Chicago, IL, USA) and MedCalc (19.1.3 MedCalc Software bv, Ostend, Belgium). The Kolmogorov-Smirnov test was used to assess normal distribution of parameters in the study population. Demographic parameters were compared by using ANOVA. Normally distributed parameters are given as mean + standard deviation. As biomarker concentrations were not normally distributed, they are given as median and inter-quartile range. Median values were compared using the Mann–Whitney-U test. Correlation analysis was performed using Spearman's rank-coefficient. Correction for multiple comparison was conducted using the Bonferroni–Holm method. ROC analysis was performed and AUCs were compared according to DeLong [18]. A $p < 0.05$ was considered as statistically significant.

3. Results

3.1. Baseline Characteristics

In total, the present study included 252 patients with a mean age of 62.6 years. While the distribution of male and female patients was quite balanced in HFpEF patients and controls, the HFrEF collective showed a significant higher number of male patients ($p < 0.001$). HFpEF patients were considerably older, compared to ICM, DCM, and controls ($p < 0.001$). Ejection fraction was significantly higher in patients with HFpEF compared to ICM and DCM patients ($p < 0.001$). BNP levels were significantly elevated in ICM ($p < 0.001$) and DCM ($p < 0.001$) compared to controls and HFpEF, while renal function was significantly impaired in the HFrEF collective ($p < 0.001$).

Regarding comorbidities, the rates of diabetes were evenly distributed in all three heart failure entities. Hypertension was present in similar rates in controls, HFpEF and ICM patients, with DCM patients showing significantly lower rates ($p < 0.001$). The rates of atrial fibrillation were significantly increased in HFpEF patients compared to all other entities ($p < 0.001$). With regards to medical therapy, HFrEF patients evidenced significantly higher rates beta-blockers, ACE-inhibitors and diuretics compared to HFpEF and controls ($p < 0.001$). Similarly, the rates of aldosterone antagonists were also higher in the HFrEF collective compared to HFpEF and controls ($p < 0.001$). Baseline characteristics are depicted in Tables 1 and 2

Table 1. Baseline Characteristics.

	Controls		HFpEF		ICM		DCM		Total		p-Value
	Mean	SD	Mean	SD	Mean	SD	Mean	SD	Mean	SD	
Age (y)	63.56	9.25	70.94	6.49	65.12	11.16	57.10	10.73	62.65	10.73	<0.0001
Height (m)	1.68	0.09	1.69	0.09	1.74	0.09	1.75	0.09	1.72	0.09	<0.0001
Weight (kg)	77.68	17.22	81.86	12.82	76.66	25.58	89.09	18.74	81.06	20.27	0.001
BMI	27.22	5.71	28.68	4.63	28.08	4.37	29.02	5.24	28.30	5.08	0.334
LVEF (%)	65.93	8.63	59.75	9.85	37.42	12.93	35.32	11.87	48.04	17.92	<0.0001
BNP (pg/mL)	73.74	86.08	165.22	162.54	435.75	488.22	684.64	866.83	430,10	646.27	<0.0001
Creatinine (µmol/L)	74.29	15.67	85.06	25.96	108.19	39.05	98.35	31.15	89.14	30.44	<0.0001
GFR (mL/min)	83.62	13.33	71.08	13.78	66.97	17.61	74.69	24.96	75.75	17.68	0.084
CRP (mg/L)	2.28	2.98	5.58	8.87	4.33	4.20	7.55	14.29	4.55	9.19	0.005
Hb (mmol/L)	8.79	0.56	8.16	0.87	8.51	0.94	8.92	0.91	8.67	0.91	0.005
LDL (mmol/L)	3.47	0.94	2.76	1.40	2.23	0.89	2.88	1.07	3.10	1.10	<0.0001
HDL (mmol/L)	1.49	0.41	1.29	0.35	0.99	0.22	1.15	0.31	1.32	0.40	<0.0001

Table 2. Concomitant diseases and medication.

	Controls	HFpEF	ICM	DCM	Total	p-Value
Sex (male)	36%	44%	86%	77%	61%	<0.0001
Diabetes	15%	39%	36%	38%	29%	0.003
Hypertension	77%	89%	78%	50%	70%	<0.001
Atrial Fibrillation	5%	50%	3%	18%	15%	<0.0001
Beta Blockers	39%	72%	100%	99%	76%	<0.0001
ACE-Inhibitors	59%	72%	96%	96%	82%	<0.0001
Loop-Diuretics	30%	56%	79%	91%	64%	<0.0001
MRA	2%	19%	61%	68%	43%	<0.0001

3.2. Biomarkers

GDF-15, evidenced a significant elevation for all heart failure entities compared to controls ($p < 0.005$) with no significant differences between the respective groups. For H-FABP, a significant elevation in all heart failure entities was observed compared to the control group ($p < 0.0001$). However, H-FABP levels were significantly higher in ICM and DCM patients compared to HFpEF ($p < 0.0001$). Levels of sST2 were significantly higher in ICM and DCM patients than in the control group ($p < 0.0001$). No significant differences between HFpEF patients and the control group were observed for sST2. Similar to sST2, levels of suPAR were significantly elevated in ICM and DCM patients compared to the control group ($p < 0.0001$) and HFpEF patients ($p < 0.01$). No significant differences between HFpEF patients and controls were observed. Biomarker levels are depicted in Table 3, comparisons of biomarker levels are depicted in Figure 1. In addition, a correction for multiple comparison was conducted by using the Bonferroni–Holm method. After correction for multiple testing, we found no changes in the statistical significance of our findings except for GDF-15 levels in controls vs. DCM. Correlation analysis of baseline characteristics and biomarkers of are given in the supplement Table S1. Results after multiple testing are given in the supplement Table S2. All biomarkers evidenced a significant correlation with BNP, Creatinine and CRP as well as an inverse correlation with ejection fraction.

Table 3. Levels of biomarkers.

	Controls		HFpEF		ICM		DCM	
	Median	Interquartile Range	Median	Interquartile Range	Median	Interquartile Range	Median	Interquartile Range
sST2 (pg/mL)	4999.00	2970.00	4318.00	2332.00	7869.00	5191.00	7010.00	5892.00
GDF-15 (pg/mL)	561.20	276.60	838.00	415.90	720.50	565.60	639.10	595.10
H-FABP (ng/mL)	0.00	0.60	0.82	0.53	1.66	3.59	1.94	1.83
suPAR (pg/mL)	2414.00	1280.00	2279.00	1753.00	3576.00	2567.00	3280.00	2349.00

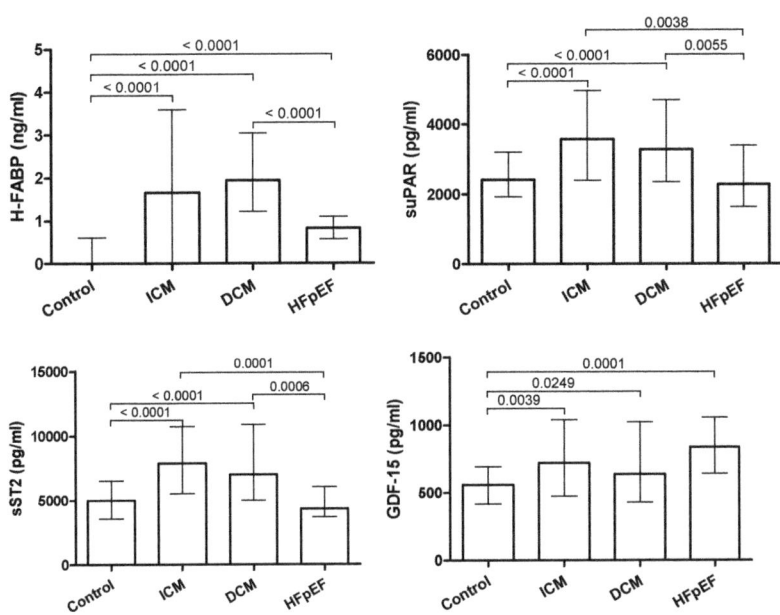

Figure 1. Comparison of biomarker levels between control group, HFpEF, ICM, and DCM patients (median + IQR).

3.3. AUC-Analysis

To evaluate the diagnostic potential of tested biomarkers in HFpEF, a ROC analysis was performed (Figure 2), and AUC was calculated for sST2, suPAR, GDF-15 and H-FABP plasma levels as diagnostic indicators for HFpEF patients. Our analysis identified H-FABP (0.792, 95% CI 0.713–0.870) and GDF-15 (0.787, 95% CI 0.696–0.878) as paramount diagnostic biom markers. In comparison, sST2 (0.567, 95%CI

0.294–0.572) and suPAR (0.543, 95% CI 0.298–0.616) evidenced a considerably lower AUC. The detailed results are depicted in Table 4. Additionally, we conducted a pairwise comparison of ROC curves according to DeLong et al. [18]. Here GDF-15 and H-FABP showed significantly higher AUCs compared to sST2 and suPAR respectively, while no significant difference between GDF-15 and H-FABP was observed. The detailed results are depicted in Table 5.

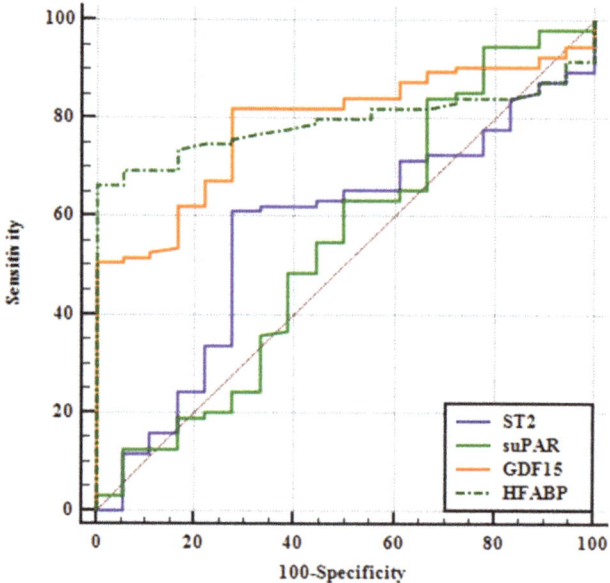

Figure 2. Receiver operating curve.

Table 4. AUC-Analysis.

Variable	AUC	SE [a]	95% CI [b]
ST2	0.567	0.0725	0.470 to 0.660
suPAR	0.543	0.0829	0.447 to 0.637
GDF15	0.787	0.0469	0.700 to 0.859
HFABP	0.792	0.0401	0.705 to 0.862

[a] DeLong et al., 1988; [b] Binomial exact

Table 5. Pairwise comparison of ROC curves.

ST2 ~ suPAR	
Difference between areas	0.0240
Standard Error [a]	0.112
95% Confidence Interval	−0.196 to 0.244
Z statistic	0.214
Significance level	$p = 0.8307$
ST2 ~ GDF15	
Difference between areas	0.220
Standard Error [a]	0.0999
95% Confidence Interval	0.0247 to 0.416
Z statistic	2.207
Significance level	$p = 0.0273$

Table 5. Cont.

ST2 ~ HFABP	
Difference between areas	0.225
Standard Error [a]	0.0830
95% Confidence Interval	0.0621 to 0.388
Z statistic	2.708
Significance level	$p = 0.0068$
suPAR ~ GDF15	
Difference between areas	0.244
Standard Error [a]	0.0996
95% Confidence Interval	0.0492 to 0.440
Z statistic	2.453
Significance level	$p = 0.0141$
suPAR ~ HFABP	
Difference between areas	0.249
Standard Error [a]	0.0983
95% Confidence Interval	0.0562 to 0.442
Z statistic	2.531
Significance level	$p = 0.0114$
GDF15 ~ HFABP	
Difference between areas	0.00439
Standard Error [a]	0.0563
95% Confidence Interval	−0.106 to 0.115
Z statistic	0.0779
Significance level	$p = 0.9379$

[a] DeLong et al., 1988.

4. Discussion

Despite the growing awareness, HFpEF remains a diagnostic and clinical challenge to date. This is partially related to its complex pathophysiology [9]. Given the increasing prevalence of HFpEF and the high rates of misdiagnosis, the need for new diagnostic tools is evident [5]. Accordingly, we aimed for a head-to-head analysis of four novel cardiovascular biomarkers and their diagnostic benefit in patients with HFpEF compared to controls to address this evident gap.

Regarding baseline characteristics we observed significant differences between the respective patient collectives. HFpEF patients were the oldest subgroup in our study, a finding that is typical for this disease entity and also matches former studies. A slow progression of myocardial fibrosis and remodeling with gradual diastolic impairment might explain the delayed onset of symptoms and consequently the higher age. Additionally, ICM and DCM patients evidenced worse renal function as well as decreased ejection fraction and significantly elevated BNP levels compared to HFpEF and controls. Moreover, HFpEF patients evidenced lower rates of a standard heart failure therapy, a finding which must be mainly attributed to the lack of an evidence-based therapy for HFpEF patients.

With regards to levels of GDF-15, a significant elevation was present in all three types of heart failure compared to controls. HFpEF patients provided the highest levels in the study collective, however without significant differences between HFpEF in comparison to HFrEF patients. While the detailed mechanisms involved in the GDF-15 pathway are not yet fully understood, it seems to be involved in the regulation of apoptosis, cell repair, and cell growth [15,19]. Accordingly, latest studies have also demonstrated a correlation between GDF-15 and atrial and myocardial fibrosis along with a prognostic impact in cardiovascular disease [20,21]. Additionally, GDF-15 is also involved in the regulatory processes of inflammatory pathways [22]. GDF-15 levels were shown to be significantly elevated in HFrEF in former studies [10]. However, the finding of an increase in GDF-15 in HFpEF patients represents a new aspect. The elevation might be attributed to the progressive myocardial fibrosis and remodeling involved in this disease entity, which could act as a trigger for the secretion of GDF-15. As GDF-15 has shown a significant prognostic impact in HFrEF patients, a similar prognostic value can be assumed for HFpEF patients. As potential surrogate for fibrosis burden, GDF-15 might also act as a monitoring parameter for HFpEF patients in the future.

H-FABP represents a highly sensitive marker for myocardial ischemia [23]. We observed a significant increase in all three heart failure entities. For HFrEF patients, an increase in H-FABP was reported in earlier studies and subclinical myocardial ischemia was proposed as the most probable cause for this finding [10]. Interestingly, based on our results it seems that subclinical ischemia is also present in HFpEF patients. A possible explanation might be a relative shortage in myocardial oxygen supply, based on various processes such as increased wall thickness of the left ventricle in this group of patients. Above all, due to the impaired ventricular filling, a relative shortage in blood supply is present [4]. Moreover, ventricular hypertrophy primarily triggered by arterial hypertension might add to this shortage [4]. Nevertheless, former studies have also shown a considerable prevalence of storage diseases such as amyloidosis and Morbus Fabry resulting in HFpEF [24]. Additionally, also an impairment in coronary microcirculation by means of coronary microvascular endothelial inflammation increasing resting tension through a reduction in nitric oxide bioavailability, cyclic guanosine monophosphate content and protein kinase G (PKG) activity found in HFpEF patients contributes to a shortage in myocardial oxygen supply [25]. Accordingly, based on these processes, H-FABP might prove a promising tool in the diagnosis and controlling the success of treatment of HFpEF patients, quantitating the amount of subclinical ischemia.

Regarding levels of sST2 we found a significant increase in ICM and DCM patients compared to controls and HFpEF, while no significant difference between HFpEF patients and the control group was observed. There are two isoforms of ST2, which both act as receptor to Interleukin-33: The membrane bound ST2L receptor responsible for potential cardioprotective effects, mediated trough IL-33 and the soluble ST2, which acts as a decoy receptor for IL-33 [26]. Due to its role as decoy receptor for the cardioprotective IL-33, sST2 constitutes a marker of increased cardiac strain and cardiac fibrosis and was also reported to be elevated in inflammatory diseases [26,27]. Moreover, studies have shown increased levels and a prognostic relevance of sST2 in HFrEF and acute coronary syndrome [14]. Accordingly, our findings regarding elevated concentrations of sST2 in ICM and DCM patients are consistent with former studies. However, contrary to our expectations, HFpEF patients evidenced low levels of sST2 similar to the control group. This finding also matches former studies, which reported lower levels of sST2 in HFpEF compared to HFrEF [28]. Further and bigger studies are required to verify these findings and help in explaining the underlying mechanisms of these results. Nevertheless, the process of fibrosis itself represents an important prognostic factor also for HFpEF patients [29]. Thus, despite the low levels, sST2 could potentially serve as monitoring parameter in HFpEF analogical to its application HFrEF patients due to the representation of fibrosis progression.

Similar to our findings on sST2, we found significantly elevated levels of suPAR in ICM and DCM patients compared to controls and HFpEF, while again no significant differences were observed between HFpEF patients and controls. The membrane bound uPAR is mainly expressed on the cell membrane of immunocompetent cells [30]. The soluble form (suPAR) is created through the cleavage and release of uPAR [30]. Correspondingly, suPAR represents a marker of inflammation and immune system activity [30,31]. A significant correlation of suPAR with myocardial infarction and HFrEF has been demonstrated [10,11]. The finding of increased suPAR levels in ICM and DCM patients might be mainly explained by a higher prevalence of inflammatory processes present in HFrEF, also triggered by further concomitant diseases. Further, especially larger studies should be performed to scrutinize for an explanation of these findings. To further analyze the diagnostic implications of biomarkers in HFpEF patients, we conducted an AUC analysis. Here we found considerably high values for GDF-15 and H-FABP in contrast to sST2 and suPAR. Additionally, to further evaluate the diagnostic potential of biomarkers in HFpEF patients, we conducted a pairwise comparison of ROCs. This further confirmed our previous findings of H-FABP and GDF-15 constituting paramount diagnostic markers for HFpEF. In contrast, sST2 and suPAR did not seem to have a major diagnostic benefit (see Table 2). Accordingly, with regards to HFpEF patients, GDF-15 and H-FABP represent the most promising markers for the future.

All biomarkers included in our study evidenced a significant correlation with creatinine, BNP and CRP as well as an inverse correlation with ejection fraction. Most importantly, the highly significant correlation with BNP and ejection fraction emphasizes their great potential as heart failure biomarkers. However, contrary to BNP, which is mainly secreted by cardiomyocytes in response to volume increase, novel biomarkers are involved in numerous different pathophysiologic processes, thus providing additive information to natriuretic peptides. These processes comprise subclinical ischemia and ischemic events (H-FABP) as well as cardiovascular remodeling and inflammatory processes (sST2, GDF-15 and suPAR) [11,12]. Since all these processes represent key factors in the development and progression of heart failure, novel biomarkers offer a promising opportunity to assess the impact of comorbidities on this regard [3,4]. Correspondingly, the involvement of novel biomarkers in inflammatory processes was also observed in our study, reflected by a significant correlation of all markers with CRP. In addition to novel biomarkers tested in our project, latest studies also proposed an analysis of micro-RNA expression patterns as a novel diagnostic approach in heart failure [32–34]. On this regard, De Rosa et al. could show, that transcoronary concentration gradients of circulating microRNAs could help to distinguish between different heart failure entities [33]. Similar to biomarkers in our study, circulating and exosomal micro-RNAs were also shown to correlate with clinical parameters such as left ventricular function in former studies [32,34]. In consequence, micro-RNA analysis might offer a great diagnostic benefit in the assessment of heart failure in the future. Moreover, micro-RNAs were also shown to provide diagnostic potential in other cardiovascular diseases as for example coronary artery disease and myocardial infarction [32,34]. However, while standardized testing kits for a clinical application of novel biomarkers are already available and their application is also represented in current guidelines, the diagnostic application of micro-RNA testing has yet to be implemented in clinical practice.

With regards to our findings, suggestions on the future role of H-FABP and GDF-15 in HFpEF are highly speculative due to the hypothesis generating character of our study. Nevertheless, since established testing kits are already available, their use in addition to already established markers such as BNP might be a useful approach for the future. Especially with regards to the pathophysiology in HFpEF, a combination of natriuretic peptides and novel markers seems reasonable, in order to target the different processes involved in this disease [9,19,23]. Taken together, novel biomarkers represent a promising diagnostic approach in HFpEF patients. Based on their expression patterns, they reflect different pathophysiological processes relevant in this disease entity and thus might enable a more precise diagnosis of HFpEF in the future.

5. Conclusions

In summary, novel cardiovascular biomarkers provide a considerable potential to add to the diagnostic process in HFpEF patients. While sST2 and suPAR did not show a relevant dynamic in HFpEF patients compared to controls, a significant difference was evident for H-FABP and GDF-15. These findings point towards a relevant role of subclinical ischemia in HFpEF patients and offer a new aspect in this complex pathophysiology. The increase in GDF-15 might be mainly induced by myocardial remodeling and fibrosis. Thus, GDF-15 could also offer a prognostic benefit in the future. However, cardiac biomarkers showed a lower overall expression in HFpEF patients compared to other heart failure entities, emphasizing the diagnostic challenges in HFpEF. Nevertheless, by combining the information of different pathophysiological processes by means of a multi-marker approach, novel biomarkers might be very useful in the identification of HFpEF patients in the future.

6. Limitations

The most important limitation of our study is the small sample size of the HFpEF cohort involved. This of course markedly limits the results of the current analyses. Moreover, the diagnostic criteria for HFpEF is a matter of ongoing debate and represents a clinical challenge as already mentioned above. Accordingly, the findings of the study must be interpreted with care. Additionally, the single-center and retrospective character must be taken into account. As no follow-up was performed, the dynamic of biomarkers in the progression of heart failure cannot be reflected. Moreover, our study does not include a comparison with already established markers as for example BNP. In consequence, direct comparison is limited. Despite the limitations mentioned above, the present study points out the potential benefits and advantages of the application of novel biomarkers in the diagnosis of heart failure and HFpEF. As our study suggests a diagnostic benefit in HFpEF patients, our results give rise to further investigation.

Supplementary Materials: The following are available online at http://www.mdpi.com/2077-0383/9/4/1130/s1, Table S1: Correlation Analysis of baseline characteristics and biomarkers; Table S2: Results after correction for multiple testing (Bonferroni-Holm).

Author Contributions: Conceptualization: All authors, Methodology: P.J., M.L., B.W., V.P., T.B.; software, P.J., B.W., V.P., M.L.; validation, P.J., L.J.M., R.R., U.C.H.; formal analysis, P.J., B.W.; investigation, C.J., D.K., R.P.; resources, R.C.B.-D., T.B., P.C.S., D.K.; data curation, M.L., T.B., P.J., P.C.S., C.J., R.P.; writing—original draft preparation, P.J., M.L., T.B.; writing—review and editing, P.J., M.L., T.B., R.C.B.-D., R.P., R.R., L.J.M., Christian Jung; visualization, M.L., B.W.; supervision, M.L., T.B., P.C.S., C.J., U.C.H.; project administration, P.J., T.B.; All authors have read and agreed to the published version of the manuscript.

Acknowledgments: We want to thank Fitore Marmullaku for performing assays and analyses in the laboratory.

Conflicts of Interest: The authors declare no conflict of interest.

Abbreviations

AUC	area under the curve
BMI	body mass index
BNP	brain natriuretic peptide
CKD-EPI	Chronic Kidney Disease Epidemiology Collaboration
CRP	C-reactive protein
DCM	dilative cardiomyopathy
ESC	European society of cardiology
ELISA	enzyme-linked immunosorbent assay
GDF-15	growth differentiation factor-15
GFR	glomerular filtration rate
Hb	haemoglobin
H-FABP	heart-type fatty acid binding protein
HFpEF	heart failure with preserved ejection fraction
HFrEF	heart failure with reduced ejection fraction
HDL	high density lipoprotein
ICM	ischemic cardiomyopathy
IL-33	interleukin 33
LDL	low density lipoprotein
LVEF	left ventricular ejection fraction
MRA	mineralocorticoid receptor antagonist
NYHA	New York heart association
PKG	protein kinase G
ROC	receiver operating curve
sST2	soluble suppression of tumorigenicity 2
suPAR	soluble urokinase-type plasminogen activator receptor

References

1. Bleumink, G.S.; Knetsch, A.M.; Sturkenboom, M.C.J.M.; Straus, S.M.J.M.; Hofman, A.; Deckers, J.W.; Witteman, J.C.M.; Stricker, B.H.C. Quantifying the heart failure epidemic: Prevalence, incidence rate, lifetime risk and prognosis of heart failure The Rotterdam Study. *Eur. Heart J.* **2004**, *25*, 1614–1619. [CrossRef] [PubMed]
2. Redfield, M.M. Heart Failure with Preserved Ejection Fraction. *N. Engl. J. Med.* **2017**, *376*, 897. [CrossRef] [PubMed]
3. Ponikowski, P.; Voors, A.A.; Anker, S.D.; Bueno, H.; Cleland, J.G.F.; Coats, A.J.S.; Falk, V.; González-Juanatey, J.R.; Harjola, V.P.; Jankowska, E.A.; et al. 2016 ESC Guidelines for the diagnosis and treatment of acute and chronic heart failure: The Task Force for the diagnosis and treatment of acute and chronic heart failure of the European Society of Cardiology (ESC). Developed with the special contribution of the Heart Failure Association (HFA) of the ESC. *Eur. J. Heart Fail.* **2016**, *18*, 891–975. [PubMed]
4. Borlaug, B.A. The pathophysiology of heart failure with preserved ejection fraction. *Nat. Rev. Cardiol.* **2014**, *11*, 507–515. [CrossRef]
5. Gevaert, A.B.; Boen, J.R.A.; Segers, V.F.; van Craenenbroeck, E.M. Heart Failure With Preserved Ejection Fraction: A Review of Cardiac and Noncardiac Pathophysiology. *Front. Physiol.* **2019**, *10*, 638. [CrossRef]
6. Packer, M. Leptin-Aldosterone-Neprilysin Axis: Identification of Its Distinctive Role in the Pathogenesis of the Three Phenotypes of Heart Failure in People with Obesity. *Circulation* **2018**, *137*, 1614–1631. [CrossRef]
7. McMurray, J.J.; Packer, M.; Desai, A.S.; Gong, J.; Lefkowitz, M.P.; Rizkala, A.R. Angiotensin-neprilysin inhibition versus enalapril in heart failure. *N. Engl. J. Med.* **2014**, *371*, 993–1004. [CrossRef]
8. Solomon, S.D.; McMurray, J.J.V.; Anand, I.S.; Ge, J.; Lam, C.S.P.; Maggioni, A.P.; Martinez, F.; Packer, M.; Pfeffer, M.A.; Pieske, B.; et al. Angiotensin-Neprilysin Inhibition in Heart Failure with Preserved Ejection Fraction. *N. Engl. J. Med.* **2019**, *381*, 1609–1620. [CrossRef]
9. Lekavich, C.L.; Barksdale, D.J.; Neelon, V.; Wu, J. Heart failure preserved ejection fraction (HFpEF): An integrated and strategic review. *Heart Fail. Rev.* **2015**, *20*, 643–653. [CrossRef]
10. Lichtenauer, M.; Jirak, P.; Wernly, B.; Paar, V.; Rohm, I.; Jung, C.; Schernthaner, C.; Kraus, J.; Motloch, L.J.; Yilmaz, A.; et al. A comparative analysis of novel cardiovascular biomarkers in patients with chronic heart failure. *Eur. J. Intern. Med.* **2017**. [CrossRef]
11. Schernthaner, C.; Lichtenauer, M.; Wernly, B.; Paar, V.; Pistulli, R.; Rohm, I.; Jung, C.; Figulla, H.R.; Yilmaz, A.; Cadamuro, J.; et al. Multibiomarker analysis in patients with acute myocardial infarction. *Eur. J. Clin. Investig.* **2017**, *47*, 638–648. [CrossRef] [PubMed]
12. Jirak, P.; Fejzic, D.; Paar, V.; Wernly, B.; Pistulli, R.; Rohm, I.; Jung, C.; Hoppe, U.C.; Schulze, P.C.; Lichtenauer, M.; et al. Influences of Ivabradine treatment on serum levels of cardiac biomarkers sST2, GDF-15, suPAR and H-FABP in patients with chronic heart failure. *Acta Pharmacol. Sin.* **2018**, *39*, 1189–1196. [CrossRef] [PubMed]
13. Otaki, Y.; Watanabe, T.; Kubota, I. Heart-type fatty acid-binding protein in cardiovascular disease: A systemic review. *Clin. Chim. Acta* **2017**, *474*, 44–53. [CrossRef] [PubMed]
14. Pascual-Figal, D.A.; Lax, A.; Perez-Martinez, M.T.; Asensio-Lopez, M.D.; Sanchez-Mas, J. Clinical relevance of sST2 in cardiac diseases. *Clin. Chem. Lab. Med.* **2016**, *54*, 29–35. [CrossRef] [PubMed]
15. Wollert, K.C.; Kempf, T.; Wallentin, L. Growth Differentiation Factor 15 as a Biomarker in Cardiovascular Disease. *Clin. Chem.* **2017**, *63*, 140–151. [CrossRef]
16. Eugen-Olsen, J.; Giamarellos-Bourboulis, E.J. suPAR: The unspecific marker for disease presence, severity and prognosis. *Int. J. Antimicrob. Agents* **2015**, *46*, 31. [CrossRef]
17. Yancy, C.W.; Jessup, M.; Bozkurt, B.; Butler, J.; Casey, D.E.; Colvin, M.M.; Drazner, M.H.; Filippatos, G.S.; Fonarow, G.C.; Givertz, M.M.; et al. 2017 ACC/AHA/HFSA Focused Update of the 2013 ACCF/AHA Guideline for the Management of Heart Failure: A Report of the American College of Cardiology/American Heart Association Task Force on Clinical Practice Guidelines and the Heart Failure Society of America. *J. Am. Coll. Cardiol.* **2017**, *70*, 776–803.
18. DeLong, E.R.; DeLong, D.M.; Clarke-Pearson, D.L. Comparing the areas under two or more correlated receiver operating characteristic curves: A nonparametric approach. *Biometrics* **1988**, *44*, 837–845. [CrossRef]
19. Xu, X.; Li, Z.; Gao, W. Growth differentiation factor 15 in cardiovascular diseases: From bench to bedside. *Biomarkers* **2011**, *16*, 466–475. [CrossRef]

20. Zhou, Y.M.; Li, M.J.; Zhou, Y.L.; Ma, L.; Yi, X. Growth differentiation factor-15 (GDF-15), novel biomarker for assessing atrial fibrosis in patients with atrial fibrillation and rheumatic heart disease. *Int. J. Clin. Exp. Med.* **2015**, *8*, 21201–21207.
21. Farhan, S.; Freynhofer, M.K.; Brozovic, I.; Bruno, V.; Vogel, B.; Tentzeris, I.; Baumgartner-Parzer, S.; Huber, K.; Kautzky-Willer, A. Determinants of growth differentiation factor 15 in patients with stable and acute coronary artery disease. A prospective observational study. *Cardiovasc. Diabetol.* **2016**, *15*, 016–0375. [CrossRef]
22. Adela, R.; Banerjee, S.K. GDF-15 as a Target and Biomarker for Diabetes and Cardiovascular Diseases: A Translational Prospective. *J. Diabetes Res.* **2015**, *490842*, 27. [CrossRef]
23. Niizeki, T.; Takeishi, Y.; Arimoto, T.; Takabatake, N.; Nozaki, N.; Hirono, O.; Watanabe, T.; Nitobe, J.; Harada, M.; Suzuki, S. Heart-type fatty acid-binding protein is more sensitive than troponin T to detect the ongoing myocardial damage in chronic heart failure patients. *J. Card. Fail.* **2007**, *13*, 120–127. [CrossRef]
24. Seferovic, P.M.; Damman, K.; Harjola, V.P.; Mebazaa, A.; Brunner-La Rocca, H.P.; Martens, P.; Testani, J.M.; Tang, W.H.W.; Orso, F.; Rossignol, P.; et al. Heart failure in cardiomyopathies: A position paper from the Heart Failure Association of the European Society of Cardiology. *Eur. J. Heart Fail.* **2019**, *21*, 553–576. [CrossRef] [PubMed]
25. Paulus, W.J.; Tschope, C. A novel paradigm for heart failure with preserved ejection fraction: Comorbidities drive myocardial dysfunction and remodeling through coronary microvascular endothelial inflammation. *J. Am. Coll. Cardiol.* **2013**, *62*, 263–271. [CrossRef] [PubMed]
26. Sanada, S.; Hakuno, D.; Higgins, L.J.; Schreiter, E.R.; McKenzie, A.N.J.; Lee, R.T. IL-33 and ST2 comprise a critical biomechanically induced and cardioprotective signaling system. *J. Clin. Investig.* **2007**, *117*, 1538–1549. [CrossRef] [PubMed]
27. Griesenauer, B.; Paczesny, S. The ST2/IL-33 Axis in Immune Cells during Inflammatory Diseases. *Front. Immunol.* **2017**, *8*, 475. [CrossRef] [PubMed]
28. Najjar, E.; Faxén, U.L.; Hage, C.; Donal, E. ST2 in heart failure with preserved and reduced ejection fraction. *Scand. Cardiovasc. J.* **2019**, *53*, 21–27. [CrossRef] [PubMed]
29. Schelbert, E.B.; Fridman, Y.; Wong, T.C.; Abu Daya, H.; Piehler, K.M.; Kadakkal, A.; et al. Temporal Relation Between Myocardial Fibrosis and Heart Failure With Preserved Ejection Fraction: Association With Baseline Disease Severity and Subsequent Outcome. *JAMA Cardiol.* **2017**, *2*, 995–1006. [CrossRef]
30. Thuno, M.; Macho, B.; Eugen-Olsen, J. suPAR: The molecular crystal ball. *Dis. Markers* **2009**, *27*, 157–172. [CrossRef]
31. Hamie, L.; Daoud, G.; Nemer, G.; Nammour, T.; el Chediak, A.; Uthman, I.W.; Kibbi, A.G.; Eid, A.; Kurban, M. SuPAR, an emerging biomarker in kidney and inflammatory diseases. *Postgrad. Med. J.* **2018**, *94*, 517–524. [CrossRef] [PubMed]
32. De Rosa, S.; Curcio, A.; Indolfi, C. Emerging role of microRNAs in cardiovascular diseases. *Circ. J.* **2014**, *78*, 567–575. [CrossRef] [PubMed]
33. De Rosa, S.; Eposito, F.; Carella, C.; Strangio, A.; Ammirati, G.; Sabatino, J.; Abbate, F.G.; Iaconetti, C.; Liguori, V.; Pergola, V.; et al. Transcoronary concentration gradients of circulating microRNAs in heart failure. *Eur. J. Heart Fail.* **2018**, *20*, 1000–1010. [CrossRef] [PubMed]
34. Iaconetti, C.; Sorrentino, S.; De Rosa, S.; Indolfi, C. Exosomal miRNAs in Heart Disease. *Physiology* **2016**, *31*, 16–24. [CrossRef]

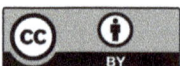

© 2020 by the authors. Licensee MDPI, Basel, Switzerland. This article is an open access article distributed under the terms and conditions of the Creative Commons Attribution (CC BY) license (http://creativecommons.org/licenses/by/4.0/).

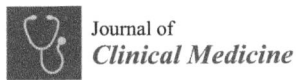 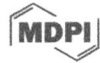

Article

Diagnosis of Non-Alcoholic Fatty Liver Disease (NAFLD) Is Independently Associated with Cardiovascular Risk in a Large Austrian Screening Cohort

David Niederseer [1,*,†], Sarah Wernly [2,†], Sebastian Bachmayer [2], Bernhard Wernly [3], Adam Bakula [1], Ursula Huber-Schönauer [2], Georg Semmler [2], Christian Schmied [1], Elmar Aigner [4] and Christian Datz [2]

[1] Department of Cardiology, University Heart Center Zurich, University of Zurich, University Hospital Zurich, 8091 Zurich, Switzerland; adam.bakula@usz.ch (A.B.); christian.schmied@usz.ch (C.S.)
[2] Department of Internal Medicine, General Hospital Oberndorf, Teaching Hospital of the Paracelsus Medical University Salzburg, 5110 Oberndorf, Austria; sarah_wernly@airpost.net (S.W.); S.Bachmayer@kh-oberndorf.at (S.B.); huber.schoenauer@gmail.com (U.H.-S.); georg.semmler@hotmail.com (G.S.); c.datz@kh-oberndorf.at (C.D.)
[3] Department of Internal Medicine II, Paracelsus Medical University Salzburg, 5020 Salzburg, Austria; bernhard@wernly.net
[4] Department of Internal Medicine I, Paracelsus Medical University Salzburg, 5020 Salzburg, Austria; e.aigner@salk.at
* Correspondence: david.niederseer@usz.ch; Tel.: +41-(0)43-253-94-71; Fax: +41-(0)44-255-44-01
† These authors contributed equally to this work.

Received: 1 March 2020; Accepted: 6 April 2020; Published: 9 April 2020

Abstract: Background: Many patients with non-alcoholic fatty liver disease (NAFLD) simultaneously suffer from cardiovascular (CV) disease and often carry multiple CV risk factors. Several CV risk factors are known to drive the progression of fibrosis in patients with NAFLD. Objectives: To investigate whether an established CV risk score, the Framingham risk score (FRS), is associated with the diagnosis of NAFLD and the degree of fibrosis in an Austrian screening cohort for colorectal cancer. Material and Methods: In total, 1965 asymptomatic subjects (59 ± 10 years, 52% females, BMI 27.2 ± 4.9 kg/m^2) were included in this study. The diagnosis of NAFLD was present if (1) significantly increased echogenicity in relation to the renal parenchyma was present in ultrasound and (2) viral, autoimmune or hereditary liver disease and excess alcohol consumption were excluded. The FRS (ten-year risk of coronary heart disease) and NAFLD Fibrosis Score (NFS) were calculated for all patients. High CV risk was defined as the highest FRS quartile (>10%). Both univariable and multivariable logistic regression models were used to calculate associations of FRS with NAFLD and NFS. Results: Compared to patients without NAFLD (n = 990), patients with NAFLD (n = 975) were older (60 ± 9 vs. 58 ± 10 years; $p < 0.001$), had higher BMI (29.6 ± 4.9 vs. 24.9 ± 3.6 kg/m^2; $p < 0.001$) and suffered from metabolic syndrome more frequently (33% vs. 7%; $p < 0.001$). Cardiovascular risk as assessed by FRS was higher in the NAFLD-group (8.7 ± 6.4 vs. 5.4 ± 5.2%; $p < 0.001$). A one-percentage-point increase of FRS was independently associated with NAFLD (OR 1.04, 95%CI 1.02–1.07; $p < 0.001$) after correction for relevant confounders in multivariable logistic regression. In patients with NAFLD, NFS correlated with FRS (r = 0.29; $p < 0.001$), and FRS was highest in patients with significant fibrosis (F3-4; 11.7 ± 5.4) compared to patients with intermediate results (10.9 ± 6.3) and those in which advanced fibrosis could be ruled-out (F0-2, 7.8 ± 5.9, $p < 0.001$). A one-point-increase of NFS was an independent predictor of high-risk FRS after correction for sex, age, and concomitant diagnosis of metabolic syndrome (OR 1.30, 95%CI 1.09–1.54; $p = 0.003$). Conclusion: The presence of NAFLD might independently improve prediction of long-term risk for CV disease and the diagnosis of NAFLD might be a clinically relevant piece in the puzzle of predicting long-term CV outcomes. Due to the significant overlap of advanced NAFLD and high CV risk, aggressive treatment of established CV risk factors could improve prognosis in these patients.

Keywords: NAFLD; cardiovascular risk; Framingham risk score; CVD; risk prediction; secondary prevention; primary prevention; metabolic syndrome; NAFLD fibrosis score

1. Introduction

With a constant increase in the incidence of metabolic syndrome, the prevalence of non-alcoholic fatty liver disease (NAFLD) is estimated to be around 25% in Europe. A steep rise in the prevalence of NAFLD from 15% in 2005 to 25% in 2010 has been observed [1]. This increase mirrors obesity rates, which nearly tripled since 1975 and reached epidemic levels [2]. Components of the metabolic syndrome such as hypertension, dyslipidemia, dysglycemia, and abdominal obesity are established risk factors for NAFLD [3]. Since they have also been established as risk factors for CVD, patients frequently suffer from both conditions.

CVD is a leading cause of death worldwide both in the general population and patients with NAFLD [4–6]. NAFLD is independently associated with several markers of subclinical atherosclerosis such as coronary artery calcification, impaired flow-mediated vasodilation, arterial stiffness, carotid artery inflammation and thickening of carotid intima-media as well as left ventricular hypertrophy and diastolic dysfunction [7,8]. Importantly, some of these studies suggest an association of these two disease entities independent from traditional risk factors. Several lines of evidence suggest that NAFLD may be causally and independently involved in CVD pathogenesis [9,10].

Different possible pathophysiological pathways link NAFLD with CVD [11]. Markers of inflammation such as cytokines, CRP, or interleukin-6 are overexpressed in these patients and also correlate with a higher degree of liver fibrosis [12]. Furthermore, patients with hepatic steatosis show elevated levels of pro-coagulant factors such as fibrinogen, von Willebrand factor and plasminogen activator inhibitor-1 [13]. Additionally, hepatic insulin resistance and atherogenic dyslipidemia seem to contribute to the development of CVD [14]. These mechanisms are possible explanations for the fact that the severity of NAFLD, especially if progressed to non-alcoholic steatohepatitis (NASH) with fibrosis, additionally contributes to CV risk [15].

In our study, we examined the prevalence of NAFLD in an Austrian screening cohort for colorectal cancer (SAKKOPI). An established non-invasive estimate of fibrosis severity i.e., the NAFLD fibrosis score (NFS) was calculated and the relation of fibrosis with CV risk as assessed by the Framingham Risk Score (FRS) evaluated.

2. Methods

2.1. Study Subjects

The study cohort consisted of 1965 Caucasians undergoing routine screening colonoscopy at a single center in Austria. All Patients were recruited between 2010 and 2014. Informed consent was obtained, and the study was approved by the local ethics committee (Ethikkommission des Landes Salzburg, approval no. 415-E/1262/2-2010).

2.2. Assessment

As previously described, participants were examined on two consecutive days [16]. On the day of admission, venous blood was drawn after an overnight fast. A whole blood count, kidney and liver tests, lipids, CRP, as well as hemoglobin A1c, an oral glucose tolerance test, and insulin levels were measured. The participants completed a detailed questionnaire including past medical history, current medical regimen, family history, smoking history ("never smokers", "former smokers", or "current smokers") dietary habits and physical activity. A standard physical examination including blood pressure, height, weight, and waist circumference) was performed. Importantly, all patients underwent abdominal ultrasonography. The liver was considered normal if echogenicity was similar to the renal parenchyma. If areas showed a significantly increased echogenicity compared to the renal parenchyma, the liver was considered steatotic. On the second day, all subjects underwent complete colonoscopy.

2.3. Definitions

The diagnosis of NAFLD was made after exclusion of viral, autoimmune and hereditary liver diseases (Wilson disease, hereditary haemochromatosis, alpha-1 antitrypsin deficiency) and excess daily alcohol consumption ≥30 g for men and ≥20 g for women according to the European clinical practice guidelines for the management of NAFLD [17]. NAFLD fibrosis score (NFS) was calculated as previously described [18]. Briefly, NFS (age, body mass index (BMI), presence of impaired fasting glucose or diabetes, aspartate-aminotransferase (AST), alanine-aminotransferase (AST), platelets and albumin) was used to stratify patients according to their risk of significant fibrosis. Specifically, patients with a NFS < −1.455 were graded as F0-2, those with NFS > 0.676 as "F3-4", and patients with a NFS between −1.455 and 0.676 as "intermediate".

Metabolic syndrome was diagnosed when three or more of the following criteria were met [19]: fasting blood glucose level ≥100 mg/dL or antidiabetic therapy, waist circumference >102 cm in males and >88 cm in females, blood pressure ≥130/85 mmHg or current antihypertensive treatment, plasma triglycerides ≥150 mg/dL, and plasma HDL <40 mg/dL in males and <50 mg/dL in females.

2.4. Cardiovascular Risk Assessment

We evaluated patients for cardiovascular disease applying the Framingham Risk Score (FRS) [20]. Although the FRS is not validated in subjects with diabetes (T2DM), we did include subjects with T2DM in our analysis and performed a separate analysis, excluding all subjects with T2DM. Since results were not changed when subjects with T2DM were excluded, we report the results including T2DM to allow for greater generalizability of our results.

2.5. Statistical Analysis

Continuous variables are expressed as mean (±standard deviation) and compared using t-test or ANOVA. Categorical data are expressed as numbers (percentage). Chi-square test was applied to calculate differences between groups. Both univariable and multivariable logistic regression was used to evaluate associations of FRS with NAFLD and NFS with CV risk. For multivariable logistic regression, elimination criteria was a p-value of < 0.10 following backward elimination. Variables were included in the multivariable model based on literature. All variables included in the multivariable models evidenced a univariable association at a p-value of $p < 0.05$. A p-value of < 0.05 was considered statistically significant. SPSS version 22.0 (IBM, USA) was used for statistical analyses.

3. Results

3.1. Analysis of the Total Study Cohort, NAFLD versus Non-NAFLD Patients

Overall, 49.6% (n = 975) of patients had NAFLD as defined by hepatic steatosis in ultrasound, while 990 patients (50.4%) did not have NAFLD. NAFLD patients were older (60 ± 9 vs. 58 ± 10 years; $p < 0.001$), evidenced higher BMI (29.6 ± 4.9 vs. 24.9 ± 3.6 kg/m^2; $p < 0.001$) and more frequently fulfilled criteria for metabolic syndrome (33% vs. 7%; $p < 0.001$). Characteristics of NAFLD versus non-NAFLD patients are shown in Table 1.

Table 1. Baseline characteristics of patients without (n = 990) and with (n = 975) non-alcoholic fatty liver disease (NAFLD).

	No NAFLD	NAFLD	Total Cohort	p-Value
	n = 990	n = 975	n = 1965	
Female	61%	43%	52%	<0.001
Age (years)	58 (10)	60 (9)	59 (10)	<0.001
Systolic RR (mmHg)	128 (18)	135 (19)	131 (18)	<0.001
Diastolic RR (mmhg)	79 (10)	83 (11)	81 (10)	<0.001
BMI (kg/m^2)	25 (4)	26 (5)	27 (4)	<0.001
Waist circumference (cm)	90 (11)	105 (12)	97 (11)	<0.001
Waist to hip ratio	1 (0.1)	1 (0.1)	1 (0.1)	<0.001
Bilirubine (mg/dL)	0.72 (0.4)	0.73 (0.4)	0.72 (0.4)	0.4
GGT (U/L)	31 (46)	48 (71)	40 (46)	<0.001
AST (U/L)	22 (12)	26 (18)	24 (12)	<0.001
INR	1.0 (0.1)	1.0 (0.1)	1.0 (0.1)	0.24
Total cholesterol (mg/dL)	219 (40)	217 (44)	218 (40)	0.25
HDL (mg/dL)	67 (18)	56 (16)	62 (18)	<0.001
LDL (mg/dL)	137 (36)	142 (39)	139 (36)	0.02
Triglycerices (mg/dL)	101 (51)	145 (85)	123 (51)	<0.001
Thrombocytes (G/L)	236 (66)	227 (65)	232 (66)	0.001
Fasting glucose (mg/dL)	97 (15)	109 (30)	103 (15)	<0.001
HbA1c (%)	5.6 (0.5)	5.9 (0.8)	5.8 (0.5)	<0.001
Metabolic syndrome	7%	33%	20%	<0.001
T2DM	9%	24%	16%	<0.001
Current smoker	19%	17%	20%	0.48
Medication				
ASS	11%	17%	14%	0.001
Statin	15%	23%	19%	<0.001
ACE-I/ARB	13%	27%	20%	<0.001
Metformin	2%	8%	5%	<0.001
CV risk score				
FRS	5.41 (5.20)	8.71 (6.38)	7.05 (5.20)	<0.001
FRS 0-2%	41%	19%	30%	<0.001
FRS >2–5%	21%	19%	20%	
FRS >5–10%	22%	30%	25%	
FRS >10%	16%	33%	24%	

NAFLD: Non-alcoholic fatty liver disease; NFS: NAFLD fibrosis score; FRS: Framingham Risk Score; RR: blood pressure; GGT: gamma-glutamyl-transferase; AST: Aspartate transaminase; INR: International normalized ratio; HDL: High-density lipoprotein; LDL: Low-density lipoprotein; HbA1c: Glycated hemoglobin; T2DM: type 2 diabetes mellitus; ASS: acetylsalicylic acid; CV: cardiovascular; OR: odds ratio.

CV risk assessed by FRS was higher in the NAFLD-group (8.7 ± 6.4 vs. 5.4 ± 5.2%; p < 0.001). After allocation of subjects to FRS into risk quartiles (Q1: FRS 0%–2%; Q2: FRS 2%–5%; Q3: FRS 5%–10%, Q4: FRS > 10%), patients with NAFLD more often were in the Q4-FRS group (33% vs. 16%; p < 0.001) compared to non-NAFLD patients.

In univariable logistic regression, this relationship corresponded to an increase of OR of 1.11, (95%CI 1.09–1.13; p < 0.001) in the likelihood for NAFLD per one-percentage-point increase of FRS. This association remained significant after correction for age, sex and metabolic syndrome (OR, 1.04 95%CI 1.02–1.07; p < 0.001) in a multivariable model (Table 2). In an additional sensitivity analysis, a one-percentage-point increase of FRS remained associated with an increased likelihood for NAFLD both in males (OR 1.08, 95%CI 1.06–1.11; p < 0.001) and females (OR 1.13, 95%CI 1.09–1.18; p < 0.001).

Table 2. Univariable and multivariable associations with the presence of NAFLD.

	Univariable			Multivariable		
	OR	95%CI	p-Value	OR	95%CI	p-Value
Age	1.03	1.02–1.04	<0.001	1.010	0.998–1.023	0.11
Female gender	0.48	0.40–0.58	<0.001	0.68	0.54–0.86	0.001
Metabolic syndrome	6.08	4.63–7.99	<0.001	5.02	3.77–6.70	<0.001
FRS	1.11	1.09–1.13	<0.001	1.06	1.04–1.08	<0.001

3.2. Analysis of Patients with NAFLD

Patients with NAFLD were grouped according to their NFS into F0-F2 (n = 604), intermediate (n = 138) and F3-4 (n = 10). The characteristics of patients according to their NFS are shown in Table 3. Over the whole NAFLD cohort, NFS correlated with FRS (r = 0.29; p < 0.001), and FRS was highest in the F3-4 group (11.7 ± 5.4%; p < 0.001 vs. F0-F2) compared to the intermediate (10.9 ± 6.3%) and the F0-F2 group (7.8 ± 5.9%). When grouping intermediate and F3-4 into an "at-risk" group (due to small sample size in F3-4), the significant differences between F0-2 essentially persisted (Table 4).

In univariable logistic regression, a one-point increase of NFS was associated with a higher likelihood of high-risk FRS (OR 1.60, 95%CI 1.41–1.83; p < 0.001). NFS remained an independent predictor of Q4-FRS after correction for sex, age, and concomitant diagnosis of metabolic syndrome (OR 1.30, 95%CI 1.09–1.54; p = 0.003). In a sensitivity analysis in both males (OR 1.84, 95%CI 1.54–2.20; p < 0.001) and females (OR 2.06, 95%CI 1.52–2.78; p < 0.001) a one-point increase of NFS remained associated with high-quartile FRS. Univariable and multivariable significant associations of age, female gender, metabolic syndrome, and FRS with the presence of high risk NFS are depicted in Table 5.

Table 3. Baseline characteristics of patients according to their NAFLD Fibrosis Score (NFS) score: F0-F2 (n = 604), intermediate (n = 138) and F3-F4 (n = 10).

	F0-F2		Intermediate		F3-F4		
	n = 604		n = 138		n = 10		
	Mean	SD	Mean	SD	Mean	SD	p-Value
Female	36%		43%		50%		0.80
Age (years)	59	9	66	8	67	9	<0.001
Systolic RR (mmHg)	134	18	139	19	148	26	<0.001
Diastolic RR (mmhg)	82	11	85	12	85	12	0.07
BMI (kg/m^2)	29	4	33	6	35	4	<0.001
Waist circumference (cm)	103	11	111	12	115	14	<0.001
Waist to hip ratio	0.96	0	0.97	0	0.97	0	0.23
Bilirubine (mg/dL)	0.70	0	0.80	1	1.57	1	<0.001
GGT (U/L)	48	76	53	70	115	145	0.02
AST (U/L)	25	15	30	24	55	61	<0.001
INR	0.99	0	1.02	0	1.17	0	<0.001
Total cholesterol (mg/dL)	221	44	202	42	221	52	<0.001
HDL (mg/dL)	57	16	53	13	57	13	0.03
LDL (mg/dL)	145	40	130	37	142	41	<0.001
Triglycerices (mg/dL)	145	84	147	101	142	68	0.97
Thrombocytes (G/L)	243	62	176	52	128	88	<0.001
Fasting glucose (mg/dL)	107	28	115	28	97	16	0.01
HbA1c (%)	5.9	1	6.0	1	5.6	0	0.08
Metabolic syndrome	30%		43%		40%		0.01
T2DM	20%		44%		20%		<0.001
Current Smoker	19%		6%		0%		0.02
Medication							
ASS	24%		31%		13%		0.21
Statin	24%		31%		13%		0.21
ACE-I/ARB	22%		38%		20%		0.02
Metformin	8%		10%		0%		0.42
FRS	7.83	5.92	10.87	6.29	11.70	5.44	<0.001

Table 4. Baseline characteristics of patients according to their NFS score: F0-F2 ($n = 604$), and intermediate or F3-F4 ($n = 148$).

	F0-F2	Intermediate or F3-F4	p-Value
	$n = 604$	$n = 148$	
Female	41%	43%	0.64
Age (years)	59 (9)	66 (9)	<0.001
Systolic RR (mmHg)	134 (18)	140 (18)	<0.001
Diastolic RR (mmhg)	82 (11)	85 (11)	0.02
BMI (kg/m^2)	29 (4)	33 (4)	<0.001
Waist circumference (cm)	103 (11)	111 (11)	<0.001
Waist to hip ratio	1 (0)	1 (0)	0.09
Bilirubine (mg/dL)	1 (0)	1 (0)	<0.001
GGT (U/L)	48 (76)	57 (76)	0.16
AST (U/L)	25 (15)	32 (15)	<0.001
INR	0.99 (0.07)	1.03 (0.07)	<0.001
Total cholesterol (mg/dL)	221 (44)	203 (44)	<0.001
HDL (mg/dL	57 (16)	53 (16)	0.01
LDL (mg/dL)	145 (40)	131 (40)	<0.001
Triglycerices (mg/dL)	145 (84)	147 (84)	0.87
Thrombocytes (G/L)	243 (62)	173 (62)	<0.001
Fasting glucose (mg/dL)	107 (28)	113 (28)	0.01
HbA1c (%)	5.9 (0.7)	6.0 (0.7)	0.12
Metabolic syndrome	30%	43%	0.003
T2DM	20%	40%	<0.001
Current Smoker	19%	6%	0.003
Medication			
ASS	16%	21%	0.11
Statin	24%	30%	0.20
ACE-I/ARB	22%	37%	0.01
Metformin	8%	10%	0.39
FRS	7.83 (5.92)	10.92 (5.92)	<0.001

Table 5. Univariable and multivariable associations with the presence of high risk NFS score.

	Univariable			Multivariable		
	OR	95%CI	p-Value	OR	95%CI	p-Value
Age	1.11	1.09–1.13	<0.001	1.17	1.14–1.21	<0.001
Female gender	0.15	0.10–0.21	<0.001	0.02	0.01–0.04	<0.001
Metabolic syndrome	2.46	1.86–3.26	<0.001	4.15	2.64–6.55	<0.001
FRS	1.60	1.41–1.83	<0.001	1.30	1.09–1.54	0.003

4. Discussion

Our study confirms that there is a "silent epidemic" of NAFLD. In the present cohort of asymptomatic individuals undergoing colonoscopy screening between 50 and 75 years of age, around 50% were diagnosed with NAFLD. In total, 14.2% of the screened patients were categorized as being intermediate and 1% of patients were at high risk for advanced fibrosis by the NFS. Importantly, patients with NAFLD had higher CV risk as defined by the FRS compared to patients without NAFLD. Finally, the CV risk was highest in patients with highest NFS scores.

The NFS does not only predict the risk for advanced liver fibrosis, but also CV risk. Interestingly, in a post-hoc analysis of the IMPROVE-IT trial the NFS identified patients who were at the highest risk for recurrent cardiovascular events. The IMPROVE-IT compared statin therapy alone to the add-on of ezetimibe in post ACS patients [21]. In this trial, higher NFS identified patients more likely to benefit from aggressive lipid-lowering therapy. Thus, although the IMPROVE-IT trial was not designed to assess the link between NAFLD and ACS, it offers important data on the potential link between fatty liver severity and atherosclerosis [21].

The most obvious link between CV risk and NFS is the fact that this score is constituted of factors like age, BMI, ALT, AST, platelets, albumin, and the presence or absence of diabetes, all of which reflect metabolic and inflammatory processes. Of note, inflammation and fibrosis are hallmarks of both liver and cardiovascular disease [18] and may therefore indicate common systemic mechanisms.

In our analysis, NAFLD was an independent risk indicator for CV risk. This is in concordance with a meta-analysis of pooled studies from European, Asian, and American countries suggesting an independent association of NAFLD with CV risk [10]. However, a British study including 17.7 million patients found that the diagnosis of NAFLD was not associated with increased risk for acute myocardial infarction or stroke after adjustment for established CV risk factors [22]. Nevertheless, in another meta-analysis of Targher et al., patients with NAFLD evidenced an increased risk of fatal and non-fatal CV disease [23]. Although the link between NAFLD and CV risk seems intuitive, the effect on CV mortality or events has not been demonstrated. Also, a role for a specific medical treatment for NAFLD in preventing CV events and mortality beyond lifestyle advice and current CV guidelines is not established [24,25]. The data in this manuscript suggests an independent relationship of CV risk and NAFLD in an Austrian cohort. Specific management strategies may be considered based on this evidence to improve liver outcomes in CV patients and CV outcomes in liver patients.

4.1. CV Risk Assessment for NALFD Patients

Considering the Joint Clinical Practice Guidelines of EASL-EASD-EASO for the management of NAFLD patients [17], a non-invasive test should be used as the first screening tool to assess disease severity. Depending on the result, patients can be graded into low, intermediate and high risk with regard to advanced fibrosis. For patients in the low risk group, their individual cardiovascular risk should be assessed by risk scores as for example by the FRS. Target goals for risk factors, e.g., for blood pressure, LDL levels, body weight or blood glucose should be treated according to primary prevention guidelines [25].

Patients with intermediate and high risk for advanced fibrosis should be referred to a hepatologist. In patients with advanced fibrosis stage or even cirrhosis CV risk should be assessed by a cardiologist as described in by Choudhary and Duseja [26]. All other patients should be clinically assessed, stratified by a CV risk score and should be managed according to respective prevention guidelines [25] (Figure 1).

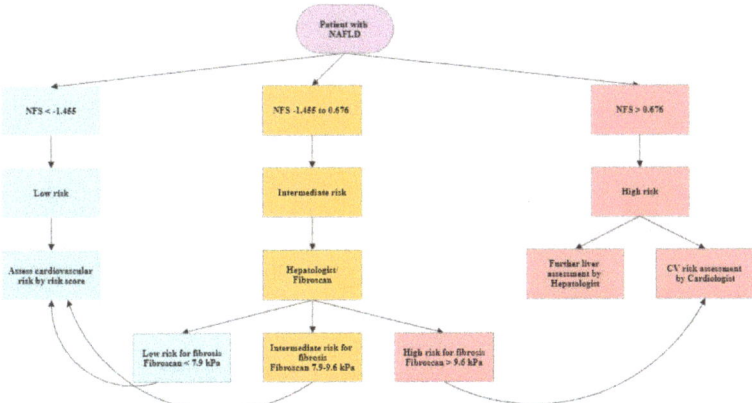

Figure 1. Cardiovascular (CV) assessment algorithm in patients with diagnosed NAFLD.

4.2. Screening for NAFLD in CV Patients

For patients after an CV event or at with a high CV risk we suggest the following approach to detect NAFLD. As a screening test the NFS could be calculated. For patients with low risk for advanced fibrosis, lifestyle modification changes could be recommended. Patients with an intermediate risk could be referred to a liver ultrasound exam and to a hepatologist with expertise in transient elastography. If these exams show no fibrosis or a low stage of fibrosis they should be managed as patients in the low risk group. For patients with intermediate risk in the NFS and advanced fibrosis or cirrhosis in the further exams as well as for patients with a high risk NFS score a hepatologist should be consulted. We are aware, that NFS was developed to estimate fibrosis in the presence of NAFLD. However, we here propose NFS as cheap and non-invasive "screening tool" for NAFLD in patients after an CV event or with a high CV risk. All patients should be treated according to the current guidelines of the European Society of Cardiology [24] (Figure 2).

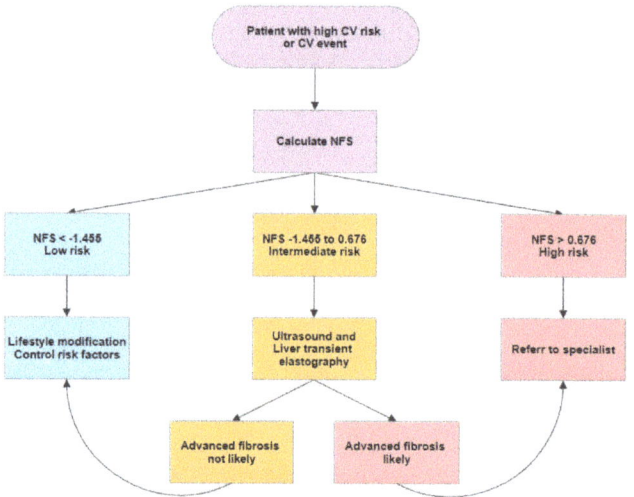

Figure 2. Liver assessment in patients with high cardiovascular risk or with a cardiovascular event in the past medical history.

5. Limitations

This study is a post-hoc analysis of a single-center prospective register and the results remain thesis-generating. However, these data mirror a real-world Austrian population and indicate a high prevalence of undetected NAFLD in the general population. Although this study cannot provide longitudinal CV outcome data, we provide data from a carefully characterized cohort in a cross-sectional study. Another limitation of this study is the linearity of the models especially in using a high number of contributing factors, an assumption that is implicit due to the design of the study.

Furthermore, ultrasound and not liver transient elastography was used to diagnose NAFLD. Finally, clinical data and established surrogate risk scores for calculation of the CV risk as well as the determination of the degree of liver fibrosis by non-invasive scores were used, even though there are other but more expensive and sometimes even more invasive methods available to determine CV risk or liver fibroses such as magnetic resonance imaging, liver biopsy, liver transient elastography, vascular ultrasound, or coronary calcium scoring.

6. Conclusions

The presence of NAFLD might independently predict long-term risk for CV disease. Therefore, patients with high risk for or known CV events should be screened for the presence of NAFLD and risk scores should be routinely applied. Non-invasive risk scores for CV risk and fibrosis could help to facilitate and optimize management of patients with NAFLD with increased CV risk. The care for patients with both NAFLD and CV disease is challenging and due to the vast overlap of patients screening for liver disease in CV patients as well as screening for NAFLD in CV patients seems reasonable [26]. Cardiologists and hepatologists should team up in the treatment of their patients [27].

Author Contributions: D.N., C.D., B.W., S.W.: Conceptualization; D.N., S.W., B.W., U.H.-S., G.S., E.A., G.S., C.S., A.B.: Data curation; B.W., S.W.: Formal analysis; C.D.: Funding acquisition; D.N., C.D.: Methodology; D.N.: Project administration; D.N., C.D.: Supervision; B.W., S.W.: Visualization; D.N., S.W.: Writing—original draft; S.B., B.W., A.B., U.H.-S., G.S., C.S., E.A., C.D.: Writing—review & editing. All authors have read and agreed to the published version of the manuscript.

Funding: Funding by SPAR AG to C.D. is greatly appreciated.

Conflicts of Interest: The authors whose names are listed immediately above certify that they have NO affiliations with or involvement in any organization or entity with any financial interest (such as honoraria; educational grants; participation in speakers' bureaus; membership, employment, consultancies, stock ownership, or other equity interest; and expert testimony or patent-licensing arrangements), or non-financial interest (such as personal or professional relationships, affiliations, knowledge or beliefs) in the subject matter or materials discussed in this manuscript.

References

1. Younossi, Z.M.; Koenig, A.B.; Abdelatif, D.; Fazel, Y.; Henry, L.; Wymer, M. Global epidemiology of nonalcoholic fatty liver disease-Meta-analytic assessment of prevalence, incidence, and outcomes. *Hepatology* **2016**, *64*, 73–84. [CrossRef] [PubMed]
2. WHO Expert Consultation. Appropriate body-mass index for Asian populations and its implications for policy and intervention strategies. *Lancet* **2004**, *363*, 157–163. [CrossRef]
3. Expert Panel on Detection, Evaluation. Treatment of High Blood Cholesterol in, A. Executive Summary of The Third Report of The National Cholesterol Education Program (NCEP) Expert Panel on Detection, Evaluation, And Treatment of High Blood Cholesterol In Adults (Adult Treatment Panel III). *JAMA* **2001**, *285*, 2486–2497. [CrossRef]
4. Roth, G.A.; Johnson, C.; Abajobir, A.; Abd-Allah, F.; Abera, S.F.; Abyu, G.; Ahmed, M.; Aksut, B.; Alam, T.; Alam, K.; et al. Global, Regional, and National Burden of Cardiovascular Diseases for 10 Causes, 1990 to 2015. *J. Am. Coll. Cardiol.* **2017**, *70*, 1–25. [CrossRef]
5. Rafiq, N.; Bai, C.; Fang, Y.; Srishord, M.; McCullough, A.; Gramlich, T.; Younossi, Z.M. Long-term follow-up of patients with nonalcoholic fatty liver. *Clin. Gastroenterol. Hepatol.* **2009**, *7*, 234–238. [CrossRef]
6. Ong, J.P.; Pitts, A.; Younossi, Z.M. Increased overall mortality and liver-related mortality in non-alcoholic fatty liver disease. *J. Hepatol.* **2008**, *49*, 608–612. [CrossRef]
7. Oni, E.T.; Agatston, A.S.; Blaha, M.J.; Fialkow, J.; Cury, R.; Sposito, A.; Erbel, R.; Blankstein, R.; Feldman, T.; Al-Mallah, M.H.; et al. A systematic review: Burden and severity of subclinical cardiovascular disease among those with nonalcoholic fatty liver; should we care? *Atherosclerosis* **2013**, *230*, 258–267. [CrossRef]
8. Mantovani, A.; Pernigo, M.; Bergamini, C.; Bonapace, S.; Lipari, P.; Pichiri, I.; Bertolini, L.; Valbusa, F.; Barbieri, E.; Zoppini, G.; et al. Nonalcoholic Fatty Liver Disease Is Independently Associated with Early Left Ventricular Diastolic Dysfunction in Patients with Type 2 Diabetes. *PLoS ONE* **2015**, *10*, e0135329. [CrossRef]
9. Targher, G.; Day, C.P.; Bonora, E. Risk of cardiovascular disease in patients with nonalcoholic fatty liver disease. *N. Engl. J. Med.* **2010**, *363*, 1341–1350. [CrossRef]
10. Wu, S.; Wu, F.; Ding, Y.; Hou, J.; Bi, J.; Zhang, Z. Association of non-alcoholic fatty liver disease with major adverse cardiovascular events: A systematic review and meta-analysis. *Sci. Rep.* **2016**, *6*, 33386. [CrossRef]
11. Byrne, C.D.; Targher, G. NAFLD: A multisystem disease. *J. Hepatol.* **2015**, *62*, S47–S64. [CrossRef]
12. Wieckowska, A.; Papouchado, B.G.; Li, Z.; Lopez, R.; Zein, N.N.; Feldstein, A.E. Increased hepatic and circulating interleukin-6 levels in human nonalcoholic steatohepatitis. *Am. J. Gastroenterol.* **2008**, *103*, 1372–1379. [CrossRef] [PubMed]

13. Targher, G.; Bertolini, L.; Zoppini, G.; Zenari, L.; Falezza, G. Increased plasma markers of inflammation and endothelial dysfunction and their association with microvascular complications in Type 1 diabetic patients without clinically manifest macroangiopathy. *Diabet. Med.* **2005**, *22*, 999–1004. [CrossRef] [PubMed]
14. Howard, G.; O'Leary, D.H.; Zaccaro, D.; Haffner, S.; Rewers, M.; Hamman, R.; Selby, J.V.; Saad, M.F.; Savage, P.; Bergman, R. Insulin sensitivity and atherosclerosis. The Insulin Resistance Atherosclerosis Study (IRAS) Investigators. *Circulation* **1996**, *93*, 1809–1817. [CrossRef] [PubMed]
15. Ekstedt, M.; Hagstrom, H.; Nasr, P.; Fredrikson, M.; Stal, P.; Kechagias, S.; Hultcrantz, R. Fibrosis stage is the strongest predictor for disease-specific mortality in NAFLD after up to 33 years of follow-up. *Hepatology* **2015**, *61*, 1547–1554. [CrossRef] [PubMed]
16. Despotovic, D.; Niederseer, D.; Brunckhorst, C. CME-EKG 60: Akut auftretende Thoraxschmerzen und Dyspnoe: Das EKG als Schlussel zur Diagnose. *Praxis* **2018**, *107*, 223–224. [CrossRef]
17. European Association for the Study of the Liver (EASL); European Association for the Study of Diabetes (EASD); European Association for the Study of Obesity (EASO). EASL-EASD-EASO Clinical Practice Guidelines for the management of non-alcoholic fatty liver disease. *J. Hepatol.* **2016**, *64*, 1388–1402. [CrossRef]
18. Angulo, P.; Hui, J.M.; Marchesini, G.; Bugianesi, E.; George, J.; Farrell, G.C.; Enders, F.; Saksena, S.; Burt, A.D.; Bida, J.P.; et al. The NAFLD fibrosis score: A noninvasive system that identifies liver fibrosis in patients with NAFLD. *Hepatology* **2007**, *45*, 846–854. [CrossRef]
19. Grundy, S.M.; Cleeman, J.I.; Daniels, S.R.; Donato, K.A.; Eckel, R.H.; Franklin, B.A.; Gordon, D.J.; Krauss, R.M.; Savage, P.J.; Smith, S.C., Jr.; et al. Diagnosis and management of the metabolic syndrome: An American Heart Association/National Heart, Lung, and Blood Institute scientific statement: Executive Summary. *Crit. Pathw. Cardiol.* **2005**, *4*, 198–203. [CrossRef]
20. Wilson, P.W.; D'Agostino, R.B.; Levy, D.; Belanger, A.M.; Silbershatz, H.; Kannel, W.B. Prediction of coronary heart disease using risk factor categories. *Circulation* **1998**, *97*, 1837–1847. [CrossRef]
21. Simon, T.G.; Corey, K.E.; Cannon, C.P.; Blazing, M.; Park, J.G.; O'Donoghue, M.L.; Chung, R.T.; Giugliano, R.P. The nonalcoholic fatty liver disease (NAFLD) fibrosis score, cardiovascular risk stratification and a strategy for secondary prevention with ezetimibe. *Int. J. Cardiol.* **2018**, *270*, 245–252. [CrossRef] [PubMed]
22. Alexander, M.; Loomis, A.K.; Van der Lei, J.; Duarte-Salles, T.; Prieto-Alhambra, D.; Ansell, D.; Pasqua, A.; Lapi, F.; Rijnbeek, P.; Mosseveld, M.; et al. Non-alcoholic fatty liver disease and risk of incident acute myocardial infarction and stroke: Findings from matched cohort study of 18 million European adults. *BMJ* **2019**, *367*, l5367. [CrossRef] [PubMed]
23. Targher, G.; Byrne, C.D.; Lonardo, A.; Zoppini, G.; Barbui, C. Non-alcoholic fatty liver disease and risk of incident cardiovascular disease: A meta-analysis. *J. Hepatol.* **2016**, *65*, 589–600. [CrossRef] [PubMed]
24. Knuuti, J.; Wijns, W.; Saraste, A.; Capodanno, D.; Barbato, E.; Funck-Brentano, C.; Prescott, E.; Storey, R.F.; Deaton, C.; Cuisset, T.; et al. 2019 ESC Guidelines for the diagnosis and management of chronic coronary syndromes. *Eur. Heart J.* **2020**, *41*, 407–477. [CrossRef]
25. Piepoli, M.F.; Hoes, A.W.; Agewall, S.; Albus, C.; Brotons, C.; Catapano, A.L.; Cooney, M.T.; Corra, U.; Cosyns, B.; Deaton, C.; et al. 2016 European Guidelines on cardiovascular disease prevention in clinical practice: The Sixth Joint Task Force of the European Society of Cardiology and Other Societies on Cardiovascular Disease Prevention in Clinical Practice (constituted by representatives of 10 societies and by invited experts)Developed with the special contribution of the European Association for Cardiovascular Prevention & Rehabilitation (EACPR). *Eur. Heart J.* **2016**, *37*, 2315–2381. [CrossRef]
26. Choudhary, N.S.; Duseja, A. Screening of Cardiovascular Disease in Nonalcoholic Fatty Liver Disease: Whom and How? *J. Clin. Exp. Hepatol.* **2019**, *9*, 506–514. [CrossRef]
27. Wernly, B.; Wernly, S.; Niederseer, D.; Datz, C. Hepatitis C virus (HCV) infection and cardiovascular disease: Hepatologists and cardiologists need to talk! *Eur. J. Intern. Med.* **2020**, *71*, 87–88. [CrossRef]

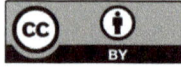

© 2020 by the authors. Licensee MDPI, Basel, Switzerland. This article is an open access article distributed under the terms and conditions of the Creative Commons Attribution (CC BY) license (http://creativecommons.org/licenses/by/4.0/).

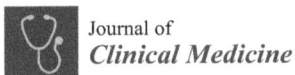

Article

Circulating miR-320a as a Predictive Biomarker for Left Ventricular Remodelling in STEMI Patients Undergoing Primary Percutaneous Coronary Intervention

Isabel Galeano-Otero [1,2,†], Raquel Del Toro [1,2,†], Agustín Guisado [3], Ignacio Díaz [2], Isabel Mayoral-González [2], Francisco Guerrero-Márquez [3], Encarnación Gutiérrez-Carretero [2,3], Sara Casquero-Domínguez [3], Luis Díaz-de la Llera [3], Gonzalo Barón-Esquivias [2,3], Manuel Jiménez-Navarro [4], Tarik Smani [1,2,*] and Antonio Ordóñez-Fernández [2,3,*]

[1] Departamento de Fisiología Médica y Biofísica, Universidad de Sevilla, 41009 Sevilla, Spain; igaleano@us.es (I.G.-O.); rdeltoro-ibis@us.es (R.D.T.)
[2] Grupo de Fisiopatología Cardiovascular, Instituto de Biomedicina de Sevilla-IBiS, Universidad de Sevilla/HUVR/Junta de Andalucía/CSIC, Sevilla 41013, CIBERCV, 28029 Madrid, Spain; nnachoddcc@hotmail.com (I.D.); isabelmayoralgon@hotmail.com (I.M.-G.); gutierrez.encarnita@gmail.com (E.G.-C.); gonzalo.baron.sspa@juntadeandalucia.es (G.B.-E.)
[3] Servicio de Cardiología, Hospital Universitario Virgen del Rocío, 41013 Sevilla, Spain; aguiras@hotmail.com (A.G.); guerreromar24@gmail.com (F.G.-M.); saracasquero@gmail.com (S.C.-D.); luissalvadordiaz@hotmail.com (L.D.-d.l.-L.)
[4] Hospital Universitario Virgen de la Victoria, Málaga 29010, CIBERCV, 28029 Madrid, Spain; mjimeneznavarro@gmail.com
* Correspondence: tasmani@us.es (T.S.); antorfernan@us.es (A.O.-F.); Tel.: +34-955-92-30-57 (T.S.)
† These authors contributed equally to this work.

Received: 22 February 2020; Accepted: 6 April 2020; Published: 8 April 2020

Abstract: Restoration of epicardial coronary blood flow, achieved by early reperfusion with primary percutaneous coronary intervention (PPCI), is the guideline recommended to treat patients with ST-segment-elevation myocardial infarction (STEMI). However, despite successful blood restoration, increasing numbers of patients develop left ventricular adverse remodelling (LVAR) and heart failure. Therefore, reliable prognostic biomarkers for LVAR in STEMI are urgently needed. Our aim was to investigate the role of circulating microRNAs (miRNAs) and their association with LVAR in STEMI patients following the PPCI procedure. We analysed the expression of circulating miRNAs in blood samples of 56 patients collected at admission and after revascularization (at 3, 6, 12 and 24 h). The associations between miRNAs and left ventricular end diastolic volumes at 6 months were estimated to detect LVAR. miRNAs were also analysed in samples isolated from peripheral blood mononuclear cells (PBMCs) and human myocardium of failing hearts. Kinetic analysis of miRNAs showed a fast time-dependent increase in miR-133a, miR-133b, miR-193b, miR-499, and miR-320a in STEMI patients compared to controls. Moreover, the expression of miR-29a, miR-29b, miR-324, miR-208, miR-423, miR-522, and miR-545 was differentially expressed even before PPCI in STEMI. Furthermore, the increase in circulating miR-320a and the decrease in its expression in PBMCs were significantly associated with LVAR and correlated with the expression of miR-320a in human failing myocardium from ischaemic origin. In conclusion, we determined the time course expression of new circulating miRNAs in patients with STEMI treated with PPCI and we showed that miR-320a was positively associated with LVAR.

Keywords: STEMI; PPCI; left ventricular adverse remodelling; circulating miRNAs

1. Introduction

ST-segment-elevation myocardial infarction (STEMI) is considered the most common and severe acute myocardial infarction (AMI) [1]. According to current guidelines, early reperfusion of coronary flow by primary percutaneous coronary intervention (PPCI) significantly mitigates cardiac cell death and cardiovascular events. PPCI has substantially reduced mortality following STEMI by decreasing the infarct size and the extent of left ventricular adverse remodelling (LVAR) [2,3]. However, increasing evidence has demonstrated that despite successful and prompt revascularization, ~25% of patients who survive STEMI develop heart failure (HF) as a consequence of LVAR [4–7]. STEMI treated with PPCI triggers a complex cascade of events associated with ischaemia and reperfusion (I/R), such as oxidative stress, neutrophil and platelet aggregation, and acute inflammatory responses [8] necessary to repair heart injuries. More specifically, peripheral blood mononuclear cells (PBMCs), mainly monocytes, participate in the acute response to heart damage. These cell populations egress from the bone marrow to the blood and infiltrate the myocardium hours after AMI [9,10]. Different studies have suggested that an exacerbated and prolonged inflammatory reaction causes irreparable damage which could be responsible for the progression of LVAR [11,12].

LVAR remains difficult to predict [13] even if there is general agreement regarding the value of troponin-I, creatine kinase (CK), and brain-derived natriuretic peptide (BNP) in post-acute coronary syndrome risk stratification [14]. However, none of the known cardiac biomarkers used today are considered reliable to predict the incidence of LVAR after PPCI in STEMI patients. Therefore, identifying new sensitive biomarkers may help to improve the early prognosis of patients with a high risk of post-infarction remodelling and dysfunction of the left ventricle after PPCI. Currently, there is great interest in the potential use of microRNAs (miRNAs) as promising novel biomarkers for the diagnosis and/or prognosis of different systemic diseases [15–17]. miRNAs are a group of small endogenous noncoding RNAs that can degrade mRNA transcripts directly, inhibit protein translation, and regulate protein expression at the post-transcriptional level [18]. miRNAs are present in blood and can be detected easily in serum or plasma due to their high stability (as reviewed previously [19]). A large number of studies have demonstrated that miRNAs are dysregulated in the blood of patients with cardiovascular diseases (CVD) compared to healthy controls. In fact, miRNAs have been suggested to be critical players in CVD since they participate in the genetic regulation of hundreds of key proteins involved in signalling pathways triggered by I/R [20–22]. Recent reports have described the expression patterns of circulating miRNAs in patients with myocardial infarction [23–25]. However, there are only a few studies describing miRNAs in STEMI patients after PPCI and their possible role as prognostic markers for the development of LVAR [26–28]. In this study, we examined the time course of the expression of miRNAs in STEMI patients after PPCI, and assessed the specific role of miR-320a as a prognostic biomarker of LVAR.

2. Materials and Methods

All procedures involving study subjects were performed according to the principles published by the declaration of Helsinki and its amendments or comparable ethical standards. The study was approved by the local Ethics Committee on Human Research at the University Hospital "Virgen del Rocio" of Seville and the University Hospital of "Virgen de la Victoria" of Málaga (approval no. 2013PI/096). Strengthening the reporting of observational studies in epidemiology (STROBE) guidelines were followed to report our findings (Figure S1).

2.1. Study Subjects and Blood Extraction

All study subjects voluntarily participated and signed an informed consent form. As depicted in Figure S1, a total of 56 participants who underwent coronary artery angiography at the above hospitals due to chest pain were selected. Patients were divided into 2 groups: (1) STEMI patients consisting of 42 patients who were diagnosed with STEMI for the first time and were treated with PPCI

1; 3 STEMI patients died before finishing this study, and (2) Control group consisting of 14 non-STEMI patients whose coronary angiogram showed no coronary lesion. The inclusion criteria were as follows: patients under 75 years old, diagnosed with AMI, presenting symptoms 2 to 6 h prior to angioplasty and exhibiting occlusion of the left anterior descending (LAD) artery with epicardial blood flow ("Thrombolysis in Myocardial Infarction" (TIMI) flow grade) of 0 in the initial angiogram. The exclusion criteria were as follows: patients with a previous history of ischaemic heart disease, a glomerular filtration rate less than 30 mL/min, TIMI flow > 0–1 at the time of angiography. Patients received standard pharmacological therapy as per current clinical guidelines. Information relative to clinical, demographical, haemodynamic, angiographic and electrocardiographic findings was prospectively registered in all cases upon admission. In some experiments, blood samples from healthy volunteers without known disease were used as a healthy control to compare the expression of miRNAs.

First, blood samples were extracted after catheter insertion in the radial artery before initiation of the PPCI procedure. These samples represented the pre-reperfusion time point 0 h. Additional blood samples were collected at 3, 6, 12 and/or 24 h after culprit vessel opening. Additional blood samples were collected 1 month after the ischaemic event. Echocardiography was performed to determine ventricular ejection fraction and systolic and diastolic left ventricular diameters and volumes before patient discharge and 6 months after PPCI to determine the possible development of LVAR. LVAR was defined as an increase of at least 20% in left ventricular end-diastolic volume (LVEDV) with left ventricular ejection fraction less than 50%, as defined according to current clinical indications [29].

Serum was obtained from whole blood samples collected without antiserum. PBMCs were isolated from blood using ethylenediaminetetraacetic acid (EDTA)-coated tubes. The lymphocyte separation media (Lymphosep; Biowest, Riverside, MO, USA) was used to isolate PBMCs from blood following the manufacturer's instructions.

2.2. Human Samples

Myocardial biopsies were obtained from the atrium of ischaemic patients with heart failure (HF) during cardiac surgery. The 7 HF patients (5 males and 2 females) had a median age of 62 years, and their ejection fraction (EF) before surgery was 52% ± 12%. Fully informed written consent was obtained from the families of all donors.

2.3. RNA Isolation and miRNA Analysis

Blood samples were collected before the start of the PPCI procedure and at multiple time points following PPCI. We used the miRNeasy Serum/Plasma kit (QIAGEN, Hilden, Germany) to extract small RNAs from serum. Briefly, 200 µL of serum was mixed with 700 µL of QIAzol Lysis Reagent included in the kit, and 10 pmol of Arabidopsis miRNA (ath-miR-159a) was added as a spike-in control. Then, we followed the manufacturer's instructions to obtain the fraction of eluted miRNAs. To obtain small RNAs from PBMCs, we used the mirVana miRNA Isolation Kit (Thermo Fisher Scientific Inc., Waltham, MA, USA). The eluted miRNAs were quantified using a fluorometer (Qubit 4 Thermo Fisher Scientific Inc., Waltham, MA, USA) through a Qubit miRNA assay (Thermo Fisher Scientific Inc., Waltham, MA, USA). We used TaqMan array miRNA card pool A (Applied Biosystems Thermo Fisher Scientific Inc., Waltham, MA, USA) to examine miRNA expression in 9 STEMI and 3 control patients. Once we had selected miRNA candidates, custom TaqMan miRNA arrays (Applied Biosystems, Thermo Fisher Scientific Inc., Waltham, MA, USA) were designed to amplify miRNAs. To validate miRNA expression, we used RT-qPCR using the TaqMan Advanced miRNA cDNA Synthesis Kit, TaqMan Advanced miRNA Assay, and TaqMan Fast Advanced Master Mix technology. To determine miRNA expression in PBMCs, we used the miScript II RT Kit (QIAGEN, Hilden, Germany) and iTaq Universal SYBR Green Supermix (Bio-Rad, Hercules, CA, USA). RT-qPCR was performed using an Applied Biosystems Viia7 7900HT thermocycler. Relative quantification analyses were performed using the software SDS2.2 and Expression Suite Software V1.0.3 (Applied Biosystems, Thermo Fisher Scientific Inc., Waltham, MA,

USA), online software ThermoFisher Cloud and QuantStudio Real Time PCR Software (Thermo Fisher Scientific Inc., Waltham, MA, USA) and Excel. Fold changes in miRNA expression were calculated using the comparative cycle threshold CT ($\Delta\Delta$CT) method. The values are expressed as the logarithm of the fold change.

2.4. In Silico miRNA Studies

We used the miRDB (miRDB v7.2, http://mirdb.org, Washington University St. Louis, MO, USA) and TargetScan (www.targetscan.org, Cambridge, MA, USA) databases to analyse miRNA targets. We found common targets between the databases through a Venn diagram. To identify microRNA target gene pathways, we used an online platform from the Gene Ontology (GO) browser PANTHER (Protein Analysis THrough Evolutionary Relationships 14.1 version, http://pantherdb.org/genelistanalysis.do, University of Southern California, Los Angeles, CA, USA).

2.5. Statistical Analysis

Data were analysed using SPSS (SPSS Inc. version 25.0 IBM, Armonk, NY, USA) and with GraphPad (GraphPad Software Inc., San Diego, CA, USA). The results are presented as the mean and standard error of the mean (SEM). The outliers were removed based on the results of QuickCalcs, an online tool of GraphPad. The Shapiro–Wilk test was used for normality. For normally distributed variables, we used an ordinary one-way ANOVA, and we performed multiple comparisons using T-test without correction (Fisher's LSD test). For non-normal distribution, we used the non-parametric Kruskal–Wallis test with multiple comparisons corrected by Dunn's test. Multivariate logistic regression analysis was performed to estimate the independent relationship between variables with significant differences ($p < 0.1$) and the appearance of LVAR. LVAR was taken as the binary dependent variable, miR-320a expression as the independent, and CK, sex and age as the covariates for adjustment. Linear regression analysis was conducted using the percentage of change in LVEDV as dependent variable. The LVAR predictive value of different parameters (miR-320a expression, CK, and age) was also evaluated using the receiver operating characteristic (ROC) curve.

3. Results

3.1. Analysis of the Clinical Data of the Subjects

Clinical information about the study subjects is shown in Table 1. A total of 42 patients with STEMI who underwent PPCI and 14 controls were included in this study. Table 1 indicates that 88% of the STEMI patients were male, and there were no significant differences between STEMI and control patients ($p > 0.05$) in terms of age, risk factors and LVEDV index at the time of admission. In contrast, we observed significant differences in cardiac markers, creatine kinase and troponin T between both groups at the onset of PPCI.

3.2. miRNA Expression Profiles in STEMI

Samples from control and STEMI patients with TIMI 0 flow were used to detect the profiles of miRNAs secreted in the serum 3 to 6 h after PPCI by a RT-qPCR-based array. Figure 1A shows volcano plot analysis indicating significant alterations in the expression of miRNAs. The hierarchical clustering analysis indicated that 25 miRNAs were differentially expressed despite the variability between STEMI patient samples compared to the control group (Figure 1B). Of these, 96 miRNAs were upregulated and 138 were downregulated. Based on this finding, we selected 5 miRNAs (miR-193b, miR-320a, miR-339-5p, miR-522, and miR-545) to examine their expression in serum taken from 8 patients with STEMI at different time points: before PPCI (0 h) and 3, 12, and 24 h after revascularization. Samples from 8 non-STEMI patients were used as controls.

Table 1. Demographic and clinical characteristics of STEMI patients ($n = 42$) and controls ($n = 14$). Data are shown as the means ± SEM and as n (%). Student's t-tests were performed. LVEDV stands for the left ventricular end-diastolic volume; (*) indicates $p < 0.05$, which is considered statistically significant; $ indicates that the variable was examined at admission.

	Controls ($n = 14$)	Patients ($n = 42$)	P Value
Age (years)	62.1 ± 11.6	58.4 ± 11.3	0.287
Male sex	7 (50.0%)	37 (88.1%)	0.002 *
Arterial hypertension	7 (50.0%)	21 (50.0%)	1.000
Smoking	7 (50.0%)	17 (40.5%)	0.541
Dyslipidaemia	8 (57.1%)	19 (45.2%)	0.449
Type 2 diabetes mellitus (%)	4 (28.6%)	10 (23.8%)	0.727
LVEDV (ml/m^2) $	50 ± 10.9	58.1 ± 12.7	0.162
Creatine kinase (mg/dL) $	96.4 ± 60.1	2502 ± 2290.6	>0.001 *
Troponin T (ng/mL) $	7.3 ± 4.9	6097.6 ± 5526.9	0.003 *

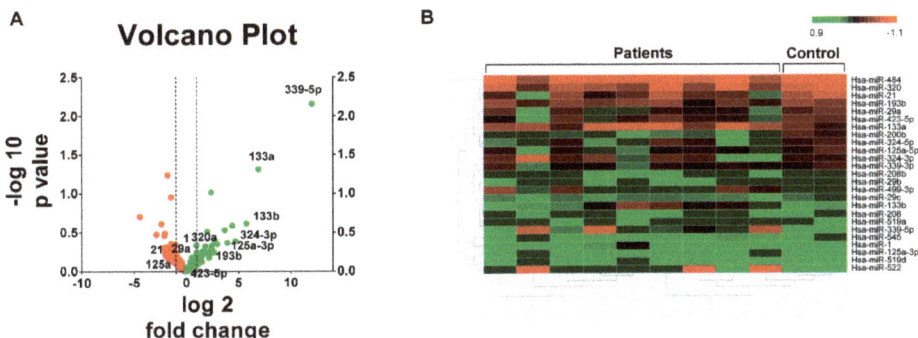

Figure 1. miRNAs differentially expressed in STEMI patients 3 h post PPCI. (**A**) Volcano plot showing miRNAs differentially expressed in STEMI patients ($n = 9$) relative to the control ($n = 3$); the x axis shows log$_2$ (fold change), and the y-axis shows –log$_{10}$ (p value). (**B**) Fragment of hierarchical clustered sample-centric heat-map analysis of the ΔCt value of differentially expressed miRNAs in STEMI patients 3 h post PPCI compared to the control. Scale bar: downregulated (red) and upregulated (green). Distance was measured by Pearson's correlation.

We also examined the levels of other miRNAs (miR-1, miR-21, miR-29a, miR-29b, miR-125, miR-133a, miR-133b, miR-208, miR-324, miR-423-5p and miR-499), selected based on a literature search focusing on their relevance in different CVD [26,30–34] using the search term "miRNA" in combination with one of the following key words: "STEMI", "ischaemia and reperfusion", "heart infarction", and "heart failure". Figure 2A–E shows a significant increase in the expression of miR-133a, miR-133b, miR-193b, miR-499, and miR-320a in STEMI patients at different time points compared to the control group. The levels of these miRNAs mainly reached a maximum increase between 3 and 12 h and returned to their basal level 24 h after PPCI. In the case of miR-423, miR-29a, miR-339-5p, and miR-324, their expression increased and remained significantly higher 24 h after PPCI (Figure 2F–I). In contrast, Figure 3A–D shows that the expression of miR-29b, miR-208, miR-522, and miR-545 was significantly downregulated soon after PPCI and continued to be downregulated at all examined time points in STEMI patients. Moreover, Figure 3E,F show that miR-1 levels were downregulated only at the time point before PPCI, while miR-21 seemed to not be sensitive to PPCI.

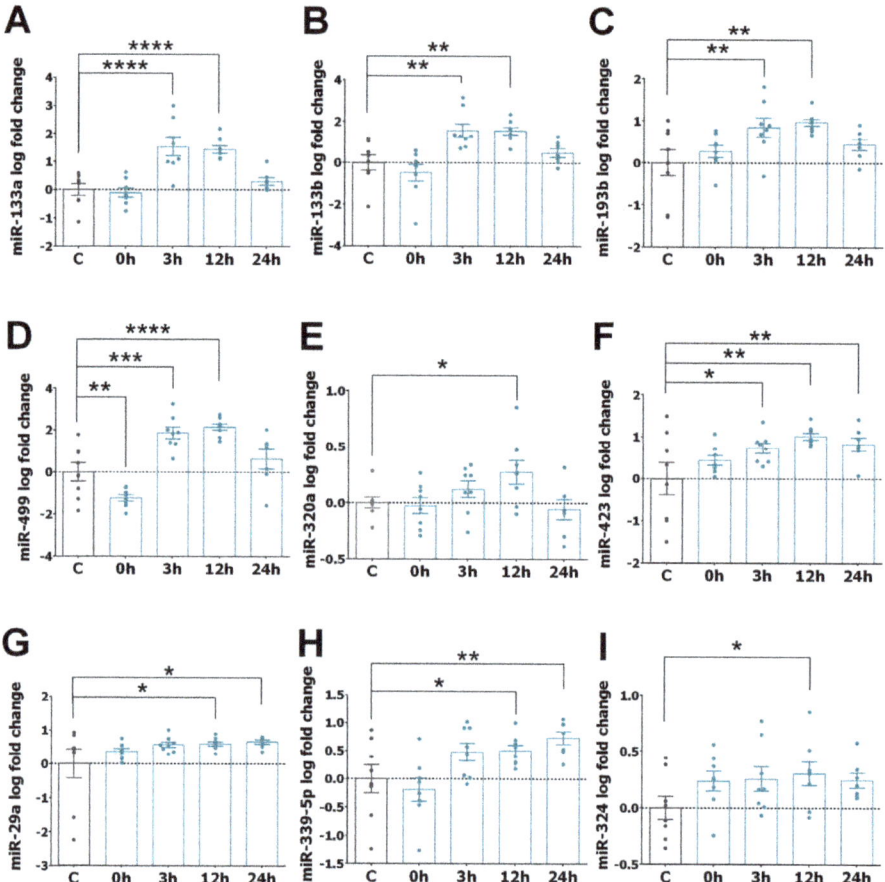

Figure 2. Upregulation of circulating miRNAs in the serum of post-STEMI patients. (**A–I**) Graphs showing the kinetics of miRNAs in serum samples of STEMI patients ($n = 8$) before PPCI (0 h) and 3, 12, and 24 h after the PPCI procedure. Bar graphs show changes in the expression of miR-133a (**A**), miR-133b (**B**), miR-193b (**C**), miR-499 (**D**), miR-320a (**E**), miR-423 (**F**), miR-29a (**G**), miR-339-5p (**H**) and miR-324 (**I**) in patients after PPCI compared to control patients ($n = 8$). Values represent the fold changes (in logarithmic scale) for each miRNA relative to controls. Data are presented as the means ± SEM. Significance is indicated by (*) for $p < 0.05$, (**) for $p < 0.01$, (***) for $p < 0.001$, and (****) for $p < 0.0001$. Ordinary one-way ANOVA with multiples comparisons using T-test without correction (Fisher's LSD test) was performed.

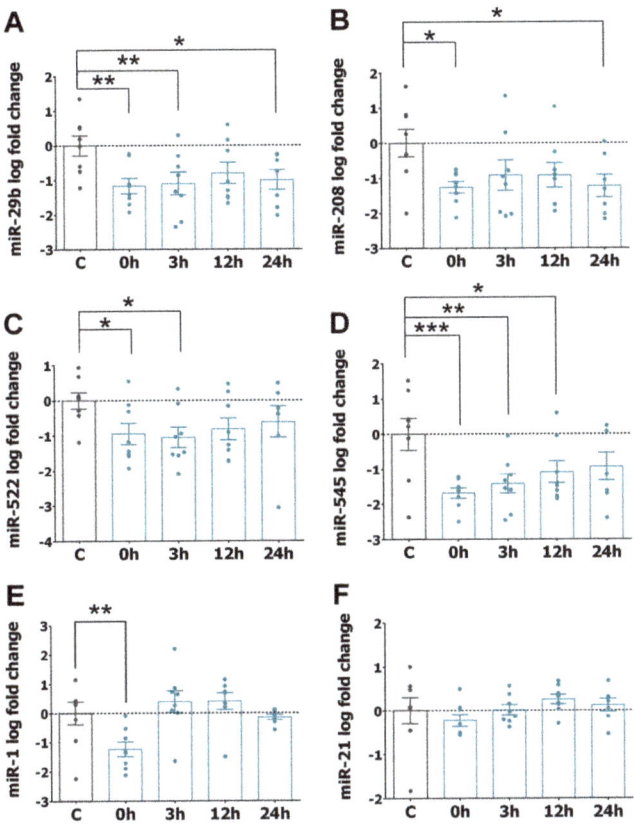

Figure 3. Downregulation of circulating miRNA levels in the serum of STEMI patients. (**A–F**) Graphs represent miRNA expression in the serum of STEMI patients ($n = 8$) compared to the control ($n = 8$) before PPCI (0 h) and 3, 12, and 24 h. Bar graphs show the expression of miR-29b (**A**), miR-208 (**B**), miR-522 (**C**), miR-545 (**D**), miR-1 (**E**) and miR-21 (**F**) in patients compared to control patients. Values are presented as the means ± SEM and represent the fold change in logarithmic scale for each miRNA relative to controls. Significance is indicated by (*) for $p < 0.05$, (**) for $p < 0.01$, and (***) for $p < 0.001$. Ordinary one-way ANOVA with multiples comparisons using T-test without correction (Fisher's LSD test) was performed.

3.3. miRNA Expression Pattern in STEMI with LVAR

To further characterize the relevance of the observed changes in the expression of miRNAs, we examined whether their levels were different in patients who developed LVAR 6 months after PPCI compared to those who did not present any adverse events after PPCI interventions. Table 2 shows that of 39 patients, 14 (22%) developed LVAR since their LVEDV index values increased significantly 6 months after PPCI compared to the values at admission. We also observed a significant difference in the level of creatine kinase, but not troponin T, at the time of admission of patients with or without LVAR. Moreover, there were no significant differences between the groups in terms of age, gender, risk factors, or pro-BNP 6 months after PPCI ($p > 0.05$).

Table 2. Demographic and clinical characteristics of STEMI patients ($n = 39$). Patients were classified into two groups: no remodelling ($n = 25$) and remodelling ($n = 14$). Data are shown as the means ± SEM and as n (%). Student's t-tests were performed. LVEDV stands for the left ventricular end-diastolic volume; (*) indicates that $p < 0.05$ is statistically significant; $ indicates that the variable was examined at admission, $$ at 1 month after PPCI and $$$ at 6 months after PPCI.

	STEMI Patients ($n = 39$)	No remodelling ($n = 25$)	Remodelling ($n = 14$)	P Value
Age (years)	57.8 ± 10.4	57.2 ± 10.6	59.1 ± 10.3	0.596
Male sex	35 (89.7%)	23 (92.0%)	12 (85.7%)	0.547
Arterial hypertension	18 (46.2%)	10 (40.0%)	8 (57.1%)	0.316
Smoking	16 (41.0%)	11 (44.0%)	5 (35.7%)	0.625
Dyslipidaemia	17 (45.2%)	12 (48.0%)	5 (35.7%)	0.471
Type 2 diabetes mellitus	9 (23.1%)	6 (24.0%)	3 (21.4%)	0.860
LVEDV (ml/m^2) $	57.9 ± 12.8	58.9 ± 12.4	55.9 ± 13.6	0.487
LVEDV (ml/m^2) $$$	67.8 ± 26.0	56.9 ± 11.2	88.8 ± 33.4	>0.001 *
Creatine kinase (mg/dL) $	3213.8 ±2209.0	2447.8 ± 1795.6	4526.9 ± 2289.9	0.004 *
Troponin T (ng/mL) $	5806.6 ± 5404.1	4853.3 ± 4414.5	7508.9 ± 6672.3	0.143
Pro-BNP (pg/mL) $$	1172.9 ± 710.7	1029.2 ± 896.2	1388.5 ± 270.4	0.466

Next, based on our previous results, we compared the expression of miR-320a, miR-193b, miR-324, miR-339-5p, miR-519a, miR-522, and miR-545 in STEMI patients ($n = 8$) with or without LVAR ($n = 8$). Figure 4A shows that the levels of miR-320a were significantly increased at 3 and 12 h after PPCI in LVAR patients compared to patients without remodelling. Moreover, no differences in the levels of the other miRNAs were observed between the groups (Figure 4B–F). To confirm that the expression levels of miR-320a were associated with the appearance of LVAR, we examined miR-320a expression in a larger cohort of patients ($n = 39$). In this case, we considered 6 h as the optimal time point to test the miRNA maximum levels after PPCI, and we also evaluated its expression 1 month after revascularization. Figure 5A confirms a transient rise of miR-320a in STEMI patients, reaching a maximum increase 6 h after PPCI, while its expression decreased significantly 1 month after patient discharge. Furthermore, the comparison of miR-320a levels between patients with or without LVAR (Figure 5B) shows that miR-320a was still significantly higher 1 month after discharge in the non-remodelling group but not in LVAR patients. This fact suggests that changes in the levels of circulating miR-320a can be associated with the appearance of LVAR. In another set of experiments, we determined the expression of miR-320a in healthy volunteers and compared it with the expression in the control group. Figure S2A shows that the levels of miR-320a were not significantly different between the two groups, and the expression of miR-320a in STEMI patients with or without LVAR compared to its levels in healthy controls (Figure S2B) was similar to those observed when compared to the clinical control (Figure 5B).

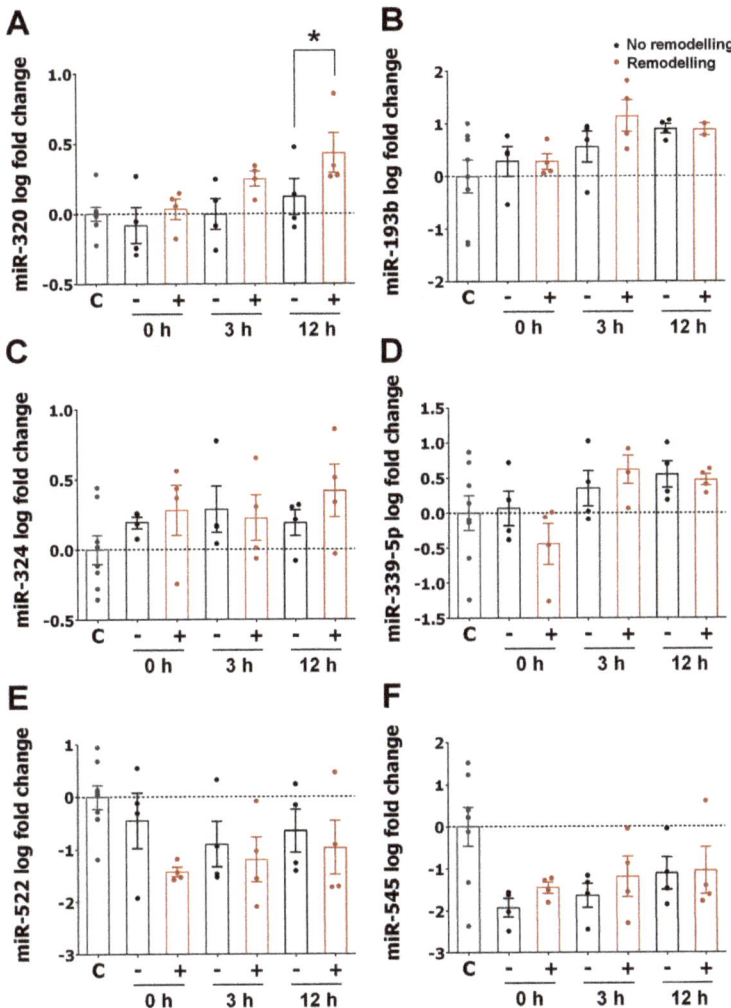

Figure 4. Comparison of the expression of miRNAs in patients with or without left ventricular adverse remodelling. (**A–F**) Bar graphs show the expression of miR-320a (**A**), miR-193b (**B**), miR-324 (**C**), miR-339-5p (**D**), miR-522 (**E**), and miR-545 (**F**) in serum samples of STEMI patients who developed left ventricular adverse remodelling (red bars, $n = 4$) or not (black bars, $n = 4$) before PPCI (0 h) and at 3, 12, and 24 h after the procedure. The values in the graphs represent the fold change in logarithmic scale for each miRNA relative to controls. Values are presented as the means ± SEM and represent the fold change in logarithmic scale for each miRNA relative to controls ($n = 8$). Significance is indicated by (*) for $p < 0.05$. Ordinary one-way ANOVA with multiples comparisons using T-test without correction (Fisher's LSD test) was performed.

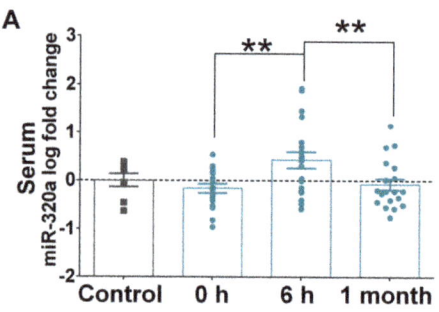
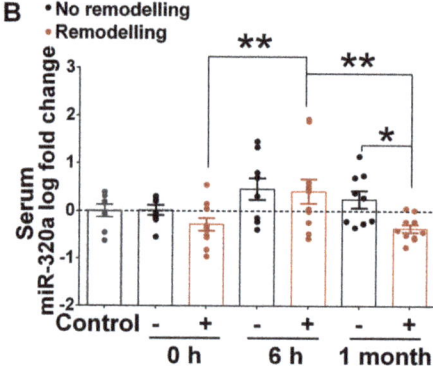

Figure 5. Comparison of the expression of miR-320a in the serum of patients with or without left ventricular adverse remodelling. (**A**) Bar graph shows miR-320a expression in serum samples of STEMI patients ($n = 20$) at 0 h, 6 h and 1 month post PPCI relative to the control ($n = 8$). (**B**) Bar graph shows the levels of miR-320a at 0 h, 6 h and 1 month after PPCI in STEMI patients who developed LVAR (red bar, $n = 11$) or not (black bar, $n = 9$). Values in the graphs represent the fold change in logarithmic scale for each miRNA relative to controls. Data are the means ± SEM. Significance is indicated by (*) for $p < 0.05$ and (**) for $p < 0.01$. Ordinary one-way ANOVA with multiples comparisons using T-test without correction (Fisher's LSD test) was performed.

3.4. Correlation of Serum Levels of miR-320a with LVAR

Linear regression and ROC analysis were performed to further confirm that changes in circulating levels of miR-320a associates with LVAR. Figure 6A shows that the levels of miR-320a at 1 month ($r = 0.651$, $p = 0.03$) correlated inversely and significantly with the percentage of changes in LVEDV, meanwhile CK ($r = 0.462$, $p = 0.053$) and age ($r = 0.085$, $p = 0.738$) showed worse association with LVEDV changes. Moreover, ROC curve analysis in Figure 6B shows that the area under the curve (AUC) of miR-320a expression was 0.889 (95% CI: 0.74–1.00; p value = 0.004), while the AUC of CK was 0.722 (95%CI: 0.463–0.981; p value = 0.102), and of age was 0.530 (95%CI: 0.251–0.809; p value = 0.819) (Figure S4). ROC analysis also indicated a sensitivity of 70% and a specificity of 88.89% for patients with the levels of miR-320a < -0.306. Furthermore, as shown in Table 3, multivariate analysis identified miR-320a as an independent predictor of LVAR ($p < 0.045$).

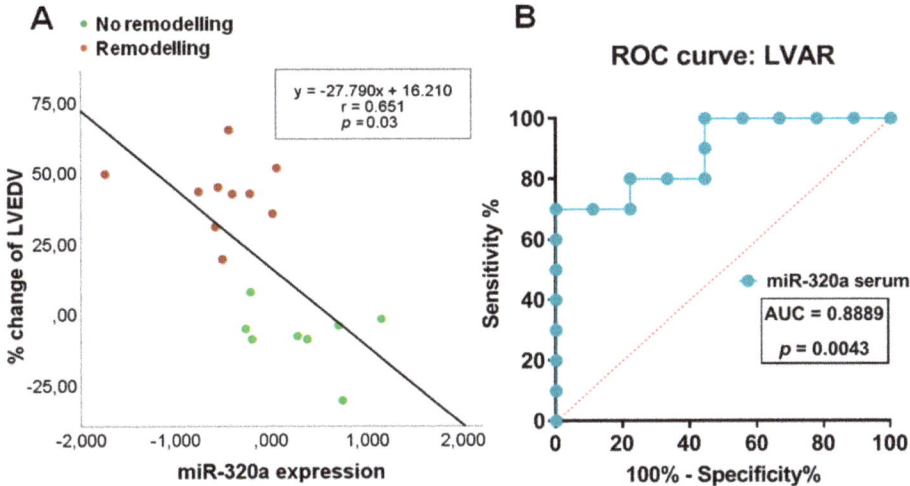

Figure 6. Correlation of serum levels of miR-320a with left ventricular adverse remodelling (LVAR) and receiver-operating characteristics (ROC) analysis. (**A**) Linear regression analysis using the percentage of change in left ventricular end-diastolic volume (LVEDV) as dependent variable and miR-320a expression 1 month post-PPCI as independent. (**B**) The area under the curve (AUC, values given on the graphs) analysis of ROC indicating sensitivity and specificity of miR-320a in predicting LVAR.

Table 3. Multivariate logistic regression to determinate independent predictors of LVAR. OR: odds ratio; CI: confidence interval. (*) indicates $p < 0.05$, which is considered statistically significant; [&] miR-320a expression in patients' serum at 1 month post-PPCI.

Factor	OR	95% CI	P Value
miR-320a [&]	0.005	0.000–0.892	0.045 *
Age	1.075	0.929–1.243	0.330
Sex	<0.001	-	0.999
Creatine Kinase	1.001	1.000–1.002	0.189

3.5. Expression of miR-320a in PBMCs Isolated from STEMI and in the Myocardium of Ischaemic Heart Failure Patients

Since AMI involves a complex cascade of events that activate acute inflammatory responses [8], we examined the possible source of the fast increase in circulating miRNAs and focused on PBMCs. Figure 7A shows that miR-320a was slightly upregulated in the PBMCs of patients suffering from STEMI even before revascularization (time point 0 h), compared to the control patients. Importantly, and in contrast to what we observed in serum samples (Figure 5A), the levels of miR-320a decreased significantly in PBMCs at 6 h after PPCI. Moreover, as shown in Figure 7B, the comparison of miR-320a in patients with or without LVAR indicated that miR-320a decreases significantly at 6 h after PPCI only in patients with LVAR, while its expression did not change in non-LVAR patients. Figure S2A also confirmed that the expression of miR-320a in PBMCs from the control group was not different than that of healthy volunteers and shows similar changes in STEMI patients with or without LVAR (Figure S3). Moreover, the multivariate analysis indicates that expression levels of miR-320a in PBMCs showed a trend association, although not significant, with LVAR (OR, 0.052; 95% CI, 0.02–1.281; $P = 0.071$ at 6 h, and OR, 0.206; 95% CI, 0.037–1.140; $P = 0.070$ at 1 month post PPCI).

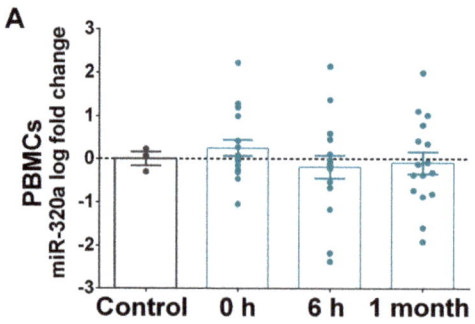

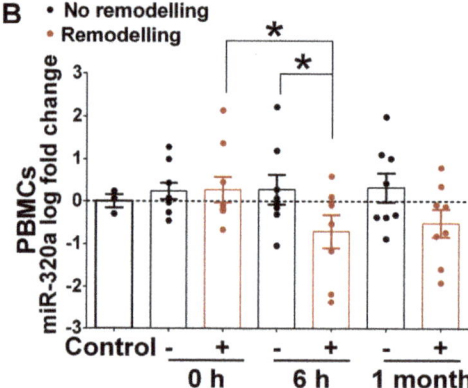

Figure 7. Expression of miR-320a in peripheral blood mononuclear cells (PBMCs) of patients with or without left ventricular adverse remodelling. (**A**) Bar graph shows miR-320a expression in PBMCs of STEMI patients ($n = 20$) at 0 h, 6 h and 1 month post PPCI relative to the control ($n = 8$). (**B**) Bar graph shows the levels of miR-320a in PBMCs at 0 h, 6 h and 1 month after PPCI in STEMI patients who developed LVAR (red bar, $n = 11$) or not (black bar, $n = 9$). Values in the graphs represent the fold change in logarithmic scale for each miRNA relative to the controls. Data are the means ± SEM. Significance is indicated by (*) for $p < 0.05$. Kruskal–Wallis test with multiple comparisons corrected by Dunn's test was performed.

Finally, we examined the expression of miR-320a and other miRNAs in patients with HF of ischaemic origin. Figure 8A shows significant expression of miR-320a in the myocardial tissue in the atrium ($n = 7$). As illustrated in Figure 8B, compared to the expression of other miRNAs, the expression of miR-320a was significantly higher than that of miR-324-5p, miR-324-3p, miR-339-5p, and miR-423 but not that of miR-29a or miR-499-5p. In contrast, miR-320a levels were lower than miR-133 levels.

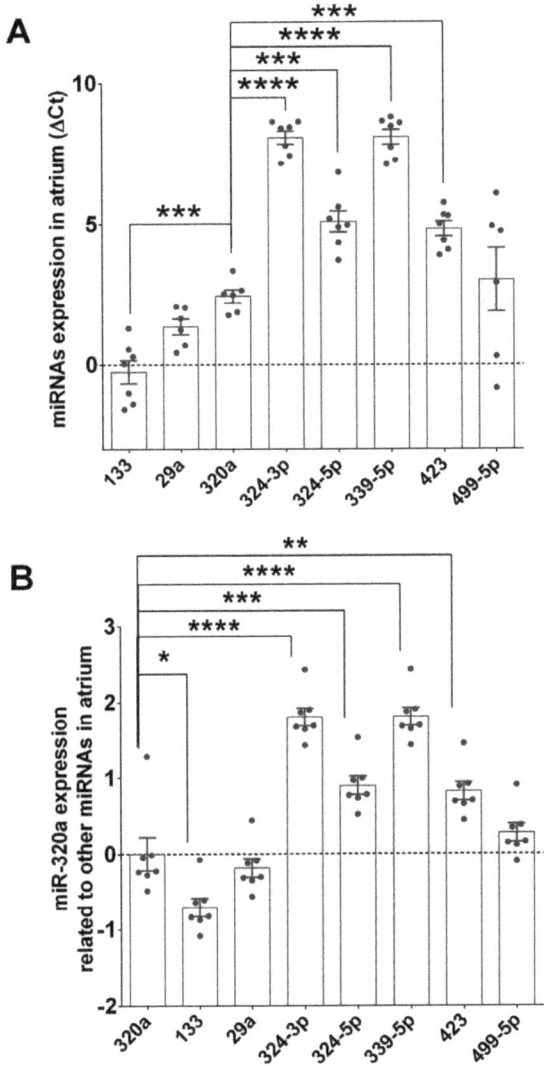

Figure 8. miR-320a is highly expressed in the atrium of patients with heart failure (HF) of ischaemic origin. (**A**) DeltaCt represents the level of Ct of different miRNAs compared to that of the endogenous control in the atrium of HF patients ($n = 7$). (**B**) Levels of expression of miR-320a related to the expression of the other miRNAs shown as fold change in logarithmic scale in the atrium of failing heart. Values are presented as the means ± SEM. Significance is indicated by (*) for $p < 0.05$, (**) for $p < 0.01$, (***) for $p < 0.001$, and (****) for $p < 0.0001$. Ordinary one-way ANOVA with multiples comparisons using T-test without correction (Fisher's LSD test) was performed.

3.6. Analysis of miR-320a Target Genes

Having confirmed the association of miR-320a with the appearance of LVAR, we next searched relevant miR-320a target genes in the context of AMI. To this end, we performed an in silico analysis using miRDB and TargetScan based on the miR-320a sequence, and compared the common genes identified in both databases. Using PANTHER software (Protein Analysis THrough Evolutionary

Relationships 14.1 version, http://pantherdb.org/genelistanalysis.do, University of Southern California, Los Angeles, CA, USA), we generated a graphic showing that 1060 genes and 520 pathways were mainly implicated in the processes regulating adverse remodelling (Figure 9). As highlighted, miR-320a was predicted to target 13 genes associated with apoptosis, 25 with the fibroblast growth factor (FGF) and tumour growth factor (TGF)-beta signalling pathways, 18 with inflammation, and 3 with oxidative stress. Altogether, these results suggest that miR-320a could have an important role in ventricular adverse remodelling through the regulation of different signalling pathways implicated in AMI.

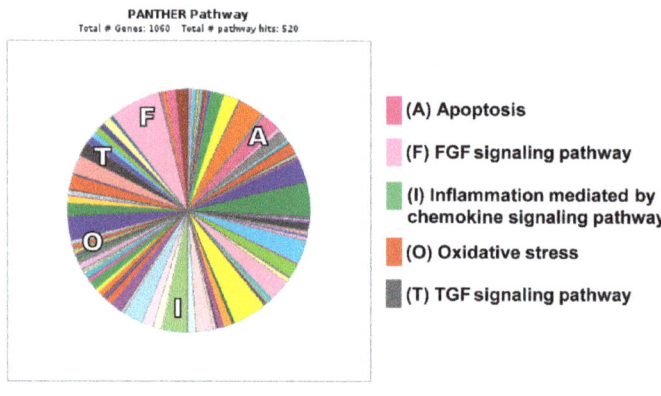

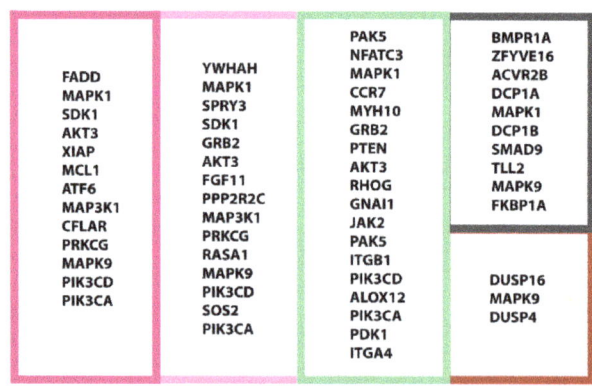

Figure 9. In silico analysis of miR-320a targets. PANTHER analysis showed the miR-320a predicted target genes involved in different pathways induced under ischaemia and reperfusion, such as apoptosis (dark pink), FGF (light pink) and TGF signalling (grey) pathways, inflammation (green) and oxidative stress (red).

4. Discussion

AMI is a complex syndrome that has become a major public health problem due to its high morbidity and mortality [35,36]. Therefore, there is an increasing need to identify new diagnostic and therapeutic biomarkers for patients with AMI, even those with successful revascularization. In fact, despite the reestablishment of coronary artery perfusion, there is still an increasing incidence of LVAR in STEMI patients who underwent successful PPCI. In agreement with the literature [4,7], almost 22% of our STEMI patients developed LVAR as early as 6 months after PPCI. Classical cardiac markers, such as troponin-T and creatine kinase, were increased in all patients suffering from STEMI at admission, confirming the severity of the infarcts. We also found that creatine kinase, but not troponin T, was significantly higher in patients who developed LVAR compared with those without LVAR, consistent with a larger infarct size, which is in agreement with other studies [37,38].

The main findings of this study are as follows: (i) miRNAs are quickly released into the circulation in different patterns following successful coronary artery revascularization in STEMI patients; (ii) a rapid increase in circulating miR-320a was observed in STEMI patients; (iii) circulating miR-320a decrease 1 month post PPCI correlates with the appearance of LVAR; (iv) the levels of miR-320a in PBMCs correlates inversely with expression in blood; and (v) higher expression of miR-320a is detected in the heart tissue of patients with HF of ischaemic origin.

In recent years, circulating miRNAs in patients with myocardial infarction have been extensively studied [23,25,39]. For instance, miR-150 [40], miR-208b, miR-34a [32], miR-328 and miR-134 [41] have been suggested as biomarkers of LVAR after AMI. However, little is known regarding miRNAs in AMI patients after revascularization. The patients selected for this study were a homogenous group of patients who were admitted to the hospital with 2 to 6 h of chest pain and no previous history of ischaemic heart disease, showing an initial TIMI flow of 0 in the LAD coronary artery after an angiogram. The inclusion criteria were rigorous to ensure consistent results related to the impact of reperfusion on miRNA expression. In contrast, other recent studies examined miRNAs in patients with a TIMI flow of 2 or 3, which may not reflect complete ischaemia [27,42]. Our study describes the expression profile of circulating miRNAs in STEMI patients examined at early time points after successful revascularization. This method provided an important assessment of how fast the levels of circulating miRNAs changed in the blood after STEMI, consistent with a recent study that nicely demonstrated monophasic and biphasic kinetic patterns of circulating miRNAs following myocardial reperfusion in STEMI patients [42]. It is well known that miRNA expression is tissue-specific and responds rapidly to changes in the body, which suggests their usability as biomarkers for the diagnosis and prognosis of diseases [23]. Here, we show that the levels of some miRNAs were significantly lower or higher at admission, indicating that these changes were triggered by ischaemia, while other miRNAs increased in a time-dependent manner after the PPCI procedure, reaching maximum levels between 3 and 12 h, which is in agreement with a recent study [42].

Recent studies on the use of PPCI described that miRNAs might also predict worse outcomes of patients who underwent PPCI. For example, miR-1 and miR-133b levels increased within 3 h of PPCI, and these miRNAs are positively associated with microvasculature obstruction and worse left ventricular functional recovery [42]. miR-1254 levels at admission predict volume changes of the left ventricle and post-STEMI left ventricular remodelling after PPCI [27]. In contrast, lower levels of miR-30e at admission are associated with no reflow in STEMI patients undergoing PPCI [43]. Here, in this study, we demonstrate for the first time that only miR-320a, which peaks at 6 h after PPCI, predicts the change in LVEDV determined at 6 months after patient discharge. According to multivariate and ROC analysis, miR-320a was independently associated with changes in LVEDV, exhibiting quite accurate sensitivity and specificity. Moreover, our data showed that miR-320a, but not CK nor age, can reliably predict the occurrence of LVAR. Nevertheless, these data deserve to be confirmed in a larger cohort of patients.

To identify the putative source of this fast increase in the level of miR-320a, we examined its expression in PBMCs since these cells have been implicated in the early inflammatory process (as reviewed elsewhere [10]). Our data indicated that miR-320a was significantly increased in PBMCs of the patients suffering from STEMI at admission before revascularization compared to the controls. Importantly, 6 h after PPCI, miR-320a levels decreased in PBMCs, which was inversely correlated with their levels in the serum of the same patients. Furthermore, the comparison of miR-320a expression in patients with or without LVAR indicated that its lower expression in PBMCs was associated with LVAR. Interestingly, we show for the first time that the human failing myocardium from ischaemic origin significantly expresses miR-320a. In these patients, we observed that the expression of miR-320a was generally higher than that of other examined miRNAs associated with heart diseases. A previous report indicated that miR-320 is likely overexpressed in human left ventricular samples of the patients with ischaemic cardiomyopathy and aortic stenosis [44], which supports our findings. Of note, miR-320a remained at a lower level both in serum and PBMCs one month after PPCI only in patients who will develop LVAR, probably because miR-320a is continuously delivered to the myocardium. Altogether, these data suggest that PBMCs from patients who will suffer adverse remodelling may express miR-320a in the blood and presumably in the myocardium, predicting a worse prognosis. This finding needs deeper investigation to demonstrate the precise mechanism by which PBMCs may release miR-320a into the bloodstream and to cardiac tissue. Emerging studies have indicated that blood contains large numbers of extracellular vesicles that transport miRNAs to different tissues in organisms [45], such as exosomes, originated from platelets, erythrocytes, leucocytes, and vascular cells, particularly the endothelium [46–48]. Recently, miR-320a has been detected in myocardial microvascular endothelial cells from a Goto–Kakizaki (GK) diabetic rat model [49]. Previous studies regarding the function of miR-320a in the myocardium have demonstrated its abnormal expression in animal heart hypertrophy and human heart disease [50–52]. miR-320 is presumably upregulated in the heart by hyperglycaemia, which acts through CD36 (fatty acid translocase) transcription [53]. Other studies determined that miR-320 overexpression is linked to cell death and apoptosis through heat-shock protein 20 [50] and insulin growth factor-1 [54], or by targeting AKIP1 and inducing the mitochondrial apoptotic pathway [55], among other mechanisms. Our results from in silico and computational miRNA target prediction algorithms revealed that miR-320a can regulate the expression of genes implicated in cardiac signalling pathways activated under ischaemia. For instance, the miR-320a predicted target genes were associated with the FGF and TGF signalling pathways, whose roles are widely known in cardiac fibrosis and wound healing [56,57]. Other target genes were associated with apoptosis and oxidative stress critical events that occur in ischaemia and reperfusion [58,59], and yet others were linked to inflammation mediated by chemokines that coincide the impact of AMI and revascularization [12]. Overall, it is clear that miR-320a upregulation may cause deleterious cellular events, and its downregulation may be involved in protection against cardiac remodelling, which will promote the improvement of heart function. Nevertheless, miR-320a-activated molecular mechanisms in the context of early revascularization are still not completely understood and deserve further investigation.

5. Conclusions

This study shows detailed miRNA release kinetics in the initial hours following PPCI. This analysis provides evidence for miR-320a as a potential prognostic biomarker for LVAR in patients who have undergone PPCI, which is promising for the preventive treatment of clinical heart failure. Further studies are needed to establish the pathophysiological and clinical significance of increased circulating miRNA-320a levels and to investigate the therapeutic efficacy of targeting miRNA-320a.

Study Limitations and Clinical Perspectives

The present study aimed to validate the proof-of-concept that circulating miRNAs can predict the outcome of STEMI patients undergoing PPCI.

In evaluating the results of this study, one must take several limitations into account:

The small sample size used in this study, due to the difficulty of recruiting patients with homogeneous criteria. Patients are only from two hospitals, therefore, a large-scale and multicentre study would be welcomed to confirm the role of miRNA-320a as a potential biomarker for STEMI patients with LVAR.

The results are limited only to patients with early revascularized STEMI with TIMI flow 0.

Our findings are essentially limited to a change in the volume of the left ventricle after revascularized STEMI up to six months, and remodelling may increase afterwards.

The specific roles of miRNAs have not been evaluated in terms of the ability to regulate gene expression in human cardiac myocytes.

It is possible that other miRNAs may also have prognostic value in this context, since RNA sequencing or microarray approaches are continuously improving in terms of sensitivity and specificity.

Supplementary Materials: The following are available online at http://www.mdpi.com/2077-0383/9/4/1051/s1, Figure S1: STROBE diagram of the subjects and the study design; Figure S2: miR-320a expression in serum and PBMCs of STEMI patients compared to healthy controls; Figure S3: miR-320a expression in PBMCs of STEMI patients compared to healthy controls; Figure S4: Receiver-operating characteristic (ROC) curves comparing sensitivity and specificity of Creatine Kinase and Age in predicting left ventricular adverse remodelling (LVAR).

Author Contributions: Conceptualization, data acquisition, analysis, and interpretation: I.G.-O., R.D.T., I.D., A.G., I.M.-G., F.G.-M., L.D.-d.l.-L., E.G.-C., M.J.-N., S.C.-D., A.O.-F. and T.S.; and investigation and methodology: I.G.-O., R.D.T., I.D., F.G.-M., G.B.-E., and T.S; writing original draft: T.S., I.G.-O., R.D.T. and A.O.-F.; revising the draft and clinical concepts: A.G., F.G.-M., L.D.-d.l.-L., G.B.-E. and A.O.-F.; funding acquisition project administration: A.O.-F. and T.S. All authors have read and agreed to the published version of the manuscript.

Funding: This research was funded by the Institute of Carlos III [grant numbers: PI18/01197; PI15/00203; CB16/11/00431]; the Spanish Ministry of Economy and Competitiveness [grant number: BFU2016-74932-C2]; and the Andalusia Government [grant number: PI-0313-2016]. This study was co-financed by FEDER Funds.

Acknowledgments: We wish to thank to Misses Elisa Bevilacqua and María Teresa Periñán Tocino for their help with some of the data processing and analysis.

Conflicts of Interest: The authors declare no conflict of interest.

Abbreviations

Acute myocardial infarction (AMI); brain-derived natriuretic peptide (BNP); cardiovascular diseases (CVD); heart failure (HF); ischaemia and reperfusion (I/R); left anterior descending (LAD); left ventricular adverse remodelling (LVAR); left ventricular end-diastolic volume (LVEDV); microRNAs (miRNAs); peripheral blood mononuclear cells (PBMCs); primary percutaneous coronary intervention (PPCI); STEMI (ST-segment-elevation myocardial infarction); thrombolysis in myocardial infarction (TIMI).

References

1. Vernon, S.T.; Coffey, S.; D'Souza, M.; Chow, C.K.; Kilian, J.; Hyun, K.; Shaw, J.A.; Adams, M.; Roberts-Thomson, P.; Brieger, D.; et al. ST-Segment-Elevation Myocardial Infarction (STEMI) Patients Without Standard Modifiable Cardiovascular Risk Factors-How Common Are They, and What Are Their Outcomes? *J. Am. Heart Assoc.* **2019**, *8*, e013296. [CrossRef] [PubMed]
2. Menees, D.S.; Peterson, E.D.; Wang, Y.; Curtis, J.P.; Messenger, J.C.; Rumsfeld, J.S.; Gurm, H.S. Door-to-balloon time and mortality among patients undergoing primary PCI. *N. Engl. J. Med.* **2013**, *369*, 901–909. [CrossRef] [PubMed]
3. Mosterd, A.; Hoes, A.W. Clinical epidemiology of heart failure. *Heart* **2007**, *93*, 1137–1146. [CrossRef] [PubMed]
4. Kelly, D.J.; Gershlick, T.; Witzenbichler, B.; Guagliumi, G.; Fahy, M.; Dangas, G.; Mehran, R.; Stone, G.W. Incidence and predictors of heart failure following percutaneous coronary intervention in ST-segment elevation myocardial infarction: The HORIZONS-AMI trial. *Am. Heart J.* **2011**, *162*, 663–670. [CrossRef]
5. Caccioppo, A.; Franchin, L.; Grosso, A.; Angelini, F.; D'Ascenzo, F.; Brizzi, M.F. Ischemia Reperfusion Injury: Mechanisms of Damage/Protection and Novel Strategies for Cardiac Recovery/Regeneration. *Int. J. Mol. Sci.* **2019**, *20*, 5024. [CrossRef]
6. Danchin, N.; Popovic, B.; Puymirat, E.; Goldstein, P.; Belle, L.; Cayla, G.; Roubille, F.; Lemesle, G.; Ferrières, J.; Schiele, F.; et al. Five-year outcomes following timely primary percutaneous intervention, late primary percutaneous intervention, or a pharmaco-invasive strategy in ST-segment elevation myocardial infarction: The FAST-MI programme. *Eur. Heart J.* **2019**, *14*, 858–866. [CrossRef]
7. Thrane, P.G.; Kristensen, S.D.; Olesen, K.K.W.; Mortensen, L.S.; Bøtker, H.E.; Thuesen, L.; Hansen, H.S.; Abildgaard, U.; Engstrøm, T.; Andersen, H.R.; et al. 16-year follow-up of the Danish Acute Myocardial Infarction 2 (DANAMI-2) trial: Primary percutaneous coronary intervention vs. fibrinolysis in ST-segment elevation myocardial infarction. *Eur. Heart J.* **2019**, *14*, 847–854. [CrossRef]
8. Ong, S.B.; Hernández-Reséndiz, S.; Crespo-Avilan, G.E.; Mukhametshina, R.T.; Kwek, X.Y.; Cabrera-Fuentes, H.A.; Hausenloy, D.J. Inflammation following acute myocardial infarction: Multiple players, dynamic roles, and novel therapeutic opportunities. *Pharmacol. Ther.* **2018**, *186*, 73–87. [CrossRef]

9. Nahrendorf, M.; Swirski, F.K.; Aikawa, E.; Stangenberg, L.; Wurdinger, T.; Figueiredo, J.L.; Libby, P.; Weissleder, R.; Pittet, M.J. The healing myocardium sequentially mobilizes two monocyte subsets with divergent and complementary functions. *J. Exp. Med.* **2007**, *204*, 3037–3047. [CrossRef]
10. Sager, H.B.; Kessler, T.; Schunkert, H. Monocytes and macrophages in cardiac injury and repair. *J. Thorac. Dis.* **2017**, *9*, S30–S35. [CrossRef]
11. Dutta, P.; Nahrendorf, M. Monocytes in myocardial infarction. *Arterioscler. Thromb. Vasc. Biol.* **2015**, *35*, 1066–1070. [CrossRef] [PubMed]
12. Liu, J.; Wang, H.; Li, J. Inflammation and inflammatory cells in myocardial infarction and reperfusion injury: A double-edged sword. *Clin. Med. Insights Cardiol.* **2016**, *10*, 79–84. [CrossRef]
13. Fertin, M.; Dubois, E.; Belliard, A.; Amouyel, P.; Pinet, F.; Bauters, C. Usefulness of circulating biomarkers for the prediction of left ventricular remodeling after myocardial infarction. *Am. J. Cardiol.* **2012**, *110*, 277–283. [CrossRef] [PubMed]
14. Chan, D.; Ng, L.L. Biomarkers in acute myocardial infarction. *BMC Med.* **2010**, *8*, 34. [CrossRef] [PubMed]
15. Zhou, S.S.; Jin, J.P.; Wang, J.Q.; Zhang, Z.G.; Freedman, J.H.; Zheng, Y.; Cai, L. MiRNAS in cardiovascular diseases: Potential biomarkers, therapeutic targets and challenges review-article. *Acta Pharmacol. Sin.* **2018**, *39*, 1073–1084. [CrossRef]
16. Yang, Y.; Huang, Q.; Luo, C.; Wen, Y.; Liu, R.; Sun, H.; Tang, L. MicroRNAs in acute pancreatitis: From pathogenesis to novel diagnosis and therapy. *J. Cell. Physiol.* **2019**, *235*, 1948–1961. [CrossRef]
17. Shoeibi, S. Diagnostic and theranostic microRNAs in the pathogenesis of atherosclerosis. *Acta Physiol.* **2019**, *288*, e13353. [CrossRef]
18. Smani, T.; Mayoral-González, I.; Galeano-Otero, I.; Gallardo-Castillo, I.; Rosado, J.A.; Ordoñez, A.; Hmadcha, A. Chapter 15: Non-coding RNAs and Ischemic Cardiovascular Diseases. Non-coding RNAs in Cardiovascular Diseases. *Adv. Exp. Med. Biol.* **2020**, *39*, 2704–2716.
19. Economou, E.K.; Oikonomou, E.; Siasos, G.; Papageorgiou, N.; Tsalamandris, S.; Mourouzis, K.; Papaioanou, S.; Tousoulis, D. The role of microRNAs in coronary artery disease: From pathophysiology to diagnosis and treatment. *Atherosclerosis* **2015**, *241*, 624–633. [CrossRef]
20. Bang, C.; Batkai, S.; Dangwal, S.; Gupta, S.K.; Foinquinos, A.; Holzmann, A.; Just, A.; Remke, J.; Zimmer, K.; Zeug, A.; et al. Cardiac fibroblast–derived microRNA passenger strand-enriched exosomes mediate cardiomyocyte hypertrophy. *J. Clin. Invest.* **2014**, *124*, 2136–2146. [CrossRef]
21. Thum, T.; Condorelli, G. Long Noncoding RNAs and MicroRNAs in Cardiovascular Pathophysiology. *Circ. Res.* **2015**, *116*, 751–762. [CrossRef] [PubMed]
22. Ye, Y.; Perez-Polo, J.R.; Qian, J.; Birnbaum, Y. The role of microRNA in modulating myocardial ischemia-reperfusion injury. *Physiol. Genomics* **2011**, *43*, 534–542. [CrossRef] [PubMed]
23. Creemers, E.E.; Tijsen, A.J.; Pinto, Y.M. Circulating microRNAs: Novel biomarkers and extracellular communicators in cardiovascular disease? *Circ. Res.* **2012**, *110*, 483–495. [CrossRef] [PubMed]
24. Condorelli, G.; Latronico, M.V.G.; Cavarretta, E. microRNAs in Cardiovascular Diseases. *J. Am. Coll. Cardiol.* **2014**, *63*, 2177–2187. [CrossRef] [PubMed]
25. Mitchell, P.S.; Parkin, R.K.; Kroh, E.M.; Fritz, B.R.; Wyman, S.K.; Pogosova-Agadjanyan, E.L.; Peterson, A.; Noteboom, J.; O'Briant, K.C.; Allen, A.; et al. Circulating microRNAs as stable blood-based markers for cancer detection. *Proc. Natl. Acad. Sci.* **2008**, *105*, 10513–10518. [CrossRef] [PubMed]
26. Liu, X.; Dong, Y.; Chen, S.; Zhang, G.; Zhang, M.; Gong, Y.; Li, X. Circulating MicroRNA-146a and MicroRNA-21 Predict Left Ventricular Remodeling after ST-Elevation Myocardial Infarction. *Cardiology* **2015**, *132*, 233–241. [CrossRef]
27. De Gonzalo-Calvo, D.; Cediel, G.; Bär, C.; Núñez, J.; Revuelta-Lopez, E.; Gavara, J.; Ríos-Navarro, C.; Llorente-Cortes, V.; Bodí, V.; Thum, T.; et al. Circulating miR-1254 predicts ventricular remodeling in patients with ST-Segment-Elevation Myocardial Infarction: A cardiovascular magnetic resonance study. *Sci. Rep.* **2018**, *8*, 15115. [CrossRef]
28. MacIejak, A.; Kostarska-Srokosz, E.; Gierlak, W.; Dluzniewski, M.; Kuch, M.; Marchel, M.; Opolski, G.; Kiliszek, M.; Matlak, K.; Dobrzycki, S.; et al. Circulating MIR-30a-5p as a prognostic biomarker of left ventricular dysfunction after acute myocardial infarction. *Sci. Rep.* **2018**, *8*, 9883. [CrossRef]

29. Lang, R.M.; Bierig, M.; Devereux, R.B.; Flachskampf, F.A.; Foster, E.; Pellikka, P.A.; Picard, M.H.; Roman, M.J.; Seward, J.; Shanewise, J.S.; et al. Recommendations for chamber quantification: A report from the American Society of Echocardiography's guidelines and standards committee and the Chamber Quantification Writing Group, developed in conjunction with the European Association of Echocardiography, a branch of the European Society of Cardiology. *J. Am. Soc. Echocardiogr.* **2005**, *18*, 1440–1463.
30. Ai, J.; Zhang, R.; Li, Y.; Pu, J.; Lu, Y.; Jiao, J.; Li, K.; Yu, B.; Li, Z.; Wang, R.; et al. Circulating microRNA-1 as a potential novel biomarker for acute myocardial infarction. *Biochem. Biophys. Res. Commun.* **2010**, *391*, 73–77. [CrossRef]
31. Wong, L.L.; Armugam, A.; Sepramaniam, S.; Karolina, D.S.; Lim, K.Y.; Lim, J.Y.; Chong, J.P.C.; Ng, J.Y.X.; Chen, Y.-T.; Chan, M.M.Y.; et al. Circulating microRNAs in heart failure with reduced and preserved left ventricular ejection fraction. *Eur. J. Heart Fail.* **2015**, *17*, 393–404. [CrossRef] [PubMed]
32. Lv, P.; Zhou, M.; He, J.; Meng, W.; Ma, X.; Dong, S.; Meng, X.; Zhao, X.; Wang, X.; He, F. Circulating miR-208b and miR-34a are associated with left ventricular remodeling after acute myocardial infarction. *Int. J. Mol. Sci.* **2014**, *15*, 5774–5788. [CrossRef] [PubMed]
33. Nabiałek, E.; Wańha, W.; Kula, D.; Jadczyk, T.; Krajewska, M.; Kowalówka, A.; Dworowy, S.; Hrycek, E.; Włudarczyk, W.; Parma, Z.; et al. Circulating microRNAs (miR-423-5p, miR-208a and miR-1) in acute myocardial infarction and stable coronary heart disease. *Minerva Cardioangiol.* **2013**, *61*, 627–637.
34. Ji, Q.; Jiang, Q.; Yan, W.; Li, X.; Zhang, Y.; Meng, P.; Shao, M.; Chen, L.; Zhu, H.; Tian, N. Expression of circulating microRNAs in patients with ST segment elevation acute myocardial infarction. *Minerva Cardioangiol.* **2015**, *63*, 397–402. [PubMed]
35. Arbab-Zadeh, A.; Nakano, M.; Virmani, R.; Fuster, V. Acute coronary events. *Circulation* **2012**, *125*, 1147–1156. [CrossRef] [PubMed]
36. Pagidipati, N.J.; Gaziano, T.A. Estimating deaths from cardiovascular disease: A review of global methodologies of mortality measurement. *Circulation* **2013**, *127*, 749–756. [CrossRef]
37. Cha, M.J.; Lee, J.H.; Jung, H.N.; Kim, Y.; Choe, Y.H.; Kim, S.M. Cardiac magnetic resonance-tissue tracking for the early prediction of adverse left ventricular remodeling after ST-segment elevation myocardial infarction. *Int. J. Cardiovasc. Imaging* **2019**, *35*, 2095–2102. [CrossRef]
38. Cuenin, L.; Lamoureux, S.; Schaaf, M.; Bochaton, T.; Monassier, J.P.; Claeys, M.J.; Rioufol, G.; Finet, G.; Garcia-Dorado, D.; Angoulvant, D.; et al. Incidence and significance of spontaneous ST segment re-elevation after reperfused anterior acute myocardial infarction—Relationship with infarct size, adverse remodeling, and events at 1 year. *Circ. J.* **2018**, *82*, 1379–1386. [CrossRef]
39. Colpaert, R.M.W.; Calore, M. MicroRNAs in Cardiac Diseases. *Cells* **2019**, *8*, 737. [CrossRef]
40. Devaux, Y.; Vausort, M.; McCann, G.P.; Zangrando, J.; Kelly, D.; Razvi, N.; Zhang, L.; Ng, L.L.; Wagner, D.R.; Squire, I.B. MicroRNA-150: A novel marker of left ventricular remodeling after acute myocardial infarction. *Circ. Cardiovasc. Genet.* **2013**, *6*, 290–298. [CrossRef]
41. He, F.; Lv, P.; Zhao, X.; Wang, X.; Ma, X.; Meng, W.; Meng, X.; Dong, S. Predictive value of circulating miR-328 and miR-134 for acute myocardial infarction. *Mol. Cell. Biochem.* **2014**, *394*, 137–144. [CrossRef] [PubMed]
42. Coelho-Lima, J.; Mohammed, A.; Cormack, S.; Jones, S.; Ali, A.; Panahi, P.; Barter, M.; Bagnall, A.; Ali, S.; Young, D.; et al. Kinetics Analysis of Circulating MicroRNAs Unveils Markers of Failed Myocardial Reperfusion. *Clin. Chem.* **2020**, *66*, 247–256. [CrossRef] [PubMed]
43. Su, Q.; Ye, Z.; Sun, Y.; Yang, H.; Li, L. Relationship between circulating miRNA-30e and no-reflow phenomenon in STEMI patients undergoing primary coronary intervention. *Scand. J. Clin. Lab. Invest.* **2018**, *78*, 318–324. [CrossRef] [PubMed]
44. Ikeda, S.; Kong, S.W.; Lu, J.; Bisping, E.; Zhang, H.; Allen, P.D.; Golub, T.R.; Pieske, B.; Pu, W.T. Altered microRNA expression in human heart disease. *Physiol. Genom.* **2007**, *31*, 367–373. [CrossRef]
45. Davidson, S.M.; Andreadou, I.; Barile, L.; Birnbaum, Y.; Cabrera-Fuentes, H.A.; Cohen, M.V.; Downey, J.M.; Girao, H.; Pagliaro, P.; Penna, C.; et al. Circulating blood cells and extracellular vesicles in acute cardioprotection. *Cardiovasc. Res.* **2019**, *115*, 1156–1166. [CrossRef]
46. Iaconetti, C.; Sorrentino, S.; De Rosa, S.; Indolfi, C. Exosomal miRNAs in heart disease. *Physiology* **2016**, *31*, 16–24. [CrossRef]
47. Quesenberry, P.J.; Aliotta, J.; Deregibus, M.C.; Camussi, G. Role of extracellular RNA-carrying vesicles in cell differentiation and reprogramming. *Stem Cell Res. Ther.* **2015**, *6*, 153. [CrossRef]

48. Mittelbrunn, M.; Sánchez-Madrid, F. Intercellular communication: Diverse structures for exchange of genetic information. *Nat. Rev. Mol. Cell Biol.* **2012**, *13*, 328–335. [CrossRef]
49. Wang, X.H.; Qian, R.Z.; Zhang, W.; Chen, S.F.; Jin, H.M.; Hu, R.M. MicroRNA-320 expression in myocardial microvascular endothelial cells and its relationship with insulin-like growth factor-1 in type 2 diabetic rats. *Clin. Exp. Pharmacol. Physiol.* **2009**, *36*, 181–188. [CrossRef]
50. Ren, X.-P.; Wu, J.; Wang, X.; Sartor, M.A.; Jones, K.; Qian, J.; Nicolaou, P.; Pritchard, T.J.; Fan, G.-C. MicroRNA-320 is involved in the regulation of cardiac ischemia/reperfusion injury by targeting heat-shock protein 20. *Circulation* **2009**, *119*, 2357–2366. [CrossRef]
51. Song, C.-L.; Liu, B.; Diao, H.-Y.; Shi, Y.-F.; Li, Y.-X.; Zhang, J.-C.; Lu, Y.; Wang, G.; Liu, J.; Yu, Y.-P.; et al. The Protective Effect of MicroRNA-320 on Left Ventricular Remodeling after Myocardial Ischemia-Reperfusion Injury in the Rat Model. *Int. J. Mol. Sci.* **2014**, *15*, 17442–17456. [CrossRef] [PubMed]
52. Thum, T.; Galuppo, P.; Wolf, C.; Fiedler, J.; Kneitz, S.; Van Laake, L.W.; Doevendans, P.A.; Mummery, C.L.; Borlak, J.; Haverich, A.; et al. MicroRNAs in the human heart: A clue to fetal gene reprogramming in heart failure. *Circulation* **2007**, *116*, 258–267. [CrossRef] [PubMed]
53. Li, H.; Fan, J.; Zhao, Y.; Zhang, X.; Dai, B.; Zhan, J.; Yin, Z.; Nie, X.; Fu, X.-D.; Chen, C.; et al. Nuclear miR-320 Mediates Diabetes-Induced Cardiac Dysfunction by Activating Transcription of Fatty Acid Metabolic Genes to Cause Lipotoxicity in the Heart. *Circ. Res.* **2019**, *125*, 1106–1120. [CrossRef] [PubMed]
54. Song, C.L.; Liu, B.; Diao, H.Y.; Shi, Y.F.; Zhang, J.C.; Li, Y.X.; Liu, N.; Yu, Y.P.; Wang, G.; Wang, J.P.; et al. Down-regulation of microRNA-320 suppresses cardiomyocyte apoptosis and protects against myocardial ischemia and reperfusion injury by targeting IGF-1. *Oncotarget* **2016**, *7*, 39740–39757. [CrossRef] [PubMed]
55. Tian, Z.Q.; Jiang, H.; Lu, Z.B. MiR-320 regulates cardiomyocyte apoptosis induced by ischemia–reperfusion injury by targeting AKIP1. *Cell. Mol. Biol. Lett.* **2018**, *23*, 41. [CrossRef] [PubMed]
56. Humeres, C.; Frangogiannis, N.G. Fibroblasts in the Infarcted, Remodeling, and Failing Heart. *JACC Basic to Transl. Sci.* **2019**, *4*, 449–467. [CrossRef]
57. Itoh, N.; Ohta, H.; Nakayama, Y.; Konishi, M. Roles of FGF signals in heart development, health, and disease. *Front. Cell Dev. Biol.* **2016**, *4*, 110. [CrossRef]
58. Kurian, G.A.; Rajagopal, R.; Vedantham, S.; Rajesh, M. The Role of Oxidative Stress in Myocardial Ischemia and Reperfusion Injury and Remodeling: Revisited. *Oxid. Med. Cell. Longev.* **2016**, *2016*, 1656450. [CrossRef]
59. Eefting, F.; Rensing, B.; Wigman, J.; Pannekoek, W.J.; Liu, W.M.; Cramer, M.J.; Lips, D.J.; Doevendans, P.A. Role of apoptosis in reperfusion injury. *Cardiovasc. Res.* **2004**, *61*, 414–426. [CrossRef]

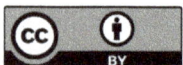

© 2020 by the authors. Licensee MDPI, Basel, Switzerland. This article is an open access article distributed under the terms and conditions of the Creative Commons Attribution (CC BY) license (http://creativecommons.org/licenses/by/4.0/).

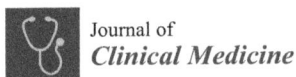

Article

Novel Biomarkers in Patients with Chronic Kidney Disease: An Analysis of Patients Enrolled in the GCKD-Study

Moritz Mirna [1], Albert Topf [1], Bernhard Wernly [1], Richard Rezar [1], Vera Paar [1], Christian Jung [2], Hermann Salmhofer [3], Kristen Kopp [1], Uta C. Hoppe [1], P. Christian Schulze [4], Daniel Kretzschmar [4], Markus P. Schneider [5], Ulla T. Schultheiss [6], Claudia Sommerer [7], Katharina Paul [8], Gunter Wolf [8], Michael Lichtenauer [1,*] and Martin Busch [8]

1. Department of Internal Medicine II, Division of Cardiology, Paracelsus Medical University of Salzburg, 5020 Salzburg, Austria; m.mirna@salk.at (M.M.); a.topf@salk.at (A.T.); b.wernly@salk.at (B.W.); r.rezar@salk.at (R.R.); v.paar@salk.at (V.P.); k.kopp@salk.at (K.K.); u.hoppe@salk.at (U.C.H.)
2. Department of Cardiology, Pulmonology and Vascular Medicine, Medical Faculty, Heinrich Heine University Duesseldorf, 40225 Duesseldorf, Germany; christian.jung@med.uni-duesseldorf.de
3. Department of Internal Medicine I, Division of Nephrology, Paracelsus Medical University of Salzburg, 5020 Salzburg, Austria; h.salmhofer@salk.at
4. Department of Internal Medicine I, Division of Cardiology, Friedrich Schiller University Jena, 07743 Jena, Germany; christian.schulze@med.uni-jena.de (P.C.S.); daniel.kretzschmar@med.uni-jena.de (D.K.)
5. Department of Nephrology and Hypertension, University Hospital Erlangen, Friedrich-Alexander University Erlangen-Nürnberg, 91054 Erlangen, Germany; markus.schneider@klinikum-nuernberg.de
6. Department of Medicine IV – Nephrology and Primary Care, Institute of Genetic Epidemiology, Medical Center–University of Freiburg, Faculty of Medicine, 79106 Freiburg, Germany; ulla.schultheiss@uniklinik-freiburg.de
7. Department of Nephrology, University of Heidelberg, 69117 Heidelberg, Germany; claudia.sommerer@med.uni-heidelberg.de
8. Department of Internal Medicine III, Friedrich Schiller University Jena, 07743 Jena, Germany; katharina.paul@med.uni-jena.de (K.P.); gunter.wolf@med.uni-jena.de (G.W.); martin.busch@med.uni-jena.de (M.B.)
* Correspondence: michael.lichtenauer@chello.at

Received: 26 January 2020; Accepted: 19 March 2020; Published: 24 March 2020

Abstract: *Background:* Chronic kidney disease (CKD) and cardiovascular diseases (CVD) often occur concomitantly, and CKD is a major risk factor for cardiovascular mortality. Since some of the most commonly used biomarkers in CVD are permanently elevated in patients with CKD, novel biomarkers are warranted for clinical practice. *Methods:* Plasma concentrations of five cardiovascular biomarkers (soluble suppression of tumorigenicity (sST2), growth differentiation factor 15 (GDF-15), heart-type fatty acid-binding protein (H-FABP), insulin-like growth factor-binding protein 2 (IGF-BP2), and soluble urokinase plasminogen activator receptor) were analyzed by means of enzyme-linked immunosorbent assay (ELISA) in 219 patients with CKD enrolled in the German Chronic Kidney Disease (GCKD) study. *Results:* Except for sST2, all of the investigated biomarkers were significantly elevated in patients with CKD (2.0- to 4.4-fold increase in advanced CKD (estimated glomerular filtration rate (eGFR) < 30 mL/min/1.73 m^2 body surface area (BSA)) and showed a significant inverse correlation with eGFR. Moreover, all but H-FABP and sST2 were additionally elevated in patients with micro- and macro-albuminuria. *Conclusions:* Based on our findings, sST2 appears to be the biomarker whose diagnostic performance is least affected by decreased renal function, thus suggesting potential viability in the management of patients with CVD and concomitant CKD. The predictive potential of sST2 remains to be proven in endpoint studies.

Keywords: CKD; CVD; biomarkers; sST2

1. Introduction

Chronic kidney disease (CKD) affects about 11.5% of the overall population with increasing age-dependent prevalence of up to 47% in persons older than 70 years [1]. Apart from old age, CKD is associated with diabetes mellitus and hypertension. Due to an increase of these precipitating and often causative diseases, the prevalence of CKD is expected to rise even further in the future [1]. Because of shared risk factors and the fact that CKD constitutes an independent risk factor itself, CKD and cardiovascular disease (CVD) often occur concomitantly [2–4]. Hence, biomarkers established in the evaluation of patients with CVD are increasingly used in patients with decreased renal function. Unfortunately, some of the most common biomarkers in this field, such as troponin or brain natriuretic peptide (BNP), are chronically elevated in patients with CKD, which may in part be due to impaired renal clearance [5–7]. Therefore, their clinical applicability in patients with CKD is limited and hence, novel biomarkers are warranted to improve diagnosis and risk stratification in these disease entities.

In the following study, plasma concentrations of novel cardiovascular biomarkers (sST2, GDF-15, H-FABP, IGF-BP2 and suPAR) were investigated in patients with various stages of CKD.

Soluble suppression of tumorigenicity (sST2; molecular mass: 36,993 Da [8]; normal reference ranges for male subjects: 4000–31,000 pg/mL; for female subjects: 2000–21,000 pg/mL [9]) is a member of the toll-like/IL-1-receptor family that acts as a scavenger-receptor for IL-33, thus attenuating the effects of this immunomodulatory cytokine [10]. sST2 is secreted in response to mechanical stress, and hence elevated plasma levels are found in patients with acute and chronic heart failure [11]. Increased plasma concentrations of sST2 have been associated with adverse outcomes in patients with coronary artery disease [12] and heart failure [11,13] in previous trials.

Growth differentiation factor 15 (GDF-15; molecular mass: 34,140 Da [14]; normal reference ranges: 310 ± 10 pg/mL [15]) is a member of the transforming growth factor ß (TGF-ß) cytokine family. GDF-15 is secreted in response to tissue injury or by the effect of proinflammatory cytokines and is involved in the regulation of inflammatory and apoptotic processes [16]. Recently, elevated plasma levels of GDF-15 have been associated with an increased risk of mortality in patients with coronary artery disease and chronic heart failure [17–19]. Furthermore, increased plasma concentrations of circulating GDF-15 were associated with a decline of renal function in patients with CKD [20].

Heart-type fatty acid-binding protein (H-FABP; molecular mass: 14,858 Da [21]; normal reference ranges for male subjects: 3.5 ± 0.4; for female subjects: 3.9 ± 0.4 ng/mL [22]) is a small cytoplasmic protein that transports long-chained fatty acids in cardiomyocytes and is considered a biomarker of myocardial ischemia [23]. In case of damage to the cell membrane, H-FABP is rapidly released into circulation and therefore was evaluated for use in diagnosis and risk stratification of coronary artery disease and acute coronary syndrome [24,25]. In fact, increased plasma levels of H-FABP are associated with an elevated risk of adverse outcomes in acute coronary syndrome and heart failure [26,27].

Insulin-like growth factor-binding protein 2 (IGF-BP2; molecular mass: 34,814 Da [28]; normal reference ranges: 321.2 ± 285.0 ng/mL [29]) is an anabolic peptide with extensive structural and functional homology to insulin. IGF-BP2 is a potent effector of growth, proliferation, and metabolism that elicits its effects via autocrine, paracrine, and endocrine mechanisms [30]. Elevated plasma concentrations of IGF-BP2 have been associated with diabetes mellitus [31], metabolic syndrome [32], and progression of CKD [33] in previous studies. Moreover, IGF-BP2 seems to be involved in the pathogenesis of atherosclerosis. In a recent trial, plasma concentrations of IGF-BP2 were inversely correlated with arterial intima-media thickness of the carotid artery in healthy participants [34,35].

Soluble urokinase plasminogen activator receptor (suPAR; molecular mass (depending on the considered isoform): 31,263–36,978 Da [36]; normal reference ranges: 2100 pg/mL, IQR: 1700–2300 pg/mL [37]) is the soluble isoform of the urokinase plasminogen activator receptor (uPAR), a membrane-bound protein in endothelial and immunological cells that plays a role in various inflammatory processes [38]. Recent evidence suggests that suPAR is involved in the formation of atherosclerotic lesions and hence, elevated plasma levels of suPAR have been associated with an increased risk for coronary artery disease and cardiovascular mortality [39]. Furthermore, elevated plasma concentrations of suPAR were recently correlated with the deterioration of renal function in patients with CKD [40,41], and an association between suPAR and primary focal segmental glomerulosclerosis (pFSGS) [42,43] was found.

2. Materials and Methods

Plasma samples from 219 of 245 patients enrolled in the regional center of Jena within the German Chronic Kidney Disease study (GCKD), Germany, were analyzed. The remaining 26 patients were excluded as serum samples were missing. The GCKD study was approved by the local ethics committee, registered in the German national registry for clinical studies (DRKS00003971) and was conducted according to the principles of the Declaration of Helsinki and Good Clinical Practice. Informed consent was obtained from all patients prior to enrollment.

2.1. Study Population

Details of the study design and the enrollment process of the GCKD study have been described previously [44]. Briefly, patients aged 18–74 years with CKD in routine nephrological care were enrolled across nine German study centers between March 2010 and March 2012. Patients were included if they had an estimated glomerular filtration rate (eGFR) of < 60mL/min/1.73m^2 body surface area (BSA) or overt proteinuria in the presence of a higher eGFR (defined as albuminuria of > 300 mg/g creatinine or proteinuria of > 500 g/g creatinine). Exclusion criteria were non-Caucasian race, history of transplantation, active malignancy, New York Heart Association (NYHA) heart failure functional class IV, and/or inability to provide written informed consent [44].

Glomerular filtration rate (GFR) was estimated using the 4-variable modification of diet in renal disease (MDRD) formula, as previously published [45,46]. CKD was categorized according to the clinical practice guidelines from the Kidney Disease: Improving Global Outcomes Initiative (KDIGO) in the following G and A-stages. G-stages: CKD stage G1: eGFR ≥ 90 mL/min/1.73 m^2 BSA, stage G2: eGFR 60–89 mL/min/1.73 m^2 BSA, stage G3a: 45–59 mL/min/1.73 m^2 BSA, stage G3b: eGFR 30–44 mL/min/1.73 m^2 BSA, and stages G4 and G5 (combined): eGFR < 30 mL/min/1.73 m^2 BSA. A-stages: urinary albumin/creatinine ratio (UACR) < 30 mg/g Crea (A1 = normo-albuminuria), 30–300 mg/g Crea (A2 = micro-albuminuria), or > 300 mg/g Crea (A3 = macro-albuminuria) [47,48]. Symptoms of heart failure were estimated by the modified Gothenburg scale, as previously published [47,49].

2.2. Blood Samples and Biomarker Analysis

Blood samples were collected upon study enrollment using a vacuum-containing system. Plasma levels of sST2, GDF-15, H-FABP, IGF-BP2, and suPAR were measured by using commercially available enzyme-linked immunosorbent assay (ELISA) kits (R&D Systems, USA). Preparation of reagents and measurements were performed according to the manufacturer's instructions. In brief, patient samples and standard protein were added to the wells of the ELISA plates (Nunc MaxiSorp flat-bottom 96 well plates, VWR International GmbH, Austria) and incubated for two hours. Plates were then washed using a Tween 20/PBS solution (Sigma Aldrich, USA). Then, a biotin-labelled antibody was added and incubated for another two hours. Plates were washed another time, and streptavidin–horseradish-peroxidase solution was added to the wells. After adding tetramethylbenzidine (TMB; Sigma Aldrich, USA) a color reaction was generated. Values of optical density (OD) were determined at 450 nm on an ELISA plate-reader (iMark Microplate Absorbance Reader, Bio-Rad Laboratories, Austria).

2.3. Statistical Analysis

Statistical analyses were performed using SPSS (Version 24.0, SPSSS Inc., USA) and GraphPad Prism software (GraphPad Software, USA). Normally distributed data was expressed as mean and standard deviation (SD); not normally distributed data was expressed as median and interquartile range (IQR). Medians were compared using a Mann–Whitney U-test or a Kruskal–Wallis test with Dunn's post-hoc test, depending on the number of groups analyzed. Bonferroni–Holm correction was conducted to adjust for multiple comparisons. To assess the association between renal function and biomarker concentrations, correlation analysis was conducted using Spearman's rank correlation test, followed by multiple linear regression analysis to adjust for parameters known for confounding with renal function (age, gender, BMI, diabetes mellitus, and arterial hypertension). Prior to multiple linear regression analysis, normal distribution was assessed by performing a Kolmogorov–Smirnov test, where applicable, and multicollinearity was excluded using the collinearity diagnostics tool by SPSS. A *p*-value < 0.05 was considered statistically significant.

3. Results

In total, 219 plasma samples of patients enrolled in the GCKD study were analyzed. The mean age was 63 ± 9 years, and the majority of patients were male (60.3%, n = 132). Regarding comorbidities, arterial hypertension was present in 90.4% (n = 198), diabetes mellitus type 2 in 39.3% (n = 86), heart failure in 26.0% (n = 57), and 49.3% had a history of smoking (n = 108) (see Table 1).

3.1. Renal Function and Causes of Renal Disease

Regarding renal function, the majority of patients was in CKD stages G3a (41.6% (n = 91), eGFR 45–59 mL/min/1.73 m^2 BSA) and G3b (32.4% (n = 71), eGFR 30–44 mL/min/1.73 m^2 BSA), followed by CKD stage 2 (13.7% (n = 30), eGFR 60–89 mL/min/1.73 m^2 BSA) and CKD stages 4 and 5 (9.6% (n = 21), eGFR < 30 mL/min/1.73 m^2 BSA); 2.7% (n = 6) of the patients had an eGFR above 90 mL/min/1.73 m^2 BSA while having proteinuria.

Regarding urinary albumin excretion, micro-albuminuria (UACR 30–300 mg/g) was observed in 32% (n = 70) of patients, whereas macro-albuminuria (UACR > 300 mg/g) was evident in 20.5% (n = 45) of the patients at the time of inclusion (see Table 1). Only two patients had an UACR above 3000 mg/g.

The median estimated glomerular filtration rate (eGFR) was 47.7 mL/min/1.73 m^2 (IQR 38.2–55.7), the median level of creatinine was 1.5 mg/dL (IQR 1.2–1.7), and the median level of cystatin-C was 1.4 mg/L (IQR 1.2–1.7). The median plasma level of serum urea was 26.5 mg/dL (IQR 20.6–33.3), the median level of uric acid was 7.1 mg/dL (IQR 6.0–8.3), and the median level of CRP was 2.4 mg/dL (IQR 1.2–4.9).

The leading cause of renal disease was nephrosclerosis (28.8%, n = 63), followed by diabetic nephropathy (diabetes mellitus type 1 and 2 combined: 17.4%, n = 38) and interstitial nephropathy (9.1%, n = 20) (see Table 1).

Table 1. Baseline characteristics, comorbidities, stages of chronic kidney disease (CKD), and causes of renal disease of the overall cohort.

General		
Age, mean (years)	63	±9
BMI, mean (kg/m^2)	30	±5.6
Serum creatinine, median (mg/dl)	1.5	IQR 1.2–1.7
eGFR, median (mL/min/1.73 m^2)	47.7	IQR 38.2–55.7
Urinary albumin/creatinine ratio (UACR), median (mg/g Crea)	44	IQR 7.4–216.7
Comorbidities	**%**	**(n)**
Hypertension	90.4	198
Diabetes mellitus	39.3	86
Heart Failure	26.0	57
CKD stages	**%**	**(n)**
Stage G1 (≥ 90 mL/min/1.73 m^2)	2.7	6
Stage G2 (eGFR 60–89 mL/min/1.73 m^2)	13.7	30
Stage G3a (eGFR 45–59 mL/min/1.73 m^2)	41.6	91
Stage G3b (eGFR 30–44 mL/min/1.73 m^2)	32.4	71
Stages G4 and G5 (eGFR <30 mL/min/1.73 m^2)	9.6	21
Urinary albumin/creatinine ratio (ACR)	**%**	**(n)**
A1 (<30 mg/g)	43.8	96
A2 (30–300 mg/g)	32.0	70
A3 (>300 mg/g)	20.5	45
Missing	4.7	8
Leading cause of renal disease	**%**	**(n)**
Vascular nephrosclerosis	28.8	63
Diabetic nephropathy	17.4	38
Interstitial nephropathy	9.1	20
IgA-nephritis	4.1	9
Autosomal dominant polycystic kidney disease	4.1	9
Membranous glomerulonephritis	2.7	6
Membranoproliferative glomerulonephritis	1.4	3
Other	17.9	40
Missing	14.6	32

BMI = body mass index, DM = diabetes mellitus.

3.2. Biomarker Concentrations

The median plasma levels of sST2, GDF-15, H-FABP, IGF-BP2, and suPAR in our study cohort are depicted in Figure 1 and Supplementary Materials, Table A1 in Appendix A.

Except for sST2, all of the investigated biomarkers showed significantly elevated plasma concentrations in the advanced stages of CKD (GDF-15: 3.6-fold increase, H-FABP: 4.4-fold increase, IGF-BP2: 3.0-fold increase, suPAR 2.0-fold increase when eGFR was <30 mL/min/1.73 m^2 BSA compared to eGFR ≥ 90 mL/min/1.73 m^2 BSA, see Figure 1 and Supplementary Materials, Table A1 in Appendix A). This finding remained statistically significant after applying Bonferroni–Holm correction for multiple comparisons (GDF-15: $p = 0.0005$, H-FABP: $p = 0.0005$, IGF-BP2: $p = 0.002$, suPAR: $p = 0.0005$).

Patients with concomitant symptoms of heart failure had significantly elevated plasma concentrations of sST2 (median 5039 pg/mL vs. 3673 pg/mL, $p = 0.008$).

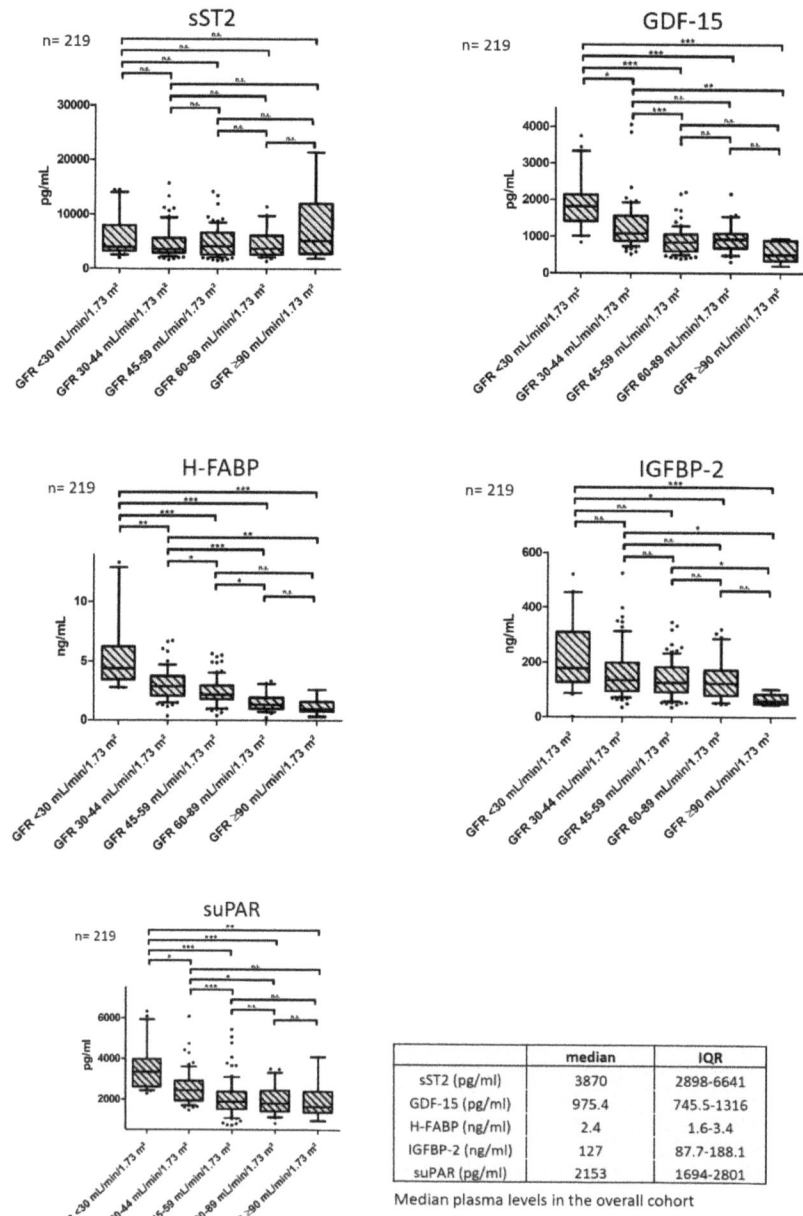

Figure 1. Biomarker concentrations throughout the stages of CKD. Median plasma levels and interquartile ranges (IQR) of the overall cohort are depicted in the additional table. * indicates a p of <0.05, ** a p of <0.01 and *** a p of <0.001, n.s.= not significant. Abbreviations: sST2 = soluble suppression of tumorigenicity, GDF-15 = growth differentiation factor 15, H-FABP = heart-type fatty acid binding protein, IGF-BP2= insulin-like growth factor binding protein 2, suPAR = soluble urokinase plasminogen activator receptor, eGFR = estimated glomerular filtration rate, IQR = interquartile range.

3.3. Correlation Analyses and Multiple Linear Regression Analyses

Plasma concentrations of GDF-15, H-FABP, suPAR, and IGF-BP2 showed a significant positive correlation with serum creatinine (GDF-15: rs = 0.566, $p < 0.0001$, H-FABP: rs = 0.584, $p < 0.0001$, suPAR: rs = 0.506, $p < 0.0001$, IGF-BP2: rs = 0.267, $p < 0.0001$; rs = correlation coefficient) and a significant inverse correlation with eGFR (GDF-15: rs = −0.493, $p < 0.0001$, H-FABP: rs = −0.550, $p < 0.0001$, suPAR: rs = −0.485, $p < 0.0001$, IGF-BP2: rs = −0.298, $p < 0.0001$), which remained statistically significant after applying Bonferroni–Holm correction. sST2 showed no correlation with renal function, neither with serum creatinine, nor with eGFR (see Figure 2 and Table 2).

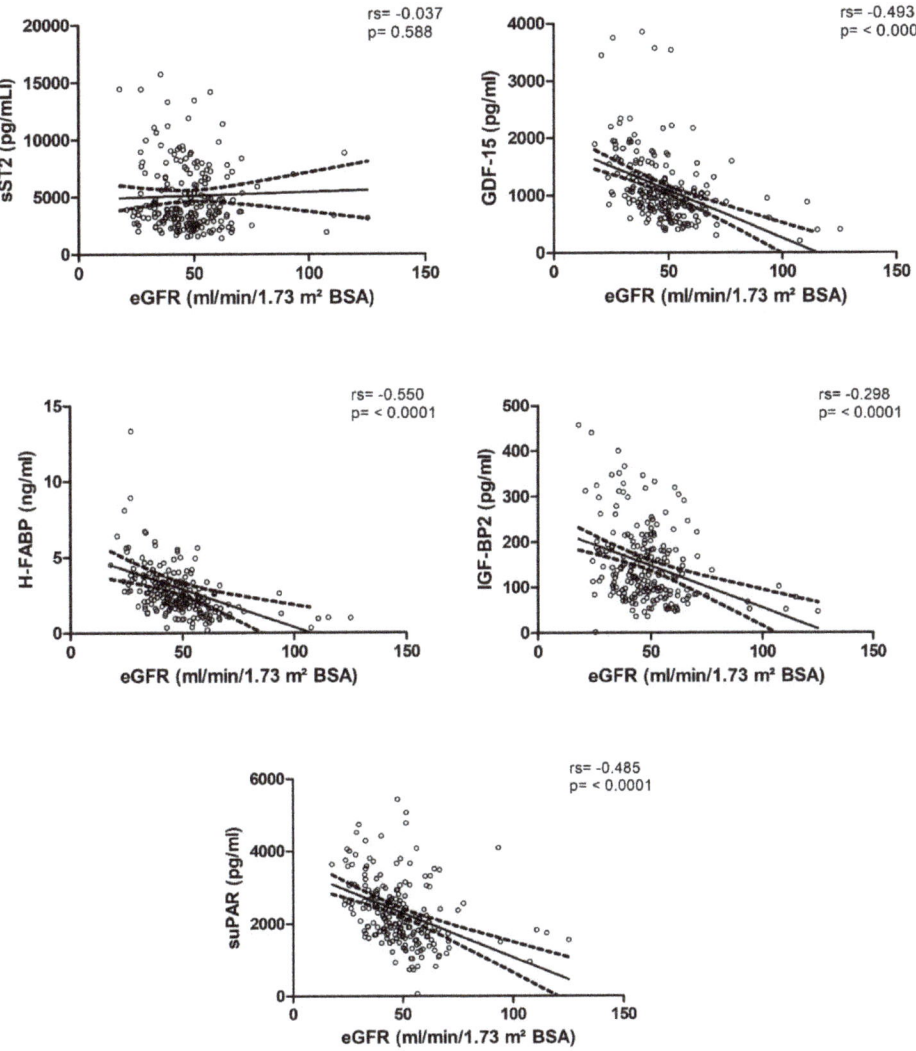

Figure 2. Visual representation of the correlation of biomarker concentrations with estimated glomerular filtration rate (eGFR).

Table 2. Correlation analysis of the investigated biomarkers.

Biomarker		BMI	Creatinine	eGFR	UACR	CRP	sST2	GDF15	H-FABP	IGF-BP2	suPAR
sST2	rs	0.890	0.125	−0.037	0.139	0.087		0.133	0.348	0.151	0.082
	p-value	0.191	0.067	0.588	0.044 *	0.200		0.049	<0.0001	0.025	0.228
GDF-15	rs	0.097	0.566	−0.493	0.251	0.240	0.133		0.491	0.266	0.614
	p-value	0.151	<0.0001	<0.0001	<0.0001	0.0004	0.049		<0.0001	<0.0001	<0.0001
H-FABP	rs	0.314	0.584	−0.550	0.100	0.162	0.348	0.491		0.194	0.516
	p-value	<0.0001	<0.0001	<0.0001	0.149	0.017	<0.0001	<0.0001		0.004	<0.0001
IGF-BP2	rs	−0.343	0.267	−0.298	0.192	−0.071	0.151	0.266	0.194		0.180
	p-value	<0.0001	<0.0001	<0.0001	0.005	0.296	0.025	<0.0001	0.004		0.007
suPAR	rs	0.243	0.506	−0.485	0.163	0.377	0.082	0.614	0.516	0.180	
	p-value	<0.0001	<0.0001	<0.0001	0.018 *	<0.0001	0.228	<0.0001	<0.0001	0.007	

* Denotes correlations that became statistically insignificant after applying a Bonferroni–Holm correction. Abbreviations: BMI = body mass index, CRP = C-reactive protein, eGFR = estimated glomerular filtration rate, rs = correlation coefficient, UACR = urinary albumin/creatinine ratio.

The correlation of biomarker concentrations with eGFR remained statistically significant in a multiple linear regression analysis after correction for parameters that are known to confound with renal function (GDF-15: B = −0.10, $p < 0.0001$; H-FABP: B = −1.187, $p < 0.0001$; IGF-BP2: B = −0.064, $p < 0.0001$; suPAR: B = −0.006, $p < 0.0001$; B = regression coefficient, see Supplementary Materials, Table A2 in Appendix A). There was still no significant correlation between plasma concentrations of sST2 and renal function (sST2: B = 0.000, 95% CI 0.000–0.001, $p = 0.643$) after adjusting for the aforementioned confounders.

Except for H-FABP, all of the biomarkers showed a weak, yet statistically significant correlation with the UACR (sST2: rs = 0.139, $p = 0.044$; GDF-15: rs = 0.251, $p < 0.0001$; IGF-BP2 rs = 0.192, $p = 0.005$; suPAR: rs = 0.163, $p = 0.018$, H-FABP: rs = 0.100, $p = 0.149$, see Table 2). Notably, the weak correlations of sST2 and suPAR with the UACR were statistically insignificant after applying the Bonferroni–Holm correction for multiple comparisons (sST2: $p = 0.088$, suPAR: $p = 0.054$).

However, after adjusting for the aforementioned confounders in another multiple linear regression model, all correlations with the UACR, except the ones with suPAR and H-FABP, remained statistically significant (sST2: B = 0.031, $p = 0.007$; GDF-15: B = 0.179, $p = 0.012$; IGF-BP2: B = 2.086, $p < 0.0001$; see Supplementary Materials, Table A2 in Appendix A).

Furthermore, the plasma concentrations of suPAR, H-FABP, and IGF-BP2 showed a significant correlation with BMI and the plasma levels of suPAR, H-FABP, and GDF-15 correlated with CRP. Additionally, the plasma concentrations of H-FABP correlated with the plasma levels of sST2, GDF-15, suPAR, and IGF-BP2, and the concentrations of suPAR correlated with the plasma levels of GDF-15 and IGF-BP2 and vice versa (see Table 2).

3.4. Biomarker Concentrations in Patients with Albuminuria

The plasma levels of GDF-15, IGF-BP2, and suPAR were significantly elevated in patients with micro-and macro-albuminuria, as defined by the UACR (Table 3). In contrast, the plasma concentrations of sST2 and H-FABP were not significantly influenced by the stage of albuminuria (see Table 3). This finding remained statistically significant after applying a Bonferroni–Holm correction for multiple comparisons (GDF-15: $p = 0.01$, IGF-BP2: $p = 0.01$, suPAR: $p = 0.012$).

Table 3. Concentrations in patients with normo-albuminuria, micro-albuminuria (UACR 30–300 mg/g, A2), and macro-albuminuria (UACR > 300 mg/g); the *p*-value represents the statistical differences between the three subgroups of albuminuria.

Biomarker	Total Cohort		Normo-albuminuria (A1)		Micro-albuminuria (A2)		Macro-albuminuria (A3)		*p*-Value
	median	IQR	median	IQR	median	IQR	median	IQR	
sST2 (pg/mL)	3870	2898–6641	3663	2726–6172	3647	2758–5793	4552	8587–3235	0.052
GDF-15 (pg/mL)	975.4	745.5–1316	892.2	675.6–1087	1035	780.9–861.7	1281	861.7–1635	0.002
H-FABP (ng/mL)	2.4	1.6–3.4	2.3	1.6–3.1	2.2	1.7–3.4	2.8	1.6–4.1	0.170
IGF-BP2 (ng/mL)	127	87.7–188.1	112.9	84.2–172.3	126.2	83.6–182.7	172.6	91.5–280.1	0.002
suPAR (pg/mL)	2153	1694–2801	1925	1653–2680	2197	1674–2723	2402	1918–2983	0.044

4. Discussion

In patients with chronic kidney disease (CKD), a high burden of cardiovascular diseases (CVD) is common, and an inverse correlation of renal function with the prevalence of coronary artery disease, congestive heart failure, and cerebrovascular disease is observed [1,50]. Moreover, the incidence of acute kidney injury has been steadily increasing in recent years, leading to higher healthcare costs and mortality and contributing to increasing prevalence rates of CKD [51,52]. With an increasing prevalence of CKD from variable causes, the number of patients with end-stage renal disease is on the rise [1,53]. Furthermore, the presence of CKD markedly increases cardiovascular mortality in a stage-dependent manner [54–56]. According to current evidence, patients with end-stage renal disease (ESRD) undergoing hemodialysis have a 10- to 30-fold higher risk of cardiovascular mortality than the general population [57].

In fact, diagnosis, risk stratification, and treatment of patients with CVD increasingly relies on cardiovascular biomarkers. Since some of the most commonly used biomarkers for these purposes (e.g., troponin or brain natriuretic peptide (BNP)) are chronically elevated in patients with CKD [57,58], novel cardiovascular biomarkers are warranted to facilitate the management of patients with decreased renal function.

In our study cohort, plasma concentrations of GDF-15, H-FABP, IGF-BP2, and suPAR were markedly elevated in patients with decreased renal function, with a 2.0- to 4.4-fold increase in biomarker levels in the advanced stages of CKD (eGFR < 30 mL/min/1.73 m^2 BSA). In contrast, we found no significant elevation of sST2 in patients with CKD. In fact, the plasma levels of sST2 even remained unaltered in advanced CKD (eGFR < 30 mL/min/1.73 m^2 BSA) and showed no correlation with estimated glomerular filtration rate (eGFR). In contrast to sST2, we found significant correlations of the plasma levels of GDF-15, H-FABP, IGF-BP2, and suPAR with serum creatinine and eGFR. Considering potential diagnostic value, it is essential to determine whether a biomarker would accumulate due to impaired renal clearance or increase due to the pathophysiologic process that it is supposed to portray (i.e., troponin in myocardial ischemia). Although the association with renal function does not preclude the predictive ability of a biomarker, its clinical applicability in the evaluation of patients with CVD and concomitant CKD appears to be somewhat limited [59]. Since some of the most commonly used conventional biomarkers in CVD are chronically elevated in patients with CKD, at least partly because of impaired renal clearance, the finding that sST2 acts independently of renal function might be of significant relevance for clinical practice. Nevertheless, this finding needs to be confirmed in large prospective endpoint trials because it to some extent contradicts the findings of a study by Alam et al. In this study, some correlation of sST2 with renal function was observed in a larger, pooled cohort, yet this relationship was very weak [60]. Furthermore, the clinical performance of biomarkers needs to be confirmed in large prospective endpoint trials. In this regard, recent trials investigated the plasma concentrations of NT-proBNP, troponin T, and IGF-BP2 in patients with CKD and reported a higher prognostic value of the investigated biomarkers in these patients [61,62]. However, it is always questionable whether such studies consistently correct their statistical models for kidney function. Hence, the adjustment for renal function may be more valid for biomarkers, which do not primarily correlate with renal function. Interestingly, although the ST2/IL-33 signaling pathway seems to be involved in various inflammatory processes [63–66], the aforementioned study by Alam et al. did not find a statistically significant association of the plasma levels of sST2 with the progression of CKD to end-stage renal disease (ESRD) [60]. Taken together with our results, it seems as if sST2, in contrast to numerous other cytokines or mediators, acts relatively independent from renal function and pathophysiologic processes affecting the kidneys.

Furthermore, all of the investigated biomarkers, except for H-FABP and sST2, were additionally elevated in patients with micro- and macro-albuminuria, as defined by the UACR. This association is of particular interest, since albuminuria is an independent cardiovascular risk factor reflecting endothelial dysfunction [67,68], which might modulate the predictive potential of the biomarkers investigated. Notably, despite no statistical significance, we observed an obvious increase in the plasma concentrations of sST2 between the different stages of albuminuria (see Table 3). This increase was accompanied by a weak, yet statistically significant correlation of sST2 with albuminuria (sST2: rs = 0.139, p = 0.044), which became statistically insignificant after applying a Bonferroni–Holm correction for multiple comparisons.

sST2 is a promising new biomarker in risk stratification and therapy guidance [69,70] in patients with acute and chronic heart failure, and was associated with an increased risk of adverse outcomes in previous trials [12,71,72]. According to our present findings, sST2 might be a useful additional biomarker in the management of patients with CVD and concomitant CKD, with or without albuminuria. Although some studies reported similar findings in the plasma levels of sST2 in patients with

CKD [73,74], the innovative value of our manuscript lies in the structured analysis and recording of five novel biomarkers, which portray different pathophysiological pathways, in a well-defined cohort. Furthermore, we investigated and described the respective plasma levels in different stages of CKD as reflected by eGFR and albuminuria.

5. Conclusions

Except for sST2, all of the investigated biomarkers were significantly elevated in patients with CKD, inversely correlating with eGFR. Based on our findings, sST2 appears to be the biomarker whose diagnostic performance is least affected by decreased renal function, hence suggesting potential viability in the management of patients with CVD and concomitant CKD. Whether this may influence its predictive potential in patients with CKD remains to be investigated by endpoint studies.

6. Limitations

A major limitation of this study is the absence of matched healthy controls, which would have further strengthened our findings. Moreover, the Gothenburg scale was found to be not ideal for reliably defining heart failure in patients with CKD in a previous trial due to shared symptoms and medications between the two disease entities [47]. However, a significant proportion of patients had concomitant heart failure, which may have acted as a bias in regard to the median concentrations of sST2. Notably, this trial did not analyze associations of the investigated biomarkers with clinical endpoints. We have to highlight that the conclusions drawn by the findings in this study are primarily of hypothesis-generating character and should be further validated in future trials. A limitation of the study may also be the applicability to populations of patients of non-Caucasian origin, since it is known that the cardiovascular risk also varies depending on ethnicity due to genetic differences. Thus, further investigative and population-specific endpoint trials, i.e., in the total GCKD cohort, seem necessary to confirm our present findings. One minor limitation is the use of estimated GFR instead of direct GFR measurement. Although more accurate, direct GFR measurement is too complex and impractical for everyday clinical use; hence, it appears unsuitable for a large multi-center trial. The use of eGFR by means of the MDRD formula does not represent a large bias regarding our current findings since only a minority of the patients had an eGFR above 60 mL/min/1.73 m^2.

Supplementary Materials: The following are available online at http://www.mdpi.com/2077-0383/9/3/886/s1, Table S1: Biomarker concentrations by estimated glomerular filtration rate (eGFR), Table S2: Multiple linear regression analysis with adjustment for age, gender, BMI, hypertension, and diabetes mellitus.

Author Contributions: M.M., A.T. and R.R. were responsible for the study design, writing and correction of the manuscript. V.P. conducted the necessary experiments and B.W. was responsible of the statistical analyses. K.K. provided English language editing, M.L. was involved in the primary design of the study, writing and correction of the manuscript. U.C.H., P.C.S., D.K., M.P.S., U.T.S., C.S., K.P., G.W., M.B., C.J. and H.S. were involved in the design of the study and provided substantial corrections and improvements to the manuscript. All authors have read and agreed to the published version of the manuscript.

Funding: This research received no external funding but the GCKD study is funded by grants from the German Ministry of Education and Research (www.gesundheitsforschung-bmbf.de; grant numbers 01ER 0804, 01ER 0818, 01ER 0819, 01ER 0820, 01ER 0821, and 01ER 0122) and the KfH Foundation for Preventive Medicine (http://www.kfh-stiftung-praeventivmedizin.de/). It is conducted under the auspices of the German Society of Nephrology (http://www.dgfn.eu).

Acknowledgments: We are very grateful for the willingness and time of all study participants of the GCKD study. The authors thank all participating patients and the physicians and nurses taking care of them. We also thank the large number of nephrologists for their support of the GCKD study (list of nephrologists currently collaborating with the GCKD study is available at http://www.gckd.org). Current GCKD investigators and collaborators with the GCKD study are: University of Erlangen-Nürnberg: K.-U.E., H.M., M.P.S., M.S., T.D., H.-U.P., B.B., A.B., D.K., A.R., A.B.E., S.A., D.B.-G., U.A.-S., B.H., A.W.; University of Freiburg: Gerd Walz, A. K., U.T.S., F. K., S. M., E. M., U. R.; RWTH Aachen University: J.F., G.S., T.S.; Charité, University Medicine Berlin: E.S., S.B.-A., K.T.; Hannover Medical School: H.H., J.M.; University of Heidelberg: M.Z., C.S., R.W.; University of Jena: G.W., M.B., R.P.; Ludwig-Maximilians University of München: T.S.; University of Würzburg: C.W., V.K., A.B.-K., B.B.; Medical University of Innsbruck, Division of Genetic Epidemiology: F.K., J.R., B.K., L.F., S.S., Hansi Weissensteiner;

University of Regensburg, Institute of Functional Genomics: P.O., W.G., H.Z.; Department of Medical Biometry, Informatics and Epidemiology (IMBIE), University Hospital of Bonn: M.S., J.N.

Conflicts of Interest: The authors declare no conflict of interest.

Appendix A

Table A1. Biomarker concentrations by estimated glomerular filtration rate (eGFR).

Biomarker	eGFR <30 mL/min/1.73 m²		eGFR 30–44 mL/min/1.73 m²		eGFR 45–59 mL/min/1.73 m²		eGFR 60–89 mL/min/1.73 m²	
	median	IQR	median	IQR	median	IQR	median	IQR
sST2 (pg/mL)	3998	3262–7949	3612	2997–5689	4167	2643–6620	3731	2660–6098
GDF-15 (pg/mL)	1816	1420–2139	1086	883.4–1567	843.8	602.5–1064	929.7	683.0–1084
H-FABP (ng/mL)	4.4	3.5–6.2	2.9	2.1–3.7	2.2	1.8–3.0	1.4	1.0–1.9
IGF-BP2 (ng/mL)	177.8	127.5–309.0	135.4	94.9–198.8	126.0	91.3–182.5	122.6	79.0–171.4
suPAR (pg/mL)	3342	2618–3977	2443	1936–2921	1898	1537–2382	1811	1422–2442

	eGFR ≥ 90 mL/min/1.73 m²		total cohort		
	median	IQR	median	IQR	p-value
sST2 (pg/mL)	5170	2820–11,952	3870	2898–6641	0.788
GDF-15 (pg/mL)	506.3	348.3–896.4	975.4	745.5–1316	<0.0001
H-FABP (ng/mL)	1.0	0.8–1.6	2.4	1.6–3.4	<0.0001
IGF-BP2 (ng/mL)	59.9	50.2–83.6	127	87.7–188.1	0.001
suPAR (pg/mL)	1648	1364–2393	2153	1694–2801	<0.0001

Table A2. Multiple linear regression analysis with adjustment for age, gender, BMI, hypertension and diabetes mellitus.

	Dependent Variable: eGFR					Dependent Variable: UACR			
	Adjustment for: Age, Gender, BMI, Hypertension, Diabetes					Adjustment for: Age, Gender, BMI, Hypertension, Diabetes			
Biomarker	r	Std. Error	95% CI	p-Value	Biomarker	r	Std. Error	95% CI	p-Value
sST2 (pg/mL)	0.000	0.000	0.000–0.001	0.643	sST2 (pg/mL)	0.031	0.011	0.008–0.053	0.007
GDF-15 (pg/mL)	−0.010	0.002	−0.013–(−0.007)	<0.0001	GDF-15 (pg/mL)	0.179	0.071	0.040–0.319	0.012
H-FABP (ng/mL)	−1.187	0.321	−1.820–(−0.555)	<0.0001	H-FABP (ng/mL)	17.542	12.923	−7.938–43.02	0.176
IGF-BP2 (ng/mL)	−0.064	0.012	−0.087–(−0.041)	<0.0001	IGF-BP2 (ng/mL)	2.086	0.464	1.170–3.001	<0.0001
suPAR (pg/mL)	−0.006	0.001	−0.008–(−0.004)	<0.0001	suPAR (pg/mL)	0.084	0.045	−0.004–0.171	0.062

Variance inflation factor (VIF): age = 1.037, gender = 1.084, BMI = 1.197, hypertension = 1.122, diabetes mellitus = 1.229. Abbreviations: eGFR = estimated glomerular filtration rate, UACR = urinary albumin/creatinine ratio, B = regression coefficient, BMI = body mass index, eGFR = estimated glomerular filtration rate, 95% CI = 95% confidence interval.

References

1. Levey, A.S.; Coresh, J. Chronic kidney disease. *Lancet* **2012**, *379*, 165–180. [CrossRef]
2. Ardhanari, S.; Alpert, M.A.; Aggarwal, K. Cardiovascular disease in chronic kidney disease: Risk factors, pathogenesis, and prevention. *Adv. Perit. Dial.* **2014**, *30*, 40–53.
3. Di Lullo, L.; House, A.; Gorini, A.; Santoboni, A.; Russo, D.; Ronco, C. Chronic kidney disease and cardiovascular complications. *Heart Fail. Rev.* **2015**, *20*, 259–272. [CrossRef] [PubMed]
4. Suckling, R.; Gallagher, H. Chronic kidney disease, diabetes mellitus and cardiovascular disease: Risks and commonalities. *J. Ren. Care* **2012**, *38*, 4–11. [CrossRef] [PubMed]
5. Kanderian, A.S.; Francis, G.S. Cardiac troponins and chronic kidney disease. *Kidney Int.* **2006**, *69*, 1112–1114. [CrossRef]
6. Stacy, S.R.; Suarez-Cuervo, C.; Berger, Z.; Wilson, L.M.; Yeh, H.-C.; Bass, E.B.; Michos, E.D. Role of Troponin in Patients With Chronic Kidney Disease and Suspected Acute Coronary Syndrome. *Ann. Intern. Med.* **2014**, *161*, 502–512. [CrossRef]
7. Takase, H.; Dohi, Y. Kidney function crucially affects B-type natriuretic peptide (BNP), N-terminal proBNP and their relationship. *Eur. J. Clin. Investig.* **2014**, *44*, 303–308. [CrossRef]
8. Universal Protein Resource (UniProt). Interleukin-1 Receptor-Like 1. Available online: https://www.uniprot.org/uniprot/Q01638#structure (accessed on 6 March 2020).
9. Dieplinger, B.; Januzzi, J.L.; Steinmair, M.; Gabriel, C.; Poelz, W.; Haltmayer, M.; Mueller, T. Analytical and clinical evaluation of a novel high-sensitivity assay for measurement of soluble ST2 in human plasma—The Presage™ ST2 assay. *Clin. Chim. Acta* **2009**, *409*, 33–40. [CrossRef]
10. Mueller, T.; Dieplinger, B. Soluble ST2 and Galectin-3: What We Know and Don't Know Analytically. *EJIFCC* **2016**, *27*, 224–237.
11. Bhardwaj, A.; Januzzi, J.L., Jr. ST2: A novel biomarker for heart failure. *Expert Rev. Mol. Diagn.* **2010**, *10*, 459–464. [CrossRef]
12. Dieplinger, B.; Egger, M.; Haltmayer, M.; Kleber, M.E.; Scharnagl, H.; Silbernagel, G.; de Boer, R.A.; Maerz, W.; Mueller, T. Increased Soluble ST2 Predicts Long-term Mortality in Patients with Stable Coronary Artery Disease: Results from the Ludwigshafen Risk and Cardiovascular Health Study. *Clin. Chem.* **2014**, *60*, 530–540. [CrossRef] [PubMed]
13. Savic-Radojevic, A.; Pljesa-Ercegovac, M.; Matic, M.; Simic, D.; Radovanovic, S.; Simic, T. Novel Biomarkers of Heart Failure. In *Advances in Clinical Chemistry*; Elsevier: Amsterdam, The Netherlands, 2017; Volume 79, pp. 93–152.
14. Universal Protein Resource (UniProt). Growth/Differentiation Factor 15. Available online: https://www.uniprot.org/uniprot/Q99988 (accessed on 6 March 2020).
15. Liu, X.; Chi, X.; Gong, Q.; Gao, L.; Niu, Y.; Chi, X.; Cheng, M.; Si, Y.; Wang, M.; Zhong, J.; et al. Association of serum level of growth differentiation factor 15 with liver cirrhosis and hepatocellular carcinoma. *PLoS ONE* **2015**, *10*, e0127518. [CrossRef] [PubMed]
16. George, M.; Jena, A.; Srivatsan, V.; Muthukumar, R.; Dhandapani, V.E. GDF 15—A Novel Biomarker in the Offing for Heart Failure. *Curr. Cardiol. Rev.* **2016**, *12*, 37–46. [CrossRef] [PubMed]
17. Zeng, X.; Li, L.; Wen, H.; Bi, Q. Growth-differentiation factor 15 as a predictor of mortality in patients with heart failure. *J. Cardiovasc. Med.* **2017**, *18*, 53–59. [CrossRef] [PubMed]
18. Wollert, K.C.; Kempf, T. Growth Differentiation Factor 15 in Heart Failure: An Update. *Curr. Heart Fail. Rep.* **2012**, *9*, 337–345. [CrossRef]
19. Zhang, S.; Dai, D.; Wang, X.; Zhu, H.; Jin, H.; Zhao, R.; Jiang, L.; Lu, Q.; Yi, F.; Wan, X.; et al. Growth differentiation factor—15 predicts the prognoses of patients with acute coronary syndrome: A meta-analysis. *BMC Cardiovasc. Disord.* **2016**, *16*, 82. [CrossRef]
20. Nair, V.; Robinson-Cohen, C.; Smith, M.R.; Bellovich, K.A.; Bhat, Z.Y.; Bobadilla, M.; Brosius, F.; de Boer, I.H.; Essioux, L.; Formentini, I.; et al. Growth Differentiation Factor-15 and Risk of CKD Progression. *J. Am. Soc. Nephrol.* **2017**, *28*, 2233–2240. [CrossRef]
21. Universal Protein Resource (UniProt). Fatty Acid-Binding Protein, Heart. Available online: https://www.uniprot.org/uniprot/P05413 (accessed on 6 March 2020).

22. Ishimura, S.; Furuhashi, M.; Watanabe, Y.; Hoshina, K.; Fuseya, T.; Mita, T.; Okazaki, Y.; Koyama, M.; Tanaka, M.; Akasaka, H.; et al. Circulating levels of fatty acid-binding protein family and metabolic phenotype in the general population. *PLoS ONE* **2013**, *8*, e81318. [CrossRef]
23. Kakoti, A.; Goswami, P. Heart type fatty acid binding protein: Structure, function and biosensing applications for early detection of myocardial infarction. *Biosens. Bioelectron.* **2013**, *43*, 400–411. [CrossRef]
24. Colli, A.; Josa, M.; Pomar, J.L.; Mestres, C.A.; Gherli, T. Heart Fatty Acid Binding Protein in the Diagnosis of Myocardial Infarction: Where Do We Stand Today? *Cardiology* **2007**, *108*, 4–10. [CrossRef]
25. Otaki, Y.; Watanabe, T.; Kubota, I. Heart-type fatty acid-binding protein in cardiovascular disease: A systemic review. *Clin. Chim. Acta* **2017**, *474*, 44–53. [CrossRef] [PubMed]
26. Boscheri, A.; Wunderlich, C.; Langer, M.; Schoen, S.; Wiedemann, B.; Stolte, D.; Elmer, G.; Barthel, P.; Strasser, R.H. Correlation of heart-type fatty acid-binding protein with mortality and echocardiographic data in patients with pulmonary embolism at intermediate risk. *Am. Heart J.* **2010**, *160*, 294–300. [CrossRef]
27. Niizeki, T.; Takeishi, Y.; Arimoto, T.; Nozaki, N. Persistently Increased Serum Concentration of Heart-Type Fatty Acid-Binding Protein Predicts Adverse Clinical Outcomes in Patients with Chronic Heart Failure. *Cric. J.* **2008**, *72*, 109–114. [CrossRef] [PubMed]
28. Universal Protein Resource (UniProt). Insulin-Like Growth Factor-Binding Protein 2. Available online: https://www.uniprot.org/uniprot/P18065 (accessed on 6 March 2020).
29. Kendrick, Z.W.; Firpo, M.A.; Repko, R.C.; Scaife, C.L.; Adler, D.G.; Boucher, K.M.; Mulvihill, S.J. Serum IGFBP2 and MSLN as diagnostic and prognostic biomarkers for pancreatic cancer. *HPB* **2014**, *16*, 670–676. [CrossRef]
30. Hoeflich, A.; Russo, V.C. Physiology and pathophysiology of IGFBP-1 and IGFBP-2—Consensus and dissent on metabolic control and malignant potential. *Best Pract. Res. Clin. Endocrinol. Metab.* **2015**, *29*, 685–700. [CrossRef] [PubMed]
31. Rajpathak, S.N.; He, M.; Sun, Q.; Kaplan, R.C.; Muzumdar, R.; Rohan, T.E.; Gunter, M.J.; Pollak, M.; Kim, M.; Pessin, J.E.; et al. Insulin-like growth factor axis and risk of type 2 diabetes in women. *Diabetes* **2012**, *61*, 2248–2254. [CrossRef]
32. Heald, A.; Kaushal, K.; Siddals, K.; Rudenski, A.; Anderson, S.; Gibson, J. Insulin-like Growth Factor Binding Protein-2 (IGFBP-2) is a Marker for the Metabolic Syndrome. *Exp. Clin. Endocrinol. Diabetes* **2006**, *114*, 371–376. [CrossRef]
33. Vasylyeva, T.L.; Ferry, R.J. Novel roles of the IGF–IGFBP axis in etiopathophysiology of diabetic nephropathy. *Diabetes Res. Clin. Pract.* **2007**, *76*, 177–186. [CrossRef]
34. Hoeflich, A.; David, R.; Hjortebjerg, R. Current IGFBP-Related Biomarker Research in Cardiovascular Disease-We Need More Structural and Functional Information in Clinical Studies. *Front. Endocrinol.* **2018**, *9*, 388. [CrossRef]
35. Martin, R.M.; Gunnell, D.; Whitley, E.; Nicolaides, A.; Griffin, M.; Georgiou, N.; Davey Smith, G.; Ebrahim, S.; Holly, J.M.P. Associations of Insulin-Like Growth Factor (IGF)-I, IGF-II, IGF Binding Protein (IGFBP)-2 and IGFBP-3 with Ultrasound Measures of Atherosclerosis and Plaque Stability in an Older Adult Population. *J. Clin. Endocrinol. Metab.* **2008**, *93*, 1331–1338. [CrossRef]
36. Universal Protein Resource (UniProt). Urokinase Plasminogen Activator Surface Receptor. Available online: https://www.uniprot.org/uniprot/Q03405 (accessed on 6 March 2020).
37. Chew-Harris, J.; Appleby, S.; Richards, A.M.; Troughton, R.W.; Pemberton, C.J. Analytical, biochemical and clearance considerations of soluble urokinase plasminogen activator receptor (suPAR) in healthy individuals. *Clin. Biochem.* **2019**, *69*, 36–44. [CrossRef] [PubMed]
38. Huai, Q.; Mazar, A.P.; Kuo, A.; Parry, G.C.; Shaw, D.E.; Callahan, J.; Li, Y.; Yuan, C.; Bian, C.; Chen, L.; et al. Structure of human urokinase plasminogen activator in complex with its receptor. *Science* **2006**, *311*, 656–659. [CrossRef] [PubMed]
39. Eapen, D.J.; Manocha, P.; Ghasemzadeh, N.; Patel, R.S.; Al Kassem, H.; Hammadah, M.; Hammadah, M.; Veledar, E.; Le, N.-A.; Pielak, T.; et al. Soluble Urokinase Plasminogen Activator Receptor Level Is an Independent Predictor of the Presence and Severity of Coronary Artery Disease and of Future Adverse Events. *J. Am. Heart Assoc.* **2014**, *3*, e001118. [CrossRef] [PubMed]
40. Hayek, S.S.; Sever, S.; Ko, Y.A.; Trachtman, H.; Awad, M.; Wadhwani, S.; Altintas, M.M.; Wei, C.; Hotton, A.L.; French, A.L.; et al. Soluble Urokinase Receptor and Chronic Kidney Disease. *N. Engl. J. Med.* **2015**, *373*, 1916–1925. [CrossRef]

41. Skorecki, K.L.; Freedman, B.I. A suPAR Biomarker for Chronic Kidney Disease. *N. Engl. J. Med.* **2015**, *373*, 1971–1972. [CrossRef]
42. Wei, C.; Trachtman, H.; Li, J.; Dong, C.; Friedman, A.L.; Gassman, J.J.; McMahan, J.L.; Radeva, M.; Heil, K.M.; Trautmann, A.; et al. Circulating suPAR in Two Cohorts of Primary FSGS. *J. Am. Soc. Nephrol.* **2012**, *23*, 2051–2059. [CrossRef]
43. Lee, J.M.; Yang, J.W.; Kronbichler, A.; Eisenhut, M.; Kim, G.; Lee, K.H.; Shin, J.I. Increased Serum Soluble Urokinase-Type Plasminogen Activator Receptor (suPAR) Levels in FSGS: A Meta-Analysis. *J. Immunol. Res.* **2019**, *2019*, 1–11. [CrossRef]
44. Eckardt, K.U.; Bärthlein, B.; Baid-Agrawal, S.; Beck, A.; Busch, M.; Eitner, F.; Ekici, A.B.; Floege, J.; Gefeller, O.; Haller, H.; et al. The German Chronic Kidney Disease (GCKD) study: Design and methods. *Nephrol. Dial. Transplant.* **2012**, *27*, 1454–1460. [CrossRef]
45. Titze, S.; Schmid, M.; Köttgen, A.; Busch, M.; Floege, J.; Wanner, C.; Kronenberg, F.; Eckardt, K.U.; Titze, S.; Prokosch, H.U.; et al. Disease burden and risk profile in referred patients with moderate chronic kidney disease: Composition of the German Chronic Kidney Disease (GCKD) cohort. *Nephrol. Dial. Transplant.* **2015**, *30*, 441–451. [CrossRef]
46. Levey, A.S.; Greene, T.; Beck, G.J.; Caggiula, A.W.; Kusek, J.W.; Hunsicker, L.G.; Klahr, S. Dietary protein restriction and the progression of chronic renal disease: What have all of the results of the MDRD study shown? Modification of Diet in Renal Disease Study group. *J. Am. Soc. Nephrol.* **1999**, *10*, 2426–2439.
47. Beck, H.; Titze, S.I.; Hübner, S.; Busch, M.; Schlieper, G.; Schultheiss, U.T.; Wanner, C.; Kronenberg, F.; Krane, V.; Eckardt, K.-U.; et al. Heart Failure in a Cohort of Patients with Chronic Kidney Disease: The GCKD Study. *PLoS ONE* **2015**, *10*, e0122552.
48. Wheeler, D.C.; Winkelmayer, W.C.; Kidney Disease: Improving Global Outcomes (KDIGO) CKD-MBD Update Work Group. KDIGO 2017 Clinical Practice Guideline Update for the Diagnosis, Evaluation, Prevention, and Treatment of Chronic Kidney Disease–Mineral and Bone Disorder (CKD-MBD). *Kidney Int. Suppl.* **2017**, *7*, 1–59.
49. Eriksson, H.; Caidahl, K.; Larsson, B.; Ohlson, L.O.; Welin, L.; Wilhelmsen, L.; Svärdsudd, K. Cardiac and pulmonary causes of dyspnea—Validation of a scoring test for clinical-epidemiological use: The Study of Men Born in 1913. *Eur. Heart J.* **1987**, *8*, 1007–1014. [CrossRef]
50. Herzog, C.A.; Asinger, R.W.; Berger, A.K.; Charytan, D.M.; Díez, J.; Hart, R.G.; Eckardt, K.-U.; Kasiske, B.L.; McCullough, P.A.; Passman, R.S.; et al. Cardiovascular disease in chronic kidney disease. A clinical update from Kidney Disease: Improving Global Outcomes (KDIGO). *Kidney Int.* **2011**, *80*, 572–586. [CrossRef]
51. Thongprayoon, C.; Kaewput, W.; Thamcharoen, N.; Bathini, T.; Watthanasuntorn, K.; Salim, S.A.; Ungprasert, P.; Lertjitbanjong, P.; Aeddula, N.R.; Torres-Ortiz, A.; et al. Acute Kidney Injury in Patients Undergoing Total Hip Arthroplasty: A Systematic Review and Meta-Analysis. *J. Clin. Med.* **2019**, *8*, 66. [CrossRef]
52. Thongprayoon, C.; Kaewput, W.; Thamcharoen, N.; Bathini, T.; Watthanasuntorn, K.; Lertjitbanjong, P.; Sharma, K.; Salim, S.A.; Ungprasert, P.; Wijarnpreecha, K.; et al. Incidence and Impact of Acute Kidney Injury after Liver Transplantation: A Meta-Analysis. *J. Clin. Med.* **2019**, *8*, 372. [CrossRef] [PubMed]
53. Salim, S.A.; Zsom, L.; Cheungpasitporn, W.; Fülöp, T. Benefits, challenges, and opportunities using home hemodialysis with a focus on Mississippi, a rural southern state. *Semin. Dial.* **2019**, *32*, 80–84. [CrossRef] [PubMed]
54. Shulman, N.B.; Ford, C.E.; Hall, W.D.; Blaufox, M.D.; Simon, D.; Langford, H.G.; Schneider, K.A. Prognostic value of serum creatinine and effect of treatment of hypertension on renal function. Results from the hypertension detection and follow-up program. The Hypertension Detection and Follow-up Program Cooperative Group. *Hypertension* **1989**, *13*, I80–I93. [CrossRef] [PubMed]
55. Foley, R.N.; Parfrey, P.S.; Sarnak, M.J. Epidemiology of cardiovascular disease in chronic renal disease. *J. Am. Soc. Nephrol.* **1998**, *9*, S16–S23. [CrossRef]
56. Go, A.S.; Chertow, G.M.; Fan, D.; McCulloch, C.E.; Hsu, C. Chronic Kidney Disease and the Risks of Death, Cardiovascular Events, and Hospitalization. *N. Engl. J. Med.* **2004**, *351*, 1296–1305. [CrossRef]
57. Sarnak, M.J.; Levey, A.S.; Schoolwerth, A.C.; Coresh, J.; Culleton, B.; Hamm, L.L.; McCullough, P.A.; Kasiske, B.L.; Kelepouris, E.; Klag, M.J.; et al. Kidney Disease as a Risk Factor for Development of Cardiovascular Disease. *Circulation* **2003**, *108*, 2154–2169. [CrossRef] [PubMed]

58. Srisawasdi, P.; Vanavanan, S.; Charoenpanichkit, C.; Kroll, M.H. The Effect of Renal Dysfunction on BNP, NT-proBNP, and Their Ratio. *Am. J. Clin. Pathol.* **2010**, *133*, 14–23. [CrossRef] [PubMed]
59. Colbert, G.; Jain, N.; de Lemos, J.A.; Hedayati, S.S. Utility of Traditional Circulating and Imaging-Based Cardiac Biomarkers in Patients with Predialysis CKD. *Clin. J. Am. Soc. Nephrol.* **2015**, *10*, 515. [CrossRef]
60. Alam, M.L.; Katz, R.; Bellovich, K.A.; Bhat, Z.Y.; Brosius, F.C.; de Boer, I.H.; Gadegbeku, C.A.; Gipson, D.S.; Hawkins, J.J.; Himmelfarb, J.; et al. Soluble ST2 and Galectin-3 and Progression of CKD. *Kidney Int. Rep.* **2019**, *4*, 103–111. [CrossRef] [PubMed]
61. Gregg, L.P.; Adams-Huet, B.; Li, X.; Colbert, G.; Jain, N.; de Lemos, A.J.; Hedayati, S.S. Effect modification of chronic kidney disease on the association of circulating and imaging cardiac biomarkers with outcomes. *J. Am. Heart Assoc.* **2017**, *6*, 7. [CrossRef] [PubMed]
62. Ravassa, S.; Beaumont, J.; Cediel, G.; Lupón, J.; López, B.; Querejeta, R.; Díez, J.; Bayés-Genís, A.; González, A. Cardiorenal interaction and heart failure outcomes. A role for insulin-like growth factor binding protein 2? *Rev. Esp. Cardiol. (Engl. Ed.)* **2020**. [CrossRef]
63. Griesenauer, B.; Paczesny, S. The ST2/IL-33 Axis in Immune Cells during Inflammatory Diseases. *Front. Immunol.* **2017**, *8*, 475. [CrossRef]
64. Stankovic, M.S.; Janjetovic, K.; Velimirovic, M.; Milenkovic, M.; Stojkovic, T.; Puskas, N.; Zaletel, I.; De Luka, S.R.; Jankovic, S.; Stefanovic, S.; et al. Effects of IL-33/ST2 pathway in acute inflammation on tissue damage, antioxidative parameters, magnesium concentration and cytokines profile. *Exp. Mol. Pathol.* **2016**, *101*, 31–37. [CrossRef]
65. Chen, W.-Y.; Tsai, T.-H.; Yang, J.-L.; Li, L.-C. Therapeutic Strategies for Targeting IL-33/ST2 Signalling for the Treatment of Inflammatory Diseases. *Cell. Physiol. Biochem.* **2018**, *49*, 349–358. [CrossRef]
66. Xu, H.; Turnquist, H.R.; Hoffman, R.; Billiar, T.R. Role of the IL-33-ST2 axis in sepsis. *Mil. Med. Res.* **2017**, *4*, 3. [CrossRef]
67. Kunimura, A.; Ishii, H.; Uetani, T.; Harada, K.; Kataoka, T.; Takeshita, M.; Harada, K.; Okumura, S.; Shinoda, N.; Kato, B.; et al. Prognostic Value of Albuminuria on Cardiovascular Outcomes after Elective Percutaneous Coronary Intervention. *Am. J. Cardiol.* **2016**, *117*, 714–719. [CrossRef] [PubMed]
68. Stephen, R.; Jolly, S.E.; Nally, J.V.; Navaneethan, S.D. Albuminuria: When urine predicts kidney and cardiovascular disease. *Cleve. Clin. J. Med.* **2014**, *81*, 41–50. [CrossRef]
69. Januzzi, J.L.; Pascual-Figal, D.; Daniels, L.B. ST2 Testing for Chronic Heart Failure Therapy Monitoring: The International ST2 Consensus Panel. *Am. J. Cardiol.* **2015**, *115*, 70B–75B. [CrossRef] [PubMed]
70. Gaggin, H.K.; Januzzi, J.L. Biomarkers and diagnostics in heart failure. *Biochim. Biophys. Acta Mol. Basis Dis.* **2013**, *1832*, 2442–2450. [CrossRef] [PubMed]
71. Aimo, A.; Vergaro, G.; Ripoli, A.; Bayes-Genis, A.; Figal, D.A.P.; de Boer, R.A.; Lassus, J.; Mebazaa, A.; Gayat, E.; Breidthardt, T.; et al. Meta-Analysis of Soluble Suppression of Tumorigenicity-2 and Prognosis in Acute Heart Failure. *JACC Heart Fail.* **2017**, *5*, 287–296. [CrossRef] [PubMed]
72. Dalal, J.J.; Digrajkar, A.; Das, B.; Bansal, M.; Toomu, A.; Maisel, A.S. ST2 elevation in heart failure, predictive of a high early mortality. *Indian Heart J.* **2018**, *70*, 822–827. [CrossRef]
73. Mueller, T.; Leitner, I.; Egger, M.; Haltmayer, M.; Dieplinger, B. Association of the biomarkers soluble ST2, galectin-3 and growth-differentiation factor-15 with heart failure and other non-cardiac diseases. *Clin. Chim. Acta* **2015**, *445*, 155–160. [CrossRef]
74. Bayes-Genis, A.; Zamora, E.; De Antonio, M.; Galán, A.; Vila, J.; Urrutia, A.; Díez, C.; Coll, R.; Altimir, S.; Lupón, J. Soluble ST2 serum concentration and renal function in heart failure. *J. Card. Fail.* **2013**, *19*, 768–775. [CrossRef]

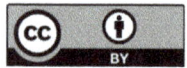

© 2020 by the authors. Licensee MDPI, Basel, Switzerland. This article is an open access article distributed under the terms and conditions of the Creative Commons Attribution (CC BY) license (http://creativecommons.org/licenses/by/4.0/).

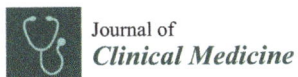
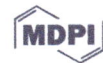

Article

Salivary Oxidative Stress Increases with the Progression of Chronic Heart Failure

Anna Klimiuk [1], Anna Zalewska [1], Robert Sawicki [2], Małgorzata Knapp [2] and Mateusz Maciejczyk [3,*]

[1] Experimental Dentistry Laboratory, Medical University of Bialystok, 24a M. Sklodowskiej-Curie Street, 15-274 Bialystok, Poland; annak04@poczta.onet.pl (A.K.); azalewska426@gmail.com (A.Z.)
[2] Department of Cardiology, Medical University of Bialystok, 24a M. Sklodowskiej-Curie Street, 15-274 Bialystok, Poland; r-sawicki@o2.pl (R.S.); malgo33@interia.pl (M.K.)
[3] Department of Hygiene, Epidemiology and Ergonomics, Medical University of Bialystok, 2c Mickiewicza Street, 15-233 Bialystok, Poland
* Correspondence: mat.maciejczyk@gmail.com

Received: 3 February 2020; Accepted: 10 March 2020; Published: 12 March 2020

Abstract: The aim of the study was to evaluate the rate of reactive oxygen species (ROS) production, antioxidant barrier, and oxidative damage in non-stimulated (NWS) and stimulated (SWS) saliva as well as plasma/erythrocytes of 50 patients with chronic heart failure (HF) divided into the two subgroups: NYHA II (33 patients) and NYHA III (17 patients). The activity of superoxide dismutase and catalase was statistically increased in NWS of HF patients as compared to healthy controls. The free radical formation, total oxidant status, level of uric acid, advanced glycation end products (AGE), advanced oxidation protein products and malondialdehyde was significantly elevated in NWS, SWS, and plasma of NYHA III patients as compared to NYHA II and controls. We were the first to demonstrate that with the progression of HF, disturbances of enzymatic and non-enzymatic antioxidant defense, and oxidative damage to proteins and lipids occur at both central (plasma/erythrocytes) and local (saliva) levels. In the study group, we also observed a decrease in saliva secretion, total salivary protein and salivary amylase activity compared to age- and gender-matched control group, which indicates secretory dysfunction of salivary glands in patients with HF. Salivary AGE may be a potential biomarker in differential diagnosis of HF.

Keywords: chronic heart failure; saliva; oxidative stress; salivary biomarkers

1. Introduction

Despite enormous progress made in the diagnosis and treatment of cardiovascular diseases, the incidence of chronic heart failure (HF) is steadily increasing and is the leading cause of death in adults. Thus, HF is not only a major clinical, but also an epidemiological and economic problem [1,2]. It is estimated that HF affects about 1%–2% of the population in developed countries, and in the age group of over 70 the disease already affects every 10th person [3]. According to the current definition, HF is a syndrome of symptoms such as dyspnea, swelling of the lower limbs, and decreased tolerance to physical activity, which may be accompanied by abnormalities in the physical examination (jugular vein dilatation, crackles over the lungs, peripheral swelling) [4]. Differentiation of HF patients based on the left ventricular ejection fraction (LVEF) is essential due to other underlying etiologies, demographic differences, co-morbidities, and responses to applied treatment [3]. Thus, we distinguish patients with normal LVEF (typically considered as ≥ 50%; HF with preserved EF (HFpEF)) as well as reduced LVEF (typically considered as < 40%; HF with reduced EF (HFrEF)) [3]. The cause of these ailments in HFrEF is a disturbed structure and/or function of the heart, which results in decreased cardiac output and increased intracardiac pressure at rest and/or during physical activity [1,2,4].

Despite varied pathogenesis (cardiac disease, pre- and post-inflammatory stress disorder, and heart arrhythmia), HF leads to impaired supply of oxygen to the body tissues depending on the current metabolic demand [1,2,4]. Importantly, many patients with HF have a history of myocardial infarction or revascularization [3].

Studies on HF indicate that an important role in its pathogenesis is played by oxidative stress [5–7]. This process creates an imbalance between the production of reactive oxygen species (ROS) and antioxidative defense, which leads to oxidative damage to proteins, lipids, and nucleic acids, causing structural damage to cells as well as disturbances in tissue integrity [8]. Indeed, the role of oxidative stress has been confirmed in the course of: Endothelial dysfunction, interstitial fibrosis of the heart, cardiomyocyte hypertrophy, and heart extracellular matrix remodeling [5,7,9,10]. Moreover, it has been demonstrated that in the early stages of HF, increased activity of antioxidant enzymes is the basic compensatory mechanism aimed at maintaining adequate blood flow and perfusion of tissues. However, HF progression leads to the depletion of antioxidant reserves and, along with increased free radical production, contributes to further progression of the disease [5,7,9,10].

Increasing attention is being paid to the use of saliva in biomedical diagnostics [11]. Unlike other bioliquids, saliva is a non-infectious laboratory material collected in a manner that is non-invasive, inexpensive, and stress-free for the patient. It is also worth noting that the composition of saliva reflects dynamic changes in the body, which makes this fluid an excellent tool for determining clinically useful biomarkers [12–15]. Salivary redox biomarkers are used in the diagnosis of diseases of affluence (obesity, insulin resistance, diabetes, chronic kidney disease) [16–18], neurodegenerative diseases (Alzheimer's disease, Parkinson's disease, dementia) [19,20], or cancer (colorectal, breast, ovarian cancer) [21,22]. However, salivary redox homeostasis has not been evaluated yet in patients with chronic heart failure. Considering that oxidative stress plays a key role in HF pathogenesis [5–7], secretory dysfunction of salivary glands may also occur in HF patients, similarly to other diseases with proven etiology of oxidative stress. Indeed, a relationship between oxidative stress and impaired salivary gland function has been demonstrated in obesity [23,24], insulin resistance [25,26], type 1 diabetes [27], and psoriasis [28]. Therefore, it is necessary to assess the salivary redox parameters in patients with HF, as well as the secretory function of the salivary glands. Because redox homeostasis cannot be characterized by a single biomarker, the aim of our work was to compare the rate of ROS production, enzymatic and non-enzymatic antioxidant barriers, and oxidative damage to proteins and lipids in non-stimulated and stimulated saliva, as well as plasma/erythrocytes of patients with chronic heart failure and healthy controls.

2. Materials and Methods

2.1. Ethical Issues

The study was approved by the Bioethics Committee of the Medical University of Bialystok, Poland (permission number R-I-002/75/2016). After a detailed explanation of the purpose of the study and presentation of possible risks, all persons involved agreed in writing to participate in the experiment.

2.2. Patients

The study group consisted of 50 patients (7 women and 43 men) treated in the Department of Cardiology with Intensive Cardiac Supervision of the Medical University of Bialystok Clinical Hospital from May 2018 to April 2019. In all patients, medical history, physical examination, resting ECG, echocardiography, chest X-ray as well as blood laboratory tests (blood count, electrolytes, glucose, hepatic and renal indicators, thyroid hormones, vitamin D, NT-proBNP, and BNP) were performed. The study included hemodynamically stable patients with chronic heart failure, qualified for the implantation of automatic cardioverter defibrillator [3]. The criterion of classification for the procedure was left ventricular ejection fraction (LVEF) ≤ 35%. Based on the classification of heart failure according to the New York Heart Association [3], the study group was divided into two subgroups of patients:

- NYHA II (n = 33)—patients with slight physical activity limitations—with no symptoms at rest, but in whom normal activity causes fatigue, palpitations, or shortness of breath;
- NYHA III (n = 17)—patients with significant physical activity limitations—with no symptoms at rest, but in whom activity lower than normal provokes symptoms.

All patients were qualified for examinations by the same experienced cardiologist (M. K.), based on the inclusion and exclusion criteria. In the study group, primary prevention has been applied to reduce the risk of sudden death and total mortality in patients with symptomatic HF (NYHA class II-III) and LVEF ≤ 35% (despite at least 3 months of optimal pharmacotherapy), who are expected to survive in good condition for more than one year, and have ischemic heart disease or dilated cardiomyopathy [3]. After classification for the study, all patients underwent coronary angiography (before the cardioverter implantation procedure).

The control group, matched to the study group by gender and age, consisted of 50 generally healthy patients (7 women and 43 men), enrolled for follow-up visits at the Restorative Dentistry Clinic of the Specialist Dental Infirmary of the Medical University of Bialystok from September 2018 to June 2019.

Only patients with a body mass index (BMI) within the range of 18.5–24.5 were qualified to both the study and control group. The exclusion criterion in both groups was the occurrence of chronic systemic and autoimmune diseases (type 1 diabetes, Sjogren's syndrome, rheumatoid arthritis, psoriasis), lung, thyroid, liver, kidney, gastrointestinal tract diseases, infectious diseases (HCV, HBV and HIV infections), and immunity disorders. Moreover, the study did not allow patients with periodontal diseases, smokers, alcohol drinkers, or patients taking antibiotics, non-steroidal anti-inflammatory drugs, glucocorticosteroids, vitamins, and dietary supplements for the last 3 months. Detailed patient characteristics are presented in Table 1.

Table 1. Clinical characteristics of chronic heart failure (HF) patients and the control group.

Patient Characteristics		Control n = 50	NYHA II n = 33	NYHA III n = 17	ANOVA p
Gender	Male n (%)	43 (86)	29 (87.88)	14 (82.35)	NA
	Female n (%)	7 (14)	4 (12.12)	3 (17.65)	NA
Age		67.57 ± 1.11	64.2 ± 1.69	69.35 ± 2.57	0.069
WBC ($\times 10^3/\mu L$)		7.4 ± 0.16	7.25 ± 0.32	8.25 ± 0.46	0.068
RBC ($\times 10^6/\mu L$)		4.5 ± 0.06	4.72 ± 0.30	4.41 ± 0.13	0.573
HGB (g/dL)		14.07 ± 0.36	13.41 ± 0.27	13.4 ± 0.34	0.494
HCT (%)		39 ± 0.43	39.77 ± 0.78	39.04 ± 0.99	0.552
MCV (fL)		91.2 ± 0.60	90.97 ± 1.15	88.86 ± 1.37	0.373
MCH (pg)		33.62 ± 0.34	30.73 ± 0.50	29.69 ± 0.56 *	<0.001
MCHC (g/dL)		34.5 ± 0.36	33.75 ± 0.96	33.39 ± 0.56	0.059
RDW-SD (fL)		45.54 ± 0.16	46.56 ± 0.94	47.52 ± 0.95	0.091
RDV-CV (%)		14.9 ± 0.19	13.99 ± 0.27	14.71 ± 0.44	0.066
PLT ($\times 10^3/\mu L$)		249 ± 1.79	187.4 ± 7.84 *	203.7 ± 15.44	<0.001
CRP (mg/L)		2.9 ± 0.2	3.2 ± 0.64	3.5 ± 0.85	0.308
Na^+ (mmol/L)		139.2 ± 0.62	138.5 ± 0.45	136.6 ± 0.85	0.229
K^+ (mmol/L)		4.2 ± 0.1	4.67 ± 0.10	4.74 ± 0.14	0.06
Creatinine (mg/dL)		0.9 ± 0.02	1.07 ± 0.06	1.32 ± 0.06	0.051

Table 1. Cont.

Patient Characteristics		Control $n = 50$	NYHA II $n = 33$	NYHA III $n = 17$	ANOVA p
GFR (ml/min)		86.03 ± 2.44	82.92 ± 0.59	72.33 ± 0.79	0.057
TSH (μIU/mL)		1.08 ± 0.03	1.03 ± 0.13	1.38 ± 0.30	0.06
FT3 (pg/mL)		2.31 ± 0.06	2.42 ± 0.11	2.29 ± 0.10	0.315
Vit. D_3 (ng/mL)		24.3 ± 0.69	18.16 ± 1.41 *	15.07 ± 2.17 *	<0.001
AST (IU/L)		20.04 ± 0.87	23.46 ± 1.36	23.8 ± 1.83	0.06
Glucose (mg/dL)		91.5 ± 2.5	99.96 ± 3.83	99.8 ± 2.35	0.08
NT-proBNP (pg/mL)		ND	1831 ± 173	4128 ± 382	<0.001 #
EF		ND	25.9 ± 1.24	19.24 ± 1.31	0.001 #
RR (mmHg)	SBP	125.3 ± 0.33	130.6 ± 3.81	123.2 ± 3.67	0.112
	DBP	71.3 ± 0.61	75.97 ± 2.16	74.94 ± 1.99	0.06
HR		ND	70.97 ± 2.20	75.94 ± 2.59	NA
Type 2 diabetes n (%)		6 (12)	2 (11.76)	4 (23.53)	NA
Cardiac dysrhythmia (atrial flutter and fibrillation) n (%)		-	10 (30.30)	10 (58.82)	NA
Coronary artery disease n (%)		-	14 (42.42)	6 (35.29)	NA
Hypercholesterolemia n (%)		-	22 (66.67)	13 (76.47)	NA
Myocardial infarction n (%)		-	5 (15.15)	1 (5.88)	NA
Hypertension n (%)		17 (34)	26 (78.79)	12 (70.59)	NA
Medications	ASA n (%)	4 (8)	16 (48.48)	6 (35.29)	NA
	Alpha receptor blocker n (%)	-	3 (9.09)	2 (11.76)	NA
	Beta receptor blocker n (%)	6 (12)	26 (78.79)	15 (88.24)	NA
	Ca^{2+} channel blocker n (%)	4 (8)	9 (27.27)	6 (35.29)	NA
	AT1- receptor blocker n (%)	-	7 (21.21)	8 (47.1)	NA
	Diuretics n (%)	10 (20)	27 (81.82)	17 (100)	NA
	ACE n (%)	7 (14)	19 (57.58)	9 (52.94)	NA
	Cardiac glycosides n (%)	-	4 (12.12)	2 (11.76)	NA
	Organic nitrate n (%)	-	1 (3.03)	0 (0)	NA
	Statins n (%)	8 (16)	19 (57.58)	9 (52.94)	NA

Abbreviations: ACE—angiotensyn converting enzyme; ALT—alanine transferase; ASA—acetylsalicylic acid; AST—aspartate aminotransferase; CRP—c-reactive protein; DBP—diastolic blood pressure; EF—ejection fraction; FT3—free fraction of triiodothyronine; FT4—free fraction of thyroxine; GFR—glomerular filtration rate; HCT—hematocrit; HGB—hemoglobin concentration; HR—heart rate; K—potassium; MCH—mean corpuscular hemoglobin; MCHC—mean corpuscular hemoglobin concentration MCV—mean corpuscular volume; MPV—mean platelet volume; Na—sodium; NT-proBNP—N-terminal fragment of prohormone B-type natriuretic peptide; NWS—non-stimulated whole saliva; NYHA II—class II in the New York Heart Association (NYHA) classification of the heart failure; NYHA III—class III in the New York Heart Association (NYHA) classification of the heart failure; PCT—procalcitonin; PDW—platelet distribution width; P-LCR—platelet large cell ratio; PLT – platelets; RBC – red blood cells; RDW-CV – red cell distribution width, coefficient of variation; RDW-SD—red cell distribution width, standard deviation; RR—blood pressure; SBP—systolic blood pressure; TSH—thyroid stimulating hormone; WBC—white blood cells. * $p < 0.05$ vs. the control group (Tukey's test); # $p < 0.05$ vs. NYHA II (Student's t-test).

2.3. Research Material

The research material consisted of venous blood as well as non-stimulated whole saliva (NWS) and stimulated whole saliva (SWS) collected from patients via the spitting method. Material for all examinations was collected before implantation of an automatic cardioverter defibrillator or a resynchronization system.

2.4. Blood Collection

Upon fasting, after an overnight rest, venous blood (10 mL) was collected using S-Monovette® K3 EDTA blood collection system (Sarstedt). Blood samples were centrifuged at 1500× g (10 min, +4 °C; MPW 351, MPW Med. Instruments, Warsaw, Poland). In order for the sample to qualify for the study, it had to reveal no hemolysis. The upper layer, i.e., the plasma, was collected and erythrocytes were rinsed three times with a cold solution of 0.9% NaCl and hemolyzed by adding 9 volumes of cold 50 mM phosphate buffer with pH 7.4 (v/v) [29]. Butylated hydroxytoluene (BHT) antioxidant was added to the samples to protect them against oxidation processes (5 µL 0.5 M BHT in acetonitrile per 0.5 mL plasma/erythrocytes) [17]. The samples were stored at -80 °C (not longer than half a year).

2.5. Saliva Collection

Saliva was collected in the morning between 8 a.m. and 10 a.m. to minimize the effect of circadian rhythm on secretion. The procedure was performed in a room where patients were not disturbed, and were rested in a sitting position with the head slightly inclined downwards, with minimized facial and lip movements. After rinsing the mouth three times with distilled water at room temperature, the patients spat out the saliva accumulated at the bottom of the mouth into a sterile Falcon-type tube placed in an ice container. Saliva collected during the first minute was discarded [18,30]. Two hours prior to saliva collection, the study/control group had not consumed any food or drinks (excluding clean water) and refrained from performing oral hygiene procedures. Moreover, at least 8 h before saliva collection, the subjects had not taken any medications. The time of NWS collection was 10 min. After a 5-min break, SWS was collected for 5 min to a maximum volume of 5 mL, upon sprinkling 10 µL of 2% citric acid at the tip of the tongue every 30 s [18,30]. The collected saliva was immediately centrifuged (3000× g, 20 min, +4 °C) [17]. BHT (5 µL 0.5 M BHT in acetonitrile per 0.5 mL supernatant saliva) was added to the obtained supernatants to protect them from oxidation, and then they were frozen to −80 °C (and stored no longer than 6 months) [17].

2.6. Dental Examination

The dental examination was conducted in accordance with the World Health Organization criteria in artificial lighting, using a mirror, an explorer, and a periodontal probe [31]. Every examination was performed by the same dentist (A. K.), immediately after the non-stimulated and stimulated saliva collection. Decay, missing, filled teeth (DMFT), Papilla Bleeding Index (PBI), Gingival Index (GI), and the occurrence of carious lesions of root cement (CR) were determined. The DMFT index is the sum of teeth with caries (D), teeth extracted due to caries (M), and teeth filled because of caries (F). The PBI showed the intensity of bleeding from the gingival papilla after probing [32]. GI criteria include qualitative changes in the gingiva [33]. Inter-rater agreements were assessed in 30 patients. The reliability for all the parameters was > 0.98.

2.7. Salivary Protein

The salivary protein concentration was determined by spectrophotometric method using bicinchoninic acid (BCA) [34]. Under the influence of protein in alkaline environment, BCA forms a stable complex with Cu^+ copper ions, that reaches its maximum absorbance at 562 nm wavelength. A commercial set of reagents (Thermo Scientific PIERCE BCA Protein Assay; Rockford, USA) was used to evaluate the salivary protein.

2.8. Salivary Amylase

The salivary amylase activity (EC 3.2.1.1) was determined spectrophotometrically using an alkaline solution of 3,5-dinitrosalicylic acid (DNS). We measured the absorbance of samples at 540 nm accompanying the increase in the concentration of reducing sugars released during the hydrolysis of starch catalyzed by salivary amylase. Salivary amylase activity was determined in duplicate samples and expressed in µmol/mg protein.

2.9. Redox Assays

Antioxidant enzymes were evaluated in erythrocytes, NWS, and SWS, while non-enzymatic antioxidants were evaluated by redox status, protein/lipid oxidation products in the plasma, NWS, and SWS [17,23,29,35,36].

2.10. Antioxidant Barrier

The activity of superoxide dismutase (SOD; E.C. 1.15.1.1) was determined by the Misra and Fridrovich method [37]. The test sample was heated to 37 °C, then adrenaline solution was added, and changes in absorbance at 480 nm wavelength were monitored. It was assumed that 1 unit of SOD corresponds to 50% inhibition of adrenaline self-oxidation to adrenochrome. SOD activity was expressed in mU/mg protein.

Catalase activity (CAT; EC 1.11.1.6) was determined by the Aebi spectrophotometric method [38]. The rate of hydrogen peroxide decomposition in the presence of a blind sample was assayed by measuring the decrease in absorbance at 240 nm wavelength. We defined 1 unit of CAT as the amount of the enzyme needed to decompose 1 mmol of hydrogen peroxide per minute. CAT activity was expressed in nmol H_2O_2/min/mg protein.

The activity of salivary peroxidase (Px; EC 1.11.1.7) was determined spectrophotometrically according to the method by Mansson-Rahemtulla et al. [39]. The method involves the reduction of 5,5'-dithiobis-(2-nitrobenzoic acid) (DTNB) to 5'-thio-2-nitrobenzoic acid (TNB). Changes in the absorbance of TNB, depending on Px activity, were measured at $\lambda = 412$ nm. The activity of Px was expressed in mU/mg protein.

The activity of glutathione peroxidase (GPx; EC 1.11.1.9) in erythrocytes was determined spectrophotometrically based on reduced nicotinamide adenine dinucleotide (NADPH) conversion to nicotinamide adenine dinucleotide cation ($NADP^+$) [40]. The absorbance of the samples was measured at 340 nm wavelength. It was assumed that 1 GPx unit catalyzes the oxidation of 1 mmol NADPH per minute. The activity was expressed in mU/mg protein.

The concentration of reduced glutathione (GSH) was determined spectrophotometrically based on the reduction of DTNB to 2-nitro-5-mercaptobenzoic acid under the influence of GSH contained in the tested sample [41]. Absorbance of the samples was measured at 412 nm. The GSH concentration was calculated from the standard curve for GSH solutions and presented as µg/mg protein.

Uric acid (UA) concentration was determined spectrophotometrically using the ability of 2,4,6-tris(2-pyridyl)-s-triazine to form a blue complex with iron ions in the presence of UA. Absorbance of the samples was measured at 490 nm. We used a commercial set of reagents (QuantiChromTMUric Acid Assay Kit DIUA-250; BioAssay Systems, Hayward, CA, USA). UA concentration was expressed in ng/mg protein (NWS, SWS) and µg/mg protein (plasma).

The activity of antioxidant enzymes was determined in NWS, SWS, and erythrocytes, and the concentrations of non-enzymatic antioxidants were determined in NWS, SWS, and plasma. All determinations were performed in duplicate samples, and the absorbance of the samples was measured with the Infinite M200 PRO Multimode Microplate Reader (Tecan).

2.11. Redox Status and ROS Production

Total antioxidant capacity (TAC) was determined spectrophotometrically according to Erel [42]. Changes in absorbance of $ABTS^{*+}$ (3-ethylbenzothiazoline-6-sulfonic acid radical cation) solution were measured at 660 nm. TAC was calculated from the standard curve for Trolox (6-hydroxy-2,5,7,8-tetramethylchroman-2-carboxylic acid). The intensity of $ABTS^{*+}$ color is proportional to the content of antioxidants in the tested sample. The TAC level was expressed in Trolox µmol/mg protein.

Total oxidant status (TOS) was determined spectrophotometrically according to Erel [43]. In the presence of oxidants contained in the sample, iron Fe^{2+} ions were oxidized to Fe^{3+} irons which then formed a colored complex with xylenol orange. Absorbance of the created complex was measured at the TOS level calculated from the standard curve for hydrogen peroxide and presented as nmol H_2O_2/min/mg protein.

The oxidative stress index (OSI) was calculated by dividing TOS by TAC, and expressed in % [28].

The rate of ROS production in saliva was determined by chemiluminescence immediately after saliva collection [44]. Luminol was used as an electron acceptor, and hydrogen peroxide as a positive control. Chemiluminescence of samples was measured in 96-well microplates with black bottoms. ROS production rate was expressed as nmol O_2./min/mg protein.

TAC, TOS, and OSI levels were evaluated in NWS, SWS, and blood plasma, while the rate of ROS production was determined only in saliva samples. All determinations were performed in duplicate samples (TOS in triplicate samples) and the absorbance/chemiluminescence of samples was measured with Infinite M200 PRO Multimode Microplate Reader (Tecan).

2.12. Protein and Lipid Oxidation Products

The content of advanced glycation end products (AGE) was determined spectrofluorimetrically according to Kalousová et al. [45]. The samples were diluted in 0.02 M PBS buffer (1:5, *v/v*), and fluorescence was measured at 350 nm excitation wavelength and 440 nm emission. AGE content was expressed in arbitrary fluorescence units (AFU) per mg of total protein.

The concentration of advanced oxidation protein products (AOPP) was determined spectrophotometrically according to Kalousová et al. [45]. The samples were diluted in 0.02 M PBS buffer (1:5, *v/v*) and the oxidative capacity of iodine ions was evaluated at 340 nm wavelength. The concentration was expressed in nmol/mg protein.

The concentration of malondialdehyde (MDA) was determined spectrophotometrically using thiobarbituric acid (TBA) [46]. The absorbance of the samples was measured at 535 nm, and 1,1,3,3-tetraethoxypropane was used as a standard. The concentration was expressed in µmol/mg protein.

The content of oxidative products of protein and lipid modifications was determined in NWS, SWS, and blood plasma. All assays were performed in duplicate samples and the absorbance/fluorescence of the samples was measured with Infinite M200 PRO Multimode Microplate Reader (Tecan).

2.13. Statistical Analysis

Statistical analysis of the results was performed using GraphPad Prism 7.0 for MacOS (GraphPad Software, La Jolla, USA). The D'Agostino-Pearson test and Shapiro–Wilk test were used to evaluate the distribution of the results. The homogeneity of variance was checked by Levine's test. The groups were compared using ANOVA analysis of variance and the Tukey's test, and where no distribution normality was obtained, ANOVA Kruskal–Wallis and Dunn's tests were used. Multiplicity adjusted *p* value was also calculated. Since most of the data showed a normal distribution, the results were presented as mean ± SEM. Correlations between redox biomarkers were assessed based on the Pearson correlation coefficient. The analysis of diagnostic usefulness of redox biomarkers was assessed by receiver operating characteristic (ROC) analysis. Statistically significant value was $p \leq 0.05$.

The number of patients was determined based on the previous pilot study, and the power of the test was assumed as 0.9.

3. Results

3.1. Dental Examination and Salivary Gland Function

The secretory activity of salivary glands was analyzed based on salivary flow rate and evaluation of total protein concentration as well as α-amylase activity in saliva. We observed a significantly lower flow of NWS and SWS in patients with NYHA II and NYHA III compared to the controls (in all cases

$p < 0.001$). The total protein content was considerably lower only in NWS in patients from both groups compared to the control group ($p = 0.04$, $p < 0.001$, respectively). The salivary amylase activity was considerably lower in NWS of NYHA II and NYHA III patients ($p < 0.001$, $p = 0.009$, respectively) and SWS of NYHA II patients ($p = 0.02$) compared to the controls. However, no significant differences in oral hygiene as well as gum and periodontal condition (DMFT, PBI, GI, and CR) were found in the study group compared to the controls (Table 2).

Table 2. Salivary gland function and stomatological characteristics of HF patients and control subjects.

Patient Characteristics	Control $n = 50$	NYHA II $n = 33$	NYHA III $n = 17$	ANOVA p
NWS flow rate (mL/min)	0.38 ± 0.01	0.27 ± 0.02 *	0.25 ± 0.02 *	<0.001
SWS flow rate (mL/min)	1.28 ± 0.02	0.79 ± 0.07 *	0.76 ± 0.07 *	<0.001
NWS total protein (μg/mL)	1352 ± 62.73	1094 ± 63.84 *	8865 ± 67.08 *	<0.001
SWS total protein (μg/mL)	1014 ± 57.36	1023 ± 56.12	1309 ± 142.8	0.09
Salivary amylase NWS (μmol/mg protein)	0.2 ± 0.01	0.08 ± 0.01 *	0.13 ± 0.01 *	<0.001
Salivary amylase SWS (μmol/mg protein)	0.27 ± 0.02	0.17 ± 0.01 *	0.18 ± 0.01	0.01
DMFT	29.32 ± 0.53	29.96 ± 0.89	30.09 ± 0.69	NS
PBI	2.09 ± 0.07	2.12 ± 0.27	2.07 ± 0.24	0.92
GI	2.05 ± 0.06	2.06 ± 0.15	2.18 ± 0.14	0.71
CR	0.78 ± 0.73	0.63 ± 0.1	0.7 ± 0.48	0.91

Abbreviations: CR—root caries; DMFT—decayed, missing, filled teeth index; GI—gingival index; n—number of patients; NWS—non-stimulated saliva; NYHA II—class II in the New York Heart Association (NYHA) classification of the heart failure; NYHA III—class III in the New York Heart Association (NYHA) classification of the heart failure; PBI—papilla bleeding index; SWS—stimulated saliva. * $p < 0.05$ vs. the control group.

3.2. Salivary Antioxidants

The antioxidant barrier was evaluated by measuring the activity of antioxidant enzymes (SOD, CAT, Px, GPx) as well as the concentration of non-enzymatic antioxidants (GSH, UA). In NWS, the activity of SOD ($p < 0.001$, $p = 0.009$, respectively), CAT (in both cases $p < 0.001$), and UA ($p = 0.03$, $p < 0.001$, respectively) was significantly higher, while GSH content (in both cases $p < 0.001$) was lower in NYHA II and NYHA III groups compared to the control group. The activity of Px ($p = 0.02$) was considerably lower in NWS of NYHA II patients than in healthy controls. Within the study group, only the concentration of UA was statistically significantly higher in NWS of NYHA II group compared to NYHA III ($p = 0.02$).

In SWS, the activity of SOD ($p < 0.001$ in both groups) and UA ($p < 0.001$ in both cases) was statistically significantly higher in NYHA II and NYHA III patients compared to the control group. On the other hand, GSH concentration was statistically considerably lower in patients with NYHA II and NYHA III compared to the controls ($p < 0.001$ in both cases), similarly to NWS (Figure 1).

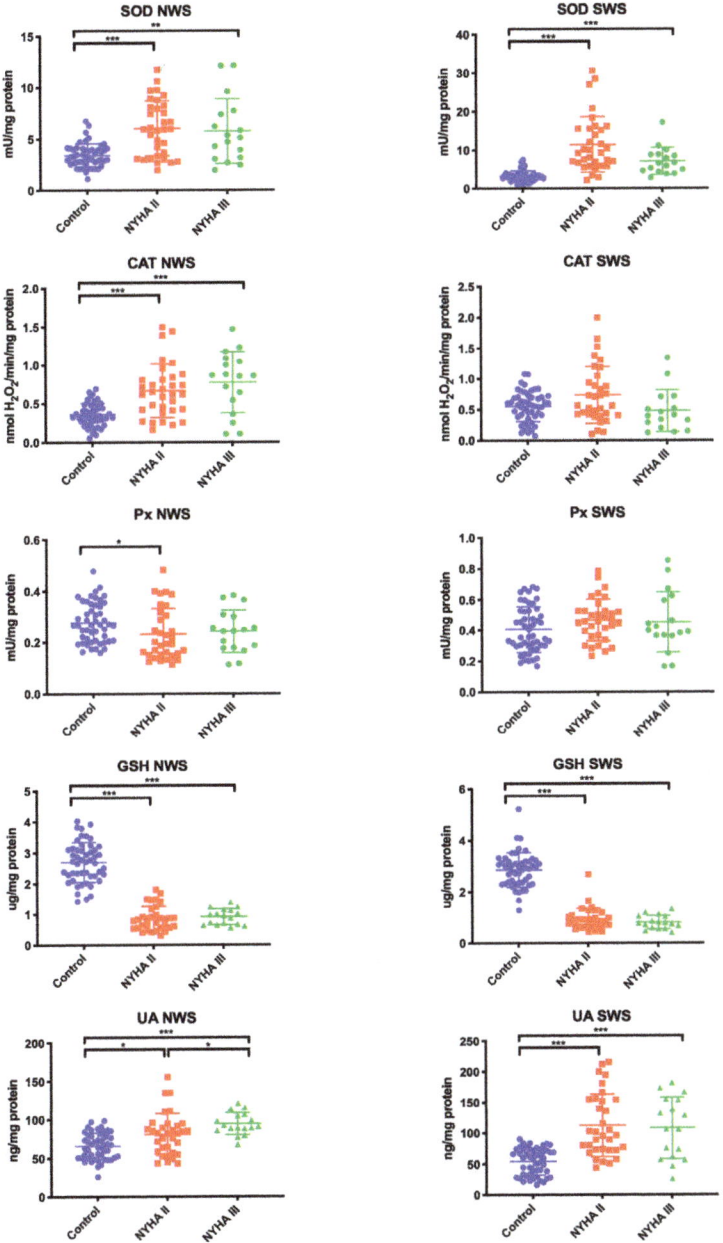

Figure 1. Enzymatic and non-enzymatic antioxidants in non-stimulated and stimulated of HF patients and the control group. Abbreviations: CAT—catalase; GPx—glutathione peroxidase; GSH—reduced glutathione; NWS—non-stimulated whole saliva; NYHA II—class II in the New York Heart Association (NYHA) classification of the heart failure; NYHA III—class III in the New York Heart Association (NYHA) classification of the heart failure; Px—salivary peroxidase; SOD—superoxide dismutase-1; SWS—stimulated whole saliva; UA—uric acid. Differences statistically important at: p *< 0.05, **< 0.01, ***< 0.001.

3.3. Salivary Total Antioxidant/Oxidant Status

The total redox status was assessed by measuring TAC, TOS, and OSI (TAC/TOS ratio), while the rate of ROS production in saliva was determined by chemiluminescence. In NWS, the mean value of TOS, OSI, and ROS was statistically significantly higher in patients with NYHA II and NYHA III compared to the control group, and in case of ROS—also within the study group (higher in NYHA III). TAC determinations revealed that the values in patients from both study groups were considerably lower than in the control group (in all cases $p < 0.001$).

In SWS, the mean value of TOS, OSI, and ROS was significantly higher in patients with NYHA II and NYHA III compared to the control group, while the mean value of TAC was lower (in all cases $p < 0.001$) (Figure 2).

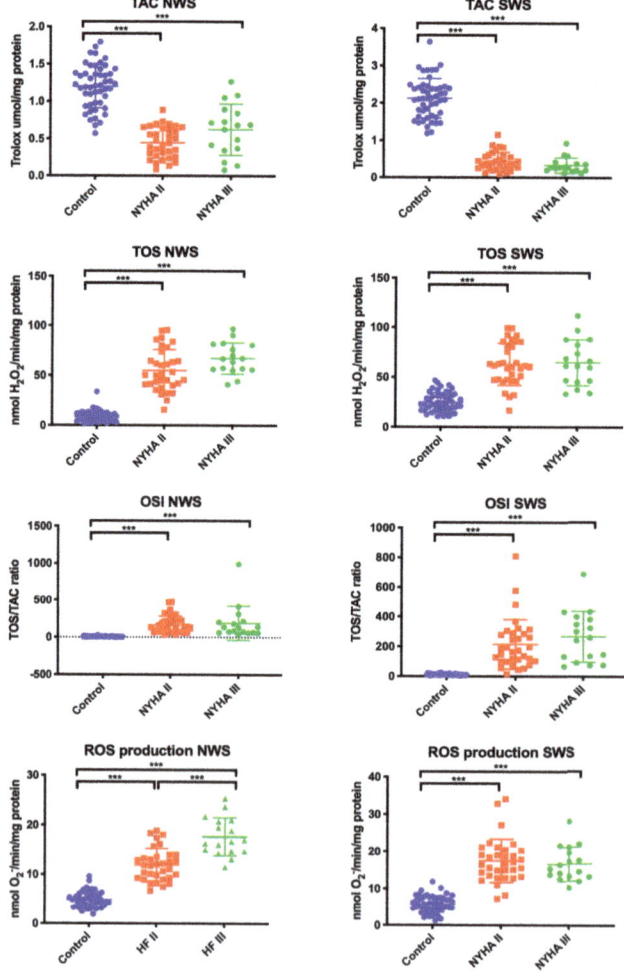

Figure 2. Total antioxidant/oxidant status in non-stimulated and stimulated saliva of HF patients and the control group. Abbreviations: NWS—non-stimulated whole saliva; NYHA II—class II in the New York Heart Association (NYHA) classification of the heart failure; NYHA III—class III in the New York Heart Association (NYHA) classification of the heart failure; OSI—oxidative stress index; SWS—stimulated whole saliva; TAC—total antioxidant capacity; TOS—total oxidant status. Differences statistically important at: p **< 0.01, ***< 0.001.

3.4. Salivary Oxidative Damage Products

Oxidative stress was assessed by measuring the oxidative damage to proteins (AGE, AOPP) and lipids (MDA). We observed a significant increase in AGE, AOPP, and MDA concentrations in patients with NYHA II and NYHA III in comparison with the control group (in all cases $p < 0.001$) and within the study group ($p = 0.04$, $p = 0.03$, $p = 0.02$, respectively).

In SWS, levels of AGE and MDA were considerably higher in NYHA II and NYHA III patients compared to healthy controls ($p < 0.001$, $p < 0.001$, $p < 0.001$, $p = 0.05$, respectively). AOPP concentration was statistically significantly higher in patients with NYHA III compared to the control group ($p < 0.001$), and in patients with NYHA III compared to those with NYHA II ($p < 0.001$) (Figure 3).

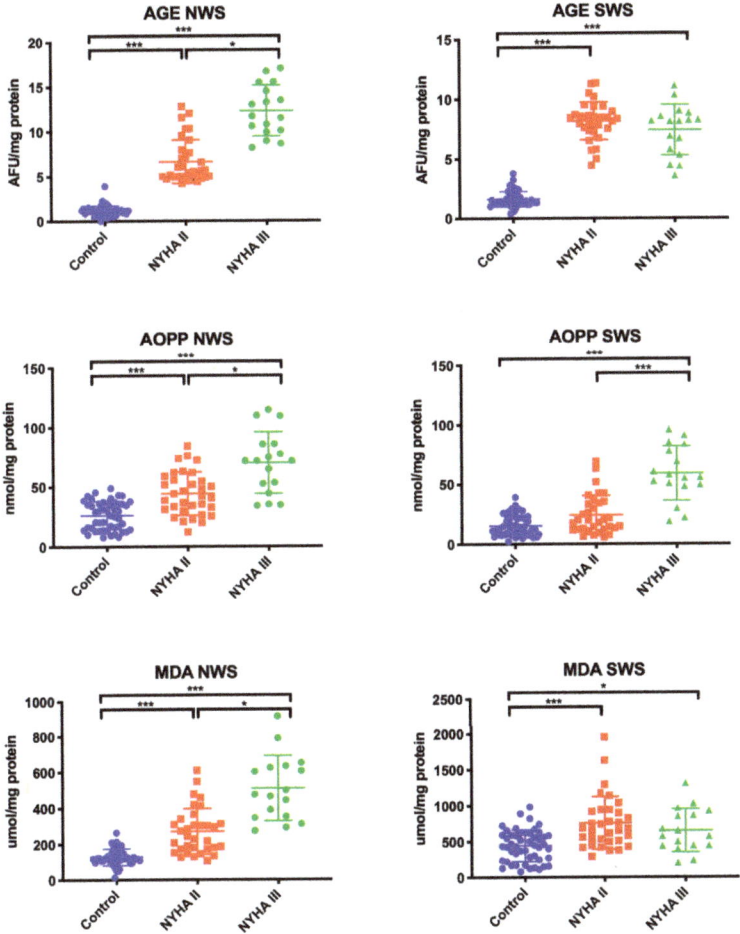

Figure 3. Oxidative damage to proteins and lipids in non-stimulated and stimulated saliva of HF patients and the control group. Abbreviations: AGE—advanced glycation end products; AOPP—advanced oxidation protein products; MDA—malondialdehyde; NWS—non-stimulated whole saliva; NYHA II—class II in the New York Heart Association (NYHA) classification of the heart failure; NYHA III—class III in the New York Heart Association (NYHA) classification of the heart failure; SWS—stimulated whole saliva. Differences statistically important at: p *< 0.05, ***< 0.001.

3.5. Erythrocytes/Plasma Redox Biomarkers

Antioxidant barrier (**A**), redox status (**B**), and oxidative damage to proteins and lipids (**C**) in the erythrocytes/plasma of HF patients and the control group are presented in Figure 4.

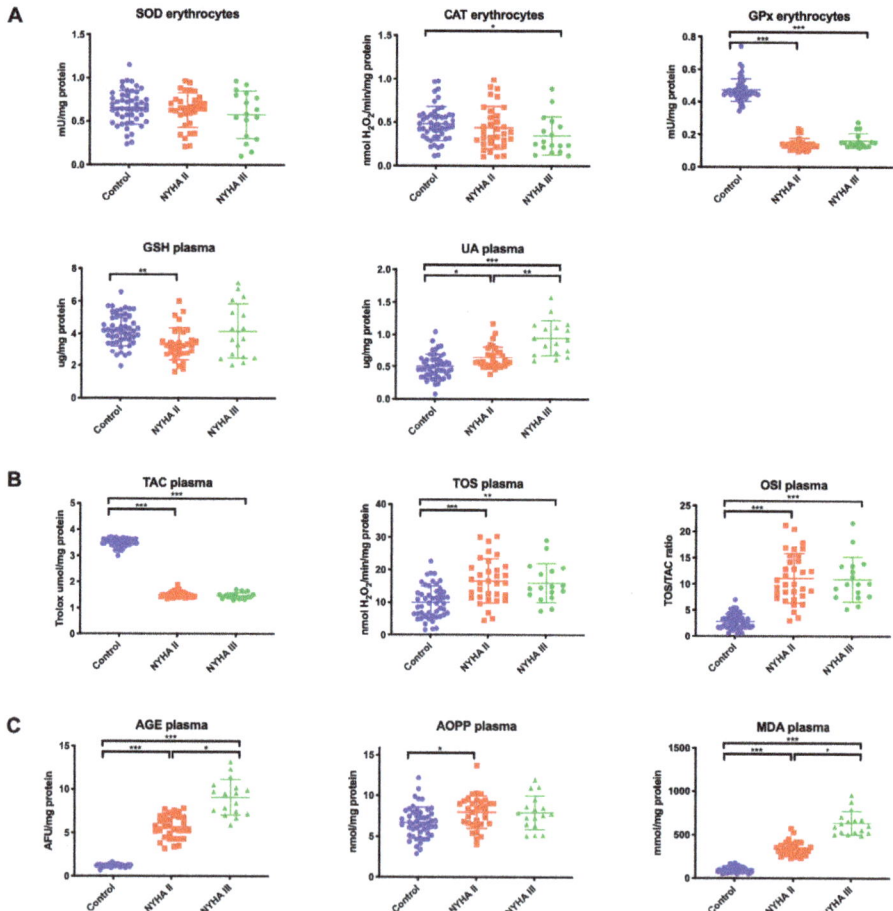

Figure 4. Antioxidant barrier (**A**), redox status (**B**), and oxidative damage to proteins and lipids (**C**) in the erythrocytes/plasma of HF patients and the control group. Abbreviations: AGE—advanced glycation end products; AOPP—advanced oxidation protein products; CAT—catalase; GPx—glutathione peroxidase; GSH—reduced glutathione; MDA—malondialdehyde; NYHA II—class II in the New York Heart Association (NYHA) classification of the heart failure; NYHA III—class III in the New York Heart Association (NYHA) classification of the heart failure; OSI—oxidative stress index; Px—salivary peroxidase; SOD—superoxide dismutase-1; TAC—total antioxidant capacity; TOS—total oxidant status; UA—uric acid. Differences statistically important at: p *< 0.05, ***< 0.001.

GPx activity ($p < 0.001$ in both study groups) in erythrocytes was significantly lower in patients with NYHA II and NYHA III compared to the control group, whereas CAT activity ($p = 0.03$) in erythrocytes was lower only in NYHA III patients, and GSH concentration ($p = 0.002$) in plasma—only in NYHA II patients. UA concentration was considerably higher both in NYHA II and NYHA III patients compared to the control and within the study group ($p = 0.02$, $p < 0.001$, $p = 0.003$, respectively) (Figure 4A).

TOS and OSI in plasma of NYHA II and NYHA III patients reached statistically significantly higher levels compared to the control group, while the level of TAC was lower (in all cases $p < 0.001$) (Figure 4B).

The plasma concentrations of AGE and MDA were considerably higher in patients with NYHA II and NYHA III than in the control group ($p < 0.001$, $p < 0.001$, $p < 0.001$, $p = 0.02$, respectively) and in patients with NYHA III compared to NYHA II ($p = 0.04$, $p = 0.02$, respectively). The content of AOPP was statistically significantly higher in NYHA II patients compared to the control group ($p = 0.01$) (Figure 4C).

3.6. Correlations

In the group of patients with chronic heart failure, we showed a positive correlation between SOD activity in saliva (both NWS and SWS) and ROS production rate ($r = 0.825$, $p < 0.0001$ and $r = 0.864$, $p < 0.0001$, respectively) and negative correlation between Px activity and ROS formation in NWS ($r = -0.836$, $p < 0.0001$). In NWS and SWS we also showed a negative correlation between GSH and AGE concentration ($r = -0.858$, $p < 0.0001$ and $r = -0.873$, $p < 0.0001$, respectively) and GSH and AOPP ($r = -0.814$, $p < 0.0001$ and $r = -0.768$, $p < 0.0001$, respectively).

We also observed a negative correlation between NWS flow rate and AGE and MDA content ($r = -0.846$, $p < 0.0001$ and $r = -0.847$, $p < 0.0001$, respectively) and a positive relationship between ROS production rate in SWS and AOPP concentration ($r = 0.892$, $p < 0.0001$). The concentration of AGE ($r = 0.84$, $p < 0.001$), AOPP ($r = 0.756$, $p < 0.001$), and MDA ($r = 0.76$, $p < 0.001$) in NWS correlated positively with their plasma content (Figure 5).

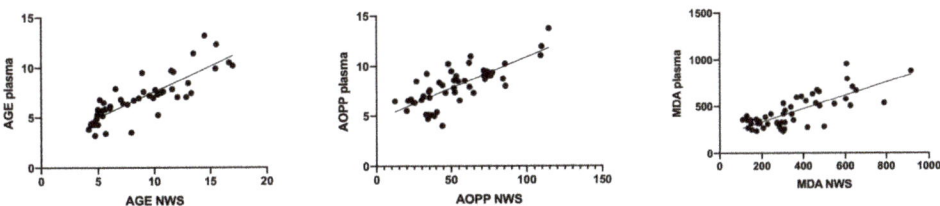

Figure 5. Correlations between salivary and plasma AGE, AOPP, and MDA in patients with heart failure. Abbreviations: AGE—advanced glycation end products; AOPP—advanced oxidation protein products; MDA—malondialdehyde; NWS—non-stimulated whole saliva.

Interestingly, we also observed positive correlation between AGE content in NWS and serum NT-proBNP ($r = 0.711$, $p < 0.0001$) and the negative relationship between the AGE content and cardiac ejection fraction ($r = -0.832$, $p < 0.0001$) (Figure 6).

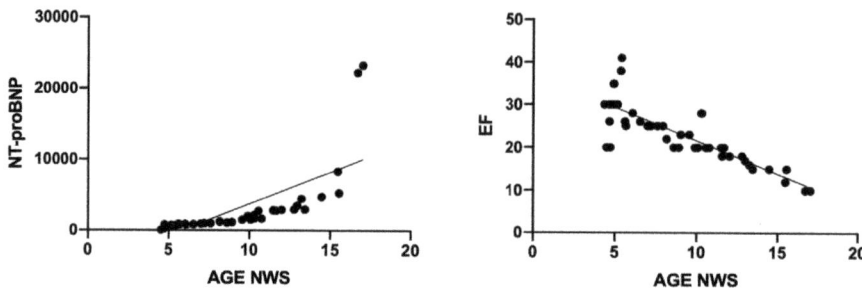

Figure 6. Correlations between salivary AGE content, serum NT-proBNP, and cardiac ejection fraction in patients with heart failure. Abbreviations: AGE—advanced glycation end products; EF—ejection fraction; NT-proBNP—N-terminal fragment of prohormone B-type natriuretic peptide; NWS—non-stimulated whole saliva.

3.7. ROC Analysis

The results of ROC analysis for redox biomarkers are presented in Table 3. UA concentration in NWS and plasma, the rate of ROS production in NWS, and the concentration of all oxidative damage products in NWS (AGE, AOPP, MDA) significantly differentiate NYHA II patients compared to NYHA III. Moreover, the assessment of AOPP concentration in SWS, as well as AGE and MDA in plasma, has a high diagnostic value in differentiating the progression of chronic heart failure (Table 3, Figure 7).

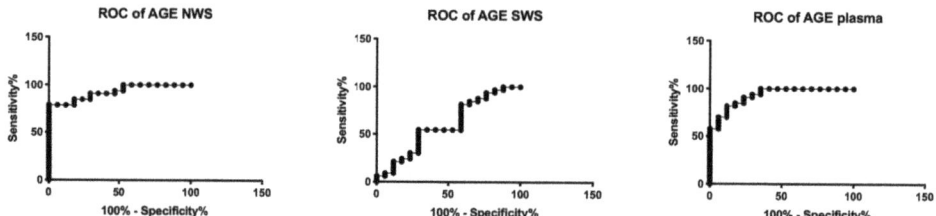

Figure 7. Receiver operating characteristic (ROC) analysis of AGE in non-stimulated and stimulated saliva as well as plasma of NYHA II and NYHA III patients. Abbreviations: AGE—advanced glycation end products; NWS—non-stimulated whole saliva; NYHA II—class II in the New York Heart Association (NYHA) classification of the heart failure; NYHA III—class III in the New York Heart Association (NYHA) classification of the heart failure; SWS—stimulated whole saliva.

Table 3. Receiver operating characteristic (ROC) analysis of oxidative stress biomarkers in non-stimulated and stimulated saliva as well as plasma/erythrocytes of NYHA II and NYHA III patients.

Parameter	NWS							SWS							Plasma/Erythrocytes					
	AUC	95% Confidence Interval	p Value	Cut-off	Sensitivity (%)	Specificity (%)		AUC	95% Confidence Interval	p Value	Cut-off	Sensitivity (%)	Specificity (%)		AUC	95% Confidence Interval	p Value	Cut-off	Sensitivity (%)	Specificity (%)
Antioxidants																				
SOD (mU/mg protein)	0.5526	0.3788 to 0.7263	0.5457	>5.616	57.58	58.82		0.6952	0.5457 to 0.8446	0.0249	>7.742	57.58	58.82		0.5544	0.3678 to 0.7409	0.5322	>0.6417	57.58	58.82
CAT (nmol H_2O_2/min/mg protein)	0.6061	0.4246 to 0.7875	0.223	<0.72	57.58	58.82		0.6894	0.5316 to 0.8472	0.033	>0.4727	63.64	62.5		0.6176	0.4517 to 0.7836	0.1765	>0.3321	57.58	58.82
Px/GPx (mU/mg protein)	0.5686	0.4024 to 0.7349	0.4304	<0.2229	57.58	58.82		0.5561	0.3737 to 0.7386	0.5189	>0.4433	57.58	58.82		0.6791	0.5257 to 0.8325	0.0396	<0.1417	63.64	64.71
GSH (ug/mg protein)	0.5918	0.4334 to 0.7502	0.2916	<0.8745	57.58	58.82		0.574	0.4062 to 0.7417	0.3954	>0.8199	57.58	58.82		0.6239	0.4368 to 0.8109	0.1546	<3.37	57.58	58.82
UA (ng/mg protein)	0.7219	0.5818 to 0.862	0.0108	<88.53	69.7	70.59		0.5152	0.34 to 0.6903	0.8618	>104.2	42.42	41.18		0.852	0.748 to 0.9561	<0.0001	<0.7263	75.76	76.47
Total antioxidant/oxidant status																				
TAC (Trolox umol/mg protein)	0.6667	0.4881 to 0.8453	0.0555	<0.5182	57.58	58.82		0.6275	0.4644 to 0.7905	0.1431	>0.3163	63.64	64.71		0.5686	0.3907 to 0.7465	0.4304	>1.475	51.52	58.82
TOS (nmol H_2O_2/min/mg protein)	0.6916	0.5459 to 0.8373	0.0277	<58.8	57.58	58.82		0.5152	0.3393 to 0.691	0.8618	<61.38	48.48	47.06		0.5205	0.354 to 0.687	0.8138	>15.14	57.58	58.82
OSI (TOS/TAC ratio)	0.5312	0.358 to 0.7044	0.72	>132.6	51.52	52.94		0.6078	0.435 to 0.7807	0.2153	<195.3	57.58	58.82		0.5116	0.3448 to 0.6784	0.8941	>10.03	51.52	52.94
ROS production (nmol O_2/min/mg protein	0.877	0.7811 to 0.9729	<0.0001	<14.49	81.82	82.35		0.5526	0.3832 to 0.7219	0.5457	>15.96	54.55	52.94		ND	ND	ND	ND	ND	ND
Oxidative damage products																				
AGE (AFU/mg protein)	0.9251	0.8565 to 0.9937	<0.0001	<9.3	81.82	82.35		0.5936	0.4192 to 0.7679	0.2823	>8.173	54.55	52.94		0.9287	0.8882 to 0.9992	<0.0001	<7.028	81.82	82.35
AOPP (nmol/mg protein)	0.7879	0.653 to 0.9228	0.0009	<52.89	69.7	70.59		0.8948	0.8039 to 0.9858	<0.0001	<38.69	81.82	82.35		0.5294	0.3548 to 0.704	0.7354	>7.937	57.58	58.82
MDA (umol/mg protein)	0.8699	0.7727 to 0.9671	<0.0001	<349.1	78.79	76.47		0.5722	0.4005 to 0.7439	0.4069	>651.3	54.55	52.94		0.9804	0.9491 to 1.012	<0.0001	<498.8	93.94	94.12

Abbreviations: AGE—advanced glycation end products; AOPP—advanced oxidation protein products; CAT—catalase; GPx—glutathione peroxidase; GSH—reduced glutathione; MDA—malondialdehyde; NWS—non-stimulated whole saliva; NYHA II—class II in the New York Heart Association (NYHA) classification of the heart failure; NYHA III—class III in the New York Heart Association (NYHA) classification of the heart failure; OSI—oxidative stress index; Px—salivary peroxidase; ROS—reactive oxygen species; SOD—superoxide dismutase; SWS—stimulated whole saliva; TAC—total antioxidant capacity; TOS—total oxidant status; UA—uric acid. Differences statistically important at: $p < 0.05$.

4. Discussion

In the presented experiment, we studied the salivary gland function as well as redox homeostasis in the saliva and blood of HF patients. Generally, the progression of HF increases oxidative stress not only at the central level (blood), but also in the NWS and SWS. Additionally, in patients with HF, there is a dysfunction of salivary glands and abnormal protein secretion to saliva. Our study was the first to characterize salivary redox profile in HF patients and evaluate the clinical usefulness of salivary biomarkers in the differential diagnosis of heart failure.

HF is a clinical disease entity of multifactorial etiology connected with hypercholesterolemia, hypertension, diabetes, smoking, unbalanced diet, and sedentary lifestyle [1,2,4]. Oxidative stress is considered both the primary and secondary cause of HF, similarly to many other systemic diseases [5–7]. Indeed, the key contribution of oxidative stress in HF has been demonstrated in the pathogenesis of genetic, neurodegenerative, neoplastic, and metabolic diseases. Therefore, redox biomarkers are gaining increasing popularity in clinical laboratory diagnostics [47–51].

Direct analysis of reactive oxygen species in the body is a very difficult task. Each of the oxidants causes specific cellular (protein/lipid) modifications. Therefore, a number of different biomarkers must be used to assess redox homeostasis [52]. In our study, we evaluated enzymatic (SOD, CAT, Px) and non-enzymatic (GSH, UA) antioxidant systems, total redox status (TAC, TOS, OSI), as well as protein (AGE, AOPP) and lipid (MDA) oxidative damage products.

An important factor influencing therapeutic success is non-invasive collection of the material for examinations, which reduces patients' anxiety and contributes to a greater desire to monitor one's health status and diagnose the disease at its early stage. An interesting alternative to blood—which is commonly used in diagnostics—is saliva. This bioliquid is produced by large salivary glands (parotid, submandibular and sublingual) as well as numerous smaller salivary glands spread throughout the oral cavity. Saliva is blood plasma filtrate, and consists of electrolytes, proteins (immunoglobulins, enzymes, mucins), hormones, and vitamins. It is also a rich source of antioxidants (Px, CAT, SOD, GSH, UA) [14,53].

Antioxidants play an important role in preventing oxidative damage to biomolecules. In the group of HF patients, we observed a significant increase in the activity of salivary antioxidant enzymes (SOD in NWS and SWS, CAT in NWS), and increased concentration of UA (in NWS, SWS, and plasma) vs. the control, which can be considered an adaptive response of the body to intensified production of free radicals. It is also confirmed by positive correlation between SOD activity in NWS and SWS and free radical production rate. It is well known that the main source of ROS in HF is the excessive activation of the renin-angiotensin-aldosterone system [5,54], which stimulates the NFkB signaling pathway and thus boosts production of proinflammatory cytokines, but also the activity of NADPH oxidase (NOX), which is the primary source of free radicals in the cell [8]. This is also evidenced by the negative correlation between Px activity in NWS and ROS production rate. Px is the only salivary enzyme produced exclusively in the salivary glands [39,55]. Thus, a decrease in Px activity may reflect the reduced activity of NWS in preventing free radical damage. Additionally, it is believed that in physiological concentrations, the main role in neutralizing hydrogen peroxide is played by Px, whereas in the conditions of ROS overproduction (extremely high levels of H_2O_2) this role is taken over by CAT [50,56]. It is therefore not surprising that we observed decreased Px activity in NWS, significantly decreased GPx activity in erythrocytes, and increased CAT activity in NWS of HF patients compared to healthy subjects.

The most important salivary antioxidant is UA, which accounts for up to 70%–80% of the antioxidant capacity of saliva [53,57]. The results of our study indicated an increased release of UA into HF patients' saliva (compared to the controls), additionally raised with the progression of the disease (significantly higher UA concentration in NYHA III group vs. NYHA II). Uric acid is formed with the participation of xanthine oxidase (XO) that transforms xanthine into hypoxanthine. The process also generates free oxygen and nitrogen radicals [58,59]. HF hypoperfusion and tissue hypoxia secondarily activate XO and are thus responsible for oxidative and nitrosative cell damage [54,60].

Interestingly, boosted XO activity increases the expression of extracellular matrix metalloproteinases, which constitutes an important factor involved in myocardial post-infarction remodeling [61,62]. These enzymes have damaging effects on the vascular endothelium, but may also disturb the remodeling of the extracellular matrix of salivary glands [63]. Thus, when in high concentrations, UA has a prooxidative effect. It was demonstrated that this compound not only generates ROS, but also produces intermediate compounds capable of alkylation of biomolecules [58,59,64]. Moreover, hyperuricemia reduces the production of nitric oxide (NO), which leads to endothelial dysfunction. It is said that oxidative stress induced by hyperuricemia is also a factor promoting the development of insulin resistance [65].

In light of the above, it is obvious that in HF patients, we observed a significant decrease in TAC (in NWS, SWS and plasma alike) compared to the control. This parameter represents the total ability to sweep free radicals [42]. Thus, decreased TAC levels suggest the exhaustion of antioxidant reserves in HF patients. However, thiol groups also have a considerable share in the antioxidant activity of saliva and blood (besides UA), which may be indirectly indicated by decreased concentration of GSH (in NWS, SWS, and plasma) in the study group.

Decreased efficiency of the antioxidant barrier increases the risk of oxidative damage to cell components. This was confirmed by raised levels of TOS and OSI, as well as significantly higher oxidative damage to proteins (↑AGE, ↑AOPP) and lipids (↑MDA) in the saliva and plasma of HF patients compared to the controls; and the negative correlation between GSH concentration in NWS as well as SWS and AGE and AOPP concentration. Interestingly, ROS production, protein glycation, and peroxidation of salivary/plasma lipids increased considerably with the progression of heart failure (higher content of AGE and MDA and increased rate of ROS production in NYHA III vs. NYHA II). This indicates the deepening of redox homeostasis disorders together with the severity/degree of disease progression.

A very common ailment in patients with HF is disturbed saliva secretion (xerostomia and hyposalivation). This was also confirmed by the results of our study. In HF patients, we observed impaired secretory function of salivary glands, as evidenced by decreased salivary secretion, significantly lower total protein content, and lowered activity of α-amylase in NWS and SWS compared to the control. A negative correlation between NWS salivary flow and AGE and MDA content, as well as a positive correlation between ROS production rate in SWS and AOPP concentration in HF patients may suggest the effect of oxidative stress on salivary gland dysfunction. It can be assumed that protein/lipid oxidation products are aggregated and accumulated in salivary glands, which—on the basis of positive feedback—boosts ROS production and leads to further oxidation of biomolecules [16,25,66]. In the end, the secretory cells of salivary glands are damaged, which is manifested by decreased production of NWS and SWS as well as disturbances in protein synthesis/secretion to saliva. Interestingly, protein oxidation products (especially AGE) also can increase the production of pro-inflammatory cytokines, which enhances damage to the salivary glands [16,25]. The impairment of salivary gland function in HF patients is evidenced not only by a decrease in salivary flow rate but also by a reduction in salivary amylase activity and total protein content. Indeed, salivary amylase is the most important salivary enzyme that has been widely recognized as a marker of salivary hypofunction [67]. Although the salivary flow rate was significantly reduced for both non-stimulated and stimulated saliva, changes in α-amylase activity as well as disturbed protein secretion to saliva were found only in NWS of HF patients. In resting conditions, 80% of saliva is secreted by submandibular glands, while in stimulation, this activity is taken over by parotid glands [29,55]. Therefore, in patients with HF, mainly submandibular dysfunction occurs. Importantly, hyposalivation can result in oral mucositis, burning of the mouth, chewing and swallowing disorders, as well as speech disorders [67]. However, the volume of saliva may also be affected by cardiovascular drugs. Medicines that reduce saliva secretion include thiazide diuretics, beta-blockers, calcium channel blockers, and ACE inhibitors [3,68].

Changes in the qualitative and quantitative composition of saliva may also predispose to dental caries and periodontal disease [67]. Therefore, patients with HF should receive an additional dental care. Nevertheless, an open question is the possibility of antioxidant supplementation to improve the condition of HF cases. Due to the high clinical relevance, this issue requires further research and observations.

An important part of our study was also the assessment of diagnostic utility of redox biomarkers. We used ROC analysis to demonstrate that numerous parameters with high sensitivity and specificity differentiate subjects with NYHA II vs. NYHA III. Particularly promising results were observed for salivary AGE (AUC = 0.93, sensitivity = 81.82%, specificity = 82.35%, NYHA II vs. NYHA III), which was additionally confirmed by a positive correlation between salivary AGE content and blood NT-proBNP concentration, as well as a negative correlation with ejection fraction. Furthermore, the AGE concentration in NWS correlated positively with their plasma content. Therefore, saliva is an alternative biological material to blood, and its collection is cheap, non-invasive, and painless. Our experiment is the first to evaluate salivary redox homeostasis in HF patients, therefore, further studies are required to evaluate the clinical value of salivary redox biomarkers in a larger group of patients.

Despite the restrictive criteria of inclusion and exclusion, our study involved elderly people diagnosed, apart from HF, with type 2 diabetes, hypercholesterolemia, or hypertension. Thus, when characterizing the redox balance of our patients, we must consider not only heart failure, but also the accompanying diseases as well as the aging process. Similarly, in human studies, the oxidative stress caused by chronic vascular disease (CVD) versus HFrEF cannot be differentiated. HF is more common in men [69–71]; however, the unequal gender distribution in our study may be due that women reach a similar HF risk as men only after the menopause [3]. In addition, we evaluated only the selected oxidative stress biomarkers, which is also a limitation of the study. The exact effect of cardiological drugs on redox parameters is also unknown.

In conclusion, in HF patients, disturbances in enzymatic and non-enzymatic antioxidant defense as well as oxidative damage to proteins and lipids occur in NWS, SWS, and plasma/erythrocytes. Redox homeostasis disorders generally worsen with HF progression, and some parameters of oxidative stress in saliva may be potential diagnostic biomarkers. In patients with HF, mainly submandibular salivary glands are affected. Due to the qualitative and quantitative changes in saliva, HF patients should be provided with additional dental care.

Author Contributions: Conceptualization, A.Z. and M.M.; Data curation, A.K. and M.M.; Formal analysis, A.K. and M.M.; Funding acquisition, A.Z. and M.M.; Investigation, A.Z. and M.M.; Methodology, A.K., A.Z. and M.M.; Project administration, A.Z. and M.M.; Resources, A.K, R.S and M.K.; Software, A.K. and R.S.; Supervision, A.Z. and M.K.; Validation, A.K and M.M.; Visualization, A.K. and M.M.; Writing – original draft, A.K. and M.M.; Writing – review & editing, A.Z. and M.M. All authors have read and agreed to the published version of the manuscript.

Funding: This research was funded by the Medical University of Bialystok, Poland (grant numbers: SUB/1/DN/20/002/1209; SUB/1/DN/20/002/3330).

Acknowledgments: The authors would like to thank Katarzyna Fejfer and Anna Skutnik for their help in collecting material for research.

Conflicts of Interest: The authors declare no conflict of interest.

References

1. Ziaeian, B.; Fonarow, G.C. Epidemiology and aetiology of heart failure. *Nat. Rev. Cardiol.* **2016**, *13*, 368–378. [CrossRef]
2. Orso, F.; Fabbri, G.; Maggioni, A. Pietro Epidemiology of heart failure. In *Handbook of Experimental Pharmacology*; Springer International Publishing AG: Berlin/Heidelberg, Germany, 2017.
3. Ponikowski, P.; Voors, A. 2016 Esc guidelines for the diagnosis and treatment of acute and chronic heart failure: The Task Force for the diagnosis and treatment of acute and chronic heart failure of the European society of cardiology (ESC): Developed with the special contribution. *Russ. J. Cardiol.* **2017**, *18*, 891–975. [CrossRef]

4. Seferovic, P.M.; Ponikowski, P.; Anker, S.D.; Bauersachs, J.; Chioncel, O.; Cleland, J.G.F.; de Boer, R.A.; Drexel, H.; Ben Gal, T.; Hill, L.; et al. Clinical practice update on heart failure 2019: Pharmacotherapy, procedures, devices and patient management. An expert consensus meeting report of the Heart Failure Association of the European Society of Cardiology. *Eur. J. Heart Fail.* **2019**, *21*, 1169–1186. [CrossRef]
5. Chen, Q.M.; Morrissy, S.; Alpert, J.S. Oxidative Stress and Heart Failure. In *Comprehensive Toxicology: Third Edition*; Elsevier Science: Amsterdam, The Netherlands, 2017; ISBN 9780081006122.
6. Bayeva, M.; Gheorghiade, M.; Ardehali, H. Mitochondria as a therapeutic target in heart failure. *J. Am. Coll. Cardiol.* **2013**, *61*, 599–610. [CrossRef]
7. Van der Pol, A.; van Gilst, W.H.; Voors, A.A.; van der Meer, P. Treating oxidative stress in heart failure: Past, present and future. *Eur. J. Heart Fail.* **2019**, *21*, 425–435. [CrossRef] [PubMed]
8. Maciejczyk, M.; Żebrowska, E.; Chabowski, A. Insulin Resistance and Oxidative Stress in the Brain: What's New? *Int. J. Mol. Sci.* **2019**, *20*, 875. [CrossRef] [PubMed]
9. Szczurek, W.; Szyguła-Jurkiewicz, B. Oxidative stress and inflammatory markers-the future of heart failure diagnostics? *Kardiochirurgia i Torakochirurgia Pol.* **2015**, *12*, 145.
10. Tsutsui, H.; Kinugawa, S.; Matsushima, S. Oxidative stress and heart failure. *Am. J. Physiol. Hear. Circ. Physiol.* **2011**, *147*, 77–81. [CrossRef] [PubMed]
11. Yoshizawa, J.M.; Schafer, C.A.; Schafer, J.J.; Farrell, J.J.; Paster, B.J.; Wong, D.T.W. Salivary biomarkers: Toward future clinical and diagnostic utilities. *Clin. Microbiol. Rev.* **2013**, *26*, 781–791. [CrossRef] [PubMed]
12. Maria, V.; Beniamino, P.; Andrea, M.; Carmen, L. Oxidative stress, plasma/salivary antioxidant status detection and health risk factors Vadalà Maria1, Palmieri Beniamino2, Malagoli Andrea3, Laurino Carmen4. *Asian J. Med. Sci.* **2017**, *8*, 32–41. [CrossRef]
13. Malathi, L.; Rajesh, E.; Aravindha Babu, N.; Jimson, S. Saliva as a diagnostic tool. *Biomed. Pharmacol. J.* **2016**, *9*. [CrossRef]
14. Javaid, M.A.; Ahmed, A.S.; Durand, R.; Tran, S.D. Saliva as a diagnostic tool for oral and systemic diseases. *J. Oral Biol. Craniofacial Res.* **2016**, *6*, 61–76. [CrossRef] [PubMed]
15. Zhang, C.Z.; Cheng, X.Q.; Li, J.Y.; Zhang, P.; Yi, P.; Xu, X.; Zhou, X.D. Saliva in the diagnosis of diseases. *Int. J. Oral Sci.* **2016**, *8*, 133–137. [CrossRef] [PubMed]
16. Zalewska, A.; Ziembicka, D.; Żendzian-Piotrowska, M.; Maciejczyk, M. The Impact of High-Fat Diet on Mitochondrial Function, Free Radical Production, and Nitrosative Stress in the Salivary Glands of Wistar Rats. *Oxid. Med. Cell. Longev.* **2019**, *2019*, 2606120. [CrossRef] [PubMed]
17. Maciejczyk, M.; Szulimowska, J.; Skutnik, A.; Taranta-Janusz, K.; Wasilewska, A.; Wiśniewska, N.; Zalewska, A. Salivary Biomarkers of Oxidative Stress in Children with Chronic Kidney Disease. *J. Clin. Med.* **2018**, *7*, 209. [CrossRef] [PubMed]
18. Świderska, M.; Maciejczyk, M.; Zalewska, A.; Pogorzelska, J.; Flisiak, R.; Chabowski, A. Oxidative stress biomarkers in the serum and plasma of patients with non-alcoholic fatty liver disease (NAFLD). Can plasma AGE be a marker of NAFLD? *Free Radic. Res.* **2019**. [CrossRef]
19. Kułak-Bejda, A.; Waszkiewicz, N.; Bejda, G.; Zalewska, A.; Maciejczyk, M. Diagnostic Value of Salivary Markers in Neuropsychiatric Disorders. *Dis. Markers* **2019**, *2019*, 1–6. [CrossRef]
20. Klimiuk, A.; Maciejczyk, M.; Choromańska, M.; Fejfer, K.; Waszkiewicz, N.; Zalewska, A. Salivary Redox Biomarkers in Different Stages of Dementia Severity. *J. Clin. Med.* **2019**, *8*, 840. [CrossRef]
21. Sawczuk, B.; Maciejczyk, M.; Sawczuk-Siemieniuk, M.; Posmyk, R.; Zalewska, A.; Car, H. Salivary Gland Function, Antioxidant Defence and Oxidative Damage in the Saliva of Patients with Breast Cancer: Does the BRCA1 Mutation Disturb the Salivary Redox Profile? *Cancers (Basel).* **2019**, *11*, 1501. [CrossRef]
22. Gornitsky, M.; Velly, A.M.; Mohit, S.; Almajed, M.; Su, H.; Panasci, L.; Schipper, H.M. Altered levels of salivary 8-oxo-7-hydrodeoxyguanosine in breast cancer. *JDR Clin. Transl. Res.* **2016**, *1*, 171–177. [CrossRef]
23. Zalewska, A.; Kossakowska, A.; Taranta-Janusz, K.; Zięba, S.; Fejfer, K.; Salamonowicz, M.; Kostecka-Sochoń, P.; Wasilewska, A.; Maciejczyk, M. Dysfunction of Salivary Glands, Disturbances in Salivary Antioxidants and Increased Oxidative Damage in Saliva of Overweight and Obese Adolescents. *J. Clin. Med.* **2020**, *9*, 548. [CrossRef] [PubMed]
24. Fejfer, K.; Buczko, P.; Niczyporuk, M.; Ładny, J.R.; Hady, H.R.; Knaś, M.; Waszkiel, D.; Klimiuk, A.; Zalewska, A.; Maciejczyk, M. Oxidative Modification of Biomolecules in the Nonstimulated and Stimulated Saliva of Patients with Morbid Obesity Treated with Bariatric Surgery. *Biomed Res. Int.* **2017**, *2017*, 4923769. [CrossRef] [PubMed]

25. Zalewska, A.; Maciejczyk, M.; Szulimowska, J.; Imierska, M.; Błachnio-Zabielska, A. High-Fat Diet Affects Ceramide Content, Disturbs Mitochondrial Redox Balance, and Induces Apoptosis in the Submandibular Glands of Mice. *Biomolecules* **2019**, *9*, 877. [CrossRef] [PubMed]
26. Kołodziej, U.; Maciejczyk, M.; Miasko, A.; Matczuk, J.; Knas, M.; Zukowski, P.; Zendzian-Piotrowska, M.; Borys, J.; Zalewska, A. Oxidative modification in the salivary glands of high fat-diet induced insulin resistant rats. *Front. Physiol.* **2017**, *8*, 20. [CrossRef]
27. Maciejczyk, M.; Kossakowska, A.; Szulimowska, J.; Klimiuk, A.; Knaś, M.; Car, H.; Niklińska, W.; Ładny, J.R.; Chabowski, A.; Zalewska, A. Lysosomal Exoglycosidase Profile and Secretory Function in the Salivary Glands of Rats with Streptozotocin-Induced Diabetes. *J. Diabetes Res.* **2017**, *2017*, 1–13. [CrossRef]
28. Skutnik-Radziszewska, A.; Maciejczyk, M.; Fejfer, K.; Krahel, J.; Flisiak, I.; Kołodziej, U.; Zalewska, A. Salivary Antioxidants and Oxidative Stress in Psoriatic Patients: Can Salivary Total Oxidant Status and Oxidative Status Index Be a Plaque Psoriasis Biomarker? *Oxid. Med. Cell. Longev.* **2020**, *2020*, 9086024. [CrossRef]
29. Maciejczyk, M.; Zalewska, A.; Ładny, J.R. Salivary Antioxidant Barrier, Redox Status, and Oxidative Damage to Proteins and Lipids in Healthy Children, Adults, and the Elderly. *Oxid. Med. Cell. Longev.* **2019**, *2019*, 1–12. [CrossRef]
30. Knaś, M.; Maciejczyk, M.; Sawicka, K.; Hady, H.R.; Niczyporuk, M.; Ładny, J.R.; Matczuk, J.; Waszkiel, D.; Żendzian-Piotrowska, M.; Zalewska, A. Impact of morbid obesity and bariatric surgery on antioxidant/oxidant balance of the unstimulated and stimulated human saliva. *J. Oral Pathol. Med.* **2016**, *45*, 455–464. [CrossRef]
31. WHO. *Oral Health Surveys—Basic Methofd*; World Health Organization: Geneva, Switzerland, 2013; p. 1.137.
32. Lobene, R.R.; Mankodi, S.M.; Ciancio, S.G.; Lamm, R.A.; Charles, C.H.; Ross, N.M. Correlations among gingival indices: A methodology study. *J Periodontol* **1989**, *60*, 159–162. [CrossRef]
33. Löe, H. The Gingival Index, the Plaque Index and the Retention Index Systems. *J. Periodontol.* **1967**, *38*, 610–616. [CrossRef]
34. Walker, J.M. The Bicinchoninic Acid (BCA) Assay for Protein Quantitation. In *The Protein Protocols Handbook*; Humana Press: Totowa, NJ, USA, 1994; pp. 5–8.
35. Maciejczyk, M.; Szulimowska, J.; Taranta-Janusz, K.; Werbel, K.; Wasilewska, A.; Zalewska, A. Salivary FRAP as A Marker of Chronic Kidney Disease Progression in Children. *Antioxidants* **2019**, *8*, 409. [CrossRef] [PubMed]
36. Borys, J.; Maciejczyk, M.; Krętowski, A.J.; Antonowicz, B.; Ratajczak-Wrona, W.; Jablonska, E.; Zaleski, P.; Waszkiel, D.; Ladny, J.R.; Zukowski, P.; et al. The redox balance in erythrocytes, plasma, and periosteum of patients with titanium fixation of the jaw. *Front. Physiol.* **2017**, *8*, 386. [CrossRef] [PubMed]
37. Misra, H.P.; Fridovich, I. The role of superoxide anion in the autoxidation of epinephrine and a simple assay for superoxide dismutase. *J. Biol. Chem.* **1972**, *247*, 3170–3175. [PubMed]
38. Aebi, H. 13Catalase in Vitro. *Methods Enzymol.* **1984**, *105*, 121–126.
39. Mansson-Rahemtulla, B.; Baldone, D.C.; Pruitt, K.M.; Rahemtulla, F. Specific assays for peroxidases in human saliva. *Arch. Oral Biol.* **1986**, *31*, 661–668. [CrossRef]
40. Paglia, D.E.; Valentine, W.N. Studies on the quantitative and qualitative characterization of erythrocyte glutathione peroxidase. *J. Lab. Clin. Med.* **1967**, *70*, 158–169.
41. Griffith, O.W. Determination of glutathione and glutathione disulfide using glutathione reductase and 2-vinylpyridine. *Anal. Biochem.* **1980**, *106*, 207–212. [CrossRef]
42. Erel, O. A novel automated direct measurement method for total antioxidant capacity using a new generation, more stable ABTS radical cation. *Clin. Biochem.* **2004**, *37*, 277–285. [CrossRef]
43. Erel, O. A new automated colorimetric method for measuring total oxidant status. *Clin. Biochem.* **2005**, *38*, 1103–1111. [CrossRef]
44. Kobayashi, H.; Gil-Guzman, E.; Mahran, A.M.; Sharma, R.K.; Nelson, D.R.; Thomas, A.J.; Agarwal, A. Quality control of reactive oxygen species measurement by luminol-dependent chemiluminescence assay. *J. Androl.* **2001**, *22*, 568–574.
45. Kalousová, M.; Skrha, J.; Zima, T. Advanced glycation end-products and advanced oxidation protein products in patients with diabetes mellitus. *Physiol. Res.* **2002**, *51*, 597–604. [PubMed]
46. Buege, J.A.; Aust, S.D. Microsomal Lipid Peroxidation. *Methods Enzymol.* **1978**, *52*, 302–310. [PubMed]

47. Tsiropoulou, S.; Dulak-Lis, M.; Montezano, A.C.; Touyz, R.M. Biomarkers of Oxidative Stress in Human Hypertension. In *Hypertension and Cardiovascular Disease*; Andreadis, E.A., Ed.; Springer International Publishing: Cham, UK, 2016; pp. 151–170. ISBN 978-3-319-39599-9.
48. Mao, P. Oxidative Stress and Its Clinical Applications in Dementia. *J. Neurodegener. Dis.* **2013**, *2013*, 319898. [CrossRef] [PubMed]
49. Peluso, I.; Raguzzini, A. Salivary and Urinary Total Antioxidant Capacity as Biomarkers of Oxidative Stress in Humans. *Patholog. Res. Int.* **2016**, *2016*, 5480267. [CrossRef] [PubMed]
50. Maciejczyk, M.; Heropolitanska-Pliszka, E.; Pietrucha, B.; Sawicka-Powierza, J.; Bernatowska, E.; Wolska-Kusnierz, B.; Pac, M.; Car, H.; Zalewska, A.; Mikoluc, B. Antioxidant Defense, Redox Homeostasis, and Oxidative Damage in Children With Ataxia Telangiectasia and Nijmegen Breakage Syndrome. *Front. Immunol.* **2019**, *10*, 2322. [CrossRef]
51. Morris, A.A.; Ko, Y.-A.; Udeshi, E.; Jones, D.P.; Butler, J.; Quyyumi, A. Novel Biomarkers of Oxidative Stress are Associated with Risk of Death and Hospitalization in Patients with Heart Failure. *J. Card. Fail.* **2018**, *24*, S21. [CrossRef]
52. Lushchak, V.I. Free radicals, reactive oxygen species, oxidative stress and its classification. *Chem Biol Interact* **2014**, *224c*, 164–175. [CrossRef]
53. Knaś, M.; Maciejczyk, M.; Waszkiel, D.; Zalewska, A. Oxidative stress and salivary antioxidants. *Dent. Med. Probl.* **2013**, *50*, 461–466.
54. Higashi, Y.; Noma, K.; Yoshizumi, M.; Kihara, Y. Endothelial function and oxidative stress in cardiovascular diseases. *Circ. J.* **2009**, *73*, 411–418. [CrossRef]
55. Żukowski, P.; Maciejczyk, M.; Waszkiel, D. Sources of free radicals and oxidative stress in the oral cavity. *Arch. Oral Biol.* **2018**, *92*, 8–17. [CrossRef]
56. Day, B.J. Catalase and glutathione peroxidase mimics. *Biochem. Pharmacol.* **2009**, *77*, 285–296. [CrossRef] [PubMed]
57. Battino, M.; Ferreiro, M.S.; Gallardo, I.; Newman, H.N.; Bullon, P. The antioxidant capacity of saliva. *J. Clin. Periodontol.* **2002**, *29*, 189–194. [CrossRef] [PubMed]
58. Glantzounis, G.; Tsimoyiannis, E.; Kappas, A.; Galaris, D. Uric Acid and Oxidative Stress. *Curr. Pharm. Des.* **2005**, *11*, 4145–4151. [CrossRef] [PubMed]
59. Sautin, Y.Y.; Johnson, R.J. Uric Acid: The Oxidant-Antioxidant Paradox. *Nucleosides, Nucleotides and Nucleic Acids* **2008**, *27*, 608–619. [CrossRef] [PubMed]
60. Hare, J.M.; Johnson, R.J. Uric acid predicts clinical outcomes in heart failure: Insights regarding the role of xanthine oxidase and uric acid in disease pathophysiology. *Circulation* **2003**, *2003*, 1951–1953. [CrossRef]
61. Cleutjens, J.P.M.; Creemers, E.E.J.M. Integration of concepts: Cardiac extracellular matrix remodeling after myocardial infarction. *J. Cardiac Fail.* **2002**, *8*, S344–S348. [CrossRef]
62. Rajagopalan, S.; Meng, X.P.; Ramasamy, S.; Harrison, D.G.; Galis, Z.S. Reactive oxygen species produced by macrophage-derived foam cells regulate the activity of vascular matrix metalloproteinases in vitro: Implications for atherosclerotic plaque stability. *J. Clin. Invest.* **1996**, *98*, 2572–2579. [CrossRef]
63. Maciejczyk, M.; Pietrzykowska, A.; Zalewska, A.; Knaś, M.; Daniszewska, I. The Significance of Matrix Metalloproteinases in Oral Diseases. *Adv. Clin. Exp. Med.* **2016**, *25*, 383–390. [CrossRef]
64. Gersch, C.; Palii, S.P.; Imaram, W.; Kim, K.M.; Karumanchi, S.A.; Angerhofer, A.; Johnson, R.J.; Henderson, G.N. Reactions of peroxynitrite with uric acid: Formation of reactive intermediates, alkylated products and triuret, and in vivo production of triuret under conditions of oxidative stress. *Nucleosides Nucleotides Nucleic Acids* **2009**, *28*, 118–149. [CrossRef]
65. Lytvyn, Y.; Perkins, B.A.; Cherney, D.Z.I. Uric Acid as a Biomarker and a Therapeutic Target in Diabetes. *Can. J. Diabetes* **2015**, *39*, 239–246. [CrossRef]
66. Maciejczyk, M.; Skutnik-Radziszewska, A.; Zieniewska, I.; Matczuk, J.; Domel, E.; Waszkiel, D.; Żendzian-Piotrowska, M.; Szarmach, I.; Zalewska, A. Antioxidant Defense, Oxidative Modification, and Salivary Gland Function in an Early Phase of Cerulein Pancreatitis. *Oxid. Med. Cell. Longev.* **2019**, *2019*, 1–14. [CrossRef] [PubMed]
67. Carpenter, G.H. The Secretion, Components, and Properties of Saliva. *Annu. Rev. Food Sci. Technol.* **2013**, *4*, 267–276. [CrossRef] [PubMed]

68. Smith, J.G.; Newton-Cheh, C.; Almgren, P.; Struck, J.; Morgenthaler, N.G.; Bergmann, A.; Platonov, P.G.; Hedblad, B.; Engstrm, G.; Wang, T.J.; et al. Assessment of conventional cardiovascular risk factors and multiple biomarkers for the prediction of incident heart failure and atrial fibrillation. *J. Am. Coll. Cardiol.* **2010**, *56*, 1712–1719. [CrossRef] [PubMed]
69. Devore, A.D.; Braunwald, E.; Morrow, D.A.; Duffy, C.I.; Ambrosy, A.P.; Chakraborty, H.; McCague, K.; Rocha, R.; Velazquez, E.J. Initiation of Angiotensin-Neprilysin Inhibition after Acute Decompensated Heart Failure: Secondary Analysis of the Open-label Extension of the PIONEER-HF Trial. *JAMA Cardiol.* **2019**, *5*, 202–207. [CrossRef]
70. Wachter, R.; Senni, M.; Belohlavek, J.; Straburzynska-Migaj, E.; Witte, K.K.; Kobalava, Z.; Fonseca, C.; Goncalvesova, E.; Cavusoglu, Y.; Fernandez, A.; et al. Initiation of sacubitril/valsartan in haemodynamically stabilised heart failure patients in hospital or early after discharge: Primary results of the randomised TRANSITION study. *Eur. J. Heart Fail.* **2019**, *21*, 998–1007. [CrossRef]
71. Greene, S.J.; Butler, J.; Albert, N.M.; DeVore, A.D.; Sharma, P.P.; Duffy, C.I.; Hill, C.L.; McCague, K.; Mi, X.; Patterson, J.H.; et al. Medical Therapy for Heart Failure With Reduced Ejection Fraction: The CHAMP-HF Registry. *J. Am. Coll. Cardiol.* **2018**, *72*, 351–366. [CrossRef]

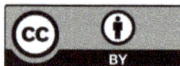
© 2020 by the authors. Licensee MDPI, Basel, Switzerland. This article is an open access article distributed under the terms and conditions of the Creative Commons Attribution (CC BY) license (http://creativecommons.org/licenses/by/4.0/).

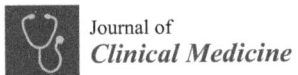 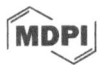

Article

Combining Novel Biomarkers for Risk Stratification of Two-Year Cardiovascular Mortality in Patients with ST-Elevation Myocardial Infarction

Naufal Zagidullin [1,2,3,4,5,*,†], Lukas J. Motloch [6,†], Diana Gareeva [1,2,3], Aysilu Hamitova [1,2,3], Irina Lakman [4,5,7], Ilja Krioni [4,5], Denis Popov [4,5], Rustem Zulkarneev [1,2,3,4,5], Vera Paar [6], Kristen Kopp [6], Peter Jirak [6], Vladimir Ishmetov [1,2,3], Uta C. Hoppe [6], Eduard Tulbaev [1,2,3] and Valentin Pavlov [1,2,3]

1. Department of Internal Diseases, Bashkir State Medical University, Lenin str., 3, 450008 Ufa, Russia; danika09@mail.ru (D.G.); musina.aisylu@mail.ru (A.H.); zurustem@mail.ru (R.Z.); ishv75@mail.ru (V.I.); tulbaev@gmail.com (E.T.); pavlov@bashgmu.ru (V.P.)
2. Department of Surgery, Bashkir State Medical University, Lenin str., 3, 450008 Ufa, Russia
3. Department of Urology, Bashkir State Medical University, Lenin str., 3, 450008 Ufa, Russia
4. Department of Electronics and Biomedical Technology, Ufa State Aviation Technical University, Karl Marx str., 12, 450077 Ufa, Russia; lackmania@mail.ru (I.L.); yogrek2@gmail.com (I.K.); popov.denis@inbox.ru (D.P.)
5. Department of Informatics and Robotics, Ufa State Aviation Technical University, Karl Marx str., 12, 450077 Ufa, Russia
6. University Clinic for Internal Medicine II, Paracelsus Medical University, Muellner Hauptstrasse 48, 5020 Salzburg, Austria; l.motloch@salk.at (L.J.M.); v.paar@salk.at (V.P.); k.kopp@salk.at (K.K.); p.jirak@salk.at (P.J.); u.hoppe@salk.at (U.C.H.)
7. Institute of Economics, Finance and Business, Bashkir State University, Validy Str. 32, 450076 Ufa, Russia
* Correspondence: znaufal@mail.ru
† These authors contributed equally to this work.

Received: 26 January 2020; Accepted: 13 February 2020; Published: 18 February 2020

Abstract: ST-elevation myocardial infarction (STEMI) is one of the main reasons for morbidity and mortality worldwide. In addition to the classic biomarker NT-proBNP, new biomarkers like ST2 and Pentraxin-3 (Ptx-3) have emerged as potential tools in stratifying risk in cardiac patients. Indeed, multimarker approaches to estimate prognosis of STEMI patients have been proposed and their potential clinical impact requires investigation. In our study, in 147 patients with STEMI, NT-proBNP as well as serum levels of ST2 and Ptx-3 were evaluated. During two-year follow-up (FU; 734.2 ± 61.2 d) results were correlated with risk for cardiovascular mortality (CV-mortality). NT-proBNP (HR = 1.64, 95% CI = 1.21–2.21, $p = 0.001$) but also ST2 (HR = 1.000022, 95% CI = 1.00–1.001, $p < 0.001$) were shown to be reliable predictors of CV-mortality, while the highest predictive power was observed with Ptx-3 (HR = 3.1, 95% CI = 1.63–5.39, $p < 0.001$). When two biomarkers were combined in a multivariate Cox regression model, relevant improvement of risk assessment was only observed with NT-proBNP+Ptx-3 (AIC = 209, BIC = 214, $p = 0.001$, MER = 0.75, MEV = 0.64). However, the highest accuracy was seen using a three-marker approach (NT-proBNP + ST2 + Ptx-3: AIC = 208, BIC = 214, $p < 0.001$, MER = 0.77, MEV = 0.66). In conclusion, after STEMI, ST2 and Ptx-3 in addition to NT-proBNP were associated with the incidence of CV-mortality, with multimarker approaches enhancing the accuracy of prediction of CV-mortality.

Keywords: myocardial infarction; STEMI; cardiovascular events; cardiovascular death; risk stratification; sST2; NT-proBNP; Pentraxin-3

1. Introduction

Despite the development of new therapeutic strategies, coronary artery disease (CAD) remains one of the main health burdens worldwide. The occurrence of ST-elevation myocardial infarction (STEMI) is especially associated with significant short- and long-term complications. Consequently, STEMI patients are at higher risk of suffering cardiovascular events (CVE), even in a long-term post-myocardial infarction (MI) period, resulting in consequent reduction of long-term survival in this population [1]. Therefore, early identification of high-risk individuals is one of the main clinical goals in daily clinical practice in these patients.

The use of biological markers has been shown to improve the accuracy of diagnosis in cardiovascular patients. Indeed, this approach promotes stratification of cardiovascular risk, both during the hospitalization period as well as in the long-term observation period. Levels of several biomarkers correlate with the severity of CVE, reflect the dynamics of disease and enhance the efficacy of therapy regimes. "Classic" biomarkers like myoglobin fraction of creatine phosphokinase (CK-MB) and Troponins correlate with the long-term outcome of STEMI patients and are integrated into daily clinical practice [1]. Indeed, high levels of N terminals pro brain natriuretic peptide (NT-proBNP) are prognostic for increased risk of sudden death, recurrence of MI or development of chronic heart failure, not only in patients with MI, but also in patients with unstable angina [2]. Nevertheless, with the exception of Troponins and especially high-sensitive Troponins (hs-Troponins), sensitivity and specificity of these biological markers of acute cardiac damage remains poor [3–6]. Therefore, additional tools are needed to promote the estimation of cardiovascular outcome.

Multimarker analytic approaches have been shown to enhance the sensitivity and specificity of prognostic assessments. Consequently, they might be a more effective tool in predicting cardiovascular mortality (CV mortality) in MI patients. "Novel" serum biomarkers like ST2 and Pentraxin-3 (Ptx-3) have recently emerged as a potentially useful tool for improving the assessment of cardiovascular disease [7–11]. Ptx-3 refers to the family of pentraxins produced locally by stromal and myeloid cells in response to proinflammatory signals. As a multifunctional protein, Ptx-3 plays an important role during vascular inflammatory processes. Consequently, it was shown to have a special role in the pathophysiology of atherosclerosis and myocardial infarction. Furthermore, it also seems to be involved in the pathology of heart failure and cardiac arrest [8]. Indeed, increased Ptx-3 levels are associated with CAD including acute coronary syndrome [7,9,12,13]. Importantly, in patients with acute coronary syndrome, elevated Ptx-3 levels were associated with a higher rate of mortality, even in long-term observational studies [14–16]. Soluble ST2 is a member of the of the interleukin 1 receptor family. Its role in cardiac pathophysiological processes including the progression of coronary atherosclerosis but also other cardiac remodeling processes was established in recent years [17]. Indeed, ST2 seems to not only participate in cardiovascular response to injury but also in myocardial remodeling processes observed in heart failure and MI [10,18]. Serum levels are associated with ischemic damage and remain high, even in the post-myocardial infarction period [19]. Consequently, serum concentrations of ST2 correlate with the outcome of MI and also heart failure patients [20–24].

Nevertheless, despite these promising results, the ability of both biomarkers to assess the outcome in MI patients still remains the matter of debate. Importantly, the question of whether combining classic biomarkers like NT-proBNP with the new biomarkers ST and Ptx-3 in a multimarker analytic approach in order to improve predictive sensitivity as well as specificity of CV mortality risk in STEMI patients remains unresolved.

Therefore, we investigated serum levels of NT-proBNP as well as ST2 and Ptx-3 in 147 STEMI patients to address this issue and evaluate mid-term cardiovascular outcome. During a two-year follow-up period (FU), initial serum concentrations were correlated with the incidence of CV mortality.

2. Methods

In this prospective, non-randomized, single-center study, we enrolled 156 consecutive patients between September 2016 and June 2017, who were hospitalized due to acute STEMI in a cardiac center of Ufa City Hospital N21 in the Russian Federation capable of performing 24/7 percutaneous catheter intervention (PCI) service. Initial diagnosis was established by twelve lead ECG at admission. ST-segment elevation was measured at the J-point at least in two contiguous leads with ST-segment elevation of 2.5 mm in men <40 years, 2 mm in men 40 years, or 1.5 mm in women in leads V2–V3 and/or 1 mm in the other leads in the absence of left ventricular hypertrophy or left bundle branch block. The diagnosis was verified during clinical FU by further ECG recordings (day two and/or day three of hospital stay), transthoracic echocardiographic (day two or day three of hospital stay), laboratory (hs-Troponin I and CK-MB at admission and during FU at day two and/or day three of hospital stay) and coronary angiography according to the 2017 ESC guidelines [1]. Dependent on the time window of STEMI diagnosis, acute coronary angiography (CAG, CAG was performed if time window estimated by primary care physician for possible primary PCI was ≤120 min) or acute thrombolysis (if time window from symptom presentation was ≤12 h and lack of contraindications for thrombolytic therapy was established by primary care physician) were performed. If patients presented with signs of failed fibrinolysis, or if there was evidence of re-occlusion or re-infarction with recurrence of ST-segment elevation indicating unsuccessful thrombolytic therapy, rescue PCI was performed as soon as possible (Table 1). Acute medical treatment, including antiplatelet regime and discharge medication after MI, were established according to the ECS guidelines (Table 1) [1]. Establishment of further relevant diagnoses was performed according to medical history, clinical findings, ECG, laboratory work up and transthoracic echocardiography.

Table 1. Characteristics of the study cohort.

Parameter	Value
n	147
Gender (male)	118 (80.3 %)
Age	60.9 ± 12.1
LVEF (%)	52.8 ± 7.2
Hx stroke (%)	5 (3.4)
Hx MI (%)	34 (23.1)
Smoker (%)	86 (58.5)
Arterial hypertension (%)	138 (93.9)
Dyslipidemia (%)	111 (75.5)
DMT2 (%)	37 (25.2)
Revascularization strategy	
Acute thrombolytic therapy (%)	35 (23.8)
Successful thrombolytic therapy (%)	17 (48.6)
Acute thrombolytic therapy followed by rescue PCI (%)	18 (51.4)
Acute PCI only (%)	112 (76.2)
Successful PCI (%)	126 (96.9)
Target vessel in acute/rescue PCA:	
LCA (%)	1 (0.7)
LAD (%)	51 (38.1)
CX (%)	12 (8.9)
RCA (%)	48 (35.8)
Multivessel approach (%)	12 (8.9)
Discharge medication	
ACE inhibitors/Angiotensin receptor blockers n (%)	143 (97.3)
Beta-blockers (%)	139 (94.6)
Diuretics (%)	51 (34.7)
Aldosterone antagonists (%)	37 (25.2)
Ivabradine (%)	12 (8.1)
Statins (%)	139 (94.6)
Acetylsalicylic acid (%)	142 (96.0)
Thienopyridines (%)	138 (93.8)
Warfarin	1 (0.7)
NOAK (%)	7 (4.8)

ACE—angiotensin converting enzymes inhibitor, CX—circumflex artery, DMT2—diabetes mellitus type 2, Hx—history of, LAD—left anterior descending artery, LCA—left main coronary artery, LVEF—left ventricle ejection fraction, NOAK—new oral anticoagulants, PCI—percutaneous coronary intervention, RCA—right coronary artery, ST2—suppression of tumorigenicity 2.

The study was performed in accordance with standards of good clinical practice and the principles of the Declaration of Helsinki. The study was approved by the Ethic committee of the Bashkir State Medical University (N1 from 23 January 2017). Prior to inclusion, all participants signed an informed consent.

The inclusion criteria were: Age > 18 years and diagnosis of STEMI according to the current guidelines (see above). The exclusion criteria were: > 48 h from start of typical symptoms of acute coronary syndrome (ACS), severe valvular dysfunction defined as severe regurgitation or stenosis of one or more of the cardiac valves, dilative cardiomyopathy, permanent atrial fibrillation and/or atrial flutter, AV block II-III according to medical history and ECG, implanted pacemaker, acute pulmonary embolism, active malignant disease defined as achieved tumor free survival under three years, severe chronic obstructive pulmonary disease (GOLD 2009 stage III-IV), uncontrolled bronchial asthma (according to Global Initiative for Asthma, GINA 2019), acute infectious diseases at the time of STEMI defined as acute pyelonephritis, community acquired pneumonia, acute bronchitis and/or flu/acute respiratory viral infection, and kidney failure defined as glomerular filtration rate (GFR) <30 mL/min1.73 m^2, as well as pregnancy or lactation.

Patient enrollment and the design of the study are presented in Figure 1. At the day of hospital admission, patients' venous blood was drawn, subsequently centrifuged and the serum was frozen for further analyses. The concentration of the biomarkers NT-proBNP, ST2 and Ptx-3 was analyzed by enzyme immunoassay as indicated by the manufacturer (for NT-porBNP: Critical diagnostics, USA, for ST2: Biomedica, Slovakia and for Ptx-3: Hycult biotech USA). In addition to the investigated biomarkers, we also evaluated the levels of hs-Troponin I and CK-MB at admission which were routinely measured to verify the diagnosis of STEMI in our center. The serum levels were investigated with the help of the electrochemiluminescence technology for immunoassay analysis as indicted by the manufacturer (Colbas e411, Roche Diagnostics, Switzerland for hs-Troponin I and CK-MB).

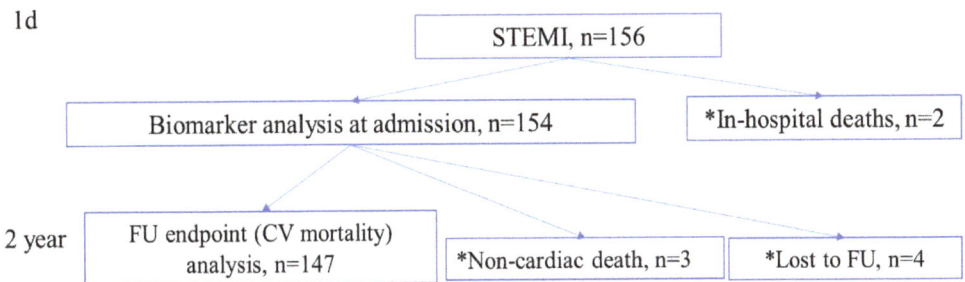

Figure 1. Patient enrollment and the design of the study. *—patients were excluded from the study. FU—follow-up, STEMI—ST-elevation myocardial infarction.

A detailed medical history was obtained at admission for all enrolled patients, including current clinical symptoms, as well as history of previous illnesses, current medications and any further relevant information. The study was carried out between September 2016 and August 2019. Follow-up analysis was conducted over two years ± four months (734.2 ± 61.2 d) from STEMI for the study endpoint with the help of the distant data approach "ProMed" program. The program in the region enables distant online monitoring of hospitalization discharge notes including death certificates. In case of absence of any notes, the patient was contacted by phone at the end of the study period to prevent loss of information due patient relocation to a region where "Promed" was not available.

The study endpoint was defined as cardiovascular mortality (termed CV mortality in this manuscript) as indicated by discharge notes and/or death certificate during the follow-up period. Patients suffering from early death during the first week of acute hospitalization for STEMI were excluded from the analysis. Furthermore, patients suffering from non-cardiovascular deaths (traumas, tumor, cancer, suicides, etc.) and patients lost to FU were also excluded. Consequently, nine patients had to be excluded from the statistical analyses. Three patients suffered from non-cardiovascular deaths during the FU (two deaths were due to trauma incidence and one patient died of cancer disease) while two patients died within one week of acute hospitalization for STEMI. Furthermore, four patients were lost to FU due to relocation and were also excluded from the analyses (Figure 1). Added together, the dropout rate was 5.8% (9/156 patients).

The mathematical model for the statistical analyses is summarized in Figure 2. The statistical analysis was carried out by our blinded statistical analytic team using SPSS software package 21 and R Studio. Data are presented as mean values (M) and standard deviation (SD) for normal distributed variables as well as interquartile range for not normal distributed variables. Mann-Whitney test was used as statistical criteria for determining differences in subgroups as having the greatest statistical power among non-parametric tests with small sample sizes. Qualitative characteristics were analyzed using the standard statistical test Chi-square. To assess cut-off points of biomarkers ROC analysis was used. Kaplan-Mayer survival curves were created after assessment of cut-off points. Log-rank and Gehan's Wilcoxon tests were applied to estimate CV-mortality and to assess the prediction ability of risk factors. To estimate the quality of multivariate proportional hazard (Cox) regression models and the prognostic ability, measure of explained randomness (MER) and measure of explained variation (MEV) were calculated. The values were estimated without nondependent variables and complete log partial likelihoods function were applied. A *p*-value <0.05 was regarded as statistically significant.

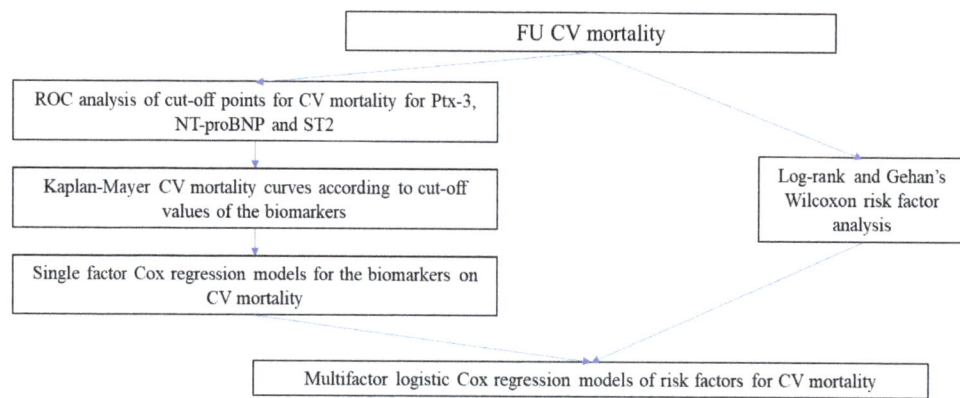

Figure 2. Mathematical model of the statistical analyses. CV mortality—cardiovascular mortality, FU—follow-up, NT-proBNP—N-terminal-pro hormone B-type natriuretic peptide, ROC—receiver operator characteristics, ST2—suppression of tumorigenicity 2.

3. Results

Table 1 presents the characteristics of the study population as well as the in-hospital treatment and discharge therapy regime. In summary, men ($n = 118$) prevailed over women ($n = 29$). Patients presented with typical comorbidities observed in the CAD population. If manageable, in-hospital treatment and discharge regime was performed according to current ECS guidelines, as indicated above [1]. 112 patients underwent primary PCI with a success rate of 97.1% (109/112), 35 patients were treated by acute thrombolytic therapy. The success rate of the thrombolytic regime was 48.6% (17/35). Consequently, in this group, 18 patients underwent rescue PCI with a successful rate of 94.4% (17/18). In summary, we observed an overall success of PCI in 126 of 130 treated patients (96.9%).

Table 2 presents the levels of routinely assessed STEMI relevant cardiac biomarkers.

Table 2. Patients' investigation data.

Parameter	Median (Q1, Q3)
n	147
CK-MB, mmol/L	100.8; (38, 175)
hs-Troponin I, ng/mL	688.4; (41, 2270)
NT-proBNP, pg/mL	518.5; (54, 2130)
ST2, ng/mL	43.8; (24.8, 56.5)
Pentraxin-3, ng/mL	131.5; (110.8, 164.3)

CK-MB—creatine kinase MB fraction, NT-proBNP—N-terminal-pro hormone B-type natriuretic peptide, ST2—suppression of tumorigenicity 2.

During a two-year FU (734.2 ± 61.2 d), CV mortality was registered in 33 (22.1%) patients. Scatter plot of the investigated biomarkers with associated survival rates are presented in Figure 3.

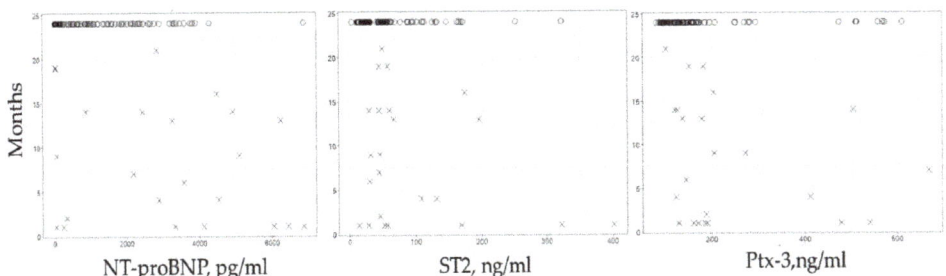

Figure 3. Scatter plots of the investigated biomarkers with associated survival rates (indicated in month) during a two-year FU after STEMI. Cases of CV mortality are indicated by a cross while cases of non-CV mortality are indicated by a circle.

The statistical analysis of the cohort was performed according to the described mathematic model. According to FU and rates of CV mortality, means of ROC analysis cut-off values for the investigated biomarkers were estimated for CV mortality (Table 3, Figure 4). Of note, log-rank and Gehan's Wilcoxon tests showed significant difference in survival functions between under and upper cut-off value for NT-proBNP (>2141 pg/mL, $\chi^2 = 24.0$, $p < 0.001$ and $\chi^2 = 23.8$, $p < 0.001$), ST2 (>27.2 ng/mL, $\chi^2 = 14.7$, $p < 0.001$ and $\chi^2 = 14.3$, $p = 0.022$) and Ptx-3 (>169 ng/mL, $\chi^2 = 7.0$, $p = 0.001$ and $\chi^2 = 7$, $p = 0.001$).

Table 3. Biomarker cut-off values for CV mortality in a two-year FU after STEMI ($p < 0.1$).

Biomarker	CV Mortality				
	Cut-Off	Sens. %	Spec. %	AUC	p-Value
Ptx-3, ng/mL	>169	68.4	82.0	0.804	0.063
NT-pro-BNP, pg/mL	>2141	73.7	80.5	0.801	0.063
ST2, ng/mL	>27.2	94.7	38.3	0.698	0.071

AUC—area under the curve, CV mortality—cardiovascular mortality, NT-proBNP—N-terminal-pro hormone B-type natriuretic peptide, Ptx-3—pentraxin 3, Sens.—sensitivity, Spec—specificity, ST2—suppression of tumorigenicity 2.

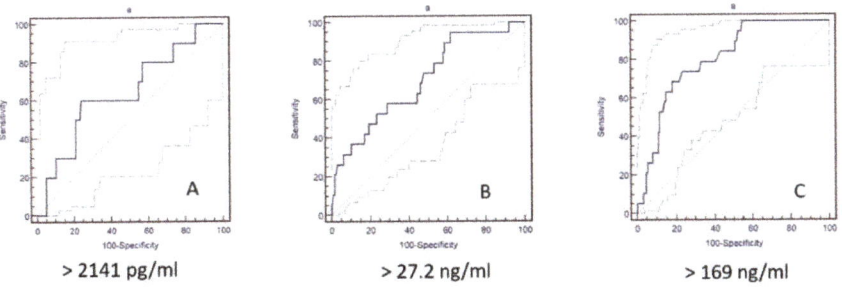

Figure 4. CV mortality cut-off values of the biomarkers NT-proBNP (**A**), ST2 (**B**) and Ptx-3 (**C**) in two-year FU after STEMI by ROC analyses.

Based on our cut-off values, the number and proportion of CV mortality/non-CV mortality (patients surviving) were evaluated (Table 4). The mean concentration of biomarkers in these subgroups are presented in Table 5.

Table 4. CV mortality/survivals according to cut-off values in a two-year FU after STEMI ($p < 0.1$).

	NT-proBNP, pg/mL		ST2, ng/mL		Ptx-3, ng/mL	
	>2141	≤2141	>27.2	≤27.2	>169.0	≤169.0
n	39	108	97	50	36	111
CV mortality, n (%)	14(35.9)	5 (4.6)	18(18.6)	1(2.0)	13(36.1)	6(5.4)
Non-CV mortality, n (%)	25(64.1)	103 (95.4)	79(81.4)	49 (98.0)	23(63.8)	105(94.6)

CV mortality—cardiovascular mortality, NT-proBNP—N-terminal-pro hormone B-type natriuretic peptide, Ptx-3—pentraxin 3, ST2—suppression of tumorigenicity 2.

Table 5. Concentration of biomarkers in CV mortality/non-CV mortality subgroups in a two-year FU after STEMI presented as mean with SD.

	n	NT-proBNP, pg/mL	ST2, ng/mL	Ptx-3, ng/mL
CV mortality	33	3019.0 ± 2270.5	93.7 ± 97.1	236.8 ± 158.5
Non-CV mortality	114	1015.8 ± 972.2	51.3 ± 47.3	158.2 ± 103.6

CV mortality—cardiovascular mortality, NT-proBNP—N-terminal-pro hormone B-type natriuretic peptide, Ptx-3—pentraxin 3.

We created Kaplan-Mayer survival curves for the incidence of CV mortality during the two-year FU comparing under and over cut-off values for the investigated biomarkers NT-ProBNP, ST2 and Ptx-3 (Figure 5). Indeed, for the incidence of CV mortality they showed prominent discrepancies in survival between under and over curve death frequency especially for the biomarker Ptx-3.

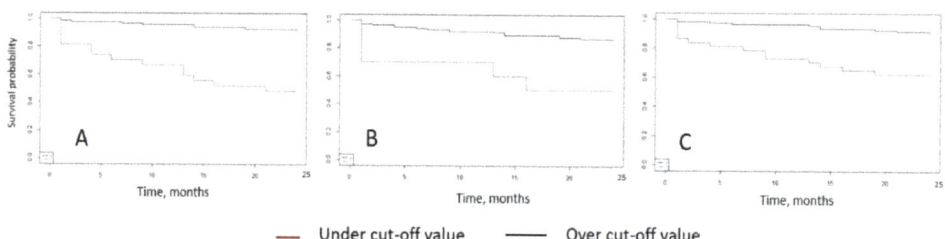

Figure 5. CV Kaplan-Mayer survival curves in two-year FU analyses under and over cut-off values for NT-pro-BNP (**A**), ST2 (**B**) and Ptx-3 (**C**).

In the next step, the endpoints of the investigated biomarkers were analyzed by univariate Cox regression. NT-pro-BNP and Ptx-3 were analyzed with linear logarithmic and ST2 in quadratic forms. Table 6 presents coefficients of univariate Cox regression for the investigated biomarkers for CV mortality. The Efron approximation of partial likelihood method was used to estimate coefficients of mortality in the Cox model. Indeed, in univariate Cox regression all investigated biomarkers (ST2, NT-proBNP and Ptx-3) were able to predict CV mortality. Of note, in this model, Ptx-3 (univariate Cox model) showed the highest hazard ratio (HR), suggesting that this biomarker may be the most accurate single marker approach for prediction of two-year mortality after STEMI.

Table 6. Univariate Cox regression for biomarkers and the incidence of CV mortality after STEMI.

Biomarker	Coefficient ± SE	Hazard Ratio	AUC	CI	p-Value
Log (NT-proBNP)	0.49 ± 0.15	1.64	0.777	1.21–2.21	0.001
$ST2^2$	0.000013 ± 0.000006	1.000022	0.800	1.00–1.001	<0.001
Log (Ptx-3)	1.12 ± 0.32	3.1	0.738	1.63–5.39	0.005

AUC—area under the curve, CI—confidential interval, NT-proBNP—N-terminal-pro hormone B-type natriuretic peptide, Ptx-3—pentraxin 3, SE—standard error, $ST2^2$—suppression of tumorigenicity 2.

Using Gehan's Wilcoxon and log-rank tests, patient characteristics (Tables 1 and 2) were analyzed to asses control variables which are associated with two-year CV mortality ($p < 0.1$; Supplemental Table S1). The following variables were shown to be associated with CV mortality during a two-year FU with $p < 0.1$: NT-proBNP, ST2, Ptx-3, age > 65 years, left ventricular ejection fraction (LVEF) < 60% on transthoracic echocardiography, male gender and high level of hs-Troponin I (Supplemental Table S1).

Biomarkers NT-proBNP, ST2 and Ptx-3 were binarized and transformed into dummy-variables, according to cut-off points, obtained above in ROC-analysis. This was done to estimate combined effects of risk factors on CV mortality in two-year FU in a relatively small amount of source data. Also, discrete variables enable more accurate interpretation of hazard ratio in the Cox model.

In the next step, the predictive power of single and multimarker approaches (different combination possibilities of NT-proBNP, ST2 and Ptx-3) were compared for CV mortality on the base of Akaike (AIC) and Schwarz (BIC) information criteria with control variables. The biomarker variables NT-proBNP, ST2 and Ptx-3 were binarized for both models. Furthermore, to confirm our results, MER and MRV values were calculated. One and two-biomarker approaches (ST + NT-proBNP, ST2 + Ptx-3 and NT-proBNP + Ptx-3) and the three-biomarker model were compared to find the most accurate combination according to the AIC and BIC information criteria as well as MER and MEV.

Table 7 presents the results of coefficients and multivariate risk by Cox model for CV mortality in the two-year FU analyses for three-/two-/one-marker models, according to AIC, BIC, MER and MEV parameters. When comparing single marker models, the application of Ptx-3 (AIC = 211, BIC = 217, $p < 0.001$, MER = 0.69, MEV = 0.56, Table 7) showed the best predictive accuracy of two-year CV mortality, as also indicated by the multivariate regression model. On the other hand, when using ST2 alone, less predictive accuracy was observed (AIC = 220, BIC = 226, $p = 0.002$, MER = 0.49, MEV = 0.39, Table 7). After adding NT-proBNP (AIC = 212, BIC = 217, $p < 0.001$, MER = 0.68, MEV = 0.57, Table 7) or Ptx-3 (AIC = 217, BIC = 222, $p < 0.001$, MER = 0.52, MEV = 0.40), the quality of the model was enhanced, when compared to the application of ST2 alone. However, only minimal improvement was achieved when these two-biomarker models were matched with the single biomarker approach using NT-proBNP or Ptx-3 alone (Table 7). Nevertheless, compared to all investigated single and two biomarker approaches, the combination of NT-proBNP and Ptx-3 (AIC = 209, BIC = 214, $p = 0.001$, MER = 0.75, MEV = 0.64) demonstrated the most powerful quality parameters, indicating this approach to be the most accurate for the prediction of two-year mortality after STEMI, when only two biomarkers are available. Of note, the most accurate combination for prediction of CV mortality after STEMI was observed with the three-biomarker model (AIC = 208, BIC = 214, $p < 0.001$, MER = 0.77, MEV = 0.66, Table 7). Consequently, our results indicate this multimarker approach using the "classic" biomarker NT-proBNP together with the "novel" biomarkers ST2 and Ptx-3 to be a promising tool for the evaluation of the risk for CV mortality during two-year FU after STEMI.

Table 7. Multivariate regression risk factors analysis for the prediction of CV mortality in two-year FU after STEMI.

Biomarker and Cut-Off Value	Coefficient ± SD	Hazard Ratio	95% CI	p-Value
ST2 (AIC = 220, BIC = 226, p = 0.002, MER = 0.49, MEV = 0.39)				
ST2 > 27.2 ng/mL	1.36 ± 0.57	3.88	1.27–11.84	0.017
Age > 65 years	1.32 ± 0.48	3.75	1.45–9.73	0.006
Male gender	0.52 ± 0.42	1.68	0.70–4.05	0.242
hs-Troponin I	0.43 ± 0.20	1.54	1.25–1.88	0.088
LVEF < 60%	−0.37 ± 0.51	0.69	0.25–1.86	0.460
Ptx-3 (AIC = 211, BIC = 217, p < 0.001, MER = 0.69, MEV = 0.56)				
Ptx-3 > 169 ng/mL	1.66 ± 0.44	5.26	2.23–12.36	0.0001
Age > 65 years	1.04 ± 0.467	2.83	1.13–7.09	0.026
Male gender	1.02 ± 0.45	2.77	1.15–6.66	0.022
hs-Troponin I	0.63 ± 0.29	1.88	1.41–2.51	0.021
LVEF < 60%	−0.28 ± 0.45	0.75	0.31–1.84	0.534
NT-proBNP (AIC = 213, BIC = 219, p < 0.001, MER = 0.66, MEV = 0.54)				
NT-proBNP > 2141 pg/mL	1.74 ± 0.52	5.67	2.05–15.61	0.0008
Age > 65 years	0.53 ± 0.54	1.70	0.59–4.88	0.322
Male gender	0.36 ± 0.45	1.43	0.59–3.44	0.427
hs-Troponin I	0.29 ± 0.22	1.34	1.07–1.66	0.208
LVEF < 60%	−0.31 ± 0.46	0,74	0.30–1.82	0.507
NT-proBNP + Ptx-3 combination (AIC = 209, BIC = 214, p = 0.001, MER = 0.75, MEV = 0.64)				
NT-proBNP > 2141 pg/mL	1.67 ± 0.51	5.32	1.95–14.46	0.001
Ptx-3 >169 ng/mL	1.19 ± 0.44	3.28	1.39–7.73	0.007
Age > 65 years	0.51 ± 0.51	1.67	0.60–4.62	0.326
Male gender	0.12 ± 0.21	1.13	0.91–1.39	0.591
hs-Troponin I	0.44 ± 0.22	1.54	1.23–1.92	0.065
LVEF < 60%	0.08 ± 0.12	1.08	0.96–1.22	0.692
NT-proBNP + ST2 combination (AIC = 212, BIC = 217, p < 0.001, MER = 0.68, MEV = 0.57)				
NT-proBNP > 2141 pg/mL	1.79 ± 0.49	5.98	2.29–15.60	0.0003
ST2 > 27.2 ng/mL	1.25 ± 0.58	3.48	1.10–10.99	0.03
age > 65 years	0.81 ± 0.51	2.25	0.83–6.10	0.111
Male gender	0.18 ± 0.22	1.20	0.96–1.49	0.281
hs-Troponin I	0.44 ± 0.23	1.54	1.23–1.96	0.058
LVEF < 60%	0.08 ± 0.12	1.08	0.96–1.22	0.696
ST2 + Ptx-3 combination (AIC = 217, BIC = 222, p < 0.001, MER = 0.52, MEV = 0.40)				
ST2 > 27.2 ng/mL	1.05 ± 0.59	2.88	0.91–9.08	0.071
Ptx-3 > 169 ng/mL	1.32 ± 0.44	3.74	1.58–8.86	0.003
Age > 65 years	1.26 ± 0.463	3.53	1.43–8.75	0.006
Male gender	0.14 ± 0.22	1.15	0.92–1.43	0.428
hs-Troponin I	0.44 ± 0.21	1.54	1.25–1.88	0.071
LVEF < 60%	0.09 ± 0.11	1.09	0.98–1.23	0.641
NT-proBNP + ST2 + Ptx-3 combination (AIC = 208, BIC = 214, p < 0.001, MER = 0.77, MEV = 0.66)				
NT-proBNP > 2141 pg/mL	1.60 ± 0.49	4.95	1.87–13.17	0.001
ST2 > 27.2 ng/mL	0.99 ± 0.59	2.70	0.84–8.69	0.095
Ptx-3 > 169 ng/mL	1.08 ± 0.44	2.94	1.24–6.99	0.055
Age > 65 years	0.73 ± 0.52	2.08	0.76–5.73	0.155
Male gender	0.11 ± 0.21	1.12	0.90–1.38	0.612
hs-Troponin I	0.43 ± 0.22	1.537	1.23–1.93	0.073
LVEF < 60%	0.07 ± 0.12	1.07	0.95–1.21	0.702

AIC—Akaike information criterion, BIC—Schwarz information criterion, LVEF—left ventricle ejection fraction, MER—measure of explained randomness, MEV—measure of explained variation, NT-proBNP—N-terminal-pro hormone B-type natriuretic peptide, Ptx-3—pentraxin 3, ST2—suppression of tumorigenicity 2.

4. Discussion

STEMI still represents a leading cause for cardiovascular morbidity and mortality worldwide and is thus also a considerable economic factor [1]. While STEMI patients show high in-hospital mortality rates, they are also at high risk for major adverse cardiovascular events and CV mortality after the acute phase [1,24]. Accordingly, the identification of high-risk patients after STEMI represents one of the main clinical goals. However, despite the evident need, tools for risk-stratification and prognosis after STEMI remain scarce, thereby giving rise to numerous investigations. Of note, numerous studies have proposed a multi-marker approach as best practice. Furthermore, to maximize diagnostic power, a combination of biomarkers from different pathogenetic backgrounds is suggested [11,25,26].

In this study, we therefore aimed to evaluate two novel cardiac biomarkers, sST2 and Ptx-3 along with the established cardiac marker NT-pro-BNP for risk stratification in STEMI patients during two-year FU. Of note, all three evaluated biomarkers represent different pathophysiological backgrounds, yet they seem to be of prognostic value for prediction of the outcome in patients suffering from myocardial infarction and associated pathologies like heart failure.

Indeed, NT-pro-BNP secreted by cardiomyocytes, constitutes a marker mainly utilized in the diagnosis and monitoring of heart failure patients [27]. However, NT-pro-BNP was also shown to be elevated in MI, showing a correlation with the extension of the infarct scar [28,29]. Given its application in routine heart failure FU, the prognostic impact of NT-pro-BNP in STEMI patients was anticipated in previous studies [27,29–31]. Ptx-3, a member of the group of pattern-recognition receptors is a marker, involved in the immune-system [7]. Its regulative function in complementary system activation has been considered as a possible mechanism involved in tissue damage after coronary ischemia and reperfusion [8]. Indeed, in larger epidemic studies, this protein was proposed as a prognostic tool showing a significant relationship with cardiovascular and all-cause mortality [32,33]. On the other hand, ST2 represents a marker of inflammation and cardiac stress. There are two known isoforms of ST2, a membrane bound ST2L and a soluble form, sST2 [10]. A ligand to both isoforms is interleukin-33 (IL-33), which is known to mediate cardioprotective effects on a molecular level through binding to the ST2L receptor [34]. In contrast, sST2 acts as a decoy receptor, binding IL-33 and making it unavailable for cardioprotective signaling through the ST2L receptor [34]. Accordingly, an increase in sST2 indicates a decrease in cardioprotective effects. Consequently, this biomarker is elevated in numerous cardiovascular pathologies, such as in heart failure, but also in myocardial infarction [10]. Indeed, several studies have demonstrated its predictive potential in patients suffering from MI [22,35,36]. However, ST2 in isolation cannot be considered as a risk factor. Its low specificity in relation to endpoints during MI was confirmed in the CLARITY-TIMI study [37]. However, as indicated by a subanalysis of this trial, when ST2 is combined with NT-proBNP, the predictive prognostic power of short-term risk stratification in this population is enhanced [37]. Nevertheless, the prognostic power during a longer observation period has not yet been evaluated.

In our trial, all tested biomarkers (ST2, Ptx-3, NT-pro-BNP) showed a promising potential for the prediction of two-year CV mortality after STEMI (Tables 6 and 7). Nevertheless, when comparing the predictive accuracy using a single marker approach, both in univariate cox regression but also in the multivariate regression model, Ptx-3 levels were associated with the highest accuracy for prediction of two-year CV mortality (Tables 6 and 7). Of note, these results are in accordance with previous data. Indeed, in MI patients (including STEMI), elevated Ptx-3 levels at hospital admission were associated with higher rate of mortality, even in long-term observational studies [14–16]. Furthermore, as already suggested by the CLARITY-TIMI results, in our trial ST2 levels at admission were associated with less predictive accuracy when matched with the other two evaluated biomarkers [37]. We were, however, inspired by further promising data from a subanalysis of CLARITY-TIMI [37] suggesting improvement of short-term risk stratification when combined with NT-proBNP. We decided to investigate its potential value when applied in multimarker models (NT-proBNP+St2 or Ptx-3+ST2). However, when matched with the application of NT-proBNP or Ptx-3 alone, only minimal improvement of predictive accuracy was observed (Table 7). Our results therefore suggest that ST2 may be of lesser value for prediction of midterm (two-year) CV mortality after STEMI when used alone but also when applied in two-biomarker approaches. Interestingly, in our study, the two-biomarker combination of NT-proBNP and Ptx-3 was able to improve the accuracy of the investigated risk assessment (Table 7). Indeed, our results are in accordance with previous trials, which revealed good predictive power for both NT-proBNP but also Ptx-3 when applied in mid- and long-term risk assessment in patients suffering from MI [14–16,27,29–31]. Nevertheless, to the best of our knowledge, our results indicate for the first time that the combined multimarker approach (NT-proBNP+Ptx-3) might be a promising tool for the prediction of two-year mortality after STEMI, when only two biomarkers are available. Despite promising results revealed by the investigation of this two-biomarker model, in our trial the most accurate combination was observed using a three-marker combination (NT-proBNP+Ptx-3+ST2, Table 7). Therefore, our results might suggest that this strategy is the most promising when utilized for midterm (two-year) risk assessment for CV mortality in a high-risk population. Indeed, these findings support previous speculations, proposing a combination of cardiac biomarkers from different pathogenetic backgrounds for improvement of risk stratification in different cardiovascular pathologies [11,21,25,38].

In our study, the CV mortality rate of 22.1% during two-year FU seems high. However, when compared to previous registry results, it is only slightly higher than cardiovascular endpoint rates in the average European population [39]. Our finding may be mainly attributed to the large rural regions with an inadequate access to medical care and FU system, also represented by the high number of patients undergoing primarily thrombolytic therapy (35/147, 23.8%) in our study. Additionally, high alcohol consumption, an unhealthy diet, a high incidence of metabolic syndrome and social-economic factors must be taken into account in this regard [40,41]. Nevertheless, when exploring high-risk populations, one must also consider potential associated advantages. Indeed, high-risk patients can be effectively identified retrospectively in the described population. Furthermore, our data emphasize the potential need for application of multimarker approaches in populations at increased risk for cardiovascular events.

Compared to previous trials, the cut-off levels for biomarkers proposed in our study are relatively divergent. Indeed, ST2 was shown to be a prognostic marker in the follow-up of heart failure patients, with a cut-off level of >35 ng/mL indicating a worse prognosis [21,23]. However, the calculated cut-off for ST2 for our study endpoint CV mortality was 27 ng/mL. The potential reasons for this finding might be diverse. First, different ELISA kits for ST2 are available, differing substantially in the results for ST2. Second, given the inclusion of patients up to 48 h after onset of symptoms, a delay in blood sampling may be a potential confounder in this regard, with ST2 levels peaking about 6–18 h after onset of symptoms in myocardial infarction [22,35]. Additionally, the young mean age of our study collective may have had an influence on the relatively low cut-off. Nevertheless, while dealing with CV mortality in a STEMI population with higher LVEF, considering the proposed cut-off value of 35 ng/mL in the FU of stable heart failure with reduced ejection fraction patients in numerous studies, our cut-off value seems reasonable [21,23]. On the other hand, regarding NT-pro-BNP, given the time between blood sampling and onset of symptoms as well as the ongoing secretion of NT-pro-BNP following myocardial infarction, these findings also seem adequate. When dealing with Ptx-3, one must consider the lack of a standardized test. Therefore, a nominal comparison to other studies should be considered invalid.

In conclusion, our study proposes a significant correlation of ST2, Ptx-3 and NT-pro-BNP with two-year CV mortality in STEMI patients. All three biomarkers have shown prognostic efficacy in prediction of two-year CV mortality. Nevertheless, when using a single marker approach at admission, the highest accuracy might be associated with Ptx-3 levels, with ST2 levels showing the lowest accuracy. When applying a two-biomarker approach in this setting, the most appropriate two-marker model seems to be the combination of the biomarkers NT-proBNP and Ptx-3 with associated improvement of risk assessment. In our trial, the three-biomarker model (NT-proBNP + ST2 + Ptx-3) was able to predict CV mortality with the highest accuracy indicating this approach to be a promising clinical tool in this risk population. This confirms previous suspicions, suggesting multimarker approaches for risk stratification and monitoring in cardiovascular diseases.

Our study suffers from several limitations. One of the limitations is the relatively small sample size investigated in a single center study. Furthermore, the dropout rate was relatively high (9/156 patients, 5.8%). One must also consider the high rate of thrombolytic therapy (35/147 patients, 23.8%), which is explained by longer patient transfer from distant rural regions to the cardiac center. While hs-Troponin I and CK-MB were applied to confirm diagnosis of STEMI, hs-Tropinin T levels were not routinely used to facilitate the diagnosis of acute MI. As already mentioned, given the inclusion of patients up to 48 h after onset of symptoms, a delay in blood sampling may be a potential confounder. However, our data represent a real-life scenario, which in daily clinical practice is often characterized by various time points of presentation after STEMI. Also, notably, fast and routine applications of measurements of ST2 and Ptx-3 levels are currently still lacking. Therefore, despite promising results, routine application of the proposed multimarker approaches may be limited.

Supplementary Materials: The following are available online at http://www.mdpi.com/2077-0383/9/2/550/s1, Table S1: Gehan's Wilcoxon and log-rank analysis of risk factors for CVD in patients with STEMI during the follow-up period.

Author Contributions: Conceptualization, N.Z., L.J.M. and V.P. (Valentin Pavlov); Data curation, R.Z.; Investigation, D.G. and A.H.; Methodology, I.L.; Resources, V.I. and E.T.; Software, I.K. and D.P.; Writing—original draft, V.P. (Vera Paar), P.J. and U.C.H.; Writing—review & editing, K.K. All authors have read and agreed to the published version of the manuscript.

Conflicts of Interest: The authors declare no conflict of interest.

References

1. Ibanez, B.; Lames, S.; Agewall, S.; Antunes, M.J.; Bucciarelli-Ducci, C.; Bueno, H.; Caforio, A.L.P.; Crea, F.; Goudevenos, J.A.; Halvorsen, S.; et al. 2017 ESC Guidelines for the management of acute myocardial infarction in patients presenting with ST-segment elevation: The Task Force for the management of acute myocardial infarction in patients presenting with ST-segment elevation of the European Society of Cardiology (ESC). *Eur. Heart J.* **2018**, *39*, 119–177. [PubMed]
2. Magnussen, C.; Blankenberg, S. Biomarkers for heart failure: Small molecules with high clinical relevance. *J. Intern. Med.* **2018**, *283*, 530–543. [CrossRef] [PubMed]
3. Sarko, J.; Pollack, C.V. Cardiac troponins. *J. Emerg. Med.* **2002**, *23*, 57–65. [CrossRef]
4. Margit, M.B.; Klaus, H.; Schröder, A.; Ebert, C.; Borgya, A.; Gerhardt, W.; Remppis, A.; Zehelein, J.; Katus, H.A. Improved troponin T ELISA specific for cardiac troponin T isoform: Assay development and analytical and clinical validation. *Clin. Chem.* **1997**, *43*, 458–466.
5. Garg, P.; Morris, P.; Fazlanie, A.L.; Vijayan, S.; Dancso, B.; Dastidar, A.G.; Plein, S.; Mueller, C.; Haaf, P. Cardiac biomarkers of acute coronary syndrome: From history to high-sensitivity cardiac troponin. *Intern. Emerg. Med.* **2017**, *12*, 147–155. [CrossRef]
6. James, S.; Lindback, J.; Tilly, J.; Siegbahn, A.; Venge, P.; Armstrong, P.; Califf, R.; Simoons, M.L.; Wallentin, L.; Lindahl, B. Troponin-T and N-terminal pro-B-type natriuretic peptide predict mortality benefit from coronary revascularization in acute coronary syndromes: A GUSTO-IV substudy. *J. Am. Coll. Cardiol.* **2006**, *48*, 1146–1154. [CrossRef]
7. Casula, M.; Montecucco, F.; Bonaventura, A.; Liberale, L.; Vecchié, A.; Dallegri, F.; Carbone, F. Update on the role of Pentraxin 3 in atherosclerosis and cardiovascular diseases. *Vasc. Pharm.* **2017**, *99*, 1–12. [CrossRef]
8. Ristagno, G.; Fumagalli, F.; Bottazzi, B.; Mantovani, A.; Olivari, D.; Novelli, D.; Latini, R. Pentraxin 3 in Cardiovascular Disease. *Front. Immunol.* **2019**, *10*, 823. [CrossRef]
9. Fornai, F.; Carrizzo, A.; Forte, M.; Ambrosio, M.; Damato, A.; Ferrucci, M.; Biagioni, F.; Busceti, C.; Puca, A.A.; Vecchione, C. The inflammatory protein Pentraxin 3 in cardiovascular disease. *Immun. Ageing* **2016**, *13*, 25. [CrossRef]
10. Ciccone, M.M.; Cortese, F.; Gesualdo, M.; Riccardi, R.; Di Nunzio, D.; Moncelli, M.; Iacoviello, M.; Scicchitano, P. A novel cardiac bio-marker: ST2: A review. *Molecules* **2013**, *18*, 15314–15328. [CrossRef]
11. Aydin, S.; Ugur, K.; Aydin, S.; Sahin, İ.; Yardim, M. Biomarkers in acute myocardial infarction: Current perspectives. *Vasc. Health Risk Manag.* **2019**, *17*, 1–10. [CrossRef] [PubMed]

12. Helseth, R.; Solheim, S.; Opstad, T.; Hoffmann, P.; Arnesen, H.; Seljeflot, I. The time profile of Pentraxin 3 in patients with acute ST-elevation myocardial infarction and stable angina pectoris undergoing percutaneous coronary intervention. *Mediat. Inflamm.* **2014**, *2014*, 608414. [CrossRef] [PubMed]
13. Morishita, T.; Uzui, H.; Nakano, A.; Fukuoka, Y.; Ikeda, H.; Amaya, N.; Kaseno, K.; Ishida, K.; Lee, J.D.; Tada, H. Association of Plasma pentraxin-3 Levels With Coronary Risk Factors and the Lipid Profile: A Cross-Sectional Study in Japanese Patients With Stable Angina Pectoris. *Heart Vessel.* **2018**, *33*, 1301–1310. [CrossRef] [PubMed]
14. Akgul, O.; Baycan, O.F.; Nakano, A.; Fukuoka, Y.; Ikeda, H.; Amaya, N.; Kaseno, K.; Ishida, K.; Lee, J.D.; Tada, H. Long-term prognostic value of elevated pentraxin 3 in patients undergoing primary angioplasty for ST-elevation myocardial infarction. *Coron. Artery Dis.* **2015**, *26*, 592–597. [CrossRef]
15. Mjelva, O.R.; Ponitz, V.; Brügger-Andersen, T.; Grundt, H.; Staines, H.; Nilsen, D.W. Long-term prognostic utility of pentraxin 3 and D-dimer as compared to high-sensitivity C-reactive protein and B-type natriuretic peptide in suspected acute coronary syndrome. *Eur. J. Prev. Cardiol.* **2016**, *23*, 1130–1140. [CrossRef]
16. Altay, S.; Cakmak, H.A.; Kemaloğlu Öz, T.; Özpamuk Karadeniz, F.; Türer, A.; Erer, H.B.; Kılıç, G.F.; Keleş, İ.; Can, G.; Eren, M. Long-term prognostic significance of pentraxin-3 in patients with acute myocardial infarction: 5-year prospective cohort study. *Anatol. J. Cardiol.* **2017**, *17*, 202–209. [CrossRef]
17. Pascual-Figal, D.A.; Januzzi, J.L. The biology of ST2: The International ST2 Consensus Panel. *Am. J. Cardiol.* **2015**, *115*, 3B–7B. [CrossRef]
18. Miñana, G.; Núñez, J.; Bayés-Genís, A.; Revuelta-López, E.; Ríos-Navarro, C.; Núñez, E.; Chorro, F.J.; López-Lereu, M.P.; Monmeneu, J.V.; Lupón, J.; et al. ST2 and Left Ventricular Remodeling After ST-segment Elevation Myocardial Infarction: A Cardiac Magnetic Resonance Study. *Int. J. Cardiol.* **2018**, *270*, 336–342. [CrossRef]
19. Weir, R.A.; Miller, A.M.; Murphy, G.E.; Clements, S.; Steedman, T.; Connell, J.M.; McInnes, I.B.; Dargie, H.J.; McMurray, J.J. Serum soluble ST2: A potential novel mediator in left ventricular and infarct remodeling after acute myocardial infarction. *J. Am. Coll. Cardiol.* **2010**, *55*, 243–250. [CrossRef]
20. Lupón, J.; de Antonio, M.; Galán, A.; Vila, J.; Zamora, E.; Urrutia, A.; Bayes-Genis, A. Combined use of the novel biomarkers high-sensitivity troponin T and ST2 for heart failure risk stratification vs conventional assessment. *Mayo Clin. Proc.* **2013**, *88*, 234–243. [CrossRef]
21. Bayes-Genis, A.; Richards, A.M.; Maisel, A.S.; Mueller, C.; Ky, B. Multimarker testing with ST2 in chronic heart failure. *Am. J. Cardiol.* **2015**, *115*, 76B–80B. [CrossRef] [PubMed]
22. Richards, A.M.; Somma, S. Di.; Mueller, T. ST2 in stable and unstable ischemic heart diseases. *Am. J. Cardiol.* **2015**, *115*, 48B–58B. [CrossRef]
23. Maisel, A.S.; Richards, A.M.; Pascual-Figal, D.; Mueller, C. Serial ST2 testing in hospitalized patients with acute heart failure. *Am. J. Cardiol.* **2015**, *115*, 32B–37B. [CrossRef] [PubMed]
24. Ponikowski, P.; Voors, A.A.; Anker, S.D.; Bueno, H.; Cleland, J.G.; Coats, A.J.; Falk, V.; González-Juanatey, J.R.; Harjola, V.P.; Jankowska, E.A.; et al. ESC Guidelines for the diagnosis and treatment of acute and chronic failure: The Task Force for the diagnosis and treatment of acute and chronic heart failure of the European Society of Cardiology (ESC). Developed with the special contribution of the Heart Failure Association (HFA) of the ESC. *Eur. J. Heart Fail.* **2016**, *18*, 891–975. [PubMed]
25. Lichtenauer, M.; Jirak, P.; Wernly, B.; Paar, V.; Rohm, I.; Jung, C.; Schernthaner, C.; Kraus, J.; Motloch, L.J.; Yilmaz, A.; et al. A comparative analysis of novel cardiovascular biomarkers in patients with chronic heart failure. *Eur. J. Intern. Med.* **2017**, *44*, 31–38. [CrossRef]
26. Jirak, P.; Fejzic, D.; Paar, V.; Wernly, B.; Pistulli, R.; Rohm, I.; Jung, C.; Hoppe, U.C.; Schulze, P.C.; Lichtenauer, M.; et al. Influences of Ivabradine treatment on serum levels of cardiac biomarkers sST2, GDF-15, suPAR and H-FABP in patients with chronic heart failure. *Acta Pharm. Sin.* **2018**, *39*, 1189–1196. [CrossRef]
27. Oremus, M.; McKelvie, R.; Don-Wauchope, A.; Santaguida, P.L.; Ali, U.; Balion, C.; Hill, S.; Booth, R.; Brown, J.A.; Bustamam, A.; et al. A systematic review of BNP and NT-proBNP in the management of heart failure: Overview and methods. *Heart Fail. Rev.* **2014**, *19*, 413–419. [CrossRef]
28. Fan, J.; Ma, J.; Xia, N.; Sun, L.; Li, B.; Liu, H. Clinical Value of Combined Detection of CK-MB, MYO, cTnI and Plasma NT-proBNP in Diagnosis of Acute Myocardial Infarction. *Clin. Lab.* **2017**, *63*, 427–433. [CrossRef]
29. Reinstadler, S.J.; Feistritzer, H.J.; Reindl, M.; Klug, G.; Metzler, B. Utility of NT-proBNP in predicting infarct scar and left ventricular dysfunction at a chronic stage after myocardial infarction. *Eur. J. Intern. Med.* **2016**, *29*, 16–18. [CrossRef]

30. Kopec, M.; Duma, A.; Helwani, M.A.; Brown, J.; Brown, F.; Gage, B.F.; Gibson, D.W.; Miller, J.P.; Novak, E.; Jaffe, A.S.; et al. Improving Prediction of Postoperative Myocardial Infarction With High-Sensitivity Cardiac Troponin T and NT-proBNP. *Anesth. Analg.* **2017**, *124*, 398–405. [CrossRef]
31. Drewniak, W.; Szybka, W.; Bielecki, D.; Malinowski, M.; Kotlarska, J.; Krol-Jaskulska, A.; Popielarz-Grygalewicz, A.; Konwicka, A.; Dąbrowski, M. Prognostic Significance of NT-proBNP Levels in Patients Over 65 Presenting Acute Myocardial Infarction Treated Invasively or Conservatively. *Biomed Res. Int.* **2015**, *2015*, 1–6. [CrossRef] [PubMed]
32. Jenny, N.S.; Arnold, A.M.; Kuller, L.H.; Tracy, R.P.; Psaty, B.M. Associations of pentraxin 3 with cardiovascular disease and all-cause death: The Cardiovascular Health Study. *Arterioscler. Thromb. Vasc. Biol.* **2009**, *29*, 594–599. [CrossRef] [PubMed]
33. Jenny, N.S.; Blumenthal, R.S.; Kuller, L.H.; Tracy, R.P.; Psaty, B.M. Associations of pentraxin 3 with cardiovascular disease: The multiethnic study of atherosclerosis. *J. Thromb. Haemost.* **2014**, *12*, 999–1005. [CrossRef] [PubMed]
34. Sanada, S.; Hakuno, D.; Higgins, L.J.; Schreiter, E.R.; McKenzie, A.N.; Lee, R.T. IL-33 and ST2 comprise a critical biomechanically induced and cardioprotective signaling system. *J. Clin. Investig.* **2007**, *117*, 1538–1549. [CrossRef] [PubMed]
35. Eggers, K.M.; Armstrong, P.W.; Califf, R.M.; Simoons, M.L.; Venge, P.; Wallentin, L.; James, S.K. ST2 and mortality in non-ST-segment elevation acute coronary syndrome. *Am. Heart J.* **2010**, *159*, 788–794. [CrossRef] [PubMed]
36. Jenkins, W.S.; Roger, V.L.; Jaffe, A.S.; Weston, S.A.; AbouEzzeddine, O.F.; Jiang, R.; Manemann, S.M.; Enriquez-Sarano, M. Prognostic Value of Soluble ST2 After Myocardial Infarction: A Community Perspective. *Am. J. Med.* **2017**, *130*, 1112. [CrossRef]
37. Sabatine, M.S.; Morrow, D.A.; Higgins, L.J.; MacGillivray, C.; Guo, W.; Bode, C.; Rifai, N.; Cannon, C.P.; Gerszten, R.E.; Lee, R.T. Complementary roles for biomarkers of biomechanical strain ST2 and N-terminal prohormone B-type natriuretic peptide in patients with ST-elevation myocardial infarction. *Circulation.* **2008**, *117*, 1936–1944. [CrossRef]
38. Jirak, P.; Mirna, M.; Wernly, B.; Paar, V.; Thieme, M.; Betge, S.; Franz, M.; Hoppe, U.; Lauten, A.; Kammler, J.; et al. Analysis of novel cardiovascular biomarkers in patients with peripheral artery disease (PAD). *Minerva Med.* **2018**, *109*, 443–450. [CrossRef]
39. Gierlotka, M.; Zdrojewski, T.; Wojtyniak, B.; Poloński, L.; Stokwiszewski, J.; Gąsior, M.; Kozierkiewicz, A.; Kalarus, Z.; Wierucki, Ł.; Chlebus, K.; et al. Incidence, treatment, in-hospital mortality and one-year outcomes of acute myocardial infarction in Poland in 2009–2012—Nationwide AMI-PL database. *Kardiol. Pol.* **2015**, *73*, 142–158. [CrossRef]
40. Nowbar, A.N.; Howard, J.P.; Finegold, J.A.; Asaria, P.; Francis, D.P. 2014 global geographic analysis of mortality from ischaemic heart disease by country, age and income: Statistics from World Health Organisation and United Nations. *Int. J. Cardiol.* **2014**, *174*, 293–298. [CrossRef]
41. Sidorenkov, O.; Nilssen, O.; Grjibovski, A.M. Metabolic syndrome in Russian adults: Associated factors and mortality from cardiovascular diseases and all causes. *BMC Public Health* **2010**, *10*, 582. [CrossRef] [PubMed]

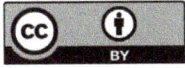

© 2020 by the authors. Licensee MDPI, Basel, Switzerland. This article is an open access article distributed under the terms and conditions of the Creative Commons Attribution (CC BY) license (http://creativecommons.org/licenses/by/4.0/).

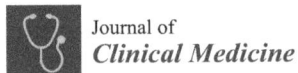 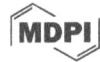

Article

Urinary Liver-Type Fatty-Acid-Binding Protein Predicts Long-Term Adverse Outcomes in Medical Cardiac Intensive Care Units

Hiroyuki Naruse [1], Junnichi Ishii [1,*], Hiroshi Takahashi [2], Fumihiko Kitagawa [1], Hideto Nishimura [3], Hideki Kawai [3], Takashi Muramatsu [3], Masahide Harada [3], Akira Yamada [3], Wakaya Fujiwara [4], Mutsuharu Hayashi [4], Sadako Motoyama [3], Masayoshi Sarai [3], Eiichi Watanabe [3], Hideo Izawa [4] and Yukio Ozaki [3]

1. Department of Joint Research Laboratory of Clinical Medicine, Fujita Health University School of Medicine, Toyoake 470-1192, Japan; hnaruse@fujita-hu.ac.jp (H.Na.); fkitaga@fujita-hu.ac.jp (F.K.)
2. Division of Statistics, Fujita Health University School of Medicine, Toyoake 470-1192, Japan; hirotaka@fujita-hu.ac.jp
3. Department of Cardiology, Fujita Health University School of Medicine, Toyoake 470-1192, Japan; hidetonishimura0621@gmail.com (H.Ni.); hidekikawai@xc4.so-net.ne.jp (H.K.); takam@fujita-hu.ac.jp (T.M.); mharada@fujita-hu.ac.jp (M.H.); a-yamada@fujita-hu.ac.jp (A.Y.); sadakom@fujita-hu.ac.jp (S.M.); msarai@fujita-hu.ac.jp (M.S.); enwatan@mtj.biglobe.ne.jp (E.W.); ozakiyuk@fujita-hu.ac.jp (Y.O.)
4. Department of Cardiology, Bantane Hospital, Nagoya 454-8509, Japan; wakayafj@fujita-hu.ac.jp (W.F.); muhayasi@med.nagoya-u.ac.jp (M.H.); izawa@fujita-hu.ac.jp (H.I.)
* Correspondence: jishii@fujita-hu.ac.jp; Tel.: +81-562-93-2312

Received: 20 January 2020; Accepted: 7 February 2020; Published: 10 February 2020

Abstract: We prospectively investigated the prognostic value of urinary liver-type fatty-acid-binding protein (L-FABP) levels on hospital admission, both independently and in combination with serum creatinine-defined acute kidney injury (AKI), to predict long-term adverse outcomes in 1119 heterogeneous patients (mean age; 68 years) treated at medical (non-surgical) cardiac intensive care units (CICUs). Patients with stage 5 chronic kidney disease were excluded from the study. Of these patients, 47% had acute coronary syndrome and 38% had acute decompensated heart failure. The creatinine-defined AKI was diagnosed according to the "Kidney Disease: Improving Global Outcomes" criteria. The primary endpoint was a composite of all-cause death or progression to end-stage kidney disease, indicating the initiation of maintenance dialysis therapy or kidney transplantation. Creatinine-defined AKI occurred in 207 patients, with 44 patients having stage 2 or 3 disease. During a mean follow-up period of 41 months after enrollment, the primary endpoint occurred in 242 patients. Multivariate Cox regression analyses revealed L-FABP levels as independent predictors of the primary endpoint ($p < 0.001$). Adding L-FABP to a baseline model with established risk factors further enhanced reclassification and discrimination beyond that of the baseline model alone, for primary-endpoint prediction (both; $p < 0.01$). On Kaplan–Meier analyses, increased L-FABP (≥4th quintile value of 9.0 ng/mL) on admission or presence of creatinine-defined AKI, correlated with an increased risk of the primary endpoint ($p < 0.001$). Thus, urinary L-FABP levels on admission are potent and independent predictors of long-term adverse outcomes, and they might improve the long-term risk stratification of patients admitted at medical CICUs, when used in combination with creatinine-defined AKI.

Keywords: liver-type fatty-acid-binding protein; long-term outcomes; cardiac intensive care units; acute kidney injury

1. Introduction

Liver-type fatty-acid-binding protein (L-FABP; molecular weight, 14,000) is expressed in the proximal tubular epithelial cells [1] and binds to free fatty acids in the cytoplasm [2,3]. During renal injury, L-FABP binds to lipid peroxidation products and is excreted into urine, protecting the proximal tubules from oxidative stress [4]. Therefore, urinary L-FABP might be a suitable marker of renal tubular injury. In a heterogeneous cohort of patients treated in medical (nonsurgical) cardiac intensive care units (CICUs), urinary L-FABP levels were found to be potent predictors of acute kidney injury (AKI) [5,6]. However, to date, the association between urinary L-FABP levels and long-term adverse outcomes in patients treated at medical CICUs remains poorly understand.

The consensus definition of AKI is currently based on acute changes in serum creatinine levels or decreases in urine output. However, the serum creatinine-defined definition for AKI has several limitations because creatinine is a muscle metabolite that is an insensitive and nonspecific marker of kidney excretory function at only steady state [7]. Combining kidney excretory function parameter with tubular injury markers has prognostic relevance. Kidney tubular injury markers can predict the need for renal replacement, length of hospital stay, and in-hospital mortality in critically ill and surgical patients [8,9]. Furthermore, "subclinical AKI", as evidenced by increased urinary tubular injury markers without serum creatinine increase, is associated with severe in-hospital clinical outcomes [10]. However, only few studies of patients after cardiac surgery have reported that tubular injury marker combined with creatinine-defined AKI status could predict the increased risk of long-term adverse outcomes [11,12].

This study prospectively investigated the prognostic value of urinary L-FABP levels on admission, both independently and in combination with creatinine-defined AKI, in patients hospitalized at medical CICUs.

2. Materials and Methods

2.1. Study Design

This prospective study was conducted at the Department of Cardiology, Fujita Health University School of Medicine (Toyoake, Japan). We enrolled patients hospitalized at medical (non-surgical) CICUs in Fujita Health University Hospital from January 2012 to December 2013. The ethics committee of Fujita Health University approved this study (study protocol number 11-053), which was in accordance with the Declaration of Helsinki. All patients individually provided written informed consent.

Patients with cardiovascular disease requiring hospitalization as determined by the attending physician of the medical CICUs were eligible for enrollment. We obtained urinary and blood samples upon admission, for baseline biomarker measurements. Meanwhile, we excluded patients who had the following characteristics—(1) under 18 years old, (2) undergoing cardiac surgery, (3) experiencing trauma, (4) having stage 5 chronic kidney disease (CKD), (5) receiving percutaneous cardiopulmonary support before admission, (6) having an active malignant disease being treated with chemotherapy or radiation, and (7) having autoimmune diseases. Independent physicians blinded to urinary L-FABP levels could freely select therapy as indicated. Clinical characteristics were obtained from patients' medical records, upon enrollment.

2.2. Definitions and Calculations

Patients were diagnosed with serum creatinine-defined AKI, according to the "Kidney Disease: Improving Global Outcomes" criteria, that is, an increase in serum creatinine by ≥0.3 mg/dL, within 48 h, or an increase in serum creatinine to ≥1.5 times the baseline, within 1 week [13]. The lowest known serum creatinine value during the past 3 months was used as baseline creatinine. For patients with unknown baseline, we used the lowest creatinine value within 7 days after admission at medical CICUs. We calculated the serum creatinine-based estimated glomerular filtration rate (eGFR), using the Modification of Diet in Renal Disease Study equation, as recommended by the Japan CKD Initiative [14].

Incident end-stage kidney disease (ESKD) indicated the initiation of maintenance dialysis therapy or kidney transplantation, whereas an eGFR <60 mL/min/1.73 m^2 indicated CKD.

Diabetes was defined as a history of or current diabetes or a fasting plasma glucose level ≥126 mg/dL, a hemoglobin A1c value ≥6.5%, or the presence of diabetic retinopathy. Hypertension was defined as having a systolic blood pressure ≥140 mmHg, a diastolic blood pressure ≥90 mmHg, or a history of antihypertensive treatment. Dyslipidemia was defined as a total cholesterol level ≥220 mg/dL or a history of lipid-lowering therapy. Patients with smoking history were classified as either current or ex-smokers. We calculated the sequential organ failure assessment (SOFA) score according to the worst value of the parameters, which include PaO_2/FiO_2, platelet count, bilirubin, mean arterial blood pressure and the use of vasoactive drugs, the Glasgow Coma Scale, and creatinine and urine output [15]. We routinely performed 2D echocardiography to calculate left ventricular ejection fraction (LVEF), using the modified Simpson's method.

All patients were clinically followed up for a mean period of 41 months after enrollment. The primary endpoint was a composite of all-cause mortality or progression to ESKD. All-cause mortality was the secondary endpoint. Data for the endpoints were obtained from hospital charts and through telephone interviews with patients. The telephone interviews were conducted by trained reviewers who were blinded to the patient L-FABP levels.

2.3. Biomarker Measurements

Immediately after admission, urinary and blood samples were collected in nonheparinized tubes and then centrifuged at 1000× g at 4 °C for 15 min, before storage at −80 °C until assayed. We measured the urinary L-FABP levels by an enzyme-linked immunosorbent assay (ELISA) using the Human L-FABP ELISA Kit (CMIC, Tokyo, Japan). Plasma B-type natriuretic peptide (BNP) levels were measured using a chemiluminesence enzyme immunoassay for human BNP (Shionogi & Co., Ltd., Osaka, Japan). We measured serum high-sensitivity troponin T (hs-TnT) levels via an electrochemiluminescence immunoassay, using a Cobas®e601 system (Roche Diagnostics, Tokyo, Japan), and serum high-sensitivity C-reactive protein (hs-CRP) levels via a latex-enhanced hs-CRP immunoassay (N-Latex CRP II, Siemens Healthineers, Tokyo, Japan). Serum creatinine levels were determined by an enzyme method, using the Liquitech®Creatinine PAP II (Roche Diagnostics, Tokyo, Japan) upon admission, daily until day 3, and then on day 7.

2.4. Statistical Analyses

We performed statistical analyses using StatFlex version 6 (Artech Co. Ltd. Osaka, Japan). Normally distributed variables are expressed as mean values ± standard deviations, whereas nonparametric data are presented as medians and interquartile ranges. Considering that the urinary L-FABP, plasma BNP, serum hs-TnT, and serum hs-CRP data were irregularly distributed, analyses were performed after log-transformation to meet the criteria for use in normalized statistical approaches (after statistical confirmation). The relationship between urinary L-FABP and other baseline valuables was studied by linear regression analysis. Intergroup differences were evaluated by one-way analysis of variance or the Kruskal–Wallis test for continuous variables and by the chi-square test for categorical variables. Moreover, we examined the intergroup differences in endpoint by the Kaplan–Meier method and compared them using the log-rank test. Hazard ratios and 95% confidence intervals were calculated for each factor via the Cox proportional hazards analysis. All baseline variables with $p < 0.05$ in univariate analyses were integrated into the Cox multivariate model to determine the independent predictors of the endpoint.

To assess whether the accuracy of predicting the endpoint would improve after adding L-FABP into a baseline model with established risk factors, we calculated the C-index, net reclassification improvement (NRI), and integrated discrimination improvement (IDI). The established risk factors were as follows—age, hypertension, diabetes mellitus, CKD, paroxysmal or persistent atrial fibrillation, acute decompensated heart failure, myocardial infarction history, coronary revascularization history, systolic blood pressure, heart rate, mechanical ventilation before admission, and BNP. The C-index was defined as the area under the receiver operating characteristic curves between individual predictive probabilities for the endpoint and the incidence of endpoint, and it was compared with the baseline model [16]. NRI was a relative indicator of how many patients had improved in the predicted probability of the endpoint, whereas IDI indicated the average improvement in the predicted probability of the endpoint, after adding variables into the baseline model [17]. We considered $p < 0.05$ as statistically significant.

3. Results

3.1. Baseline Characteristics and Outcomes

We enrolled 1119 patients with a mean age of 68 years (23–83 years) and summarized their demographics and clinical characteristics in Tables 1 and 2. These patients were admitted due to the following diagnoses—acute coronary syndrome (529 (47%)), acute decompensated heart failure (424 (38%)), arrhythmia (51 (5%)), primary pulmonary hypertension (32 (3%)), acute aortic syndrome (24 (2%)), infective endocarditis (14 (1%)), takotsubo cardiomyopathy (11 (1%)), and others (34 (3%)). Of these patients, 497 (44%) were diagnosed with CKD, with no case of kidney transplantation. Urinary L-FABP levels correlated with age ($r = 0.06$, $p = 0.03$), and eGFR ($r = -0.25$, $p < 0.001$). Among the 1119 patients, 207 (18.5%) developed creatinine-based AKI in which 44 had stage 2 or 3 disease.

Table 1. Primary diagnosis.

Acute coronary syndrome, n (%)	529 (47)
STEMI, n	217
NSTEM, n	264
Unstable angina, n	48
Acute decompensated heart failure, n (%)	424 (38)
With reduced ejection fraction (LVEF < 40%), n	217
With mid-range ejection fraction (40% ≤ LVEF < 50%), n	67
With preserved ejection fraction (LVEF ≥ 50%), n	140
Arrhythmia, n (%)	51 (5)
Supraventricular tachycardia, n	6
Ventricular tachycardia, n	14
Sick sinus syndrome, n	13
Second- or third-degree atrioventricular block, n	18
Primary pulmonary hypertension, n (%)	32 (3)
Acute aortic syndrome, n (%)	24 (2)
Infective endocarditis, n (%)	14 (1)
Takotsubo cardiomyopathy, n (%)	11 (1)
Others, n (%)	34 (3)

Data are expressed as numbers (%). STEMI, ST-segment elevation myocardial infarction; NSTEMI, non-ST-segment elevation myocardial infarction; LVEF, left ventricular ejection fraction.

Table 2. Baseline characteristics of study population according to primary endpoint.

	All Patients	Primary Endpoint (+)	Primary Endpoint (−)	p Value
Number	1119	242	877	
Age (year)	68 ± 12	73 ± 9	67 ± 13	<0.001
Male, n (%)	732 (65)	157 (65)	575 (66)	0.84
Hypertension, n (%)	724 (65)	158 (65)	566 (65)	0.83
Dyslipidemia, n (%)	520 (47)	97 (40)	423 (48)	0.02
Diabetes, n (%)	420 (38)	88 (36)	332 (38)	0.67
Current or ex-smoker, n (%)	324 (29)	70 (29)	254 (29)	0.99
Previous myocardial infarction, n (%)	214 (19)	61 (25)	153 (17)	0.007
Prior hospitalization for worsening heart failure, n (%)	215 (19)	53 (22)	162 (19)	0.23
Previous coronary revascularization, n (%)	213 (19)	59 (24)	154 (18)	0.02
Paroxysmal or persistent AF, n (%)	248 (22)	77 (32)	171 (20)	<0.001
Acute decompensated heart failure, n (%)	424 (38)	143 (59)	281 (32)	<0.001
SOFA score	2 (1–4)	4 (2–5)	2 (1–4)	<0.001
Systolic blood pressure, mmHg	141 ± 31	135 ± 32	143 ± 31	<0.001
Heart rate, beats per minutes	86 ± 25	90 ± 24	85 ± 26	0.001
Emergent CAG or PCI before admission, n (%)	405 (36)	69 (29)	336 (38)	0.005
Mechanical ventilation before admission, n (%)	20 (1.8)	6 (2.5)	14 (1.6)	0.36
IABP before admission, n (%)	96 (8.6)	20 (8.3)	76 (8.7)	0.84
White blood cell count, $\times 10^3/\mu L$	8.7 ± 3.6	8.4 ± 3.9	8.7 ± 3.4	0.19
Hemoglobin, g/dL	12.7 ± 2.3	11.7 ± 2.3	13.0 ± 2.2	<0.001
eGFR, mL/min/1.73 m^2	66.6 ± 26.6	54.2 ± 25.2	70.0 ± 26.0	<0.001
Glucose, mg/dL	159 ± 70	170 ± 75	156 ± 68	0.006
hs-CRP, mg/L	2.32 (0.75–10.3)	4.50 (1.09–24.3)	1.99 (0.69–8.18)	<0.001
BNP, pg/mL	186 (53–631)	581 (158–1210)	133 (43–479)	<0.001
hs-TnT, pg/mL	59 (17–445)	56 (24–290)	62 (15–51)	0.43
Urinary L-FABP, ng/mL	5.8 (2.4–16.9)	9.2 (3.1–27.0)	5.2 (2.2–14.5)	<0.001
LVEF, %	47.3 ± 13.8	42.4 ± 14.4	48.7 ± 13.3	<0.001
Treatment at enrollment, n (%)				
Antiplatelet drugs	387 (35)	111 (46)	276 (32)	<0.001
Statins	355 (32)	70 (29)	285 (33)	0.29
RAAS inhibitors	469 (42)	110 (46)	359 (41)	0.21
Beta-blockers	301 (27)	84 (35)	217 (25)	0.002
Diuretics	305 (27)	103 (43)	202 (23)	<0.001
Anticoagulant drugs	163 (15)	52 (22)	111 (13)	<0.001
Creatinine-defined AKI, n (%)	207 (18.5)	68 (28.1)	139 (15.8)	<0.001

Data are presented as number (%), mean ± standard deviation, or median (25th–75th percentile). AF, atrial fibrillation; SOFA, Sequential Organ Failure Assessment; CAG, coronary angiography; PCI, percutaneous coronary intervention; IABP, intra-aortic balloon pump; eGFR, creatinine-based estimated glomerular filtration rate; hs-CRP, high-sensitivity C-reactive protein; BNP, B-type natriuretic peptide; hs-TnT, high-sensitivity cardiac troponin T; L-FABP, liver-type fatty-acid-binding protein; LVEF, left ventricular ejection fraction; RAAS, renin–angiotensin–aldosterone system; AKI, acute kidney injury.

During a mean follow-up period of 41 months, the primary endpoint occurred in 242 patients, of which 17 developed ESKD. All-cause death was manifested in 228 patients, of which 141 experienced cardiovascular deaths. Cardiovascular deaths were caused by heart failure in 85, myocardial infarction in 23, stroke in 17, sudden death in 10, and arrhythmia in 6 patients.

Patients who developed the primary endpoint were older and had higher SOFA score, higher heart rate, higher levels of glucose, hs-CRP, BNP, hs-TnT, and L-FABP, and lower levels of hemoglobin, eGFR, and LVEF than those who did not. Many patients who developed the primary endpoint had the following characteristics—coronary revascularization history; paroxysmal or persistent atrial fibrillation; acute decompensated heart failure; antiplatelet drugs; β blockers; diuretics; anticoagulant drugs; and AKI. The median length of medical CICUs stay in patients with primary endpoint (4.0 (3.0–6.0) days) was longer than those without (3.0 (2.0–4.0) days) ($p < 0.001$).

3.2. Prognostic Value of Urinary L-FABP

When patients were divided into quintiles according to the L-FABP levels (1st, <1.7 ng/mL; 2nd, 1.7–4.1 ng/mL; 3rd, 4.2–8.9 ng/mL; 4th, 9.0–22.8 ng/mL; and 5th, >22.8 ng/mL), the Kaplan–Meier primary-endpoint free survival rate in the 1st, 2nd, 3rd, 4th, and 5th L-FABP quintiles were 81.7%, 85.8%, 80.3%, 73.9%, and 70.1%, respectively ($p < 0.001$; Figure 1). Given that the Kaplan–Meier primary-endpoint free survival curves for the 1st, 2nd, and 3rd quintiles were relatively similar, as well as those for the 4th and 5th quintiles, we used the 4th quintile value for L-FABP (9.0 ng/mL) as the cutoff value for endpoint prediction.

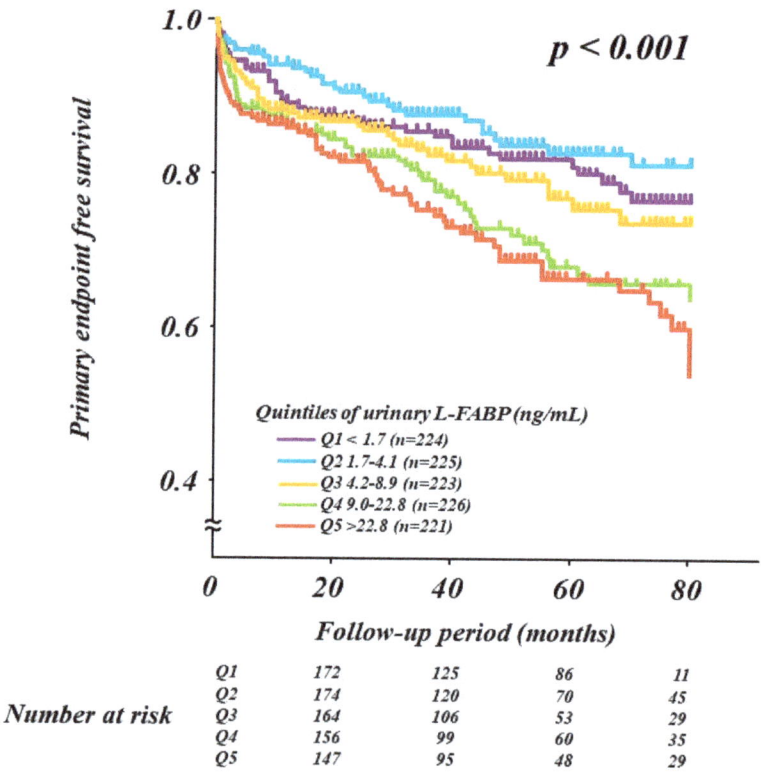

Figure 1. Kaplan–Meier curves for the primary endpoint according to the L-FABP level quintiles. L-FABP, liver-type fatty-acid-binding protein.

As revealed in the Cox multivariate analysis, L-FABP was the independent predictor of the primary endpoint when assessed as either continuous variables ($p < 0.001$) or variables categorized by the 4th quintile value of 9.0 ng/mL ($p < 0.001$) (Table 3). Age, systolic blood pressure, hemoglobin, BNP, and LVEF also remained significantly associated with the primary endpoint. Similar results were obtained for all-cause mortality (Table 3).

Table 3. Multivariate predictors of primary endpoint and all-cause mortality.

(A) Primary Endpoint	Model 1		Model 2	
Variables	HR (95% CI)	p Value	HR (95% CI)	p Value
Age (per 10 years increment)	1.54 (1.32–1.81)	<0.001	1.54 (1.32–1.80)	<0.001
Previous myocardial infarction	0.81 (0.56–1.18)	0.27	0.86 (0.59–1.25)	0.43
Paroxysmal or persistent AF	1.16 (0.87–1.55)	0.32	1.16 (0.87–1.56)	0.31
Previous coronary revascularization	1.09 (0.75–1.59)	0.66	1.06 (0.73–1.55)	0.76
Acute decompensated heart failure	1.03 (0.74–1.42)	0.87	1.06 (0.77–1.47)	0.72
Systolic blood pressure (per 10 mmHg increment)	0.94 (0.90–0.98)	0.004	0.93 (0.89–0.97)	0.002
Heart rate (per 10 beats per minutes increment)	1.03 (0.98–1.08)	0.26	1.03 (0.98–1.09)	0.26
Hemoglobin (per 1 g/dL increment)	0.88 (0.83–0.94)	<0.001	0.88 (0.83–0.94)	<0.001
CKD	1.14 (0.85–1.54)	0.38	1.18 (0.88–1.58)	0.28
hs-CRP (per 10-fold increment)	1.08 (0.91–1.27)	0.40	1.09 (0.93–1.29)	0.29
BNP (per 10-fold increment)	1.84 (1.37–2.49)	<0.001	1.80 (1.34–2.44)	<0.001
Urinary L-FABP (per 10-fold increment)	1.47 (1.22–1.76)	<0.001		
Urinary L-FABP (ng/mL)				
< 9.0 (1st + 2nd + 3rd quintile)			Reference	
≥ 9.0 (4th + 5th quintile)			1.63 (1.25–2.12)	<0.001
LVEF (per 10% increment)	0.86 (0.78–0.96)	0.005	0.87 (0.79–0.97)	0.01
(B) All-cause Mortality	**Model 1**		**Model 2**	
Variables	HR (95% CI)	p Value	HR (95% CI)	p Value
Age (per 10 years increment)	1.66 (1.41–1.96)	<0.001	1.66 (1.40–1.96)	<0.001
Previous myocardial infarction	0.85 (0.58–1.24)	0.40	0.89 (0.61–1.31)	0.56
Paroxysmal or persistent AF	1.20 (0.89–1.61)	0.24	1.20 (0.89–1.62)	0.24
Previous coronary revascularization	1.11 (0.75–1.63)	0.60	1.08 (0.73–1.59)	0.70
Acute decompensated heart failure	1.00 (0.71–1.39)	0.99	1.02 (0.73–1.43)	0.90
Systolic blood pressure (per 10 mmHg increment)	0.93 (0.89–0.97)	0.002	0.92 (0.88–0.97)	<0.001
Heart rate (per 10 beats per minutes increment)	1.03 (0.97–1.08)	0.35	1.02 (0.97–1.08)	0.37
Hemoglobin (per 1 g/dL increment)	0.90 (0.85–0.96)	0.002	0.91 (0.85–0.97)	0.004
CKD	1.02 (0.75–1.37)	0.92	1.05 (0.78–1.42)	0.74
hs-CRP (per 10-fold increment)	1.13 (0.95–1.35)	0.17	1.15 (0.97–1.37)	0.10
BNP (per 10-fold increment)	1.89 (1.39–2.57)	<0.001	1.86 (1.36–2.53)	<0.001
Urinary L-FABP (per 10-fold increment)	1.43 (1.18–1.72)	<0.001		
Urinary L-FABP (ng/mL)				
< 9.0 (1st + 2nd + 3rd quintile)			Reference	
≥ 9.0 (4th + 5th quintile)			1.50 (1.14–1.97)	0.003
LVEF (per 10% increment)	0.87 (0.78–0.97)	0.009	0.88 (0.79–0.98)	0.02

Multivariate model adjusted for all baseline variables with $p < 0.05$ by univariate analysis. L-FABP levels were assessed as either continuous variables (Model 1) or variables categorized into quintiles (Model 2). HR, hazard ratio; CI, confidence interval; AF, atrial fibrillation; CKD, chronic kidney disease; hs-CRP, high-sensitivity C-reactive protein; BNP, B-type natriuretic peptide; L-FABP, liver-type fatty-acid-binding protein; LVEF, left ventricular ejection fraction.

3.3. Discrimination and Reclassification of L-FABP for Adverse Outcomes

We assessed the effect of adding L-FABP to a baseline model of established risk factors. As shown in Table 4, adding L-FABP significantly improved the reclassification of patients beyond that of the baseline model alone ($p < 0.001$); IDI improved similarly after adding L-FABP ($p = 0.002$). Conversely, the C-index did not improve beyond the baseline model alone, considering that the C-statistic is insensitive for comparing the models [18]. Similar results were seen for all-cause death (Table 4).

Table 4. Discrimination and reclassification of L-FABP.

(A) Primary Endpoint						
	C-index	p Value	NRI	p Value	IDI	p Value
Established risk factor model	0.756	Reference		Reference		Reference
Established risk factor model + L-FABP	0.763	0.76	0.252	<0.001	0.013	0.002
(B) All-cause Mortality						
	C-index	p Value	NRI	p Value	IDI	p Value
Established risk factor model	0.760	Reference		Reference		Reference
Established risk factor model + L-FABP	0.766	0.80	0.222	0.001	0.012	0.004

Established risk factors included age, hypertension, diabetes mellitus, chronic kidney disease, atrial fibrillation, acute decompensated heart failure, previous myocardial infarction, previous coronary revascularization, systolic blood pressure, heart rate, mechanical ventilation before admission, and B-type natriuretic peptide. L-FABP, liver-type fatty-acid-binding protein; NRI, net reclassification improvement; IDI, integrated discrimination improvement.

3.4. Combination of L-FABP and Creatinine-Defined AKI

We classified the patients into four groups according to the L-FABP increment (≥4th quintile value of 9.0 ng/mL) or creatinine-defined AKI status. The Kaplan–Meier primary-endpoint free survival rates were 83.5% in patients without increased L-FABP or creatinine-defined AKI ($n = 612$), 75.7% in patients without creatinine-defined AKI who had increased L-FABP ($n = 300$), 77.3% in patients with creatinine-defined AKI who did not have increased L-FABP ($n = 75$), and 61.4% in patients with both increased L-FABP and creatinine-defined AKI ($n = 132$) ($p < 0.001$; Figure 2). Increased L-FABP without creatinine-defined AKI was identified in 59% ($n = 300$) of patients with AKI, indicating subclinical AKI, compared with creatinine-defined AKI only, and these patients were at a greater risk of the primary endpoint than those without increased L-FABP or creatinine-defined AKI ($p = 0.02$). Similar results were observed for all-cause death (Figure 2).

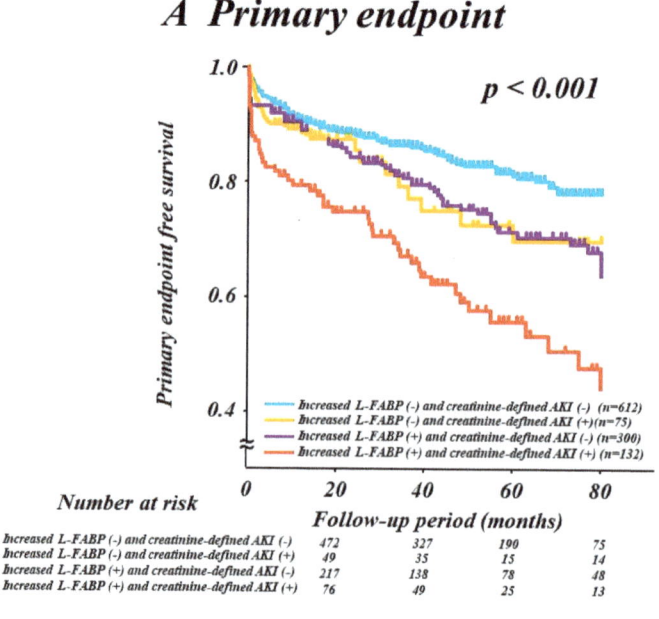

Figure 2. Cont.

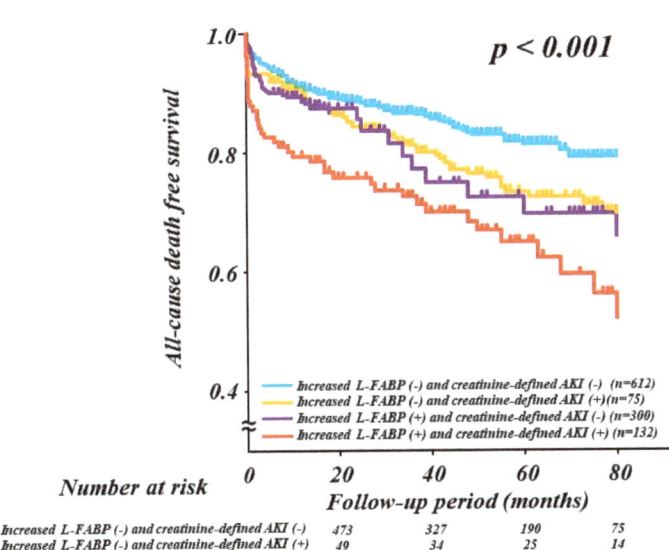

Figure 2. Kaplan–Meier curves for the primary endpoint (**A**) and all-cause mortality (**B**) according to L-FABP increment (≥9 ng/mL) or serum creatinine-defined AKI status. AKI, acute kidney injury; L-FABP, liver-type fatty-acid-binding protein.

4. Discussion

The prospective study obtained the following main findings. First, urinary L-FABP levels upon admission were significantly independent predictors of both the primary endpoint and all-cause mortality in patients treated at medical CICUs. Second, urinary L-FABP improved the predictive value for both the primary endpoint and all-cause mortality beyond that achieved with baseline model with established risk factors, as demonstrated by NRI and IDI. Third, the combination of increased L-FABP levels and creatinine-defined AKI status correlated with an increased risk of both the primary endpoint and all-cause mortality. Thus, urinary L-FABP levels on admission are potential and independent predictors of long-term adverse outcomes, and when used in combination with creatinine-defined AKI, they might improve the long-term risk stratification of patients hospitalized at medical CICUs. As supported by our results, the novel AKI definition that considers the urinary tubular injury biomarker concentrations, might be preferable to current definitions that are limited to changes in serum creatinine alone [7,10–12].

Although AKI is a common complication in patients treated at medical CICUs [19,20], urinary L-FABP levels in such patients has rarely been investigated, compared to those treated at ICUs after surgery (particularly cardiac) and those with septic patients [21,22]. The present study has demonstrated that urinary L-FABP on admission predicts long-term adverse outcomes in a large ($n = 1119$), heterogeneous cohort of patients treated at medical CICUs and that the combination of increased L-FABP and creatinine-defined AKI status improves the long-term risk stratification of patients hospitalized at medical CICUs.

Considering that urinary tubular injury markers provide information different from that provided by creatinine-defined AKI, the combined assessment of urinary tubular injury marker and creatinine-defined AKI status can be clinically beneficial. According to the present study, the combination of increased L-FABP on admission and the presence of creatinine-defined AKI could stratify the long-term prognostic risk of patients treated at medical CICUs, as shown in patients after cardiac surgery [21]. As expected, severe long-term outcomes were found in patients with both increased L-FABP and creatinine-defined AKI (tubular damage with kidney excretory dysfunction), whereas favorable outcomes were observed in patients without increased L-FABP or creatinine-defined AKI (no tubular damage and no excretory dysfunction). Urinary L-FABP identified approximately 60% more patients with increased L-FABP but without creatinine-defined AKI (tubular damage without excretory dysfunction)—an indicator of subclinical AKI—than those with creatinine-defined AKI status alone. This outcome was intermediate in severity. A smaller group (6.7%) of patients had creatinine-defined AKI but no increased L-FABP, implying the loss of renal function without the evidence of acute tubular injury and showing an intermediate outcome. These findings are consistent with recent reports involving patients after cardiac surgery, suggesting that the urinary tubular marker complements creatinine-defined AKI in long-term prognosis [11,12].

Urinary renal tubular injury markers have been investigated in critically ill patients, for an earlier identification of AKI, improved AKI diagnosis, and aid in risk stratification [9,22–24]. However, the association of urinary tubular injury markers with long-term mortality has been seldom studied [11,12]. In the Translation Research Investigating Biomarker Endpoints for Acute Kidney Injury (TRIBE-AKI) study involving 1,199 adult patients who underwent cardiac surgery, Coca et al. showed that higher urinary interleukin 18 (IL-18) and kidney injury molecule 1 (KIM-1) levels were independently associated with 3-year mortality, regardless of the creatinine-defined AKI status [11]. Moreover, in 200 adult patients who also underwent cardiac surgery, Albert et al. reported that the combined assessment of urinary neutrophil gelatinase-associated lipocalin (NGAL) with creatinine-defined AKI status could stratify the risk of mortality within a median follow-up period of 5.6 years [12]. The authors also confirmed an increased risk of long-term mortality in subclinical AKI patients. These two studies did not evaluate BNP and high-sensitivity troponin levels, markers of left ventricular overload and myocardial injury, respectively, even though these markers are also prognostic markers in patients with cardiovascular disease. Thus, urinary L-FABP levels were independent predictors in the multivariate Cox regression model of clinical and laboratory parameters including BNP, in a heterogeneous cohort of 1119 patients treated at medical CICUs. Given that the hs-TnT levels were not significantly associated with long-term adverse outcomes in a univariate Cox regression analysis, it was not integrated in the Cox multivariate model. Furthermore, adding urinary L-FABP improved the predictive value for long-term adverse outcomes beyond that achieved with the baseline model of established risk factors, including BNP, as demonstrated by NRI and IDI.

The mechanisms that emphasize the association between increased L-FABP and long-term adverse outcomes are still unclear. Kidneys are an excellent barometer of cardiac and vascular function [25]. Recently, in 968 adult post-cardiac surgery patients from the TRIBE-AKI cohort, Parikh et al. found that the plasma markers for cardiac injury (high-sensitivity troponin and heart-type fatty-acid-binding protein) or left ventricular overload (N-terminal pro-BNP), but not urinary tubular injury markers (IL-18, NGAL, KIM-1, L-FABP, and albumin), were independently associated with increased long-term risk of cardiovascular events [25]. Thus, higher urinary L-FABP levels might reflect a more severe AKI but might not be on the casual pathway to long-term adverse outcomes. Patients who manifest a more severe AKI might be at a greater risk for long-term complications, such as death, caused by a worse functioning of other organs rather than the episode of AKI [11].

In the present study, we used ELISA, which requires approximately 3 hours to measure the urinary L-FABP levels. Recently, a latex-enhanced immunoturbidimetric assay has been established using an autoanalyzer, which was simple, speedy (within 30 min) [26], and relatively inexpensive to assay, for quantifying urinary L-FABP. Thus, the easy and rapid assay system is expected to facilitate urinary L-FABP analysis in clinical practice.

Our study had several limitations. First, this study was conducted at a single institution. Second, we evaluated urinary L-FABP as an absolute concentration; we did not use urinary creatinine correction because the urinary creatinine excretion rate might change over time under nonsteady state conditions [27]. When the L-FABP values were analyzed using urinary creatinine correction, no association was found between the L-FABP levels and outcomes (data not shown). Finally, AKI was only defined according to serum creatinine increase, because of the inconsistent data recorded and the potential alterations in urine volume induced by medical therapy. This limitation might lead to the neglect of a part of the renal insult, which might be determined by urine output.

5. Conclusions

Urinary L-FABP levels on admission are potent and independent predictors of long-term adverse outcomes in patients treated at medical CICUs. When used in combination with creatinine-defined AKI, urinary L-FABP might substantially improve the long-term risk stratification of patients admitted at medical CICUs.

Author Contributions: Conceptualization, H.N. (Hiroyuki Naruse) and J.I.; methodology, H.N. (Hiroyuki Naruse) and J.I.; software, H.T.; validation, H.N. (Hiroyuki Naruse); formal analysis, H.T.; investigation, F.K., H.N. (Hideto Nishimura), H.K., T.M., M.H. (Masahide Harada), A.Y., S.M., and M.S.; resources, J.I.; data curation, H.N. (Hiroyuki Naruse) and H.N. (Hideto Nishimura); writing—original draft preparation, H.N. (Hiroyuki Naruse); writing—review and editing, all authors; supervision, E.W., H.I. and Y.O.; funding acquisition, J.I. All authors have read and agreed to the published version of the manuscript.

Funding: This work was supported by JSPS KAKENHI (17K08995).

Acknowledgments: We thank the staff of the Department of Cardiology at Fujita Health University School of Medicine for their assistance in recruiting the participants.

Conflicts of Interest: All authors declare that they have no conflict of interest.

References

1. Portilla, D. Energy metabolism and cytotoxicity. *Semin. Nephrol.* 2003, 23, 432–438. [CrossRef]
2. Yamamoto, T.; Noiri, E.; Ono, Y.; Doi, K.; Negishi, K.; Kamijo, A.; Kimura, K.; Fujita, T.; Kinukawa, T.; Taniguchi, H.; et al. Renal L-type fatty acid-binding protein in acute ischemic injury. *J. Am. Soc. Nephrol.* 2007, 18, 2894–2902. [CrossRef] [PubMed]
3. Xu, Y.; Xie, Y.; Shao, X.; Ni, Z.; Mou, S. L-FABP: a novel biomarker of kidney disease. *Clin. Chim. Acta* 2015, 445, 85–90. [CrossRef] [PubMed]
4. Nakamura, K.; Ito, K.; Kato, Y.; Sugaya, T.; Kubo, Y.; Tsuji, A. L-type fatty acid binding protein transgenic mouse as a novel tool to explore cytotoxicity to renal proximal tubules. *Drug Metab. Pharmacokinet.* 2008, 23, 271–278. [CrossRef] [PubMed]
5. Naruse, H.; Ishii, J.; Takahashi, H.; Kitagawa, F.; Nishimura, H.; Kawai, H.; Muramatsu, T.; Harada, M.; Yamada, A.; Motoyama, S.; et al. Predicting acute kidney injury using urinary liver-type fatty-acid binding protein and serum N-terminal pro-B-type natriuretic peptide levels in patients treated at medical cardiac intensive care units. *Crit. Care.* 2018, 22, 197. [CrossRef]
6. Naruse, H.; Takahashi, H.; Ishii, J. Authors' response to letter "Prediction of acute kidney injury in intensive care unit patients". *Crit. Care.* 2019, 23, 58. [CrossRef]
7. De Oliveira, B.D.; Xu, K.; Shen, T.H.; Callahan, M.; Kiryluk, K.; D'Agati, V.D.; Tatonetti, N.P.; Barasch, J.; Devarajan, P. Molecular nephrology: types of acute tubular injury. *Nat. Rev. Nephrol.* 2019, 15, 599–612.
8. Doi, K.; Negishi, K.; Ishizu, T.; Katagiri, D.; Fujita, T.; Matsubara, T.; Yahagi, N.; Sugaya, T.; Noiri, E. Evaluation of new acute kidney injury biomarkers in a mixed intensive care unit. *Crit. Care. Med.* 2011, 39, 2464–2469. [CrossRef]
9. McIlroy, D.R.; Farkas, D.; Matto, M.; Lee, H.T. Neutrophil gelatinase-associated lipocalin combined with delta serum creatinine provides early risk stratification for adverse outcomes after cardiac surgery: A prospective observational study. *Crit. Care. Med.* 2015, 43, 1043–1052. [CrossRef]
10. Haase, M.; Devarajan, P.; Haase-Fielitz, A.; Bellomo, R.; Cruz, D.N.; Wagener, G.; Krawczeski, C.D.; Koyner, J.L.; Murray, P.; Zappitelli, M.; et al. The outcome of neutrophil gelatinase-associated lipocalin-positive subclinical acute kidney injury: A multicenter pooled analysis of prospective studies. *J. Am. Coll. Cardiol.* 2011, 57, 1752–1761. [CrossRef]

11. Coca, S.G.; Garg, A.X.; Thiessen-Philbrook, H.; Koyner, J.L.; Patel, U.D.; Krumholz, H.M.; Shlipak, M.G.; Parikh, C.R. Urinary biomarkers of AKI and mortality 3 years after cardiac surgery. *J. Am. Soc. Nephrol.* **2014**, *25*, 1063–1071. [CrossRef] [PubMed]
12. Albert, C.; Albert, A.; Kube, J.; Bellomo, R.; Wettersten, N.; Kuppe, H.; Westphal, S.; Haase, M.; Haase-Fielitz, A. Urinary biomarkers may provide prognostic information for subclinical acute kidney injury after cardiac surgery. *J. Thorac. Cardiovasc. Surg.* **2018**, *155*, 2441–2452. [CrossRef] [PubMed]
13. Kidney Disease: Improving global outcomes (KDIGO) acute kidney injury work group (2012) KDIGO clinical practice guideline for acute kidney injury. *Kidney Int. Suppl.* **2012**, *2*, 1–138.
14. Matsuo, S.; Imai, E.; Horio, M.; Yasuda, Y.; Tomita, K.; Nitta, K.; Yamagata, K.; Tomino, Y.; Yokoyama, H.; Hishida, A. Revised equations for estimated GFR from serum creatinine in Japan. *Am. J. Kidney Dis.* **2009**, *53*, 982–992. [CrossRef]
15. Vincent, J.L.; Moreno, R.; Takala, J.; Willatts, S.; De Mendonça, A.; Bruining, H.; Reinhart, C.K.; Suter, P.M.; Thijs, L.G. The SOFA (Sepsis-related Organ Failure Assessment) score to describe organ dysfunction/failure. On behalf of the Working Group on Sepsis-Related Problems of the European Society of Intensive Care Medicine. *Intensive Care Med.* **1996**, *22*, 707–710. [CrossRef]
16. DeLong, E.R.; DeLong, D.M.; Clarke-Pearson, D.L. Comparing the areas under two or more correlated receiver operating characteristic curves: a nonparametric approach. *Biometrics.* **1998**, *44*, 837–845. [CrossRef]
17. Pencina, M.J.; D'Agostino, R.B., Sr.; D'Agostino, R.B., Jr.; Vasan, R.S. Evaluating the added predictive ability of a new marker from area under the ROC curve to reclassification and beyond. *Stat Med.* **2008**, *27*, 157–172. [CrossRef]
18. Cook, N.R. Use and misuse of the receiver operating characteristic curve in risk prediction. *Circulation* **2007**, *115*, 928–935. [CrossRef]
19. Holland, E.M.; Moss, T.J. Acute Noncardiovascular Illness in the Cardiac Intensive Care Unit. *J. Am. Coll. Cardiol.* **2017**, *69*, 1999–2007. [CrossRef] [PubMed]
20. Iwagami, M.; Yasunaga, H.; Noiri, E.; Horiguchi, H.; Fushimi, K.; Matsubara, T.; Yahagi, N.; Nangaku, M.; Doi, K. Choice of renal replacement therapy modality in intensive care units: data from a Japanese Nationwide Administrative Claim Database. *J. Crit. Care* **2015**, *30*, 381–385. [CrossRef]
21. Katagiri, D.; Doi, K.; Honda, K.; Negishi, K.; Fujita, T.; Hisagi, M.; Ono, M.; Matsubara, T.; Yahagi, N.; Iwagami, M.; et al. Combination of two urinary biomarkers predicts acute kidney injury after adult cardiac surgery. *Ann. Thorac. Surg.* **2012**, *93*, 577–583. [CrossRef] [PubMed]
22. Doi, K.; Noiri, E.; Maeda-Mamiya, R.; Ishii, T.; Negishi, K.; Hamasaki, Y.; Fujita, T.; Yahagi, N.; Koide, H.; Sugaya, T.; et al. Urinary L-type fatty acid-binding protein as a new biomarker of sepsis complicated with acute kidney injury. *Crit. Care Med.* **2010**, *38*, 2037–2042. [CrossRef] [PubMed]
23. Cho, E.; Yang, H.N.; Jo, S.K.; Cho, W.Y.; Kim, H.K. The role of urinary liver-type fatty acid-binding protein in critically ill patients. *J. Korean Med. Sci.* **2013**, *28*, 100–105. [CrossRef]
24. Parr, S.K.; Clark, A.J.; Bian, A.; Shintani, A.K.; Wickersham, N.E.; Ware, L.B.; Ikizler, T.A.; Siew, E.D. Urinary L-FABP predicts poor outcomes in critically ill patients with early acute kidney injury. *Kidney Int.* **2015**, *87*, 640–648. [CrossRef] [PubMed]
25. Parikh, C.R.; Puthumana, J.; Shlipak, M.G.; Koyner, J.L.; Thiessen-Philbrook, H.; McArthur, E.; Kerr, K.; Kavsak, P.; Whitlock, R.P.; Garg, A.X.; et al. Relationship of Kidney Injury Biomarkers with Long-Term Cardiovascular Outcomes after Cardiac Surgery. *J. Am. Soc. Nephrol.* **2017**, *28*, 3699–3707. [CrossRef] [PubMed]
26. Kamijo-Ikemori, A.; Sugaya, T.; Yoshida, M.; Hoshino, S.; Akatsu, S.; Yamazaki, S.; Kimura, K.; Shibagaki, Y. Clinical utility of urinary liver-type fatty acid binding protein measured by latex-enhanced turbidimetric immunoassay in chronic kidney disease. *Clin. Chem. Lab. Med.* **2016**, *54*, 1645–1654. [CrossRef] [PubMed]
27. Waikar, S.S.; Sabbisetti, V.S.; Bonventre, J.V. Normalization of urinary biomarkers to creatinine during changes in glomerular filtration rate. *Kidney Int.* **2010**, *78*, 486–494. [CrossRef]

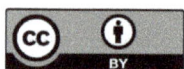

© 2020 by the authors. Licensee MDPI, Basel, Switzerland. This article is an open access article distributed under the terms and conditions of the Creative Commons Attribution (CC BY) license (http://creativecommons.org/licenses/by/4.0/).

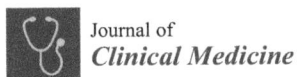 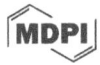

Article

Pregnancy Associated Plasma Protein-A as a Cardiovascular Risk Marker in Patients with Stable Coronary Heart Disease During 10 Years Follow-Up—A CLARICOR Trial Sub-Study

Erik Nilsson [1,2,*], Jens Kastrup [3], Ahmad Sajadieh [4], Gorm Boje Jensen [5], Erik Kjøller [6,11], Hans Jørn Kolmos [7], Jonas Wuopio [8], Christoph Nowak [9], Anders Larsson [10], Janus Christian Jakobsen [11,12], Per Winkel [11], Christian Gluud [11], Kasper K Iversen [6], Johan Ärnlöv [9,13] and Axel C. Carlsson [9]

[1] Department of Medical Epidemiology and Biostatistics, Karolinska Institutet, 17177 Stockholm, Sweden
[2] School of Medical Sciences, Örebro University, 70182 Örebro, Sweden
[3] Department of Cardiology, Rigshospitalet University of Copenhagen, 2100 Copenhagen, Denmark; jens.kastrup@regionh.dk
[4] Department of Cardiology, Copenhagen University Hospital of Bispebjerg and Frederiksberg, 2000 Frederiksberg, Denmark; ahmad.sajadieh@regionh.dk
[5] Department of Cardiology, Hvidovre Hospital University of Copenhagen, 2650 Hvidovre, Denmark; gorm.boje.jensen.01@regionh.dk
[6] Department of Cardiology S, Herlev Hospital University of Copenhagen, 2730 Herlev, Denmark; kjoller@dadlnet.dk (E.K.); kasper.karmark.iversen@regionh.dk (K.K.I.)
[7] Department of Clinical Microbiology, Odense University Hospital, 5000 Odense, Denmark; h.j.kolmos@dadlnet.dk
[8] Department of Medicine, Mora County Hospital, 79251 Mora, Sweden; jonas.wuopio@ltdalarna.se
[9] Division for Family Medicine and Primary Care, Department of Neurobiology, Care Sciences and Society, Karolinska Institutet, 14183 Huddinge, Sweden; christoph.nowak@ki.se (C.N.); axelcefam@hotmail.com (A.C.C.)
[10] Department of Medical Sciences, Uppsala University, 75185 Uppsala, Sweden; anders.larsson@akademiska.se
[11] Copenhagen Trial Unit, Centre for Clinical Intervention Research, Rigshospitalet, Copenhagen University Hospital, 2100 Copenhagen, Denmark; janus.jakobsen@ctu.dk (J.C.J.); per.winkel@ctu.dk (P.W.); christian.gluud@ctu.dk (C.G.)
[12] Department of Cardiology, Holbæk Hospital, 4300 Holbæk, Denmark
[13] School of Health and Social Studies, Dalarna University, 79131 Falun, Sweden; johan.arnlov@ki.se
* Correspondence: erik.alfred.nilsson@gmail.com

Received: 5 December 2019; Accepted: 15 January 2020; Published: 20 January 2020

Abstract: Elevated pregnancy-associated plasma protein A (PAPP-A) is associated with mortality in acute coronary syndromes. Few studies have assessed PAPP-A in stable coronary artery disease (CAD) and results are conflicting. We assessed the 10-year prognostic relevance of PAPP-A levels in stable CAD. The CLARICOR trial was a randomized controlled clinical trial including outpatients with stable CAD, randomized to clarithromycin versus placebo. The placebo group constituted our discovery cohort ($n = 1.996$) and the clarithromycin group the replication cohort ($n = 1.975$). The composite primary outcome was first occurrence of cardiovascular event or death. In the discovery cohort, incidence rates (IR) for the composite outcome were higher in those with elevated PAPP-A (IR 12.72, 95% Confidence Interval (CI) 11.0–14.7 events/100 years) compared to lower PAPP-A (IR 8.78, 8.25–9.34), with comparable results in the replication cohort. Elevated PAPP-A was associated with increased risk of the composite outcome in both cohorts (discovery Hazard Ratio (HR) 1.45, 95% CI 1.24–1.70; replication HR 1.29, 95% CI 1.10–1.52). In models adjusted for established risk factors, these trends were attenuated. Elevated PAPP-A was associated with higher all-cause mortality in both cohorts. We conclude that elevated PAPP-A levels are associated with increased long-term mortality in stable CAD, but do not improve long-term prediction of death or cardiovascular events when added to established predictors.

Keywords: pregnancy-associated plasma protein-A; coronary artery disease; cohort studies; biomarkers

1. Introduction

Pregnancy-associated plasma protein-A (PAPP-A) is a cell membrane-bound metalloproteinase which regulates local availability of insulin-like growth factor 1 (IGF-1) [1]. It has been evaluated as a prognostic biomarker in acute coronary syndromes [2–11], where elevated levels are associated with increased risk of death. However, this association may be confounded by heparin treatment causing elevated PAPP-A levels in vivo through release of PAPP-A attached to cell membranes [12]. Further, PAPP-A levels predict cardiovascular events in troponin-negative patients with suspected acute coronary syndrome [3] and higher levels of circulating PAPP-A are associated with more extensive coronary artery disease [13] as well as with plaque inflammation and echogenicity [14]. In chronic stable angina pectoris PAPP-A has been less extensively studied and is associated with outcomes in some studies [15–18] but not all [19]. Studies with long-term follow-up are scarce.

PAPP-A regulates downstream growth hormone effects in the paracellular environment by cleaving insulin-like growth factor binding protein 4 (IGFBP4) bound to insulin-like growth factor 1 (IGF-1), thereby making IGF-1 available to its receptor. Since PAPP-A is normally bound to the cell membrane and not abundantly expressed, increased plasma levels in the absence of heparin treatment may represent up-regulation due to inflammation or tissue damage, in combination with escape into the circulation [20–22].

The present study is part of the larger PREdictors for MAjor Cardiovascular outcomes in stable ischemic heart disease (PREMAC) study, which aimed to identify biochemical predictors of cardiovascular events and all-cause mortality in persons with stable coronary artery disease (CAD) utilizing data originating from the CLARICOR (clarithromycin for patients with stable coronary heart disease) trial [23]. In the CLARICOR Trial, patients were randomized to clarithromycin or placebo and the main outcomes consisted of myocardial infarction (AMI), unstable angina pectoris (UAP), cardiovascular mortality, and all-cause mortality. In a previous report on the same cohort, elevated PAPP-A, defined as values ≥ 4 µ/mL, was found to predict risk of death and myocardial infarction during medium term (median 2.8 years) follow up [17]. The aim of the present study was to assess the predictive power of elevated PAPP-A levels for the 10-year outcomes in stable CAD.

2. Experimental Section

The PREMAC study focused on the presence of predictors of cardiovascular events and all-cause mortality in persons with stable CAD and included a detailed statistical analysis plan [23]. Biomarker assessment was performed using stored biobank samples from the CLARICOR trial [24] and outcome data was retrieved from public registers. The CLARICOR trial was approved by local ethics committees and regulatory authorities (Regional Ethics Committee HB 2009/015 and KF 01-076/99; the Danish Data Protection Agency 1999–1200–174 and 2012–41–0757; and the Danish Medicines Agency 2612–975).

2.1. Patient Selection

The CLARICOR trial was a randomized, placebo-controlled trial with blinded outcome assessment including outpatients with stable CAD. All patients discharged from wards or outpatient clinics in the Copenhagen area in Denmark with a diagnosis of acute myocardial infarction or unstable angina pectoris during the years 1993–1999 who were alive and aged 18–85 years old in 1999 (n = 13.702) were invited to a screening interview at one of five cardiology centers. Of the 6116 (44.6%) patients accepting the invitation, 1567 (25.6%) were excluded, 177 (2.9%) chose not to participate, and the remaining 4372 (71.5%) were randomized to oral clarithromycin 500 mg once daily for 2 weeks (n = 2.172) vs. placebo (n = 2.200) during the winter 1999–2000. Exclusion criteria of the CLARICOR trial were: AMI or UAP within the previous 3 months, percutaneous transluminal coronary angioplasty and coronary bypass surgery within the previous 6 months, impaired renal or hepatic function, congestive heart failure (New York Heart Association (NYHA) IV classification of heart failure), active malignancy, incapacity to manage own affairs, breast feeding, and possible pregnancy. In the CLARICOR trial, clarithromycin was found to increase both the risk of cardiovascular and all-cause mortality [24–27].

The patients randomized to placebo in the CLARICOR study were included as the discovery cohort in the present study, while those randomized to clarithromycin formed the replication cohort. We excluded participants with missing data in any of the variables, leaving n = 1.996 (92%) in the discovery cohort, and n = 1.975 (90%) in the replication cohort.

2.2. Baseline Data

During enrollment interviews, smoking status, current medication, and known hypertension or diabetes were noted. Information concerning sex, age, and history of myocardial infarction or unstable angina pectoris were extracted from local hospital files. Blood samples were collected at each of the study sites immediately before randomization, using blood collection tubes without additives. Serum was prepared according to normal hospital routine with approximately coagulation for 30 min and centrifugation at 1500 g for 10 min. Serum was frozen on the day of collection at −20 °C and at −80 °C after transportation to the central laboratory facility. Storage problems were the only noteworthy cause of missing data. Estimated glomerular filtration rate (eGFR) was calculated using the creatinine-based Chronic Kidney Disease Epidemiology Collaboration (CKD-EPI) formula [28]. Smoking status was categorized as never, former, or current smoker. No physical investigations were made at randomization interview; nor were any longitudinal predictor information collected during follow-up.

2.3. Pregnancy-Associated Plasma Protein A Levels

The PAPP-A levels measured in a previous study were used in the present study [17]. The enzyme-linked immunosorbent assay used for quantification of PAPP-A has been described in detail previously [17,29]. The detection limit was 4 mIU/L. The intra-assay coefficient of variation was 2.0% at 71.7 mIU/L and 5.7% at 10.4 mIU/L, with corresponding inter-assay coefficients of variation of 6.4% and 8.7%, respectively. Elevated serum PAPP-A was defined as values at or above 4 mIU/L, based on levels in healthy blood donors [29]. Note that although the CLARICOR trial data did not include information on heparin use, study participants were outpatients with stable CAD and heparin is not used in this setting.

2.4. Outcomes

Follow-up was until 31 December 2009 where the official permissions expired. Outcome data was procured from national patient registries. These are mandatory for inpatient care and all events diagnosed and coded during hospital admission are therefore detected, resulting in virtually no loss to follow-up. Vital status was retrieved from the Danish Central Civil Register, cause of death from the National Register of Causes of Death, and hospital admissions from the Danish National Patient Register (NPR), which covers all hospital admissions. These registries have almost complete coverage [30]. By trial protocol, events during the first 2.6 years of follow-up were adjudicated by a blinded committee, previously described in detail [23,24]. For the 10-year studies, registry outcomes were used after verifying that the results were consistent with those based on adjudication data [30,31].

The Danish 10-digit central person registration (CPR) number is used at all contacts with the health care system. At discharge from hospital, at least one action diagnosis (A diagnosis) specifying the main reason for the admission is noted in the NPR. These A diagnoses, and in case of death the 'underlying cause of death' code (in the official terminology of the National Register of Causes of Death), was used for classifying outcomes according to the 10th revision of the International Statistical Classification of Diseases and Related Health Problems (ICD-10) coding system as follows: AMI (I21.0–23.9), UAP (I20.0 and I24.8–24.9), cerebrovascular disease (CeVD) (I60.0–64.9 and G45.0–46.8), cardiovascular death (I00.0–99.9 unless already covered), and death due to non-cardiovascular disease (A00.0–T98.3 unless already covered). A composite outcome was defined as AMI, UAP, CeVD, or death due to any cause. Follow-up time was censored at occurrence of an outcome, death, or end of follow-up (31st December 2009 giving a median possible survival time of 10 years ± 3 months after randomization).

2.5. Statistical Analysis

Incidence rates (IR) were calculated using only the first occurrence of an event and the time to event or censoring at end of study was used in the denominator. We used Cox proportional hazards model for the statistical analysis. Multivariable models were adjusted according to the pre-specified analysis plan, for clinical predictors (sex, age at randomization, smoking history, history of myocardial infarction, hypertension, and diabetes), medical treatment (acetylsalicylic acid, beta-blocker, calcium-antagonist, angiotensin-converting enzyme (ACE)-inhibitor, long lasting nitrate, diuretic, digoxin, statin, and anti-arrhythmic drugs), and standard biochemical predictors (log-transformed high-sensitivity-reactive protein (CRP), glomerular filtration rate (GFR) estimated by creatinine, triglycerides, total cholesterol, high-density lipoprotein (HDL) cholesterol, low-density lipoprotein (LDL) cholesterol, apolipoprotein A1, and apolipoprotein B). Standard predictors adjusted for in multivariable models are listed in Appendix A. Triglycerides and total cholesterol were log transformed.

As the proportional hazard's assumption was violated for age at entry for all-cause death and the composite outcome (Bonferroni adjusted $p < 0.0044$ for all-cause mortality; and $p < 0.00056$ for the composite outcome), we excluded age from all models for these two outcomes. In order to provide additional insights into the potential influence of age on these associations, we conducted multivariable logistic regression models (including age as a co-variate since the proportional hazard assumption is not a requisite for these analyses).

3. Results

Baseline characteristics of the discovery and replication cohorts are presented in Table 1 They showed no major differences between the cohorts. The proportion of participants with elevated PAPP-A levels was 13% ($n = 263$) in the discovery cohort and 12% ($n = 244$) in the replication cohort.

Table 2 displays outcomes by PAPP-A level. In the discovery cohort, the composite outcome was more common among those who elevated PAPP-A, compared to those with low PAPP-A levels (72% compared to 59%), with a corresponding difference in incidence rates ($p < 0.0001$). The same pattern was seen in the replication cohort.

Table 1. Baseline characteristics of the two study cohorts.

Variable	Discovery Cohort	Replication Cohort
Number of participants	1996	1975
PAPP-A ≥ 4 mIU/L	263 (13)	244 (12)
Female	623 (31)	602 (30)
Age at entry, years	65 ± 10	65 ± 10
CRP, mg/L	5.25 ± 7.7	5.76 ± 9.3
Apolipoprotein A1, mg/dL	1.70 ± 0.34	1.70 ± 0.36
Apolipoprotein, mg/dL	1.21 ± 0.32	1.21 ± 0.33
eGFR, mL/min	76.3 ± 20	76.5 ± 19
Diabetes mellitus	299 (15)	301 (15)
Hypertension	805 (40)	790 (40)
Never smoked	394 (20)	339 (17)
Former smoker	925 (46)	903 (46)
Current smoker	677 (34)	735 (37)
History of myocardial infarction	635 (32)	640 (32)
Statin treatment	822 (41)	812 (41)
Aspirin treatment	1763 (88)	1733 (88)
Beta blocker treatment	619 (31)	589 (30)
Calcium antagonist treatment	702 (35)	680 (34)
ACE inhibitor treatment	522 (26)	552 (28)
Long-acting nitrate treatment	412 (21)	411 (21)
Diuretics treatment	690 (35)	698 (35)
Digoxin treatment	115 (6)	138 (7)
Antiarrhythmic treatment	42 (2)	46 (2)

Baseline characteristics in the discovery (placebo) and replication (clarithromycin) cohorts, presented as mean ± standard deviation for continuous variables and n (%) for categorical variables. Abbreviations: PAPP-A: pregnancy-associated plasma protein A; CRP: high sensitivity C-reactive protein; eGFR: estimated glomerular filtration rate; ACE: angiotensin converting enzyme.

Table 2. Incidence rates of the composite outcome by PAPP-A level.

PAPP-A Category	Variable	Discovery Cohort	Replication Cohort
PAPP-A ≥ 4 mIU/L	N	263	244
	Outcomes, N (%)	189 (72)	168 (69)
	IR, per 100 years	12.72	12.04
	95% CI	11.0–14.7	10.35–14.01
PAPP-A < 4 mIU/L	N	1733	1731
	Outcomes, N (%)	1015 (59)	1052 (61)
	IR per 100 years	8.78	9.38
	95% CI	8.25–9.34	8.83–9.96

The composite outcome was defined as acute myocardial infarction, unstable angina pectoris, cerebrovascular disease, or death due to any cause. Outcomes (with % of participants at risk) is the number of persons experiencing the composite outcome during 10-years follow-up. Incidence rates (IR) were calculated using only the first occurrence of the outcome during follow-up. Abbreviations: PAPP-A: pregnancy-associated plasma protein A; CI, Confidence Interval.

In the survival analysis (Table 3), Cox proportional hazards models adjusted for sex (model A) showed that PAPP-A ≥ 4 µ/mL was associated with an increased risk of the composite outcome in the discovery cohort and, less markedly, in the replication cohort; with adjustment for a large number of other risk factors (model B, see Table 3), comprising comorbidities and biochemical markers, these risk trends were attenuated in the discovery cohort and disappeared in the replication cohort.

Table 3. Risk of composite outcome associated with the binary covariate elevated PAPP-A.

Variable	Discovery Cohort		Replication Cohort	
	Model A	Model B	Model A	Model B
Hazard ratio	1.45	1.29	1.28	1.06
95% CI	1.24–1.70	1.10–1.52	1.08–1.50	0.89–1.25
p-value	< 0.001	< 0.001	0.003	0.51

Cox proportional hazards models are applied to the composite outcome defined as acute myocardial infarction, unstable angina pectoris, cerebrovascular disease, or death due to any cause. Model A was adjusted for sex. Model B was adjusted for established risk factors and co-morbidities, standard biochemical predictors, and treatments as listed in Appendix A. All models in this table are shown without adjustments for age at entry. Abbreviations: PAPP-A, pregnancy-associated plasma protein A.

Comparable results, with elevated PAPP-A being associated with increased risk of the composite outcome in the discovery cohort, but not in the replication cohort, were found in adjusted logistic regression models (Table S1) where age was also included in the multivariable model. We found no interaction between sex and PAPP-A on mortality ($p = 0.22$) or on the composite outcome ($p = 0.17$).

The association between PAPP-A ≥ 4 mIU/L and other outcomes is shown in Table S2. Elevated PAPP-A was associated with higher all-cause mortality in the discovery cohort, an association that remained in the fully adjusted analysis as well as in a logistic regression that included age as a predictor variable (Table S1). These findings were reproduced in the replication cohort.

Interestingly, these secondary analyses suggest that PAPP-A elevation is at least as strong a predictor for non-cardiovascular as for cardiovascular death (Table S2).

We also evaluated the predictive utility of PAPP-A in the group of placebo-treated patients when added to a large number of standard predictors (Table S3). Adding elevated PAPP-A as a predictor produced no visible improvements (apart from a slight numerical instability).

4. Discussion

Our main finding is that PAPP-A levels ≥ 4 mIU/L are associated with increased long-term risk of composite adverse outcome as well as all-cause mortality in patients with stable CAD. Although the association to all-cause mortality remained after extensive multivariable adjustment, the association to the composite outcome was not reproduced in our replication cohort when adjusted for many other risk factors. This may indicate that the placebo group and the clarithromycin treated group (the replication group) are not completely compatible in that clarithromycin was found to increase mortality [24–27]. It may also indicate that the association between PAPP-A and outcomes is confounded by some of these other risk factors, for example diabetes [20,32]. Over-adjustment may also be a problem in this context [33]. Our choice of covariates in the various multivariate analyses was mandated by the choice made for the Cox analyses of the placebo-treated patients described in the pre-specified analysis plan.

The growth hormone (GH) axis and PAPP-A has been implicated in the progression of atherosclerosis. Locally, insulin-like growth factor 1 (IGF-1) promotes multiple mechanisms involved in plaque formation and an association between PAPP-A and atherosclerosis has been demonstrated [2,34]. PAPP-A is found in atherosclerotic plaques on cell-types involved in the atherosclerotic process, including vascular smooth muscle cells, endothelial cells and macrophages [1], its expression is elevated in vulnerable plaques [2]. PAPP-A activity is related to atherosclerotic lesion size in rodents [35,36] and higher levels of circulating PAPP-A are associated with more extensive coronary artery disease in humans [13].

Reduced PAPP-A activity is associated with diminished vascular cell proliferation in response to injury, reduced plaque area and less luminal occlusion in atherosclerosis [37]. Conversely, increased PAPP-A activity is associated with proliferation of vascular smooth muscle cells [34]. Regulation of vascular smooth muscle cell proliferation could therefore be a mechanism by which PAPP-A influences the atherosclerotic process. PAPP-A could also be linked to atherosclerosis through modulating the effects of IGF-1 on lipid-, glucose-, and protein metabolism [38,39].

However, the exact mechanism by which PAPP-A is involved (causally or as a by-product) in the promotion of atherosclerosis remains elusive, in part as a result of conflicting findings on the effects of IGF-1 action on the vasculature [40]. Notably, the relationship between serum levels of IGF-1 and PAPP-A and local IGF-1 activity is unclear and may for example be dependent on body composition, inflammation, or conditions such as diabetes mellitus or obesity [40]. Circulating levels are therefore not necessarily directly related to the hypothesized pathophysiological mechanisms by which IGF-1 and PAPP-A are implicated in development of coronary artery disease. Consequently, the association between PAPP-A and mortality described in the present study may be related to other factors than cardiovascular disease progression. Indeed, we did not find any clear association with cardiovascular outcomes and it should be noted that the IGF-1 system including PAPP-A may for example be related to development of cancer [41]. There was in our results consistently no association between elevated PAPP-A and myocardial infarction, UAP, or stroke, although there was an association to cardiovascular mortality in the minimally adjusted analysis in the replication cohort.

The association between PAPP-A levels and outcomes in stable CAD has been studied previously. In 103 stable CAD patients, with a median follow-up of 4.9 years, higher PAPP-A was associated with increased mortality as well as the composite outcome of death and acute coronary syndrome [15]. Interestingly, but potentially problematic [33], those authors adjusted their estimates for the extent of coronary atherosclerosis, which could be considered an intermediate in the hypothesized causal pathway between PAPP-A and cardiovascular events. In another cohort study, including 534 patients with stable CAD and 393 patients with acute coronary syndrome, with a median follow-up time of 5.0 years, the authors found no association to cardiovascular mortality in the subgroup stable CAD, but higher PAPP-A was associated with increased cardiovascular mortality in the overall cohort as well as in the acute coronary syndrome (ACS) subgroup [19]. Although these results were adjusted for several conventional predictors, there was no adjustment for age. In a previous study on the CLARICOR cohort participants, PAPP-A levels were studied in relation to medium-term outcomes [17]. Important differences in that study from the present study include a shorter follow-up (median 2.8 years), joining of the placebo and the treatment group in a single cohort, and differing definitions of the composite outcome. In line with our present results, the previous study found that elevated PAPP-A was associated with the composite outcome of myocardial infarction and death as well as all-cause mortality in adjusted analyses [17].

PAPP-A has also been studied in ACS, but there is limited generalizability from these studies to the context of stable CAD. In troponin-negative patients with suspected ACS, PAPP-A predicted future cardiovascular events [3], although we are uncertain if PAPP-A was sampled before administration of heparin. Others found that PAPP-A predicted cardiovascular events in ACS and it seems that PAPP-A was sampled after heparin infusion, indicating that the PAPP-A levels included PAPP-A released from the cell membrane during heparin treatment [6]. In that study, PAPP-A predicted outcomes in TnT-negative patients. Furthermore, differences in stable versus acute CAD may have support in PAPP-A physiology since chronic and transient PAPP-A expression may have differing effects on neointimal formation following vascular injury [42].

Our present study has several strengths: a large study sample, detailed characterization of the participants, longitudinal study design, 10 years follow-up, and a replication of all analyses in the clarithromycin group of the trial. As far as we know, there are no other large cohort studies on associations between PAPP-A levels in patients with stable CAD. National Danish registers are known to be of high completeness and accuracy [30], but a small number of non-fatal events can be missed when participants are hospitalized abroad. Results in our study are likely valid for patients with stable CAD as ascertained at the baseline interview and it remains to be shown if similar risks are seen for other relevant patient groups, such as patients with acute symptoms or patients during recovery from a major event.

Limitations are the unknown generalizability to other ethnic groups and to those unlikely to volunteer to participate in studies. Distortion by the active intervention with clarithromycin cannot be excluded, although we saw similar associations as to those in the placebo cohort. As regards the replication cohort, with its previously described surplus of unfavorable cardiovascular outcomes [26,27,43], we noted that elevated PAPP-A here tended to lose its unfavorable implications. Such interaction, if present, would imply that the harmful effect of clarithromycin was more marked in those with low PAPP-A levels. However, the trend nowhere came close to statistical significance. Nor do we have any theoretical arguments in favor thereof. Another limitation is that there was no data on heparin treatment at baseline. However, as the participants in our study had no indication for heparin, it is unlikely that this lack of data would have any substantial influence on our results and conclusions. In addition, there was no data on left ventricular ejection fraction, although this may be partially or completely compensated by other covariables included in the analyses, as age, sex, hypertension, prior acute myocardial infarction, creatinine, diuretics, and digoxin are related to left ventricular ejection fraction [44].

5. Conclusions

Elevated PAPP-A levels are associated with increased long-term mortality in stable CAD, but they do not improve long-term prediction of composite outcome of death or cardiovascular events when added to established predictors.

Supplementary Materials: The following are available online at http://www.mdpi.com/2077-0383/9/1/265/s1, Table S1: Logistic regression analyses of risk associated with elevated PAPP-A $\geq$ 4 mIU/L, Table S2: Risk of specific outcomes associated with elevated PAPP-A, Table S3: The role of elevated PAPP-A when used in combination with 'standard predictors' in the prediction of outcome status. All pertinent anonymized data will be uploaded at ZENODO (http://zenodo.org/) when the individual manuscripts have been published.

Author Contributions: Conceptualization, C.G. and A.S.; methodology, C.G., J.C.J., C.N., A.L., E.N., J.Ä., J.K., P.W., E.K., and J.W.; validation, C.G.; formal analysis, E.N., A.C.C., and P.W.; investigation, C.G., J.K., G.B.J., and K.K.I.; resources, C.G.; data curation, C.G. and P.W.; supervision, C.G., J.C.J. and J.Ä.; project administration, C.G. and G.B.J.; funding acquisition, C.G. and K.K.I.; software, P.W.; visualization, not applicable; writing—original draft preparation, E.N., A.C.C., and J.Ä.; writing—review and editing, All authors. All authors have read and agreed to the published version of the manuscript.

Funding: This study was funded by the Copenhagen Trial Unit, Centre for Clinical Intervention Research. The original funders of the CLARICOR trial were: The Danish Heart Foundation, grant numbers 01-1-5-21-22894, 99-2-5-103-22773, 99-1-5-87-22712, and 97-2-5-70-22537; The Copenhagen Hospital Corporation, grant date 7 October 1997; The Danish Research Council, grant numbers 9702122 and 22-00-0261; The 1991 Pharmacy Foundation, grant number HPN/ld/71-97; The Copenhagen Hospital Corporation and the Copenhagen Trial Unit. Abbott Laboratories, IDC, Queensborough, UK supplied the clarithromycin and placebo tablets.

Acknowledgments: We thank the CLARICOR trial participants. We thank the investigators and other staff involved in the first phases of the CLARICOR trial: Bodil Als-Nielsen, Morten Damgaard, Jørgen Fischer Hansen, Stig Hansen, Olav H. Helø, Per Hildebrandt, Jørgen Hilden, Inga Lind, Henrik Nielsen, Lars Petersen, Christian M. Jespersen, Maria Skoog, and Jane Lindschou.

Conflicts of Interest: The authors declare no conflict of interest. The funders had no role in the design of the study; in the collection, analyses, or interpretation of data; in the writing of the manuscript, or in the decision to publish the results.

Appendix A

Predictors Adjusted for in Multivariable Models

Predictors were pre-specified in the study protocol. Standard predictors adjusted for in multivariable models are listed below. Note that age at entry was omitted from Cox regression analyses due to violation of proportional hazard assumption when all-cause mortality and the composite outcome was analyzed.

Clinical predictors were: sex, age at entry, smoking history, history of myocardial infarction as opposed to angina only, hypertension, and diabetes.

Standard biochemical predictors were: Log-transformed high-sensitivity C-reactive protein (CRP), estimated glomerular filtration rate (eGFR) estimated by creatinine, triglycerides and lipoproteins (total cholesterol, high density lipoprotein (HDL) cholesterol, low density lipoprotein (LDL) cholesterol, apolipoprotein A1, and apolipoprotein B).

The current medical treatment was included as proxy predictors because information about post infarction heart failure and post-infarction angina pectoris are not available to us: Aspirin (Yes/No), beta-blocker (Yes/No), calcium antagonist (Yes/No), ACE inhibitor (Yes/No), long lasting nitrate (Yes/No), diuretic (Yes/No), digoxin (Yes/No), statin (Yes/No), and anti-arrhythmic drugs (Yes/No).

References

1. Steffensen, L.B.; Conover, C.A.; Oxvig, C. PAPP-A and the IGF system in atherosclerosis: what's up, what's down? *Am. J. Physiol. Heart Circ. Physiol.* **2019**, *317*, H1039–H1049. [CrossRef]
2. Bayes-Genis, A.; Conover, C.A.; Overgaard, M.T.; Bailey, K.R.; Christiansen, M.; Holmes, D.R.J.; Virmani, R.; Oxvig, C.; Schwartz, R.S. Pregnancy-associated plasma protein A as a marker of acute coronary syndromes. *N. Engl. J. Med.* **2001**, *345*, 1022–1029. [CrossRef]
3. Lund, J.; Qin, Q.-P.; Ilva, T.; Pettersson, K.; Voipio-Pulkki, L.-M.; Porela, P.; Pulkki, K. Circulating pregnancy-associated plasma protein a predicts outcome in patients with acute coronary syndrome but no troponin i elevation. *Circulation* **2003**, *108*, 1924–1926. [CrossRef]
4. Qin, Q.-P.; Kokkala, S.; Lund, J.; Tamm, N.; Voipio-Pulkki, L.-M.; Pettersson, K. Molecular distinction of circulating pregnancy-associated plasma protein a in myocardial infarction and pregnancy. *Clin. Chem.* **2005**, *51*, 75–83. [CrossRef] [PubMed]
5. Heeschen, C.; Dimmeler, S.; Hamm, C.W.; Fichtlscherer, S.; Simoons, M.L.; Zeiher, A.M. Pregnancy-associated plasma protein-a levels in patients with acute coronary syndromes: Comparison with markers of systemic inflammation, platelet activation, and myocardial necrosis. *J. Am. Coll. Cardiol.* **2005**, *45*, 229–237. [CrossRef]
6. Armstrong, E.J.; Morrow, D.A.; Sabatine, M.S. Inflammatory biomarkers in acute coronary syndromes: Part IV: Matrix metalloproteinases and biomarkers of platelet activation. *Circulation* **2006**, *113*, e382–e385. [CrossRef]
7. Body, R.; Ferguson, C. Towards evidence-based emergency medicine: Best bets from the manchester royal infirmary. Pregnancy-associated plasma protein A: A novel cardiac marker with promise. *Emerg. Med. J.* **2006**, *23*, 875–877. [CrossRef] [PubMed]
8. Lund, J.; Qin, Q.-P.; Ilva, T.; Nikus, K.; Eskola, M.; Porela, P.; Kokkala, S.; Pulkki, K.; Pettersson, K.; Voipio-Pulkki, L.-M. Pregnancy-associated plasma protein A: A biomarker in acute ST-elevation myocardial infarction (STEMI). *Ann. Med.* **2006**, *38*, 221–228. [CrossRef]
9. Bonaca, M.P.; Scirica, B.M.; Sabatine, M.S.; Jarolim, P.; Murphy, S.A.; Chamberlin, J.S.; Rhodes, D.W.; Southwick, P.C.; Braunwald, E.; Morrow, D.A. Prospective evaluation of pregnancy-associated plasma protein-a and outcomes in patients with acute coronary syndromes. *J. Am. Coll. Cardiol.* **2012**, *60*, 332–338. [CrossRef]
10. Parveen, N.; Subhakumari, K.N.; Krishnan, S. Pregnancy associated plasma protein-a (PAPP-A) levels in acute coronary syndrome: A case control study in a tertiary care centre. *Indian J. Clin. Biochem.* **2015**, *30*, 150–154. [CrossRef]
11. Daidoji, H.; Takahashi, H.; Otaki, Y.; Tamura, H.; Arimoto, T.; Shishido, T.; Miyashita, T.; Miyamoto, T.; Watanabe, T.; Kubota, I. A combination of plaque components analyzed by integrated backscatter intravascular ultrasound and serum pregnancy-associated plasma protein a levels predict the no-reflow phenomenon during percutaneous coronary intervention. *Catheter. Cardiovasc. Interv.* **2015**, *85*, 43–50. [CrossRef] [PubMed]
12. Iversen, K.; Teisner, A.; Dalager, S.; Olsen, K.E.; Floridon, C.; Teisner, B. Pregnancy associated plasma protein-a (PAPP-A) is not a marker of the vulnerable atherosclerotic plaque. *Clin. Biochem.* **2011**, *44*, 312–318. [CrossRef] [PubMed]
13. Cosin-Sales, J.; Kaski, J.C.; Christiansen, M.; Kaminski, P.; Oxvig, C.; Overgaard, M.T.; Cole, D.; Holt, D.W. Relationship among pregnancy associated plasma protein-a levels, clinical characteristics, and coronary artery disease extent in patients with chronic stable angina pectoris. *Eur. Heart J.* **2005**, *26*, 2093–2098. [CrossRef] [PubMed]
14. Consuegra-Sanchez, L.; Fredericks, S.; Kaski, J.C. Pregnancy-associated plasma protein-a (PAPP-A) and cardiovascular risk. *Atherosclerosis* **2009**, *203*, 346–352. [CrossRef] [PubMed]

15. Elesber, A.A.; Conover, C.A.; Denktas, A.E.; Lennon, R.J.; Holmes, D.R.J.; Overgaard, M.T.; Christiansen, M.; Oxvig, C.; Lerman, L.O.; Lerman, A. Prognostic value of circulating pregnancy-associated plasma protein levels in patients with chronic stable angina. *Eur. Heart J.* **2006**, *27*, 1678–1684. [CrossRef] [PubMed]
16. Consuegra-Sanchez, L.; Petrovic, I.; Cosin-Sales, J.; Holt, D.W.; Christiansen, M.; Kaski, J.C. Prognostic value of circulating pregnancy-associated plasma protein-a (PAPP-A) and proform of eosinophil major basic protein (pro-MBP) levels in patients with chronic stable angina pectoris. *Clin. Chim. Acta* **2008**, *391*, 18–23. [CrossRef]
17. Iversen, K.K.; Teisner, B.; Winkel, P.; Gluud, C.; Kjøller, E.; Kolmos, H.J.; Hildebrandt, P.R.; Hilden, J.; Kastrup, J. Pregnancy associated plasma protein-a as a marker for myocardial infarction and death in patients with stable coronary artery disease: A prognostic study within the claricor trial. *Atherosclerosis* **2011**, *214*, 203–208. [CrossRef]
18. Schulz, O.; Reinicke, M.; Kramer, J.; Berghofer, G.; Bensch, R.; Schimke, I.; Jaffe, A. Pregnancy-associated plasma protein A values in patients with stable cardiovascular disease: Use of a new monoclonal antibody-based assay. *Clin. Chim. Acta* **2011**, *412*, 880–886. [CrossRef]
19. Zengin, E.; Sinning, C.; Zeller, T.; Rupprecht, H.-J.; Schnabel, R.B.; Lackner, K.-J.; Blankenberg, S.; Westermann, D.; Bickel, C. The utility of pregnancy-associated plasma protein A for determination of prognosis in a cohort of patients with coronary artery disease. *Biomark. Med.* **2015**, *9*, 731–741. [CrossRef]
20. Oxvig, C. The role of PAPP-A in the IGF system: Location, location, location. *J. Cell Commun. Signal.* **2015**, *9*, 177–187. [CrossRef]
21. Bayes-Genis, A.; Schwartz, R.S.; Lewis, D.A.; Overgaard, M.T.; Christiansen, M.; Oxvig, C.; Ashai, K.; Holmes, D.R.J.; Conover, C.A. Insulin-like growth factor binding protein-4 protease produced by smooth muscle cells increases in the coronary artery after angioplasty. *Arterioscler. Thromb. Vasc. Biol.* **2001**, *21*, 335–341. [CrossRef] [PubMed]
22. Conover, C.A. Key questions and answers about pregnancy-associated plasma protein-A. *Trends Endocrinol. Metab.* **2012**, *23*, 242–249. [CrossRef] [PubMed]
23. Winkel, P.; Jakobsen, J.C.; Hilden, J.; Lange, T.; Jensen, G.B.; Kjøller, E.; Sajadieh, A.; Kastrup, J.; Kolmos, H.J.; Larsson, A.; et al. Predictors for major cardiovascular outcomes in stable ischaemic heart disease (Premac): Statistical analysis plan for data originating from the Claricor (clarithromycin for patients with stable coronary heart disease) trial. *Diagn. Progn. Res.* **2017**, *1*, 10. [CrossRef] [PubMed]
24. Jespersen, C.M.; Als-Nielsen, B.; Damgaard, M.; Hansen, J.F.; Hansen, S.; Helø, O.H.; Hildebrandt, P.; Hilden, J.; Jensen, G.B.; Kastrup, J.; et al. Randomised placebo controlled multicentre trial to assess short term clarithromycin for patients with stable coronary heart disease: Claricor trial. *BMJ* **2006**, *332*, 22–27. [CrossRef]
25. Gluud, C.; Als-Nielsen, B.; Damgaard, M.; Fischer Hansen, J.; Hansen, S.; Helø, O.H.; Hildebrandt, P.; Hilden, J.; Jensen, G.B.; Kastrup, J.; et al. Clarithromycin for 2 weeks for stable coronary heart disease: 6-year follow-up of the CLARICOR randomized trial and updated meta-analysis of antibiotics for coronary heart disease. *Cardiology* **2008**, *111*, 280–287. [CrossRef]
26. Winkel, P.; Hilden, J.; Fischer Hansen, J.; Hildebrandt, P.; Kastrup, J.; Kolmos, H.J.; Kjøller, E.; Jespersen, C.M.; Gluud, C.; Jensen, G.B.; et al. Excess sudden cardiac deaths after short-term clarithromycin administration in the CLARICOR trial: Why is this so, and why are statins protective? *Cardiology* **2011**, *118*, 63–67. [CrossRef]
27. Winkel, P.; Hilden, J.; Hansen, J.F.; Kastrup, J.; Kolmos, H.J.; Kjøller, E.; Jensen, G.B.; Skoog, M.; Lindschou, J.; Gluud, C.; et al. Clarithromycin for stable coronary heart disease increases all-cause and cardiovascular mortality and cerebrovascular morbidity over 10years in the CLARICOR randomised, blinded clinical trial. *Int. J. Cardiol.* **2015**, *182*, 459–465. [CrossRef]
28. Levey, A.S.; Stevens, L.A.; Schmid, C.H.; Zhang, Y.L.; Castro, A.F.; Feldman, H.I.; Kusek, J.W.; Eggers, P.; Van Lente, F.; Greene, T.; et al. A new equation to estimate glomerular filtration rate. *Ann. Intern. Med.* **2009**, *150*, 604–612. [CrossRef]
29. Rossen, M.; Iversen, K.; Teisner, A.; Teisner, B.; Kliem, A.; Grudzinskas, G. Optimisation of sandwich ELISA based on monoclonal antibodies for the specific measurement of pregnancy-associated plasma protein (PAPP-A) in acute coronary syndrome. *Clin. Biochem.* **2007**, *40*, 478–484. [CrossRef]
30. Kjøller, E.; Hilden, J.; Winkel, P.; Galatius, S.; Frandsen, N.J.; Jensen, G.B.; Fischer Hansen, J.; Kastrup, J.; Jespersen, C.M.; Hildebrandt, P.; et al. Agreement between public register and adjudication committee outcome in a cardiovascular randomized clinical trial. *Am. Heart J.* **2014**, *168*, 197–204. [CrossRef]

31. Kjoller, E.; Hilden, J.; Winkel, P.; Frandsen, N.J.; Galatius, S.; Jensen, G.; Kastrup, J.; Hansen, J.F.; Kolmos, H.J.; Jespersen, C.M.; et al. Good interobserver agreement was attainable on outcome adjudication in patients with stable coronary heart disease. *J. Clin. Epidemiol.* **2012**, *65*, 444–453. [CrossRef] [PubMed]
32. Pellitero, S.; Reverter, J.L.; Granada, M.L.; Pizarro, E.; Pastor, M.C.; Tassies, D.; Reverter, J.C.; Salinas, I.; Sanmarti, A. Association of the IGF1/pregnancy-associated plasma protein-a system and adipocytokine levels with the presence and the morphology of carotid plaques in type 2 diabetes mellitus patients with stable glycaemic control. *Eur. J. Endocrinol.* **2009**, *160*, 925–932. [CrossRef] [PubMed]
33. Schisterman, E.F.; Cole, S.R.; Platt, R.W. Overadjustment bias and unnecessary adjustment in epidemiologic studies. *Epidemiology* **2009**, *20*, 488–495. [CrossRef] [PubMed]
34. Resch, Z.T.; Simari, R.D.; Conover, C.A. Targeted disruption of the pregnancy-associated plasma protein-a gene is associated with diminished smooth muscle cell response to insulin-like growth factor-i and resistance to neointimal hyperplasia after vascular injury. *Endocrinology* **2006**, *147*, 5634–5640. [CrossRef]
35. Conover, C.A.; Mason, M.A.; Bale, L.K.; Harrington, S.C.; Nyegaard, M.; Oxvig, C.; Overgaard, M.T. Transgenic overexpression of pregnancy-associated plasma protein-a in murine arterial smooth muscle accelerates atherosclerotic lesion development. *Am. J. Physiol. Heart Circ. Physiol.* **2010**, *299*, H284–H291. [CrossRef]
36. Conover, C.A.; Bale, L.K.; Oxvig, C. Targeted inhibition of pregnancy-associated plasma protein-a activity reduces atherosclerotic plaque burden in mice. *J. Cardiovasc. Trans. Res.* **2016**, *9*, 77–79. [CrossRef]
37. Swindell, W.R.; Masternak, M.M.; Bartke, A. In vivo analysis of gene expression in long-lived mice lacking the pregnancy-associated plasma protein A (PappA) gene. *Exp. Gerontol.* **2010**, *45*, 366–374. [CrossRef]
38. Root, A. Growth hormone. *Pediatrics* **1965**, *36*, 940–950.
39. Palmeiro, C.R.; Anand, R.; Dardi, I.K.; Balasubramaniyam, N.; Schwarcz, M.D.; Weiss, I.A. Growth hormone and the cardiovascular system. *Cardiol. Rev.* **2012**, *20*, 197–207. [CrossRef]
40. Hjortebjerg, R. IGFBP-4 and PAPP-A in normal physiology and disease. *Growth Horm. IGF Res.* **2018**, *41*, 7–22. [CrossRef]
41. Guo, Y.; Bao, Y.; Guo, D.; Yang, W. Pregnancy-associated plasma protein a in cancer: Expression, oncogenic functions and regulation. *Am. J. Cancer. Res.* **2018**, *8*, 955–963. [PubMed]
42. Bale, L.K.; Resch, Z.T.; Harstad, S.L.; Overgaard, M.T.; Conover, C.A. Constitutive expression of pregnancy-associated plasma protein-a in arterial smooth muscle reduces the vascular response to injury in vivo. *Am. J. Physiol. Endocrinol. Metab.* **2013**, *304*, E139–E144. [CrossRef] [PubMed]
43. Mosholder, A.D.; Lee, J.Y.; Zhou, E.H.; Kang, E.M.; Ghosh, M.; Izem, R.; Major, J.M.; Graham, D.J. Long-term risk of acute myocardial infarction, stroke, and death with outpatient use of clarithromycin: A retrospective cohort study. *Am. J. Epidemiol.* **2018**, *187*, 786–792. [CrossRef] [PubMed]
44. Solomon, S.D.; Claggett, B.; Desai, A.S.; Packer, M.; Zile, M.; Swedberg, K.; Rouleau, J.L.; Shi, V.C.; Starling, R.C.; Kozan, Ö.; et al. Influence of ejection fraction on outcomes and efficacy of sacubitril/valsartan (LCZ696) in heart failure with reduced ejection fraction: The prospective comparison of arni with acei to determine impact on global mortality and morbidity in heart failure (PARADIGM-HF) trial. *Circ. Heart Fail.* **2016**, *9*, e002744. [CrossRef] [PubMed]

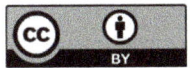 © 2020 by the authors. Licensee MDPI, Basel, Switzerland. This article is an open access article distributed under the terms and conditions of the Creative Commons Attribution (CC BY) license (http://creativecommons.org/licenses/by/4.0/).

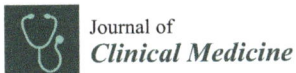 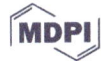

Article

Circulating Biomarkers of Cell Adhesion Predict Clinical Outcome in Patients with Chronic Heart Failure

Elke Bouwens [1], Victor J. van den Berg [1], K. Martijn Akkerhuis [1], Sara J. Baart [1], Kadir Caliskan [1], Jasper J. Brugts [1], Henk Mouthaan [2], Jan van Ramshorst [3], Tjeerd Germans [3], Victor A. W. M. Umans [3], Eric Boersma [1] and Isabella Kardys [1,*]

1 Erasmus MC, 3000CA Rotterdam, The Netherlands
2 Olink Proteomics, SE-751 83 Uppsala, Sweden
3 Northwest Clinics, 1815JD Alkmaar, The Netherlands
* Correspondence: i.kardys@erasmusmc.nl

Received: 15 November 2019; Accepted: 7 January 2020; Published: 10 January 2020

Abstract: Cardiovascular inflammation and vascular endothelial dysfunction are involved in chronic heart failure (CHF), and cellular adhesion molecules are considered to play a key role in these mechanisms. We evaluated temporal patterns of 12 blood biomarkers of cell adhesion in patients with CHF. In 263 ambulant patients, serial, tri-monthly blood samples were collected during a median follow-up of 2.2 (1.4–2.5) years. The primary endpoint (PE) was a composite of cardiovascular mortality, HF hospitalization, heart transplantation and implantation of a left ventricular assist device and was reached in 70 patients. We selected the baseline blood samples in all patients, the two samples closest to a PE, or, for event-free patients, the last sample available. In these 567 samples, associations between biomarkers and PE were investigated by joint modelling. The median age was 68 (59–76) years, with 72% men and 74% New York Heart Association class I–II. Repeatedly measured levels of Complement component C1q receptor (C1qR), Cadherin 5 (CDH5), Chitinase-3-like protein 1 (CHI3L1), Ephrin type-B receptor 4 (EPHB4), Intercellular adhesion molecule-2 (ICAM-2) and Junctional adhesion molecule A (JAM-A) were independently associated with the PE. Their rates of change also predicted clinical outcome. Level of CHI3L1 was numerically the strongest predictor with a hazard ratio (HR) (95% confidence interval) of 2.27 (1.66–3.16) per SD difference in level, followed by JAM-A (2.10, 1.42–3.23) and C1qR (1.90, 1.36–2.72), adjusted for clinical characteristics. In conclusion, temporal patterns of C1qR, CDH5, CHI3L1, EPHB4, ICAM2 and JAM-A are strongly and independently associated with clinical outcome in CHF patients.

Keywords: biomarkers; cell adhesion molecule; heart failure; repeated measurements

1. Introduction

In recent decades, chronic heart failure (CHF) has emerged as a complex syndrome that involves a broad array of biological pathways [1,2]. In this context, CHF has been associated with endothelial dysfunction and low-grade inflammation [3]. Moreover, the role of the immune system in the development and progression of CHF has received considerable attention in recent years [4]. An essential step in this process is the adherence of circulating mononuclear cells to the vascular endothelium through binding of cell adhesion molecules (CAMs) that are expressed on the surface of these mononuclear cells, or on the endothelial cells, or on both [5]. Binding of the mononuclear cells to the endothelium leads to extravasation of these cells into the involved tissue [5], promoting structural deterioration, which eventually contributes to reduced cardiac function. Interestingly, enhanced expression of CAMs has been found within the myocardial microvasculature of patients with severe

CHF as compared to healthy subjects [6], providing further support that vascular inflammation might be involved in the propagation and progression of CHF.

Different classes of CAMs have been identified, and among them are selectins, integrins, cadherins and the immunoglobulin superfamily [7]. In addition, several other molecules are involved in the cell adhesion processes. In more detail, selectins such as platelet (P)-selectin (SELP) are involved in the adhesion of leucocytes to activated endothelium and are known for the typical "rolling" of leucocytes on the surface of the endothelium. Other selectins such as endothelial (E)-selectin (SELE) are involved in the cell extravasation process. Integrins mediate the leucocyte adherence to the vascular endothelium and other cell–cell interactions [8]. Cadherins are an important family of calcium dependent cell–cell adhesion molecules. In addition to their structural role, they have been implicated in the regulation of signaling events [7]. For example, cadherin 5 (CDH5) is a major cell–cell adhesion molecule that forms adherens junctions [9]. Lastly, the immunoglobulin superfamily comprises a diverse group of proteins including intracellular adhesion molecule-1 (ICAM-1), ICAM-2 and ICAM-3, vascular adhesion molecule-1 (VCAM-1), platelet endothelial cell adhesion molecule 1 (PECAM-1) and others, which are expressed on the surface of the endothelial cells and are known for firm adhesion of leucocytes and transendothelial migration [10].

Shedding of CAMs from the cell surface results in measurable levels in peripheral blood [11], which can reflect overexpression of their membrane-bound forms. Since CAMs may thus reflect processes involved in CHF, the association of these circulating biomarkers with clinical outcome provokes interest. Temporal patterns of biomarkers of cell adhesion in CHF, and their associations with an adverse disease course, have not yet been examined. Therefore, in this study, we investigated 12 cell adhesion-related biomarkers repeatedly measured with the Olink Multiplex panel, which contains 92 known human cardiovascular biomarkers that have previously been extensively investigated in the literature as well as exploratory candidates that are thought to carry potential as new biomarkers. Specifically, here, we examined biomarkers from this panel related to the above-described mechanisms (SELP, SELE, CDH5, ICAM-2, and PECAM-1) and other potentially interesting biomarkers related to cell adhesion processes (complement component C1q receptor (C1qR), chitinase-3-like protein 1 (CHI3L1), contactin-1 (CNTN1), ephrin type-B receptor 4 (EPHB4), epithelial cell adhesion molecule (Ep-CAM), integrin beta-2 (ITGB2), and junctional adhesion molecule A (JAM-A). The aim of the present study was to evaluate the association between temporal patterns of these biomarkers of cell adhesion and clinical outcomes in stable patients with CHF.

2. Methods

2.1. Patient Selection

A total of 263 patients enrolled in the 'Serial Biomarker Measurements and New Echocardiographic Techniques in Chronic Heart Failure Patients Result in Tailored Prediction of Prognosis' (Bio-SHiFT) study were included in the Netherlands. The Bio-SHiFT study is a prospective, observational cohort study of stable patients with CHF. Patients used for the current investigation were enrolled during the first study inclusion period from October 2011 until June 2013, while follow-up lasted until 2015. Patients were recruited during their regular outpatient clinic visit, in the Erasmus MC in Rotterdam or in the Northwest Clinics in Alkmaar. To be eligible for this study, CHF had to be diagnosed ≥3 months ago according to European Society of Cardiology guidelines [12,13]. Also, patients had to be ambulatory and stable, i.e., they should not have been hospitalized for HF in the past three months. The study design of the Bio-SHiFT study (including detailed inclusion and exclusion criteria) has been described in detail previously [14,15]. The study was approved by the medical ethics committees, conducted in accordance with the Declaration of Helsinki, and registered in ClinicalTrials.gov (NCT01851538, https://clinicaltrials.gov/ct2/show/NCT01851538). Written informed consent was obtained from all patients.

2.2. Study Procedures

All patients underwent standard care at the outpatient clinic by their treating physicians, who were blinded for biomarker results. Additionally, study follow-up visits were predefined and scheduled every 3 months (±1 month). At the moment of enrolment and at each study follow-up visit, a short medical evaluation was performed, blood samples were collected and occurrence of cardiovascular events since last study visit was recorded. Blood samples were processed and stored at −80 °C within two hours after collection. As biomarkers were measured after completion of follow-up, this information did not lead to change of treatment strategies since treating physicians were unaware of the study results.

2.3. Study Endpoints

The primary endpoint (PE) was a composite of cardiac death, heart transplantation, left ventricular assist device implantation, and hospitalization for the management of acute or worsened HF, whichever occurred first. A clinical event committee, blinded for the biomarker results, reviewed hospital records and discharge letters and adjudicated the study endpoints [14,15].

2.4. Blood Sample Selection

In this first inclusion period of the Bio-SHiFT study, we collected a total of 1984 samples in 263 patients before occurrence of the PE or censoring (median of 9 (25th–75th percentile: 5–10) blood samples per patient). For reasons of efficiency, we made a selection from these samples: we selected all samples at enrolment, the last sample available in patients in whom the PE did not occur during follow-up, and the two samples available closest in time prior to the PE (which, by design, were 3 months apart). Previous investigations in this cohort have demonstrated that levels of several biomarker change in the months prior to the incident adverse event [14,15]. Thus, by selecting the last two samples prior to the endpoint, we aimed to capture this change. In event-free patients however, our previous investigations showed stable biomarker levels, in which case one additional biomarker sample suffices. In total, this selection amounted to 567 samples for the current analysis.

2.5. Biomarker Measurements

To investigate new biomarkers, the cardiovascular panel III of the Olink Multiplex platform (Olink Proteomics AB, Uppsala, Sweden) was used for a batch-wise analysis. This multiplexing assay is based on proximity extension assay technology [16]. The assay uses two oligonucleotide-labelled antibodies to bind to their respective target proteins in the sample. When the two antibodies are in close proximity, a new polymerase chain reaction target sequence is formed. The resulting sequence is detected and quantified using standard real-time PCR. The proteins/biomarkers are delivered in Normalized Protein Expression (NPX) Units, which are relative units that result from the polymerase chain reaction. The NPX units are expressed on a log2 scale where one unit higher NPX represents a doubling of the measured protein concentrations. This arbitrary unit can thus be used for relative quantification of proteins and comparing the fold changes between groups. In the 567 selected samples, we measured C1qR, CDH5, CHI3L1, CNTN1, EPHB4, Ep-CAM, ICAM2, ITGB2, JAM-A, PECAM-1, SELE and SELP. In Appendix A Table A1, an overview is given of the adhesion molecule biomarkers included in this study, including abbreviations, synonyms and function.

Additionally, in all patients, N-terminal pro–B-type natriuretic peptide (NT-proBNP) and high-sensitive troponin T (hsTnT) were measured using electrochemiluminescence immunoassays (Elecsys 2010; Roche Diagnostics, Indianapolis, IN, USA) as described before [14].

2.6. Statistical Analysis

Variables with a normal distribution are presented as the mean ± standard deviation (SD), whereas the median and 25th–75th percentile are used in case of non-normality. Differences between groups were tested with Student t-tests (for normally distributed variables) or with Mann Whitney tests (non-normally distributed variables). Categorical variables were presented as counts and percentages and differences between groups were tested with chi square tests. We used linear mixed effect models to plot the average temporal pattern of each adhesion molecule biomarker for patients with and without a PE during study follow-up.

To estimate the associations between patient-specific repeated biomarker measurements and the hazard of the PE, we applied joint modelling (JM) analyses. JM combines linear mixed effect models for temporal evolution of the repeated measurements with time-to event relative risk models for the time-to-event data [17]. By using the JM technique, analyses inherently accounted for different follow-up durations between patients [18]. We studied the predictive value of biomarker levels, as well as their rates of change (i.e., the slopes of the longitudinal biomarker trajectories). The latter analysis is of particular interest in situations where, for example, at a specific time point two patients show similar marker levels, but differed in rate of change of the marker [19]. First, all JM analyses were performed univariably. Subsequently, we considered a 'clinical model' and an 'established biomarker model', to adjust for potential confounders. The clinical model was adjusted for age, gender, diabetes mellitus, atrial fibrillation, New York Heart Association (NYHA) class, use of diuretics and systolic blood pressure, while the established cardiac biomarker model was adjusted for NT-proBNP and hsTnT (measured at study enrolment). For all the JM analyses, we used the Z-score (i.e., the standardized form) of the log2-transformed biomarkers to allow for direct comparisons of different biomarkers. Results are given as hazard ratios (HR) with their 95% confidence intervals (CI) per SD change of the biomarker's level or slope.

We used the conventional $p < 0.05$ threshold to conclude significance for the relation between patient characteristics and the occurrence of the PE during follow-up (Table 1). For the other analyses, we corrected for multiple testing using the Bonferonni correction ($n = 12$), which resulted in a corrected significance level of $p < 0.004$. Analyses were performed with SPSS Statistics 24 (IBM Inc., Chicago, IL, USA) and R Statistical Software using packages nlme [20] and JMbayes [17].

3. Results

3.1. Baseline Characteristics and Study Endpoints

During a median (25th–75th percentile) follow-up of 2.2 (1.4–2.5) years, a total of 70 (27%) patients reached the PE: 56 patients were re-hospitalized for acute or worsened HF, three patients underwent heart transplantation, two patients underwent left ventricular assistant device implantation, and nine patients died of cardiovascular causes. Table 1 displays the patients' characteristics at enrolment and the differences in these characteristics between patients who reached the PE during follow-up and patients who did not. The median age was 68 (25th–75th percentile: 59–76), years, with 72% men and 74% NYHA class I–II. The median duration of HF was 4.6 (1.7–9.9) years. Patients who reached the endpoint during follow-up were older and more often in a higher NYHA-class (III or IV), compared to patients who did not reach the PE. They also had a longer duration of HF, lower systolic blood pressures, higher levels of NT-proBNP and hsTNT, were more likely to have atrial fibrillation and diabetes mellitus, and had a higher prevalence of diuretics use. Baseline levels of C1qR, CDH5, CHI3L1, EPHB4 and JAM-A were significantly higher in patients who later experienced the endpoint compared to patients who remained event-free.

Table 1. Patients characteristics in relation to the occurrence of the primary endpoint (PE).

Variable	Total	PE Reached during Follow-Up		p-Value
		Yes	No	
	263 (100)	70 (27)	193 (73)	
Demographics				
Age—years	68 (59–76)	72 (60–80)	67 (58–75)	0.021 *
Men	189 (72)	53 (76)	136 (71)	0.40
Clinical characteristics				
Body Mass Index (kg/m^2)	26 (24–30)	27 (24–30)	26 (24–30)	0.80
Heart rate (eats/min)	67 ± 12	69 ± 13	67 ± 11	0.22
Systolic blood pressure (mmHg)	122 ± 20	117 ± 17	124 ± 21	0.020 *
Diastolic blood pressure (mmHg)	72 ± 11	70 ± 10	73 ± 11	0.06
Features of heart failure				
Duration of HF (years)	4.6 (1.7–9.9)	6.8 (2.8–12.5)	3.8 (1.1–8.2)	0.002 *
NYHA class III or IV	69 (26)	31 (44)	38 (20)	<0.001 *
HF with reduced ejection fraction	250 (95)	66 (94)	184 (95)	0.75
HF with preserved ejection fraction	13 (5)	4 (6)	9 (5)	
Left ventricular ejection fraction	31 ± 11	28 ± 11	31 ± 11	0.108
Established biomarkers				
NT-proBNP (pmol/L)	137 (52–273)	282 (176–517)	95 (32–208)	<0.001 *
HsTnT (ng/L)	18 (10–33)	32 (21–50)	14 (8–27)	<0.001 *
eGFR (mL/min per 1.73m^2)	58 (43–76)	53 (40–73)	59 (44–77)	0.20
Etiology of heart failure				
Ischemic	117 (45)	36 (51)	81 (42)	0.17
Hypertension	34 (13)	10 (14)	24 (12)	0.69
Secondary to valvular disease	12 (5)	5 (7)	7 (4)	0.31
Cardiomyopathy	68 (26)	15 (21)	53 (28)	0.32
Unknown or Others	32 (12)	4 (6)	28 (15)	
Medical history				
Prior Myocardial infarction	96 (37)	32 (46)	64 (33)	0.060
Prior Percutaneous coronary intervention	82 (31)	27 (39)	55 (29)	0.12
Prior Coronary artery bypass grafting	43 (16)	13 (19)	30 (16)	0.56
Prior CVA/TIA	42 (16)	15 (21)	27 (14)	0.15
Atrial fibrillation	106 (40)	36 (51)	70 (36)	0.027 *
Diabetes Mellitus	81 (31)	32 (46)	49 (25)	0.002 *
Hypercholesterolemia	96 (37)	30 (43)	66 (34)	0.20
Hypertension	120 (46)	38 (54)	82 (43)	0.090
COPD	31 (12)	12 (17)	19 (10)	0.11
Medication use				
Beta-blocker	236 (90)	61 (87)	175 (91)	0.40
ACE-I or ARB	245 (93)	63 (90)	182 (94)	0.22
Diuretics	237 (90)	68 (97)	169 (88)	0.021 *
Loop diuretics	236 (90)	68 (97)	168 (87)	0.017 *
Thiazides	7 (3)	3 (4)	4 (2)	0.39
Aldosterone antagonist	179 (68)	53 (76)	126 (65)	0.11
Biomarker level at baseline in arbitrary unit (NPX values)				
C1qR	8.88 (8.56–9.27)	9.16 (8.78–9.50)	8.78 (8.50–9.20)	<0.001 *
CDH5	2.29 (2.00–2.67)	2.36 (2.12–2.84)	2.27 (1.96–2.60)	0.010 *
CHI3L1	7.68 (6.88–8.39)	8.08 (7.53–8.72)	7.47 (6.68–8.20)	<0.001 *
CNTN1	2.01 (1.72–2.25)	2.00 (1.68–2.22)	2.01 (1.75–2.27)	0.58
EpCAM	5.11 (4.38–5.82)	4.91 (4.40–5.71)	5.18 (4.36–5.90)	0.41
EPHB4	1.35 (1.08–1.66)	1.55 (1.19–1.95)	1.31 (1.05–1.58)	<0.001 *

Table 1. Cont.

Variable	Total	PE Reached during Follow-Up		p-Value
		Yes	No	
	263 (100)	70 (27)	193 (73)	
Biomarker level at baseline in arbitrary unit (NPX values)				
ICAM-2	4.20 (3.88–4.59)	4.35 (4.00–4.64)	4.18 (3.85–4.51)	0.061
ITGB2	4.65 (4.39–4.90)	4.64 (4.41–4.96)	4.67 (4.39–4.89)	0.86
JAM-A	5.22 (4.64–5.80)	5.41 (4.79–6.02)	5.08 (4.56–5.71)	0.024 *
PECAM-1	4.74 (4.36–5.17)	4.77 (4.36–5.39)	4.70 (4.35–5.10)	0.32
SELE	2.89 (2.46–3.28)	3.06 (2.51–3.32)	2.84 (2.45–3.28)	0.40
SELP	8.84 (8.46–9.38)	8.98 (8.54–9.58)	8.78 (8.42–9.28)	0.087

Variables with a normal distribution are presented as the mean ± SD, whereas non-normally distributed continuous variables are expressed as the median (25th–75th percentile). Categorical variables are expressed as counts (percentages). Missing values < 5% if applicable, except for systolic blood pressure (5.3%). * p-value < 0.05. ACE-I: angiotensin-converting enzyme inhibitors, ARB: angiotensin II receptor blockers, C1qR: complement component C1q receptor, CDH5: cadherin 5, CHI3L1: chitinase-3-like protein 1, CNTN1: contactin-1, COPD: chronic obstructive pulmonary disease, CVA: cerebrovascular accident, eGFR: estimated glomerular filtration rate, Ep-CAM: epithelial cell adhesion molecule, EPHB4: Ephrin type-B receptor 4, HF: heart failure, HsTnT: high-sensitive troponin T, ICAM-2: intercellular adhesion molecule-2, ITGB2: integrin beta-2, JAMA: junctional adhesion molecule A, NPX: Normalized Protein Expression, NT-proBNP: N-terminal pro–B-type natriuretic peptide, NYHA: New York Heart Association, PECAM-1: Platelet endothelial cell adhesion molecule 1, SELE: E-selectin, SELP: P-selectin and TIA: transitory ischemic attack.

3.2. Temporal Patterns of Circulating Biomarkers of Cell Adhesion in Relation to Study Endpoints

Figure 1 depicts the average temporal evolutions of biomarkers of cell adhesion from twenty-four months before the PE or before last sample moment (for patients who remained event-free) onwards, based on linear mixed effect models. As the endpoint or last sample moment approached, biomarkers C1qR, CDH5, CHI3L1, EPHB4, ICAM-2 and JAM-A showed higher levels in patients who experienced the PE versus those who remained event-free. Some were already higher 24 months before the endpoint, while others were not but diverged as the end-point drew closer. On the other hand, CNTN1, EpCAM, ITGB2, PECAM-1, SELE and SELP did not show a clear difference between both groups.

Table 2 shows the associations of the repeatedly measured levels of biomarkers of cell adhesion with the PE based on JM analyses. C1qR showed the strongest association in univariate analysis with a HR of 2.22 (95% CI: 1.62–3.10) per SD change at any point in time during follow-up. After adjustment for clinical characteristics, CHI3L1 remained the strongest predictor of the PE, with a HR of 2.27 (95% CI: 1.66–3.16). CHI3L1 was followed by JAM-A (HR 2.10, 95% CI: 1.42–3.23) and C1qR (HR 1.90, 95% CI: 1.36–2.72). In addition, the risk estimates of CHI3L1 (HR 1.68, 95% CI: 1.23–2.35) and JAM-A (HR 1.75, 95% CI: 1.25–2.49) remained significant after adjustment for baseline established cardiac biomarkers NT-proBNP and hsTNT.

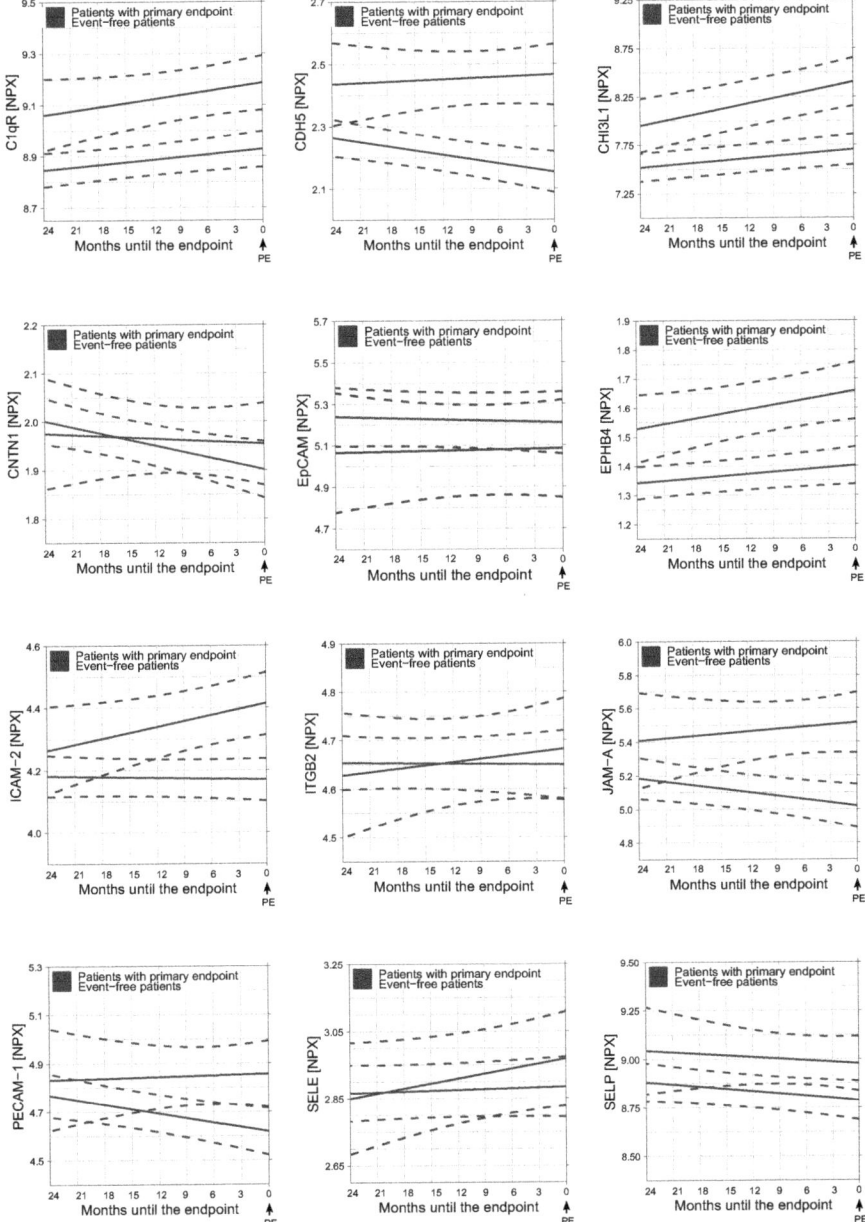

Figure 1. Average temporal patterns of adhesion molecule biomarkers during follow-up approaching the primary endpoint (PE) or last sample moment. X-axis: time remaining to the PE (for patients who experienced incident adverse events) or time remaining to last sample moment (for patients who remained event-free). Therefore, 'time zero' is defined as the occurrence of the endpoint or last sample moment and is depicted on the right side of the x-axis, so that the average marker trajectory can be visualized as the endpoint approaches. Y-axis: biomarker levels in arbitrary, relative units (Normalized Protein Expression, NPX). Solid red line: Average temporal pattern of biomarker levels in patients who

reached the primary endpoint during follow-up. Solid blue line: Average temporal pattern of biomarker levels in patients who remained endpoint free (solid blue line). Dashed lines: 95% confidence interval. Abbreviations: Complement component C1q receptor: C1qR, Cadherin 5: CDH5, Chitinase-3-like protein 1: CHI3L1, CNTN1: Contactin-1, Ep-CAM: Epithelial cell adhesion molecule, EPHB4: Ephrin type-B receptor 4, ICAM2: Intercellular adhesion molecule-2, ITGB2: Integrin beta-2, JAM-A: Junctional adhesion molecule A, NPX: Normalized Protein Expression, PE: primary endpoint, PECAM-1: Platelet endothelial cell adhesion molecule 1, SELE: E-selectin, and SELP: P-selectin.

Table 2. Associations between the levels of biomarkers of cell adhesion and the primary endpoint.

Biomarker	Crude Model HR (95% CI)	p-Value	Clinical Model HR (95% CI)	p-Value	Biomarker Model HR (95% CI)	p-Value
C1qR	2.22 (1.62–3.10)	<0.001 *	1.90 (1.36–2.72)	<0.001 *	1.47 (1.04–2.14)	0.028
CDH5	2.01 (1.47–2.77)	<0.001 *	1.79 (1.30–2.50)	<0.001 *	1.56 (1.14–2.14)	0.004
CHI3L1	2.11 (1.60–2.84)	<0.001 *	2.27 (1.66–3.16)	<0.001 *	1.68 (1.23–2.35)	0.002 *
CNTN1	0.93 (0.66–1.32)	0.70	0.98 (0.67–1.45)	0.92	0.93 (0.66–1.31)	0.66
EpCAM	0.86 (0.66–1.11)	0.27	0.90 (0.67–1.20)	0.46	0.90 (0.69–1.17)	0.46
EPHB4	1.90 (1.48–2.44)	<0.001 *	1.77 (1.35–2.33)	<0.001 *	1.37 (1.03–1.80)	0.031
ICAM2	2.08 (1.51–2.94)	<0.001 *	1.79 (1.29–2.53)	0.001 *	1.53 (1.12–2.12)	0.005
ITGB2	1.07 (0.77–1.47)	0.70	0.95 (0.65–1.37)	0.77	1.04 (0.75–1.42)	0.83
JAM-A	1.86 (1.34–2.63)	<0.001 *	2.10 (1.42–3.23)	<0.001 *	1.75 (1.25–2.49)	0.001 *
PECAM-1	1.39 (1.00–1.94)	0.050	1.60 (1.10–2.35)	0.013	1.47 (1.04–2.08)	0.031
SELE	1.11 (0.86–1.44)	0.43	1.07 (0.81–1.40)	0,66	1.11 (0.86–1.44)	0.43
SELP	1.34 (0.98–1.86)	0.071	1.45 (1.01–2.10)	0.044	1.49 (1.08–2.06)	0.018

Hazard ratios (HRs) and 95% confidence intervals (CIs) are given per standard deviation change at any point in time during follow-up, which were estimated by joint modelling (JM) analysis. JM combines linear mixed effect (LME) models for the temporal evolution of the repeated measurements with Cox proportional hazard models for the time-to-event data. Thus, all available measurements are simultaneously taken into account in the current analyses (i.e., all baseline samples, the last sample available in patients in whom the PE did not occur during follow-up, and the two samples available closest in time prior to the primary endpoint). Crude model: Cox model unadjusted, LME model unadjusted; Clinical model: Cox and LME models adjusted for age, sex, diabetes, atrial fibrillation, baseline New York Heart Association class, diuretics, and systolic blood pressure; Established cardiac biomarker model: Cox and LME models adjusted for baseline NT-proBNP and hsTnT. Data for systolic blood pressure was missing in >5% of patients. Imputations were applied using the patients' clinical and outcome data. * p-value below the corrected significance level for multiple testing (p-value < 0.004).

Apart from evaluating the predictive value of repeatedly assessed biomarker levels, we also evaluated their rates of change (i.e., the slopes of the longitudinal biomarker trajectories) and concurrent HRs. Although the trajectories plotted by using linear mixed effect models (Figure 1) have already provided an impression of temporal evolution of biomarker level in those with and without incident PEs, evaluating slope by means of the JM provides the possibility to evaluate instantaneous slope, which may render additional insights. In these analyses, the same biomarkers remained significant predictors of the PE, i.e., CDH5, CD93, CHI3L1, EPHB4, ICAM-2 and JAM-A, even after adjusting for clinical factors (Table 3). JAM-A showed numerically the strongest association with the PE with a HR of 1.64 (95% CI: 1.23–2.24) per 0.1SD change of the annual slope, followed by CHI3L1 (HR 1.58, 95% CI: 1.36–1.93) and CDH5 (HR 1.47, 95% CI: 1.17–2.00).

Table 3. Associations between the slope of biomarkers of cell adhesion and the primary endpoint.

Biomarker	Crude Model		Clinical Model		Biomarker Model	
	HR (95% CI)	p-Value	HR (95% CI)	p-Value	HR (95% CI)	p-Value
C1qR	1.34 (1.16–1.56)	<0.001 *	1.43 (1.13–1.92)	0.002 *	1.12 (1.02–1.24)	0.019
CDH5	1.36 (1.18–1.60)	<0.001 *	1.47 (1.17–2.00)	<0.001 *	1.16 (1.07–1.27)	<0.001 *
CHI3L1	1.41 (1.29–1.57)	<0.001 *	1.58 (1.36–1.93)	<0.001 *	1.27 (1.18–1.39)	<0.001 *
CNTN1	1.04 (0.94–1.17)	0.45	1.04 (0.92–1.18)	0.53	1.06 (0.98–1.15)	0.13
EpCAM	1.01 (0.88–1.16)	0.92	1.01 (0.88–1.17)	0.88	1.01 (0.92–1.11)	0.83
EPHB4	1.33 (1.19–1.51)	<0.001 *	1.34 (1.15–1.68)	<0.001 *	1.14 (1.04–1.25)	0.005
ICAM2	1.32 (1.22–1.45)	<0.001 *	1.44 (1.27–1.72)	<0.001 *	1.22 (1.15–1.31)	<0.001 *
ITGB2	1.07 (0.94–1.21)	0.32	0.99 (0.83–1.16)	0.90	1.05 (0.97–1.15)	0.23
JAM-A	1.34 (1.12–1.62)	0.002 *	1.64 (1.23–2.24)	0.001 *	1.10 (0.99–1.24)	0.085
PECAM-1	1.15 (0.98–1.40)	0.088	1.09 (0.86–1.72)	0.80	1.06 (0.97–1.18)	0.21
SELE	1.21 (1.05–1.41)	0.015	1.19 (0.99–1.41)	0.060	1.10 (0.96–1.23)	0.15
SELP	1.29 (1.13–1.49)	0.020	1.45 (1.22–1.84)	<0.001 *	1.12 (0.94–1.27)	0.15

Hazard ratios (HRs) and 95% confidence intervals (CIs) are given per 0.1 standard deviation of the annual slope at any point in time during follow-up, which were estimated by joint modelling (JM) analysis. JM combines linear mixed effect (LME) models for the temporal evolution of the repeated measurements with Cox proportional hazard models for the time-to-event data. Thus, all available measurements are simultaneously taken into account in the current analyses (i.e., all baseline samples, the last sample available in patients in whom the PE did not occur during follow-up, and the two samples available closest in time prior to the primary endpoint). Crude model: Cox model unadjusted, LME model unadjusted; Clinical model: Cox and LME models adjusted for age, sex, diabetes, atrial fibrillation, baseline New York Heart Association class, diuretics and systolic blood pressure; Established cardiac biomarker model: Cox and LME models adjusted for baseline NT-proBNP and hsTnT. Data for systolic blood pressure was missing in >5% of patients. Imputations were applied using the patients' clinical and outcome data.
* p-value below the corrected significance level for multiple testing (p-value < 0.004).

4. Discussion

In the present study, we found that biomarkers of cell adhesion C1qR, CDH5, CHI3L1, EPHB4, ICAM-2 and JAM-A were associated with clinical outcomes in 263 stable patients with CHF. At baseline, levels of biomarkers C1qR, CDH5, CHI3L1, EPHB4 and JAM-A were higher in patients who later experienced the PE compared to patients who remained event-free. Furthermore, the average biomarker evolutions over time of these markers, and additionally of ICAM-2, showed higher levels as the PE approached. Even more important, repeatedly measured levels of these biomarkers of cell adhesion were independently associated with the PE. Even adjusted for clinical factors, biomarkers of cell adhesion served as predictors of clinical adverse events.

Recent studies suggest a pivotal role of CAMs in the processes of HF. Until now, however, research on CAMs in relation to adverse clinical outcomes in patients with CHF is limited. Previous studies have mostly described the value of single measurements of adhesion molecules (e.g., at admission) for prognosis, and studies were relatively small. Our study, which was based on repeated measurements, demonstrates a promising role for several adhesion biomarkers for individual prognostication in CHF patients Temporal patterns shortly before an adverse event occurs have not yet been investigated in detail previously, while this might be a crucial time window for therapeutic interventions.

In our study, CHI3L1 was the biomarker whose association with the PE was numerically the strongest after adjustment for clinical factors. CHI3L1 is a glycoprotein secreted in vitro by cells such as activated macrophages and neutrophils in different tissues with inflammation. Studies on patients with acute myocardial infarction, stable coronary artery disease, atrial fibrillation and CHF have demonstrated elevated levels of CHI3L1 compared with healthy controls [21]. Moreover, several studies have previously examined CHI3L1 in relation to clinical outcome in CHF; but repeated measurements were never used. Some of these studies showed that CHI3L1 is associated with all-cause mortality [22] and that it is able to detect patients at high risk for adverse outcomes as well [23,24]. Other studies failed to demonstrate such associations. Rathcke at al. examined CHI3L1 levels in patients with CHF and in age-matched controls without cardiovascular disease [25]. They found higher levels of CHI3L1 at baseline in patients with CHF, but these levels did not predict cardiovascular events or overall mortality. Mathiasen et al. [21] suggested that, most likely, elevated levels of CHI3L1 in CHF patients are explained by the presence of concomitant diseases. CHF is a complex disorder, often complicated by other comorbidities in which CHI3L1 is known to be elevated, such as arrhythmias, renal dysfunction, diabetes mellitus and hypertension. These concomitant diseases could thus possibly explain the differences in CHI3L1 levels when compared to healthy individuals. Conversely, in our study, we not only adjusted for age, but also for clinical factors, and still we found an association between CHI3L1 and clinical adverse events.

The barrier formed by endothelial cells allows regulated passage of immune cells in the normal state and during inflammatory conditions. This passage is mediated through junctional molecules, such as ICAM-2, CDH5, JAMA, and PECAM-1 [26,27]. ICAM-2 participates in the docking of leukocytes to the endothelium, and is likely to be relevant for leukocyte diapedesis [28]. For example, former research showed that endothelial cell activation leads to neutrophil transmigration, supported by the sequential roles of ICAM-2, JAM-A and PECAM-1 [26]. We are not aware of previous investigations that link ICAM-2 to prognosis of stable CHF patients. We show that rate of change of ICAM-2 independently predicts adverse clinical outcome. This suggests that prognosis differs between patients with stable ICAM-2 values and patients with increasing ICAM-2 values. CDH5 is an endothelial transmembrane glycoprotein and is the major molecule for cell–cell adhesion that forms adherens junctions [9]. Shedding of CDH5 into the circulation is associated with severe acute kidney injury and with more severe organ dysfunction in patients with sepsis [29] and increased levels of soluble CDH5 were associated with poor outcome in severe sepsis [30]. In cardiovascular research, elevated levels of CDH5 have also been reported to be associated with coronary atherosclerosis [31]. Based on our results, CDH5 may be of use as a biomarker that reflects on-going inflammation and indicates impending adverse events in CHF patients. JAM-A is involved in the regulation of vascular permeability [27] and genetic deletion and blockade of JAM-A generally results in increased permeability of endothelial cells [32]. JAM-A is also thought to be required for movement of leukocytes toward sites of inflammation [33] and it may be considered as a marker of acute endothelial activation and dysfunction [34]. This is in line with our findings; we demonstrate that repeatedly measured levels of JAM-A show a numerically strong independent association with the PE. The significant role of PECAM-1 in platelet aggregation and migration of leukocytes through the endothelium [35] is interesting in the context of CHF. PECAM-1 has been suggested as a sensitive marker providing early diagnostic aid in acute coronary syndromes [36]. In heart failure research, soluble PECAM-1 was found to be elevated in the majority of patients with severe CHF [37]. However, we did not find an association of PECAM-1 with prognosis in our CHF cohort.

SELP is of great interest because of its key role in interactions between platelets, leucocytes, and endothelium [38]. Abnormal surface SELP expression [39,40] and soluble SELP levels [41] have been reported in decompensated heart failure, suggesting persistent platelet activation. Regarding their prognostic value, however, levels of soluble SELP, platelet surface SELP, and total platelet SELP did not determine prognosis [42] and our results support these findings. Ep-CAM, CNTN1, ITGB2, and SELE also showed negative results in our study.

Less is known about the other biomarkers in relation to CHF. For example, C1qR is a transmembrane receptor once thought to be only a receptor for C1q, but is now thought to play a role in endothelial cell adhesion [43]. The up-regulation of this receptor by inflammatory mediators and the ability of complement component C1q itself to increase ICAM-1 expression suggest a potential role for the receptor in vascular inflammation and immune injury [44]. To the best of our knowledge, C1qR has never been linked directly to prognostication in CHF patients. In our study, repeatedly measured levels of this marker were independently associated with the PE. EPHB4 serves as receptor for its transmembrane ligand ephrin-B2. Both are specifically expressed on arterial and venous endothelial cells. Hamada et al. concluded ephrin-B2 forward signaling and EPHB4 reverse signaling differentially affect cell adhesion and migration between arterial and venous endothelial cells [45]. We found that both level and slope analysis of EPHB4 were significantly associated with the endpoint, even after adjusting for clinical factors.

While the 263 patients included in our investigation were ambulatory and stable, it has been advocated that grouping of HF patients should not be approached only based on symptoms [46], nor on ejection fraction solely [47]. Definitions have been described to identify more advanced disease HF (AdHF), i.e., patients with worsening clinical condition, high rates of re-hospitalization and mortality (meaning a condition where standard treatments are inadequate and additional interventions must be applied; these patients are suitable for LVAD), as well as end-stage heart failure (patients for which advanced therapies, such as LVAD, is contraindicated and palliative cares should be pursued) [48]. In post-hoc analyses, based on our available data, we identified at least 57 patients who might be categorized into these two groups at baseline; given their ambulant condition most likely the AdHF group. Thirty of them eventually experienced an endpoint during follow-up. Compared to the other 206 patients, these 57 patients were older, had a higher heart rate, lower systolic and diastolic blood pressure, had higher NT-proBNP, hsTnT and eGFR levels, and were more likely to have prior CVA/TIA and diabetes mellitus. Malfunction of other organs could affect prognosis [49], and, therefore, differences in such risk factors should be taken into account (as for example also highlighted in a recent study about the role of oxidative stress and vascular inflammation in diabetic patients which could result in myocardial infarction [50]). Since we adjusted our current analyses of the association between circulating biomarkers of cell adhesion and clinical outcomes for variables such as diabetes mellitus and atrial fibrillation, we believe we have accounted for this type of confounding as much as we could in this observational study.

Our study has some limitations. First, because of efficiency reasons, we did not use all 1984 available trimonthly samples, but selected 3 samples for patients with a PE (baseline and last 2 prior to the PE), and 2 samples for event-free patients, resulting in 567 samples. Our previous investigations using all samples demonstrated that most of the examined biomarkers show an increase shortly prior to the incident adverse event. Thus, we believe that with our approach we retain the most informative measurements while enhancing efficiency. Second, as described before [15,51], our cohort comprised mainly HF patients with a reduced ejection fraction. This can most likely be attributed to the fact that in the Netherlands, most HF patients with a preserved ejection fraction are treated in secondary referral centers or by the general practitioner. Finally, we used biomarker values in Normalized Protein Expression (NPX) Units, i.e., relative units. While these values can be used for comparing patients and changes over time within a patient, for clinical applications absolute concentrations are recommended.

In conclusion, the present study demonstrates that serial measurements of C1qR, CDH5, CHI3L1, EPHB4, ICAM-2 and JAM-A are independently associated with clinical adverse events in patients with CHF, suggesting that markers of cell adhesion could be useful for individual risk profiling. These biomarkers are also interesting for future therapeutic purposes, as CAMs may be used as targets to inhibit vascular inflammation and endothelial dysfunction. Further studies are warranted to confirm these associations, to investigate whether a combination of different markers (for example C1qR, CHI3L1 and JAM-A) may improve prognostication and to better elucidate the pathophysiological role of cell adhesion in CHF.

Author Contributions: Conceptualization, K.M.A., V.A.W.M.U., E.B. (Eric Boersma) and I.K.; methodology, E.B. (Elke Bouwens), S.J.B., and I.K.; formal analysis, E.B. (Elke Bouwens); investigation, E.B. (Elke Bouwens), V.J.v.d.B., K.M.A., S.J.B., K.C., J.J.B., H.M., J.v.R., T.G., V.A.W.M.U., E.B. (Eric Boersma) and I.K.; resources, E.B. (Elke Bouwens), V.J.v.d.B., K.M.A., S.J.B., K.C., J.J.B., H.M., J.v.R., T.G., V.A.W.M.U., E.B. (Eric Boersma), and I.K.; data curation, E.B. (Elke Bouwens) and I.K.; writing—original draft preparation, E.B. (Elke Bouwens); writing—review and editing, E.B. (Elke Bouwens), V.J.v.d.B., K.M.A., S.J.B., K.C., J.J.B., H.M., J.v.R., T.G., V.A.W.M.U., E.B. (Eric Boersma) and I.K.; visualization, E.B. (Elke Bouwens) and I.K.; supervision, I.K.; project administration, E.B. (Elke Bouwens) and I.K.; funding acquisition, E.B. (Eric Boersma) and I.K. All authors have read and agreed to the published version of the manuscript

Funding: This work was supported by the Jaap Schouten Foundation and the Noordwest Academie.

Conflicts of Interest: One of the co-authors, Henk Mouthaan, is employed by Olink Proteomics.

Appendix A

Table A1. Overview of the assessed biomarkers of cell adhesion.

Abbreviation	Full Name	Synonyms	Function
C1qR	Complement component C1q receptor	CD93	Stimulates endothelial expression of adhesion molecules/C1q-mediated endothelial cell adhesion
CDH5	Cadherin 5	VE cadherin	Major cell–cell adhesion molecule that forms adherens junctions
CHI3L1	Chitinase-3-like protein 1	YKL-40, HC gp39, brp-39, gp38k, and MGP-40	Endothelial activation and dysfunction
CNTN1	Contactin-1	GP130	Expressed in neuronal tissues, associates with other cell surface proteins and believed to participate in signal transduction pathways and cell functions
Ep-CAM	Epithelial cell adhesion molecule	CD326	Cell–cell adhesion molecule and part of diverse processes such as signaling, cell migration, proliferation, and differentiation
EPHB4	Ephrin type-B receptor 4	HTK and Tyro11	Essential role in vascular development
ICAM-2	Intercellular adhesion molecule-2	CD102	Adherence and transmigration of leucocytes
ITGB2	Integrin beta-2	CD18	Ligands for ICAM-1, and critical for the migration of leucocytes to sites of inflammation
JAM-A	Junctional adhesion molecule A	F11R	Involved in the migration of leukocytes through the endothelial cell barrier
PECAM-1	Platelet endothelial cell adhesion molecule 1	CD31	Platelet/endothelial interaction, adherence and transmigration of leucocytes
SELE	E-selectin	CD62E, ELAM-1, and LECAM2	Leucocyte rolling
SELP	P-selectin	CD154	Platelet/endothelial interaction and leucocyte rolling

References

1. Doehner, W.; Frenneaux, M.; Anker, S.D. Metabolic impairment in heart failure: The myocardial and systemic perspective. *J. Am. Coll. Cardiol.* **2014**, *64*, 1388–1400. [CrossRef] [PubMed]
2. Yndestad, A.; Damas, J.K.; Oie, E.; Ueland, T.; Gullestad, L.; Aukrust, P. Systemic inflammation in heart failure–the whys and wherefores. *Heart Fail. Rev.* **2006**, *11*, 83–92. [CrossRef] [PubMed]
3. Chong, A.Y.; Blann, A.D.; Lip, G.Y.H. Assessment of endothelial damage and dysfunction: Observations in relation to heart failure. *QJM Int. J. Med.* **2003**, *96*, 253–267. [CrossRef] [PubMed]
4. Zhang, Y.; Bauersachs, J.; Langer, H.F. Immune mechanisms in heart failure. *Eur. J. Heart Fail.* **2017**, *19*, 1379–1389. [CrossRef]
5. Yin, W.H.; Chen, J.W.; Young, M.S.; Lin, S.J. Increased endothelial monocyte adhesiveness is related to clinical outcomes in chronic heart failure. *Int. J. Cardiol.* **2007**, *121*, 276–283. [CrossRef]
6. Wilhelmi, M.H.; Leyh, R.G.; Wilhelmi, M.; Haverich, A. Upregulation of endothelial adhesion molecules in hearts with congestive and ischemic cardiomyopathy: Immunohistochemical evaluation of inflammatory endothelial cell activation. *Eur. J. Cardiothorac. Surg.* **2005**, *27*, 122–127. [CrossRef]
7. Juliano, R.L. Signal transduction by cell adhesion receptors and the cytoskeleton: Functions of integrins, cadherins, selectins, and immunoglobulin-superfamily members. *Annu. Rev. Pharmacol. Toxicol.* **2002**, *42*, 283–323. [CrossRef]
8. Anker, S.D.; von Haehling, S. Inflammatory mediators in chronic heart failure: An overview. *Heart* **2004**, *90*, 464–470. [CrossRef]

9. Breviario, F.; Caveda, L.; Corada, M.; Martin-Padura, I.; Navarro, P.; Golay, J.; Introna, M.; Gulino, D.; Lampugnani, M.G.; Dejana, E. Functional properties of human vascular endothelial cadherin (7B4/cadherin-5), an endothelium-specific cadherin. *Arterioscler. Thromb. Vasc. Biol.* **1995**, *15*, 1229–1239. [CrossRef]
10. Granger, D.N.; Senchenkova, E. Inflammation and the Microcirculation. San Rafael (CA): Morgan & Claypool Life Sciences, 2010. Chapter 7, Leukocyte–Endothelial Cell Adhesion. Available online: https://www.ncbi.nlm.nih.gov/books/NBK53380/ (accessed on 2 January 2020).
11. Price, D.T.; Loscalzo, J. Cellular adhesion molecules and atherogenesis 1. *Am. J. Med.* **1999**, *107*, 85–97.
12. McMurray, J.J.; Adamopoulos, S.; Anker, S.D.; Auricchio, A.; Bohm, M.; Dickstein, K.; Falk, V.; Filippatos, G.; Fonseca, C.; Gomez-Sanchez, M.A.; et al. ESC Guidelines for the diagnosis and treatment of acute and chronic heart failure 2012: The Task Force for the Diagnosis and Treatment of Acute and Chronic Heart Failure 2012 of the European Society of Cardiology. Developed in collaboration with the Heart Failure Association (HFA) of the ESC. *Eur. Heart J.* **2012**, *33*, 1787–1847. [PubMed]
13. Paulus, W.J.; Tschope, C.; Sanderson, J.E.; Rusconi, C.; Flachskampf, F.A.; Rademakers, F.E.; Marino, P.; Smiseth, O.A.; De Keulenaer, G.; Leite-Moreira, A.F.; et al. How to diagnose diastolic heart failure: A consensus statement on the diagnosis of heart failure with normal left ventricular ejection fraction by the Heart Failure and Echocardiography Associations of the European Society of Cardiology. *Eur. Heart J.* **2007**, *28*, 2539–2550. [CrossRef] [PubMed]
14. Van Boven, N.; Battes, L.C.; Akkerhuis, K.M.; Rizopoulos, D.; Caliskan, K.; Anroedh, S.S.; Yassi, W.; Manintveld, O.C.; Cornel, J.H.; Constantinescu, A.A.; et al. Toward personalized risk assessment in patients with chronic heart failure: Detailed temporal patterns of NT-proBNP, troponin T, and CRP in the Bio-SHiFT study. *Am. Heart J.* **2018**, *196*, 36–48. [CrossRef] [PubMed]
15. Brankovic, M.; Akkerhuis, K.M.; van Boven, N.; Anroedh, S.; Constantinescu, A.; Caliskan, K.; Manintveld, O.; Cornel, J.H.; Baart, S.; Rizopoulos, D.; et al. Patient-specific evolution of renal function in chronic heart failure patients dynamically predicts clinical outcome in the Bio-SHiFT study. *Kidney Int.* **2018**, *93*, 952–960. [CrossRef]
16. Solier, C.; Langen, H. Antibody-based proteomics and biomarker research—Current status and limitations. *Proteomics* **2014**, *14*, 774–783. [CrossRef]
17. Rizopoulos, D. The R package JMbayes for fitting joint models for longitudinal and time-to-event data using MCMC. *arXiv* **2014**, arXiv:14047625. Available online: http://CRANR-projectorg/package=nlme (accessed on 8 August 2018).
18. Rizopoulos, D. Dynamic predictions and prospective accuracy in joint models for longitudinal and time-to-event data. *Biometrics* **2011**, *67*, 819–829. [CrossRef]
19. Rizopoulos, D. *Joint Models for Longitudinal and Time-to-Event Data: With Applications in R*; Chapman and Hall/CRC: Boca Raton, FL, USA, 2012.
20. Pinheiro, J.; Bates, D.; DebRoy, S.; Sarkar, D. R Core Team (2014) nlme: Linear and Nonlinear Mixed Effects Models. R Package Version 3.1-117. Available online: http://CRAN.R-project.org/package=nlme (accessed on 8 August 2018).
21. Mathiasen, A.B.; Henningsen, K.M.; Harutyunyan, M.J.; Mygind, N.D.; Kastrup, J. YKL-40: A new biomarker in cardiovascular disease? *Biomark. Med.* **2010**, *4*, 591–600. [CrossRef]
22. Harutyunyan, M.; Christiansen, M.; Johansen, J.S.; Kober, L.; Torp-Petersen, C.; Kastrup, J. The inflammatory biomarker YKL-40 as a new prognostic marker for all-cause mortality in patients with heart failure. *Immunobiology* **2012**, *217*, 652–656. [CrossRef]
23. Bilim, O.; Takeishi, Y.; Kitahara, T.; Ishino, M.; Sasaki, T.; Suzuki, S.; Shishido, T.; Kubota, I. Serum YKL-40 predicts adverse clinical outcomes in patients with chronic heart failure. *J. Card Fail.* **2010**, *16*, 873–879. [CrossRef]
24. Arain, F.; Gullestad, L.; Nymo, S.; Kjekshus, J.; Cleland, J.G.; Michelsen, A.; McMurray, J.J.; Wikstrand, J.; Aukrust, P.; Ueland, T. Low YKL-40 in chronic heart failure may predict beneficial effects of statins: Analysis from the controlled rosuvastatin multinational trial in heart failure (CORONA). *Biomarkers* **2017**, *22*, 261–267. [CrossRef] [PubMed]
25. Rathcke, C.N.; Kistorp, C.; Raymond, I.; Hildebrandt, P.; Gustafsson, F.; Lip, G.Y.; Faber, J.; Vestergaard, H. Plasma YKL-40 levels are elevated in patients with chronic heart failure. *Scand. Cardiovasc. J.* **2010**, *44*, 92–99. [CrossRef] [PubMed]

26. Woodfin, A.; Voisin, M.B.; Imhof, B.A.; Dejana, E.; Engelhardt, B.; Nourshargh, S. Endothelial cell activation leads to neutrophil transmigration as supported by the sequential roles of ICAM-2, JAM-A, and PECAM-1. *Blood* **2009**, *113*, 6246–6257. [CrossRef] [PubMed]
27. Reglero-Real, N.; Colom, B.; Bodkin, J.V.; Nourshargh, S. Endothelial Cell Junctional Adhesion Molecules: Role and Regulation of Expression in Inflammation. *Arterioscler. Thromb. Vasc. Biol.* **2016**, *36*, 2048–2057. [CrossRef]
28. Vestweber, D. Adhesion and signaling molecules controlling the transmigration of leukocytes through endothelium. *Immunol. Rev.* **2007**, *218*, 178–196. [CrossRef]
29. Yu, W.K.; McNeil, J.B.; Wickersham, N.E.; Shaver, C.M.; Bastarache, J.A.; Ware, L.B. Vascular endothelial cadherin shedding is more severe in sepsis patients with severe acute kidney injury. *Crit Care.* **2019**, *23*, 18. [CrossRef]
30. Zhang, R.Y.; Liu, Y.Y.; Li, L.; Cui, W.; Zhao, K.J.; Huang, W.C.; Gu, X.W.; Liu, W.; Wu, J.; Min, D.; et al. Increased levels of soluble vascular endothelial cadherin are associated with poor outcome in severe sepsis. *J. Int. Med. Res.* **2010**, *38*, 1497–1506. [CrossRef]
31. Soeki, T.; Tamura, Y.; Shinohara, H.; Sakabe, K.; Onose, Y.; Fukuda, N. Elevated concentration of soluble vascular endothelial cadherin is associated with coronary atherosclerosis. *Circ. J.* **2004**, *68*, 1–5. [CrossRef]
32. Luissint, A.C.; Nusrat, A.; Parkos, C.A. JAM-related proteins in mucosal homeostasis and inflammation. *Semin. Immunopathol.* **2014**, *36*, 211–226. [CrossRef]
33. Nourshargh, S.; Krombach, F.; Dejana, E. The role of JAM-A and PECAM-1 in modulating leukocyte infiltration in inflamed and ischemic tissues. *J. Leukoc. Biol.* **2006**, *80*, 714–718. [CrossRef]
34. Curaj, A.; Wu, Z.; Rix, A.; Gresch, O.; Sternkopf, M.; Alampour-Rajabi, S.; Lammers, T.; van Zandvoort, M.; Weber, C.; Koenen, R.R.; et al. Molecular Ultrasound Imaging of Junctional Adhesion Molecule A Depicts Acute Alterations in Blood Flow and Early Endothelial Dysregulation. *Arterioscler Thromb Vasc Biol.* **2018**, *38*, 40–48. [CrossRef] [PubMed]
35. Newman, P.J.; Newman, D.K. Signal transduction pathways mediated by PECAM-1: New roles for an old molecule in platelet and vascular cell biology. *Arterioscler. Thromb. Vasc. Biol.* **2003**, *23*, 953–964. [CrossRef] [PubMed]
36. Soeki, T.; Tamura, Y.; Shinohara, H.; Sakabe, K.; Onose, Y.; Fukuda, N. Increased soluble platelet/endothelial cell adhesion molecule-1 in the early stages of acute coronary syndromes. *Int. J. Cardiol.* **2003**, *90*, 261–268. [CrossRef]
37. Serebruany, V.L.; Murugesan, S.R.; Pothula, A.; Atar, D.; Lowry, D.R.; O'Connor, C.M.; Gurbel, P.A. Increased soluble platelet/endothelial cellular adhesion molecule-1 and osteonectin levels in patients with severe congestive heart failure. Independence of disease etiology, and antecedent aspirin therapy. *Eur. J. Heart Fail* **1999**, *1*, 243–249. [CrossRef]
38. Blann, A.D.; Nadar, S.K.; Lip, G.Y. The adhesion molecule P-selectin and cardiovascular disease. *Eur. Heart J.* **2003**, *24*, 2166–2179. [CrossRef] [PubMed]
39. O'Connor, C.M.; Gurbel, P.A.; Serebruany, V.L. Usefulness of soluble and surface-bound P-selectin in detecting heightened platelet activity in patients with congestive heart failure. *Am. J. Cardiol.* **1999**, *83*, 1345–1349. [CrossRef]
40. Stumpf, C.; Lehner, C.; Eskafi, S.; Raaz, D.; Yilmaz, A.; Ropers, S.; Schmeisser, A.; Ludwig, J.; Daniel, W.G.; Garlichs, C.D. Enhanced levels of CD154 (CD40 ligand) on platelets in patients with chronic heart failure. *Eur. J. Heart Fail.* **2003**, *5*, 629–637. [CrossRef]
41. Gibbs, C.R.; Blann, A.D.; Watson, R.D.; Lip, G.Y. Abnormalities of hemorheological, endothelial, and platelet function in patients with chronic heart failure in sinus rhythm: Effects of angiotensin-converting enzyme inhibitor and beta-blocker therapy. *Circulation* **2001**, *103*, 1746–1751. [CrossRef]
42. Chung, I.; Choudhury, A.; Patel, J.; Lip, G.Y. Soluble, platelet-bound, and total P-selectin as indices of platelet activation in congestive heart failure. *Ann. Med.* **2009**, *41*, 45–51. [CrossRef]
43. Ghebrehiwet, B.; Feng, X.; Kumar, R.; Peerschke, E.I. Complement component C1q induces endothelial cell adhesion and spreading through a docking/signaling partnership of C1q receptors and integrins. *Int. Immunopharmacol.* **2003**, *3*, 299–310. [CrossRef]
44. Guo, W.X.; Ghebrehiwet, B.; Weksler, B.; Schweitzer, K.; Peerschke, E.I. Up-regulation of endothelial cell binding proteins/receptors for complement component C1q by inflammatory cytokines. *J. Lab. Clin. Med.* **1999**, *133*, 541–550. [CrossRef]

45. Hamada, K.; Oike, Y.; Ito, Y.; Maekawa, H.; Miyata, K.; Shimomura, T.; Suda, T. Distinct roles of ephrin-B2 forward and EphB4 reverse signaling in endothelial cells. *Arterioscler. Thromb. Vasc. Biol.* **2003**, *23*, 190–197. [CrossRef] [PubMed]
46. Severino, P.; Mariani, M.V.; Fedele, F. Futility in cardiology: The need for a change in perspectives. *Eur. J. Heart Fail.* **2019**, *21*, 1483–1484. [CrossRef] [PubMed]
47. Severino, P.; Maestrini, V.; Mariani, M.V.; Birtolo, L.I.; Scarpati, R.; Mancone, M.; Fedele, F. Structural and myocardial dysfunction in heart failure beyond ejection fraction. *Heart Fail. Rev.* **2019**. [CrossRef]
48. Severino, P.; Mather, P.J.; Pucci, M.; D'Amato, A.; Mariani, M.V.; Infusino, F.; Birtolo, L.I.; Maestrini, V.; Mancone, M.; Fedele, F. Advanced Heart Failure and End-Stage Heart Failure: Does a Difference Exist. *Diagnostics* **2019**, *9*, 170. [CrossRef]
49. Severino, P.; D'Amato, A.; Netti, L.; Pucci, M.; Infusino, F.; Maestrini, V.; Mancone, M.; Fedele, F. Myocardial Ischemia and Diabetes Mellitus: Role of Oxidative Stress in the Connection between Cardiac Metabolism and Coronary Blood Flow. *J. Diabetes Res.* **2019**, *2019*, 9489826. [CrossRef]
50. Fedele, F.; Severino, P.; Calcagno, S.; Mancone, M. Heart failure: TNM-like classification. *J. Am. Coll. Cardiol.* **2014**, *63*, 1959–1960. [CrossRef]
51. Bouwens, E.; Brankovic, M.; Mouthaan, H.; Baart, S.; Rizopoulos, D.; van Boven, N.; Caliskan, K.; Manintveld, O.; Germans, T.; van Ramshorst, J.; et al. Temporal Patterns of 14 Blood Biomarker candidates of Cardiac Remodeling in Relation to Prognosis of Patients With Chronic Heart Failure-The Bio- SH i FT Study. *J. Am. Heart Assoc.* **2019**, *8*, e009555. [CrossRef]

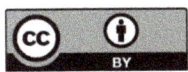

© 2020 by the authors. Licensee MDPI, Basel, Switzerland. This article is an open access article distributed under the terms and conditions of the Creative Commons Attribution (CC BY) license (http://creativecommons.org/licenses/by/4.0/).

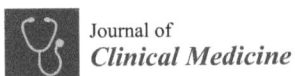 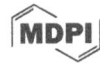

Article

Left Ventricular Function and Myocardial Triglyceride Content on 3T Cardiac MR Predict Major Cardiovascular Adverse Events and Readmission in Patients Hospitalized with Acute Heart Failure

Kuang-Fu Chang [1,2,†], Gigin Lin [2,3,4,†], Pei-Ching Huang [2], Yu-Hsiang Juan [2], Chao-Hung Wang [5], Shang-Yueh Tsai [6], Yu-Ching Lin [1], Ming-Ting Wu [7], Pen-An Liao [2], Lan-Yan Yang [8], Min-Hui Liu [5], Yu-Chun Lin [2,3], Jiun-Jie Wang [2,3], Koon-Kwan Ng [1,*] and Shu-Hang Ng [2,*]

1. Department of Radiology, Chang Gung Memorial Hospital, Keelung and Chang Gung University, Keelung 20401, Taiwan; kc1116@cgmh.org.tw (K.-F.C.); yuching1221@cgmh.org.tw (Y.-C.L.)
2. Department of Medical Imaging and Intervention, Chang Gung Memorial Hospital, Linkou and Chang Gung University, Taoyuan 33305, Taiwan; giginlin@cgmh.org.tw (G.L.); spookie@cgmh.org.tw (P.-C.H.); 8801131@cgmh.org.tw (Y.-H.J.); wakefield1006@gmail.com (P.-A.L.); jack805@gmail.com (Y.-C.L.); jiunjie.wang@gmail.com (J.-J.W.)
3. Imaging Core Lab, Institute for Radiological Research, Chang Gung University, Taoyuan 333, Taiwan
4. Clinical Metabolomics Core Lab, Chang Gung Memorial Hospital, Taoyuan 333, Taiwan
5. Department of Cardiology and Heart Failure Center, Chang Gung Memorial Hospital, Keelung 20401, Taiwan; bearty54@gmail.com (C.-H.W.); khfoffice@gmail.com (M.-H.L.)
6. Graduate Institute of Applied Physics, National Chengchi University, Taipei 11605, Taiwan; syytsai@gmail.com
7. Department of Radiology, Kaohsiung Veterans General Hospital, Kaohsiung 81362, Taiwan; wu.mingting@gmail.com
8. Clinical Trial Center, Chang Gung Memorial Hospital at Linkou, Taoyuan 333, Taiwan; lyyang0111@gmail.com
* Correspondence: ngkk@ms14.hinet.net (K.-K.N.); shuhangng@gmail.com (S.-H.N.); Tel.: +886-2431-3131 (ext. 2214) (K.-K.N.); +886-3328-1200 (ext. 2575) (S.-H.N.); Fax: +886-2433-2869 (K.-K.N.); +886-3397-1936 (S.-H.N.)
† These authors contributed equally to this work.

Received: 30 December 2019; Accepted: 7 January 2020; Published: 8 January 2020

Abstract: Background: This prospective study was designed to investigate whether myocardial triglyceride (TG) content from proton magnetic resonance spectroscopy (MRS) and left ventricular (LV) function parameters from cardiovascular magnetic resonance imaging (CMR) can serve as imaging biomarkers in predicting future major cardiovascular adverse events (MACE) and readmission in patients who had been hospitalized for acute heart failure (HF). Methods: Patients who were discharged after hospitalization for acute HF were prospectively enrolled. On a 3.0 T MR scanner, myocardial TG contents were measured using MRS, and LV parameters (function and mass) were evaluated using cine. The occurrence of MACE and the HF-related readmission served as the endpoints. Independent predictors were identified using univariate and multivariable Cox proportional hazard regression analyses. Results: A total of 133 patients (mean age, 52.4 years) were enrolled. The mean duration of follow-up in surviving patients was 775 days. Baseline LV functional parameters—including ejection fraction, LV end-diastolic volume, LV end-diastolic volume index (LVEDVI), and LV end-systolic volume ($p < 0.0001$ for all), and myocardial mass ($p = 0.010$)—were significantly associated with MACE. Multivariable analysis revealed that LVEDVI was the independent predictor for MACE, while myocardial mass was the independent predictor for 3- and 12-month readmission. Myocardial TG content (lipid resonances δ 1.6 ppm) was significantly associated with readmission in patients with ischemic heart disease. Conclusions: LVEDVI and myocardial mass are potential imaging biomarkers that independently predict MACE and readmission, respectively, in patients discharged after hospitalization for acute HF. Myocardial TG predicts readmission in patients with a history of ischemic heart disease.

Keywords: cardiac magnetic resonance imaging; heart failure; left ventricular systolic function; magnetic resonance spectroscopy; myocardial triglyceride content

1. Introduction

Heart failure (HF) is a complex clinical syndrome that results from a variety of conditions preventing the left ventricle (LV) from supporting physiological circulation [1]. Patients with HF are at an increased risk of major adverse cardiovascular events (MACE)—including death, myocardial infarction, stroke, and hospitalizations [2,3]—which pose a significant public health burden globally. The 3-month readmission rates of patients with acute HF remains as high as 25–50%, with 5-year survival rates <50% [4]. Optimized risk sFCtratification would help to prioritize the surveillance for those who are prone to experience MACE.

Cardiomyocytes primarily depend on the oxidation of fatty acids as their source of energy [5]. Because the heart does not serve as a storage depot for fat, the concentration of triglycerides (TG) in the myocardium is low under physiological conditions. However, cardiac steatosis may develop as a result of abnormal regulation of fatty acids uptake or alterations in lipid metabolism. TG accumulation in the heart has been recognized as a risk factor for cardiovascular (CV) disease [6–8]. Vilahur et al. have shown that intramyocardial lipids impaired myofibroblast-related collagen synthesis with resultant poor healing of the myocardial scar post-myocardial infarction, while excess cardiac lipids exacerbated apoptosis and led to extensive myocardial infarcts [9]. Proton magnetic resonance spectroscopy (^{1}H-MRS) has been used to obtain in vivo quantitative measures of myocardial TG content in patients with CV disorders [10–12]. We have previously used 3.0 T CMR to analyze the association between myocardial unsaturated fatty acids (UFA) content and left ventricular (LV) function in patients who had been hospitalized for acute HF [13]. Furthermore, cardiac magnetic resonance imaging (CMR) is well established as the gold standard in the assessment of cardiac structure and function, with incremental diagnostic and prognostic information in HF [14–16]. We, therefore, hypothesize that the quantitative information about myocardial TG content from ^{1}H-MRS and LV function parameters from CMR may help predict the occurrence of future MACE and readmission in patients who have been hospitalized for acute HF.

This prospective study was designed to investigate whether myocardial TG content from ^{1}H-MRS (primary aim) and LV function parameters from CMR (secondary aim) can serve as imaging biomarkers in predicting future MACE and readmission in patients who have been hospitalized for acute HF.

2. Methods

2.1. Ethics Approval and Consent to Participate

Ethical approval was granted by the Institutional Review Board of the Keelung Chang Gung Memorial Hospital (IRB 102-2772A3). The study is reported in accordance with the STROBE (STrengthening the Reporting of OBservational studies in Epidemiology) statement and has been registered at ClinicalTrials.gov (Identifier: NCT02378402) on 21 February 2015. All patients provided their written informed consent.

2.2. Study Design and Patient Population

Between March 2014 and June 2016, we prospectively screened 200 patients and enrolled a total of 147 patients who were hospitalized with acute HF at a tertiary referral hospital with a dedicated HF center (IRB 102-2772A3, ClinicalTrial.gov: NCT02378402). Patients were scanned whose medical condition had become stable after treatment, specifically when they (1) had an oral medication regimen stable for at least 24 h; (2) had no intravenous vasodilator or inotropic agents for at least 24 h; and (3) were ambulatory before discharge to assess functional capacity. Patients aged between 20 and 70 years with acute HF, with initial HF stage C, classified according to the American College of Cardiology (ACC) and the American Heart Association (AHA) HF classification system [4], were eligible. Patients who were unwilling to participate or presenting with general contraindications to CMR (e.g., claustrophobia, metal-containing implants, cardiac pacemakers, or unable to comply with the examiners) were excluded. Additional exclusion criteria were as follows: Positive history of open cardiac surgery; pregnancy or breastfeeding; and inability to adhere to treatment and/or follow-up. All of the medical records underwent a central review by a multidisciplinary team to confirm that the identified patients were suitable for inclusion. The following variables were collected at baseline: Demographic data (age, sex, height, and weight), cardiovascular risk factors (smoking, hypertension, diabetes), previous history of cardiovascular disease (angina, myocardial infarction, dilated cardiomyopathy, myocarditis), and medication use. Serum lipid levels (total cholesterol, very-low-density lipoprotein cholesterol, low-density lipoprotein cholesterol, high-density lipoprotein cholesterol, and TG) were measured 1 month before CMR imaging. Patients with a previous history of angina or myocardial infarction were defined as an ischemic group, while the others as non-ischemic group. Previously, 48 of the 133 patients have been reported in a cross-sectional interim report to study the association of LV function and myocardial TG on CMR [13]. In this study, we further evaluated their predictive value in a longitudinal observational study. The patient flow diagram is present in Figure 1.

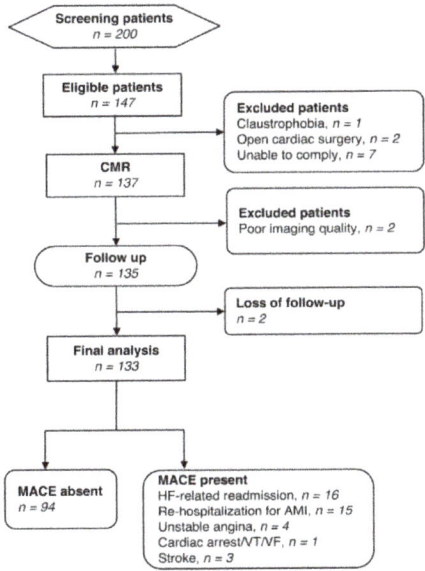

Figure 1. Flow diagram of the study cohort. Note.—AMI, acute myocardial infarction; CMR, cardiac magnetic resonance; HF, heart failure; MACE, major cardiovascular event; VT, ventricular tachycardia; VF, ventricular fibrillation.

2.3. H-MRS

Clinical MRS was acquired before contrast administration using the same settings and anatomical localizations as previously reported [13]. In brief, respiratory-triggered cardiac-gated point-resolved spectroscopy (PRESS) [17] was implemented to acquire localized ^{1}H MRS voxels to a $2 \times 2 \times 1$ cm^3 spectroscopic volume within the interventricular septum during the end-systolic phase. The MRS acquisition parameters were as follows: Nominal TR (repetition time)/TE (echo time), 550 ms/33 ms;

64 averages; window size, 1024 points; bandwidth, 2000 Hz [18–21]. Spectra with and without water suppression were used to obtain water and myocardial TG signals, respectively [22].

2.4. CMR Imaging

Patients were required to fast overnight before undergoing CMR examinations on a 3.0-Tesla Siemens Skyra MR scanner (Siemens, Erlangen, Germany). No pre-medications were used. The scanner was equipped with an 18-channel phased-array receiver body coil and operated on a VD13 platform. Steady-state free precession (SSFP) cine imaging was used to produce images with both short-axis (contiguous 8 mm slice thickness) and standard long-axis views (2-, 3- and 4-chamber views). Late gadolinium enhancement (LGE) at 10 min after gadolinium injection in the short-axis (9 to 13 images covering the entire LV), 2-chamber, and 4-chamber planes. The following settings were employed: Echo time, 1.2 ms; repetition time, 3.4 ms; field of view, 34–40 cm; matrix, 256 × 256.

2.5. Image Analysis

Left ventricular ejection fraction (LVEF) was measured on short-axis cine LV images with post-processing software (VB17, Argus Viewer and Function, Siemens, Erlangen, Germany) on a separate workstation. LV endocardial and epicardial borders were manually drawn at end-diastole and end-systole on short-axis cine images and LVEF and end-diastolic LV mass from each slice were measured accordingly. Papillary muscles were not included in the LV mass. Left ventricular end-diastolic volume (LVEDV) and end-systolic volume (LVESV) were calculated using the same methodology. The left ventricular end-diastolic volume index (LVEDVI) was determined by dividing the LVEDV by the body surface area (BSA). The LV global function index (LVGFI) was calculated with the following formula:

$$\text{LVGFI} = [\text{LVESV}/(\text{LVEDV}+\text{LVESV})/2 + (\text{LV mass}/1.05)] \times 100 \tag{1}$$

LCModel 6.2 software package (http://s-provencher.com/pages/lcmodel.shtml) was used for the quantification of TG by fitting the time-domain ^{1}H-MRS spectra (Figure 2). Multiple resonance peaks of fat including methyl (–(CH$_2$)$_n$–CH$_3$) peak δ 0.9 ppm, methylene (–(CH$_2$)$_n$–) peaked at 1.3 ppm, beta-carboxyl (–CO-CH$_2$-CH$_2$–) at 1.6 ppm, alpha-allylic (–CH$_2$–CH=CH–CH$_2$–) peaked at 2.02 ppm (denote by Lip2.1), alpha-carboxyl (–CO-CH$_2$-CH$_2$–) peaked at 2.24 ppm (denote by Lip2.3), diacyl (–CH=CH–CH$_2$–CH=CH–) peaked at 2.75 ppm (denote by Lip2.8), olefinic (–CH=CH–) at 5.29 ppm (denote by Lip5.3) were fitted. Water-suppressed spectra were used to quantify the total myocardial TG resonance and its—including FA (lipid resonances δ 0.9, 1.3 and 1.6 ppm) and UFA (lipid resonance δ 2.02 ppm, 2.24 ppm, 2.75 ppm, and 5.29 ppm), i.e., the ratio of the metabolite resonance area to the unsuppressed water resonance area. Water resonance (~δ 4.7 ppm) without water suppression was also determined for normalization. Cramer-Rao lower bound (CRLB) of TG provided by the LCModel was served as a goodness-of-fit, and used for the evaluation of the spectra quality.

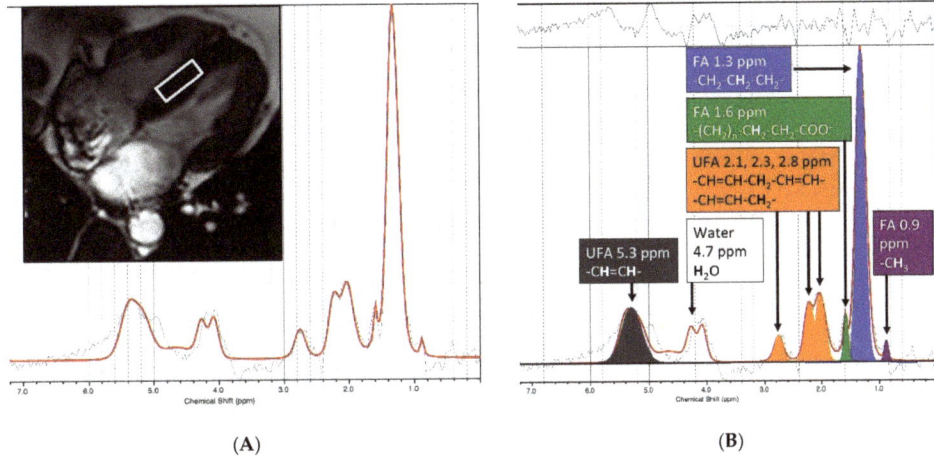

Figure 2. Example myocardial CMR spectroscopy. (**A**) A $2 \times 2 \times 1$ cm^3 spectroscopic volume (white box) was acquired from the interventricular septum during the systolic phase to generate an input spectrum. (**B**) ^{1}H-CMR spectra were fitted and analyzed using the LCModel 6.2 software package (right). We quantified the components of myocardial triglyceride resonances, i.e., fatty acids (FA, lipid resonances δ 0.9, 1.3, and 1.6 ppm) and unsaturated fatty acids (UFA, lipid resonance δ 2.1 and 2.3, 2.8, 5.3 ppm).

2.6. Treatment and Definition of the Study Outcomes

Patients were clinically followed on a monthly basis by a dedicated HF team, who were aware of conventional CMR but blinded to the MRS results. MACE is a composite of clinical events without standard definition, because individual outcomes used to make this composite endpoint vary by study [2,3,23]. According to our study endpoints, we used the term MACE to comprise the composite of the events including HF worsening, HF-related readmissions, cardiac catheterization, unstable angina, stroke, cardiac arrest/ventricular tachycardia (VT)/ventricular fibrillation (VF), and cardiac death. However, the HF related-readmission rates were not included in MACE and, thus, were separately considered. The appropriate length of the 2-year follow-up was determined based on our previous heart failure cohort study [24].

2.7. Data Analysis

Univariate and stepwise multivariable regression analyses (Wald statistics) were used to assess CMR parameters. A complete-case analysis was implemented (missing data were not excluded). Survival curves were plotted with the Kaplan-Meier method (log-rank test). Two-group comparisons of continuous and categorical variables were performed with the Student's *t*-test (two-group comparisons) and chi-square test, respectively. Continuous variables were determined by the recursive partitioning method to obtain the optimal cut-off values. Independent predictors of MACE and readmission rates were identified using univariate and multivariable Cox proportional hazard regression analyses. A Bonferroni posthoc correction was conducted to reduce Type I Error by dividing the original α-value by the number of analyses on the dependent variable. Data correlation was evaluated based on the Spearman rank test. Data analyses were performed using the following software: SPSS (version 11; SPSS Inc., Chicago, IL, USA), MedCalc (version 9.2.0.0; MedCalc Software, Mariakerke, Belgium), and R (version 3.5.3, R Foundation for Statistical Computing, Vienna, Austria, www.r-project.org).

3. Results

3.1. Patient Characteristics

A total of 133 consecutive patients (mean age, 52.4 years) entered the final analysis, with the mean follow-up time for surviving patients being 775 days. Table S1 details the baseline LV functional parameters. The baseline LVEF of this patient population was 52.2 (52.2 ± 21.7%). There were more patients with preserved EF ≥55% ($n = 71$) than reduced EF <55% ($n = 62$). MACE was observed in 39 cases (29.3%). The MACE with their distribution being as follows: HF-related readmission ($n = 16$; ischemic/non-ischemic 6/10), re-hospitalization for acute myocardial infarction ($n = 15$; 15/0), unstable angina ($n = 4$; 4/0), cardiac arrest ($n = 1$; 1/0), and stroke ($n = 3$; 0/3). There were no cases of cardiac death. The baseline clinical characteristics of the study participants are summarized in Table 1. Patients who experienced MACE did not differ from those who did not in terms of baseline clinical characteristics. As far as HF-related events are concerned, 6 patients (4.5%) were readmitted within 3 months and 18 patients (13.5%) within 12 months. Only one patient (0.8%) was readmitted within 30 days. Ischemic heart disease was identified in 50 patients, with the involvement of the left main ($n = 2$), left anterior descending ($n = 36$), left circumflex ($n = 26$), and right coronary artery ($n = 23$), verified by the presence of a myocardial scar on LGE. The remaining 83 patients had no history of ischemic heart disease and had no myocardial scar on LGE.

Table 1. Baseline characteristics of the study patients ($n = 133$).

Variable	MACE ($n = 39$)	Non-MACE ($n = 94$)	p Value
Clinical profile			
Male sex (%)	74.2%	57.5%	0.088
Age (years)	52.3 ± 10.0	52.7 ± 10.3	0.846
Height (m)	1.7 ± 0.1	1.7 ± 0.1	0.656
Weight (kg)	70.5 ± 13.8	69.6 ± 15.9	0.751
BMI (kg/m^2)	25.7 ± 3.9	25.6 ± 5.3	0.953
Heart rate	73.8 ± 14.2	71.3 ± 13.2	0.350
SBP (mmHg)	125.3 ± 19.5	131.9 ± 21.1	0.087
DBP (mmHg)	73.0 ± 11.7	76.4 ± 10.2	0.116
Smoking	53.8%	42.5%	0.316
Comorbidities			
Hypertension	47.3%	45.0%	0.956
DM	23.7%	20.0%	0.813
Angina	36.6%	32.5%	0.802
MI	36.6%	32.5%	0.802
DCM	16.1%	10.0%	0.512
Myocarditis	2.2%	5.0%	0.742
CAD	35.5%	32.5%	0.894
Medications			
DM drugs	16.1%	20.0%	0.771
Anti-platelets	39.8%	37.5%	0.957
Statins	23.7%	17.5%	0.576
Thrombolytic agents	6.5%	0.0%	0.235
Antiarrhythmic drugs	14.0%	10.0%	0.729
Diuretics	39.8%	30.0%	0.381
Calcium channel blockers	10.8%	7.5%	0.794
Beta blockers	68.8%	62.5%	0.611
ACEI/ARB	68.8%	57.5%	0.289
Vasodilators	16.1%	5.0%	0.139
Iron supplements	5.4%	2.5%	0.781

Table 1. Cont.

Variable	MACE (n = 39)	Non-MACE (n = 94)	p Value
Laboratory data			
AST (U/L)	31.4 ± 28.5	27.9 ± 24.3	0.556
ALT (U/L)	28.1 ± 16.5	39.8 ± 49.3	0.187
HDL (mg/dL)	43.5 ± 12.4	43.5 ± 12.1	0.988
VLDL (mg/dL)	30.3 ± 15.7	28.6 ± 13.0	0.598
LDL (mg/dL)	106.2 ± 53.2	109.7 ± 38.4	0.737
Total cholesterol/HDL	5.1 ± 5.3	4.4 ± 1.1	0.449
LDL/HDL	2.8 ± 1.2	2.7 ± 1.0	0.663
Total cholesterol (mg/dL)	189.3 ± 49.4	185.2 ± 35.7	0.672
Triglyceride (mg/dL)	165.5 ± 129.1	151.2 ± 86.2	0.564
Non-HDL (mg/dL)	145.8 ± 45.0	141.7 ± 35.4	0.662
Glucose (mg/dL)	113.2 ± 31.2	123.5 ± 51.2	0.210
HbA1c (mg/dL)	6.2 ± 1.2	6.4 ± 1.6	0.421
TIBC (ug/dL)	377.9 ± 85.8	346.7 ± 52.2	0.413
Troponin (ng/mL)	2.0 ± 8.9	0.3 ± 0.7	0.428
BNP (pg/mL)	342.9 ± 583.0	450.4 ± 569.7	0.470
Neutrophil count (%)	62.7 ± 12.6	57.5 ± 12.4	0.078
Hemoglobin (g/dL)	14.4 ± 3.5	13.5 ± 1.5	0.129
MCV (fl)	87.7 ± 6.7	86.4 ± 8.0	0.322
MCH (pg)	29.6 ± 2.7	29.0 ± 3.1	0.240
MCHC (%)	33.7 ± 1.0	41.0 ± 47.5	0.337

Note—Categorical data are expressed as numbers (%), whereas continuous variables are given as means ± standard deviations unless otherwise specified. Abbreviations: BMI, body mass index; CAD, coronary artery disease; SBP, systolic blood pressure; DBP, diastolic blood pressure; MACE, major adverse cardiac events; DM, diabetes mellitus; MI, myocardial infarction; DCM, dilated cardiomyopathy; ACEI, angiotensin-converting enzyme inhibitors; ARB, angiotensin receptor blockers; AST, aspartate aminotransferase; ALT, alanine transaminase; HDL, high-density lipoprotein; VLDL, very-low-density lipoprotein; LDL, low-density lipoprotein; TIBC, total iron-binding capacity; BNP, B-type natriuretic peptide; MCV, mean corpuscular volume; MCH, mean corpuscular hemoglobin; MCHC, mean corpuscular hemoglobin concentration.

3.2. Associations between CMR, and ^{1}H-MRS Parameters with MACE and HF-Related Readmission

All of the CMR parameters (EF, LVEDV, LVEDVI, LVESV, LV mean cavity volume, LV global volume, and LVGFI) were reciprocally correlated with one another ($p < 0.0001$). The results of univariate Cox regression analysis for MACE and HF-related readmission are shown in Tables 2 and 3. After allowance for potential confounders in multivariable analysis, LVEDVI was identified as an independent predictor for MACE, whereas myocardial mass independently predicted 3- and 12-month readmission rates. Kaplan-Meier survival analysis (Figure 3) demonstrated that patients with low LVEDVI (≤ 90.2 mL/m^2) had a lower probability for MACE than those with high LVEDVI (>90.2 mL/m^2, log-rank test, $p < 0.0001$).

Table 2. Univariate and stepwise multivariable Cox regression analysis of CMR and ^{1}H-MRS factors associated with major adverse cardiovascular events.

CMR & MRS Parameters	Overall (n = 133)				Ischemia (n = 50)				Non-Ischemia (n = 83)			
	Univariate		Stepwise Multivariable		Univariate		Stepwise Multivariable		Univariate		Stepwise Multivariable	
Variable	HR	p Value	HR	p Value	HR	p Value	HR	p Value	HR	p Value	HR	p Value
EF (%)	0.97	<0.001			0.99	0.456			0.95	0.001		
LV EDV (mL)	1.01	<0.001	1.01	<0.001 *	1.00	0.099			1.01	<0.001		
LV EDVI (mL/m^2)	1.01	<0.001			1.01	0.041			1.02	<0.001		
LV ESV (mL)	1.01	<0.001			1.00	0.189			1.01	<0.001		
Cardiac output (L/min)	1.08	0.463			1.25	0.067			0.95	0.768		
Myocardial mass (g)	1.01	0.001			1.01	0.144	1.32	0.044	1.01	<0.001	1.32	0.044
LV stroke volume (mL)	1.00	0.635			1.01	0.341			1.01	0.836		
LV mean cavity volume (mL)	1.01	<0.001			1.00	0.132			1.01	<0.001		
LV myocardial volume (mL)	1.01	0.001			1.01	0.144			1.01	<0.001		
LV global volume (mL)	1.00	<0.001			1.00	0.103			1.00	<0.001		
LVGFI (%)	0.97	0.001			0.99	0.562			0.95	<0.001		
FA 0.9 ppm	1.00	0.508			1.00	0.573			1.00	0.671		
FA 1.3 ppm	1.00	0.599			1.00	0.697			1.00	0.764		
FA 1.6 ppm	1.00	0.967			1.00	0.472			1.00	0.706		
UFA 2.1 ppm	1.00	0.557			1.00	0.938			1.00	0.779		
UFA 2.3 ppm	1.00	0.796			1.00	0.876			0.94	0.604		
UFA 2.8 ppm	1.00	0.796			1.00	0.753			0.18	0.772		
FA (09,13,16)	1.00	0.617			1.00	0.701			1.00	0.748		
UFA (21,23,28,53)	1.00	0.881			1.00	0.640			1.00	0.722		
TG (FA+UFA)	1.00	0.592			1.00	0.643			1.00	0.740		
FA/TG	1.68	0.219			1.89	0.292			1.60	0.605		
UFA/TG	0.60	0.219			0.53	0.292			0.62	0.605		
FA/UFA	1.00	0.089			1.01	0.023	1.01	0.022	0.98	0.426		

Note.—Abbreviations: HR, hazard ratio; CI, confidence interval; BMI, body mass index; SBP, systolic blood pressure; DBP, diastolic blood pressure; EF, ejection fraction; LV, left ventricular; EDV, end-diastolic volume; EDVI, end-diastolic volume index; ESV, end-systolic volume; FA, fatty acid; LVGFI, left ventricular global volume index; TG, triglycerides; UFA, unsaturated fatty acids. * significant after Bonferroni correction.

Table 3. Univariate and stepwise multivariable Cox regression analysis of CMR and ^{1}H-MRS factors associated with heart failure-related readmission.

CMR& MRS Parameters	Overall (n = 133)				Ischemia (n = 50)				Non-Ischemia (n = 83)			
	Univariate		Stepwise Multivariable		Univariate		Stepwise Multivariable		Univariate		Stepwise Multivariable	
Variable	HR	p Value	HR	p Value	HR	p Value	HR	p Value	HR	p Value	HR	p Value
EF (%)	0.96	<0.001			0.97	0.184			0.94	0.001		
LV EDV (mL)	1.01	<0.001			1.01	0.152			1.01	<0.001		
LV EDVI (mL/m^2)	1.02	<0.001	1.02	<0.001 *	1.02	0.106			1.02	0.001	1.01	<0.001 *
LV ESV (mL)	1.01	<0.001			1.01	0.119			1.01	<0.001		
Cardiac output (L/min)	0.85	0.348			0.92	0.781			0.81	0.326		
Myocardial mass (g)	1.01	<0.001			1.01	0.177			1.01	0.001		
LV stroke volume (mL)	0.99	0.447			0.99	0.699			0.99	0.408		
LV mean cavity volume (mL)	1.01	<0.001			1.01	0.130			1.01	<0.001		
LV myocardial volume (mL)	1.01	<0.001			1.01	0.177			1.01	0.001		
LV global volume (mL)	1.01	<0.001	1.01	<0.001 *	1.01	0.107	1.02	0.001 *	1.01	<.001	1.01	0.002 *
LVGFI (%)	0.94	<0.001			0.95	0.148			0.94	<0.001		
FA 0.9 ppm	0.70	0.523			0.86	0.708			0.00	0.555		
FA 1.3 ppm	1.00	0.746			0.96	0.832			1.00	0.769		
FA 1.6 ppm	0.68	0.635				0.006		0.003 *	0.22	0.735		
UFA 2.1 ppm	0.34	0.629			0.50	0.723			0.16	0.766		
UFA 2.3 ppm	0.65	0.718			0.82	0.737			0.24	0.770		
UFA 2.8 ppm	0.04	0.619			0.71	0.780				0.487		
FA (09,13,16)	0.99	0.589			0.96	0.0718			1.00	0.795		
UFA (21,23,28,53)	0.93	0.581			0.77	0.708			0.96	0.635		
TG (FA+UFA)	0.99	0.589			0.99	0.851			0.99	0.680		
FA/TG	2.72	0.183			56.41	0.095			1.21	0.818		
UFA/TG	0.37	0.183			0.02	0.095			0.83	0.818		
FA/UFA	1.01	0.396			1.01	0.318			1.00	0.858		

Note.—Abbreviations: HR, hazard ratio; CI, confidence interval; BMI, body mass index; SBP, systolic blood pressure; DBP, diastolic blood pressure; EF, ejection fraction; LV, left ventricular; EDV, end-diastolic volume; EDVI, end-diastolic volume index; ESV, end-systolic volume; FA, fatty acid; LVGFI, left ventricular global volume index; TG, triglycerides; UFA, unsaturated fatty acids. * significant after Bonferroni correction.

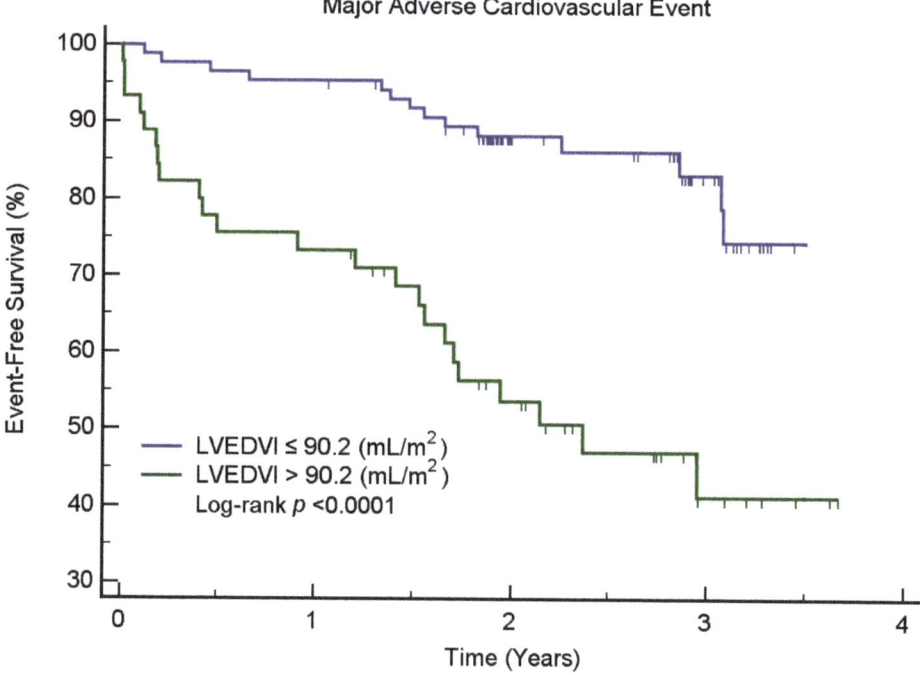

Figure 3. Kaplan-Meier curves for MACE-free survival in patients stratified according to the left ventricular end-diastolic volume index (LVEDVI) on CMR. Note—Kaplan-Meier survival analysis demonstrated that all patients with low LVEDVI ($\leq$90.2 mL/m^2) had a lower probability for MACE than those with high LVEDVI (>90.2 mL/m^2, log-rank test, $p < 0.0001$). MACE, major cardiovascular event.

We found that baseline myocardial TG content—FA/UFA ratio—was significantly associated with the MACE, whilst the level of lipid resonances δ 1.6 ppm was significantly associated with HF-related readmission for those patients with ischemic heart disease. Kaplan-Meier survival analysis (Figure 4) demonstrated that ischemic patients with a low level of lipid resonance δ 1.6 ppm ($\leq$0.99) had a lower probability for HF-related readmission than those with a high lipid resonance δ 1.6 ppm (>0.99, log-rank test, $p < 0.0001$). In non-ischemic patients, Kaplan-Meier survival analysis (Figure 5) demonstrated that patients with low LV global volume ($\leq$231 mL) had a lower probability for HF-related readmission than those with high LV global volume (>231 mL, log-rank test, $p < 0.0001$). Myocardial TG content was not associated with MACE or HF-related readmission in non-ischemic patients. The levels of lipid resonances δ 1.6 ppm inversely correlated with the myocardial mass ($r = -0.290$, $p = 0.009$) and LV global volume ($r = -0.282$, $p = 0.011$) in non-ischemic patients. No correlations between the myocardial TG content and CMR functional parameters were found in the ischemic patient group.

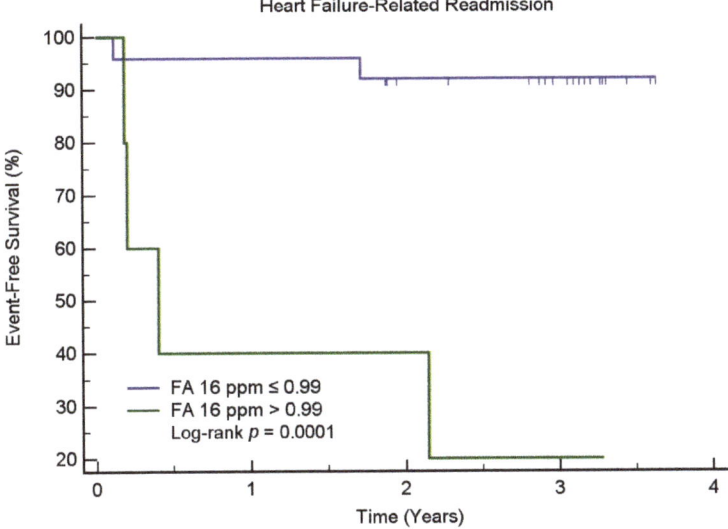

Figure 4. Kaplan-Meier curves for readmission-free survival in ischemic patients stratified according to the level of lipid resonances δ 1.6 ppm on ^{1}H-MRS. Note—Kaplan-Meier survival analysis demonstrated that ischemic patients with low levels of lipid resonances δ 1.6 ppm (≤0.99) had a lower probability for heart failure-related readmission than those with high levels of lipid resonances δ 1.6 ppm (>0.99, log-rank test, $p < 0.0001$). Note.—Abbreviations: FA, fatty acid.

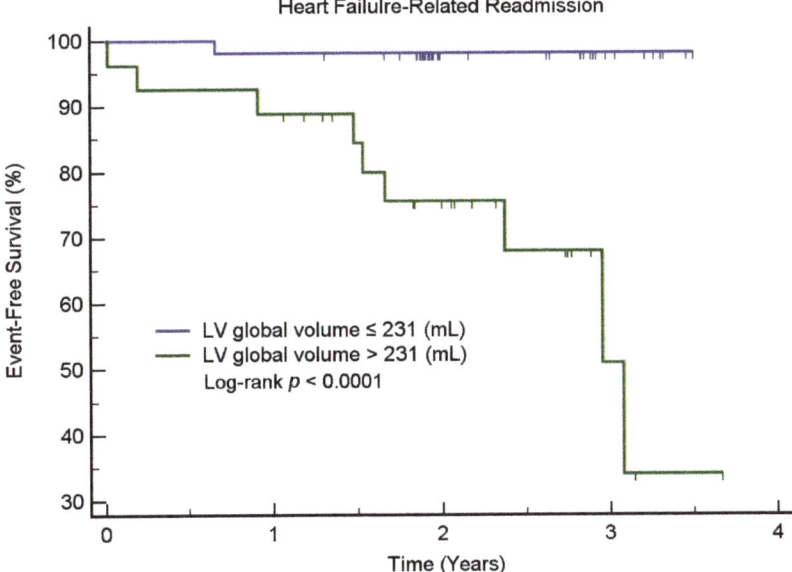

Figure 5. Kaplan-Meier curves for readmission-free survival in non-ischemic patients stratified according to LV (left ventricular) global volume on CMR. Note—Kaplan-Meier survival analysis showed that non-ischemic patients with low LV global volume (≤231 mL) had a lower probability for heart failure-related readmission than those with high LV global volume (>231 mL, log-rank test, $p < 0.0001$).

4. Discussion

This study was designed to simultaneously assess the prognostic significance of myocardial TG content (assessed by ^{1}H-MRS) and LV function parameters (measured on CMR) in the prediction of MACE and readmission in patients hospitalized for acute HF. Our main results can be summarized as follows. First, an increased LVEDVI was identified as an independent predictor of reduced MACE-free survival. Second, myocardial mass was independently associated with 3- and 12-month readmission rates. Finally, we found myocardial TG content—FA/UFA ratio—was significantly associated with MACE, whilst the level of lipid resonances δ 1.6 ppm was significantly associated with HF-related readmission for patients with ischemic heart disease. Taken together, these data indicate that assessment of LV function on CMR may improve the risk stratification of patients who have been hospitalized for acute HF. ^{1}H-MRS assessment might be reserved for patients with a history of ischemic heart disease.

In patients with HF, diastolic wall strain has been reported as an independent predictor of MACE [25], and the global circumferential strain may improve the prognostic stratification [26]. However, both diastolic wall strain and global circumferential strain require expertise for post-processing from cine CMR, and were not performed in the present study. In contrast, LVEDVI (defined as the volume of blood in the LV at end load filling indexed for body surface area) is easier to integrate in the clinical routine. Mewton et al. [27] have reported that LVGFI—a CMR parameter that integrates LV structure with global function—has a strong predictive value of MACE in a multiethnic population of men and women without a history of CVD at baseline. However, in the current study, LVGFI was a significant prognostic predictor in univariate but not in multivariable analysis. It is possible that the weaker predictor value of LVGFI—as compared with LVEDVI—observed in our study could reflect compensatory modifications in LV mass and volumes aimed at preserving systolic function during HF. Because HF is a complex clinical syndrome that results from a variety of conditions preventing the LV from supporting the physiological circulation. Our study explored the possibility of linking the dysregulation of myocardial TG with the future MACE, based on evidence showing the associations of myocardial TG and CV disease [6–8], plus the potential of quantitative readout of MRS in differentiating various lipid species in the myocardium [10]. Using this technique, we have previously shown that patients hospitalized for acute HF are characterized by increased myocardial UFA content [13]. The predictive value of myocardial TG contents—FA/UFA ratio and levels of lipid resonances δ 1.6 ppm, were further validated in the current case-control study. Indeed, increased myocardial TG content is a prerequisite of cardiac steatosis, which may ultimately result in lipotoxicity and heart dysfunction [6–8,10]. In line with our results, Wei et al. [28] demonstrated that myocardial steatosis is mechanistically linked to diastolic dysfunction in women with coronary microvascular dysfunction. The early alterations of myocardial TG measured by using ^{1}H-MRS might be supplementary to the diastolic dysfunction to improve the stratification for patients with ischemic heart disease.

Readmissions are frequent in patients with acute HF and served as a secondary outcome measure in the current study. A previous report demonstrated that diabetes mellitus, hyperlipidemia, CAD, length of stay at the index admission, and prescription of beta-blockers were significant predictors of readmission rates [29]. The 30-day, 3-month, and 12-month readmission rates observed in our study were 0.8%, 4.5%, 13.5%, respectively, being markedly lower than those observed in Western countries [30,31]. Interestingly, we identified myocardial mass measured on CMR as an independent predictor of readmission rates. The present study supports the concept that LV mass measured by CMR is a viable predictor of adverse cardiovascular events [27], either from the MESA (Multi-Ethnic Study of Atherosclerosis) study [32] or the Cardiovascular Health Study [33]. Further independent studies in larger sample sizes are needed to confirm this pilot observation.

Our data should be interpreted in the context of some limitations. First, the single-center of our study may bring into question its generalizability, as the study population was highly selected for those with medical conditions becoming stable and ready to discharge. The number of HF-related readmissions might be too small for meaningful multivariable analyses. However, it is noteworthy that patients were recruited regardless of the underlying cause of HF. The data should be interpreted carefully because pathophysiologically diverse endpoints were included in this study. Second, the resonance δ 1.6 ppm sometimes overlaps with the main CH_2 resonance δ 1.3 ppm. The sum of the signal intensities δ 0.9, 1.3 and 1.6 ppm would have been more reliably extracted from an in vivo cardiac ^{1}H-MRS. Nonetheless, the quantitative analysis was carried out using well-established LC Model software to enhance the generalizability of the current study. Third, longitudinal 3-T CMR and ^{1}H-MRS examinations were not performed and changes in LVEDVI and/or myocardial TG content were not investigated over time. A validation cohort for our findings would help to elucidate the clinical value of such imaging biomarkers, however, it was outside of the pre-specified analysis for this study.

5. Conclusions

Our results indicate that LVEDVI and myocardial mass are potential imaging biomarkers that independently predict MACE and readmission, respectively, in patients discharged after hospitalization for acute HF. Myocardial TG predicts readmission in patients with a history of ischemic heart disease. Further studies are needed to determine whether LVEDVI and myocardial mass, as well as myocardial TG, may serve as therapeutic targets to improve prognoses in targeted patient populations.

Supplementary Materials: The following are available online at http://www.mdpi.com/2077-0383/9/1/169/s1, Table S1: CMR and 1H-MRS parameters in the study patients with and without MACE (n = 133).

Author Contributions: K.-F.C., K.-K.N., C.-H.W., J.-J.W., S.-H.N., and G.L. drafted the manuscript. C.-H.W., M.-H.L., M.-T.W., J.-J.W., S.-H.N., and G.L. designed the study. K.-F.C., P.-A.L., P.-C.H., K.-K.N., Y.-H.J., Y.-C.L. (Yu-Ching Lin), Y.-C.L. (Yu-Chun Lin), J.-J.W., S.-H.N., and G.L. analyzed the data, prepared the Tables and Figures. S.-Y.T. and G.L. carried out the analysis of magnetic resonance spectroscopy data. L.-Y.Y. and G.L. performed the statistical analysis. All authors have read and agreed to the published version of the manuscript.

Funding: This study was supported by Chang Gung Medical Foundation CMRPG2C0511-3, CMRPD3D0011-3, CMRPG3C1861-3, CMRPG3C1871-3 and CPRPG3G0021-3. The funding body has no role in the design of the study and collection, analysis, and interpretation of data and in writing the manuscript. The authors acknowledge the assistance provided by the Cancer Center and Clinical Trial Center (Statistician Lan-Yan Yang), Chang Gung Memorial Hospital, Linkou, Taiwan, which was founded by the Ministry of Health and Welfare of Taiwan MOHW106-TDU-B-212-113005. The funding body has no role in the design of the study and collection, analysis, and interpretation of data and in writing the manuscript.

Acknowledgments: We appreciate statistician Lan-Yan Yang and Hsin-Ying Lu for their assistance in data analysis.

Conflicts of Interest: The authors of this manuscript declare no relationships with any companies whose products or services may be related to the subject matter of the article.

References

1. Ponikowski, P.; Voors, A.A.; Anker, S.D.; Bueno, H.; Cleland, J.G.F.; Coats, A.J.S.; Falk, V.; Gonzalez-Juanatey, J.R.; Harjola, V.P.; Jankowska, E.A.; et al. 2016 ESC Guidelines for the diagnosis and treatment of acute and chronic heart failure: The Task Force for the diagnosis and treatment of acute and chronic heart failure of the European Society of Cardiology (ESC) Developed with the special contribution of the Heart Failure Association (HFA) of the ESC. *Eur. Heart J.* **2016**, *37*, 2129–2200. [PubMed]
2. Tsutsui, H.; Tsuchihashi, M.; Takeshita, A. Mortality and readmission of hospitalized patients with congestive heart failure and preserved versus depressed systolic function. *Am. J. Cardiol.* **2001**, *88*, 530–533. [CrossRef]
3. Yancy, C.W.; Jessup, M.; Bozkurt, B.; Butler, J.; Casey, D.E., Jr.; Drazner, M.H.; Fonarow, G.C.; Geraci, S.A.; Horwich, T.; Januzzi, J.L.; et al. 2013 ACCF/AHA guideline for the management of heart failure: Executive summary: A report of the American College of Cardiology Foundation/American Heart Association Task Force on practice guidelines. *Circulation* **2013**, *128*, 1810–1852. [CrossRef] [PubMed]
4. Hunt, S.A.; Abraham, W.T.; Chin, M.H.; Feldman, A.M.; Francis, G.S.; Ganiats, T.G.; Jessup, M.; Konstam, M.A.; Mancini, D.M.; Michl, K.; et al. ACC/AHA 2005 Guideline Update for the Diagnosis and Management of Chronic Heart Failure in the Adult: A report of the American College of Cardiology/American Heart Association Task Force on Practice Guidelines (Writing Committee to Update the 2001 Guidelines for the Evaluation and Management of Heart Failure): Developed in collaboration with the American College of Chest Physicians and the International Society for Heart and Lung Transplantation: Endorsed by the Heart Rhythm Society. *Circulation* **2005**, *112*, e154–e235. [PubMed]

5. Taegtmeyer, H.; McNulty, P.; Young, M.E. Adaptation and maladaptation of the heart in diabetes: Part I: General concepts. *Circulation* **2002**, *105*, 1727–1733. [CrossRef]
6. Wright, J.J.; Kim, J.; Buchanan, J.; Boudina, S.; Sena, S.; Bakirtzi, K.; Ilkun, O.; Theobald, H.A.; Cooksey, R.C.; Kandror, K.V.; et al. Mechanisms for increased myocardial fatty acid utilization following short-term high-fat feeding. *Cardiovasc. Res.* **2009**, *82*, 351–360. [CrossRef]
7. Turkbey, E.B.; McClelland, R.L.; Kronmal, R.A.; Burke, G.L.; Bild, D.E.; Tracy, R.P.; Arai, A.E.; Lima, J.A.; Bluemke, D.A. The impact of obesity on the left ventricle: The Multi-Ethnic Study of Atherosclerosis (MESA). *JACC Cardiovasc. Imaging* **2010**, *3*, 266–274. [CrossRef]
8. Wende, A.R.; Abel, E.D. Lipotoxicity in the heart. *Biochim. Biophys. Acta* **2010**, *1801*, 311–319. [CrossRef]
9. Vilahur, G.; Casani, L.; Juan-Babot, O.; Guerra, J.M.; Badimon, L. Infiltrated cardiac lipids impair myofibroblast-induced healing of the myocardial scar post-myocardial infarction. *Atherosclerosis* **2012**, *224*, 368–376. [CrossRef]
10. Faller, K.M.; Lygate, C.A.; Neubauer, S.; Schneider, J.E. (1) H-MR spectroscopy for analysis of cardiac lipid and creatine metabolism. *Heart Fail. Rev.* **2013**, *18*, 657–668. [CrossRef]
11. Bizino, M.B.; Hammer, S.; Lamb, H.J. Metabolic imaging of the human heart: Clinical application of magnetic resonance spectroscopy. *Heart* **2014**, *100*, 881–890. [CrossRef] [PubMed]
12. Mahmod, M.; Bull, S.; Suttie, J.J.; Pal, N.; Holloway, C.; Dass, S.; Myerson, S.G.; Schneider, J.E.; De Silva, R.; Petrou, M.; et al. Myocardial steatosis and left ventricular contractile dysfunction in patients with severe aortic stenosis. *Circ. Cardiovasc. Imaging* **2013**, *6*, 808–816. [CrossRef] [PubMed]
13. Liao, P.A.; Lin, G.; Tsai, S.Y.; Wang, C.H.; Juan, Y.H.; Lin, Y.C.; Wu, M.T.; Yang, L.Y.; Liu, M.H.; Chang, T.C.; et al. Myocardial triglyceride content at 3 T cardiovascular magnetic resonance and left ventricular systolic function: A cross-sectional study in patients hospitalized with acute heart failure. *J. Cardiovasc. Magn. Reson.* **2016**, *18*, 9. [CrossRef] [PubMed]
14. Aljizeeri, A.; Sulaiman, A.; Alhulaimi, N.; Alsaileek, A.; Al-Mallah, M.H. Cardiac magnetic resonance imaging in heart failure: Where the alphabet begins! *Heart Fail. Rev.* **2017**, *22*, 385–399. [CrossRef] [PubMed]
15. Todiere, G.; Marzilli, M. Role of cardiac imaging in heart failure. *Minerva Cardioangiol.* **2012**, *60*, 347–362. [PubMed]
16. Partington, S.L.; Cheng, S.; Lima, J.A. Cardiac magnetic resonance imaging for stage B heart failure. *Heart Fail. Clin.* **2012**, *8*, 179–190. [CrossRef]
17. Bottomley, P.A. Spatial localization in NMR spectroscopy in vivo. *Ann. N. Y. Acad. Sci.* **1987**, *508*, 333–348. [CrossRef]
18. Liu, C.Y.; Bluemke, D.A.; Gerstenblith, G.; Zimmerman, S.L.; Li, J.; Zhu, H.; Lai, S.; Lai, H. Myocardial steatosis and its association with obesity and regional ventricular dysfunction: Evaluated by magnetic resonance tagging and 1H spectroscopy in healthy African Americans. *Int. J. Cardiol.* **2014**, *172*, 381–387. [CrossRef]
19. Reingold, J.S.; McGavock, J.M.; Kaka, S.; Tillery, T.; Victor, R.G.; Szczepaniak, L.S. Determination of triglyceride in the human myocardium by magnetic resonance spectroscopy: Reproducibility and sensitivity of the method. *Am. J. Physiol. Endocrinol. Metab.* **2005**, *289*, E935–E939. [CrossRef]
20. van der Meer, R.W.; Doornbos, J.; Kozerke, S.; Schar, M.; Bax, J.J.; Hammer, S.; Smit, J.W.; Romijn, J.A.; Diamant, M.; Rijzewijk, L.J.; et al. Metabolic imaging of myocardial triglyceride content: Reproducibility of 1H MR spectroscopy with respiratory navigator gating in volunteers. *Radiology* **2007**, *245*, 251–257. [CrossRef]
21. O'Connor, R.D.; Xu, J.; Ewald, G.A.; Ackerman, J.J.; Peterson, L.R.; Gropler, R.J.; Bashir, A. Intramyocardial triglyceride quantification by magnetic resonance spectroscopy: In vivo and ex vivo correlation in human subjects. *Magn. Reson. Med.* **2011**, *65*, 1234–1238. [CrossRef] [PubMed]
22. Weiss, K.; Summermatter, S.; Stoeck, C.T.; Kozerke, S. Compensation of signal loss due to cardiac motion in point-resolved spectroscopy of the heart. *Magn. Reson. Med.* **2014**, *72*, 1201–1207. [CrossRef] [PubMed]
23. Kip, K.E.; Hollabaugh, K.; Marroquin, O.C.; Williams, D.O. The problem with composite end points in cardiovascular studies: The story of major adverse cardiac events and percutaneous coronary intervention. *J. Am. Coll. Cardiol.* **2008**, *51*, 701–707. [CrossRef]
24. Cheng, M.L.; Wang, C.H.; Shiao, M.S.; Liu, M.H.; Huang, Y.Y.; Huang, C.Y.; Mao, C.T.; Lin, J.F.; Ho, H.Y.; Yang, N.I. Metabolic disturbances identified in plasma are associated with outcomes in patients with heart failure: Diagnostic and prognostic value of metabolomics. *J. Am. Coll. Cardiol.* **2015**, *65*, 1509–1520. [CrossRef] [PubMed]

25. Minamisawa, M.; Miura, T.; Motoki, H.; Ueki, Y.; Shimizu, K.; Shoin, W.; Harada, M.; Mochidome, T.; Yoshie, K.; Oguchi, Y.; et al. Prognostic Impact of Diastolic Wall Strain in Patients at Risk for Heart Failure. *Int. Heart J.* **2017**, *58*, 250–256. [CrossRef] [PubMed]
26. Mordi, I.; Bezerra, H.; Carrick, D.; Tzemos, N. The Combined Incremental Prognostic Value of LVEF, Late Gadolinium Enhancement, and Global Circumferential Strain Assessed by CMR. JACC. *Cardiovasc. Imaging* **2015**, *8*, 540–549.
27. Mewton, N.; Opdahl, A.; Choi, E.Y.; Almeida, A.L.; Kawel, N.; Wu, C.O.; Burke, G.L.; Liu, S.; Liu, K.; Bluemke, D.A.; et al. Left ventricular global function index by magnetic resonance imaging—A novel marker for assessment of cardiac performance for the prediction of cardiovascular events: The multi-ethnic study of atherosclerosis. *Hypertension* **2013**, *61*, 770–778. [CrossRef]
28. Wei, J.; Nelson, M.D.; Szczepaniak, E.W.; Smith, L.; Mehta, P.K.; Thomson, L.E.; Berman, D.S.; Li, D.; Bairey Merz, C.N.; Szczepaniak, L.S. Myocardial steatosis as a possible mechanistic link between diastolic dysfunction and coronary microvascular dysfunction in women. *Am. J. Physiol. Heart Circ. Physiol.* **2016**, *310*, H14–H19. [CrossRef]
29. Deeka, H.; Skouri, H.; Noureddine, S. Readmission rates and related factors in heart failure patients: A study in Lebanon. *Collegian* **2016**, *23*, 61–68. [CrossRef]
30. Butler, J.; Kalogeropoulos, A. Worsening heart failure hospitalization epidemic we do not know how to prevent and we do not know how to treat! *J. Am. Coll. Cardiol.* **2008**, *52*, 435–437. [CrossRef]
31. Desai, A.S.; Stevenson, L.W. Rehospitalization for heart failure: Predict or prevent? *Circulation* **2012**, *126*, 501–506. [CrossRef] [PubMed]
32. Bluemke, D.A.; Kronmal, R.A.; Lima, J.A.; Liu, K.; Olson, J.; Burke, G.L.; Folsom, A.R. The relationship of left ventricular mass and geometry to incident cardiovascular events: The MESA (Multi-Ethnic Study of Atherosclerosis) study. *J. Am. Coll. Cardiol.* **2008**, *52*, 2148–2155. [CrossRef] [PubMed]
33. de Simone, G.; Gottdiener, J.S.; Chinali, M.; Maurer, M.S. Left ventricular mass predicts heart failure not related to previous myocardial infarction: The Cardiovascular Health Study. *Eur. Heart J.* **2008**, *29*, 741–747. [CrossRef] [PubMed]

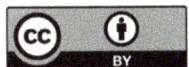

© 2020 by the authors. Licensee MDPI, Basel, Switzerland. This article is an open access article distributed under the terms and conditions of the Creative Commons Attribution (CC BY) license (http://creativecommons.org/licenses/by/4.0/).

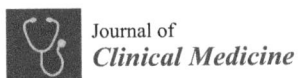
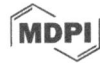

Article

Ceruloplasmin, NT-proBNP, and Clinical Data as Risk Factors of Death or Heart Transplantation in a 1-Year Follow-Up of Heart Failure Patients

Ewa Romuk [1,*], Wojciech Jacheć [2], Ewa Zbrojkiewicz [3], Alina Mroczek [3], Jacek Niedziela [4], Mariusz Gąsior [4], Piotr Rozentryt [3,4] and Celina Wojciechowska [2]

1. Department of Biochemistry, Faculty of Medical Sciences in Zabrze, Medical University of Silesia, 40-055 Katowice, Poland
2. Second Department of Cardiology, Faculty of Medical Sciences in Zabrze, Medical University of Silesia, 40-055 Katowice, Poland; wjachec@interia.pl (W.J.); wojciechowskac@wp.pl (C.W.)
3. Department of Toxicology and Health Protection, Faculty of Health Sciences in Bytom, Medical University of Silesia, 40-055 Katowice, Poland; ezbrojkiewicz@op.pl (E.Z.); alina.mroczek@wp.pl (A.M.); prozentryt@sum.edu.pl (P.R.)
4. 3rd Department of Cardiology, Faculty of Medical Sciences in Zabrze, Medical University of Silesia, Silesian Centre for Heart Disease, 41-800 Zabrze, Poland; jacek.niedziela@gmail.com (J.N.); m.gasior@op.pl (M.G.)
* Correspondence: eromuk@gmail.com; Tel.: +48-322-722-318

Received: 28 November 2019; Accepted: 30 December 2019; Published: 3 January 2020

Abstract: We investigated whether the additional determination of ceruloplasmin (Cp) levels could improve the prognostic value of N-terminal pro-B-type natriuretic peptide (NT-proBNP) in heart failure (HF) patients in a 1-year follow-up. Cp and NT-proBNP levels and clinical and laboratory parameters were assessed simultaneously at baseline in 741 HF patients considered as possible heart transplant recipients. The primary endpoint (EP) was a composite of all-cause death (non-transplant patients) or heart transplantation during one year of follow-up. Using a cut-off value of 35.9 mg/dL for Cp and 3155 pg/mL for NT-proBNP (top interquartile range), a univariate Cox regression analysis showed that Cp (hazard ratio (HR) = 2.086; 95% confidence interval (95% CI, 1.462–2.975)), NT-proBNP (HR = 3.221; 95% CI (2.277–4.556)), and the top quartile of both Cp and NT-proBNP (HR = 4.253; 95% CI (2.795–6.471)) were all risk factors of the primary EP. The prognostic value of these biomarkers was demonstrated in a multivariate Cox regression model using the top Cp and NT-proBNP concentration quartiles combined (HR = 2.120; 95% CI (1.233–3.646)). Lower left ventricular ejection fraction, VO_2max, lack of angiotensin-converting enzyme inhibitor or angiotensin receptor blocker therapy, and nonimplantation of an implantable cardioverter-defibrillator were also independent risk factors of a poor outcome. The combined evaluation of Cp and NT-proBNP had advantages over separate NT-proBNP and Cp assessment in selecting a group with a high 1-year risk. Thus multi-biomarker assessment can improve risk stratification in HF patients.

Keywords: ceruloplasmin; NT-proBNP; heart failure

1. Introduction

Systolic heart failure (HF) is a complex disease caused by reduced ejection fraction of the left ventricle, often leading to the worsening of symptoms and poor quality of life, despite proper diagnosis and treatment according to current guidelines. All-cause mortality in these patients remains high and heart transplantation is a therapeutic option in end-stage HF. Adverse outcomes for HF patients are associated with many contributing factors. Stratification of risk factors is a great challenge in out-patient clinic cohorts, in which patients still undergo significant mortality and morbidity, despite stable HF. Different clinical and laboratory parameters can be helpful to identify patients at higher risk of adverse outcomes. Biological markers reflecting several pathophysiological abnormalities of HF have become powerful and convenient noninvasive tools for the stratification of HF patients [1–3]. Brain natriuretic peptide (BNP) and N-terminal pro-BNP (NT-proBNP) are secreted by cardiomyocytes in response to hemodynamic overload or neurohormonal disturbances. In clinical practice, NT-proBNP is recommended as a marker over BNP, because of its longer plasma half-life and lower levels of biological variation. NT-proBNP is the best-known diagnostic biomarker [4]. The usefulness of NT-proBNP for risk stratification varies depending on the stage of HF, time of assessment (onset of hospitalization, pre-discharge, or out-patient clinic evaluation), and duration of follow-up. However, there is no conclusive evidence that plasma NT-proBNP concentration is a guide for more effective therapy [5–8]. Ceruloplasmin (Cp) is an acute-phase reactant that is synthesized and secreted by the liver and monocyte/macrophages. It is elevated in conditions of acute inflammation. Cp contains seven copper atoms per molecule, participates in copper transport and metabolism, and has ferroxidase activity [9,10]. Furthermore, Cp is involved in the modulation of coagulation and angiogenesis and the inactivation of biogenic amines [11,12]. It is possible that increased levels of Cp may decrease available plasma NO, thus increasing reactive oxygen species formation and oxidative cell injury [13]. Several recent reports have indicated that Cp levels are elevated in patients with heart failure, regardless of its etiology [14–16].

Different pathobiological processes are involved in heart failure; thus, it is not surprising that single biomarkers, even natriuretic peptides, fail to predict all risks associated with HF.

The aim of this study was to examine the prognostic value of clinical factors, with special consideration of Cp, in a large cohort of HF patients and to investigate whether the combination of Cp and NT-proBNP could provide additional prognostic information in HF patients in a 1-year follow-up.

2. Materials and Methods

2.1. Clinical Assessment

We analyzed data in a subgroup of patients included in the Prospective Registry of Heart Failure (PR-HF) and Studies Investigating Co-morbidities Aggravating Heart Failure (SICA-HF) studies described elsewhere [17]. A cohort of patients with chronic systolic HF were prospectively recruited from patients referred to our inpatients clinic as potential candidates for heart transplantation. The main inclusion criteria were reduced left ventricular ejection fraction (LVEF ≤ 40%) and symptomatic HF, despite pharmacological treatment according to the current published ESC guidelines, at least 3 months before inclusion. The exclusion criteria included acute myocardial infarction; pulmonary thromboembolism; constrictive pericarditis; infectious pericarditis; prior heart transplantation; noncardiac conditions resulting in an expected mortality of less than 12 months, as judged by the treating physician; and a history of alcohol abuse or known antioxidant supplementation. These criteria were fulfilled in the 1216 PR-HF and SICA-HF studies. We analyzed data from 741 participants (aged 48–59 years) who had completed clinical and laboratory assessments.

A detailed description of the clinical echocardiographic evaluation of patients included in the study has been presented elsewhere [18].

The primary outcome was a composite of death from all causes (nontransplant patients) or heart transplantation. In the case of heart transplantation, the endpoint was reached and the patient was not followed up further. Patients were followed for a year via direct or phone contact. In some cases, the exact data regarding patient death were obtained from family members or the national identification number database by dedicated research personnel. Prior to enrolment in the study, all participants provided written informed consent. The local ethics committee of Silesian Medical University approved the study protocol (NN-6501-12/I/04). All procedures were performed in accordance with the 1975 Declaration of Helsinki and its revision in 2008.

2.2. Biochemical Methods

Venous blood samples obtained at enrollment were processed, separated by centrifugation at 1500× g for 10 min, frozen at −70 °C, and partially stored at −70 °C until assayed. Serum protein, albumin, fibrinogen, CRP, alanine aminotransferase, aspartate aminotransferase, gamma-glutamyl-transferase (GGTP), alkaline phosphatase, bilirubin, and lipid parameters and serum iron, sodium, creatinine, glucose, and uric acid concentrations were measured by colorimetric methods (Cobas 6000 e501; Roche, Basel, Switzerland). Hemoglobin, leukocytes, and platelets were measured using a MEDONIC M32C analyzer (Alpha Diagnostics, Warsaw, Poland). NT-proBNP was measured using a chemiluminescence method (Cobas 6000 e501).

Serum Cp concentration was determined spectrophotometrically, according to the Richterich reaction with p-phenyl-diamine [19]. Cp catalyzes the oxidation of colorless p-phenylenediamine, resulting in a blue-violet dye. Twenty microliters of serum was added to the test sample, while 20 μL of serum and 200 μL of sodium azide solution were added to the control sample to stop the reaction. Then, 1 mL of p-phenylenediamine dihydrochloride in acetate buffer was added to both test and control samples. After a 15-min incubation, 200 μL of sodium azide was added to the test sample. Finally, after a 15-min incubation, the absorbance of test and control samples was measured at 560 nm using a PerkinElmer VICTOR-X3 plate reader. The samples were not previously thawed before Cp assays. The intra-assay coefficient of variation was 3.7% and the intra-assay precision was 4%.

2.3. Statistical Analysis

Study participants were divided into subgroups based on Cp concentration quartiles (Table 1). Moreover, two subgroups, firstly, both Cp and NT-proBNP in the top quartile and, secondly, remaining patients (Cp or NT-proBNP in I–III quartiles including patients with Cp in I–III quartiles and NT-proBNP in I–IV quartiles or NT-proBNP in I–III quartiles and Cp in I–IV quartiles), were also compared (Table 2). The Shapiro–Wilk test was used to evaluate the distribution of all continuous variables. Continuous data are presented as the median, with the first and fourth quartiles (because of non-normal distribution of the data). Categorical data are presented as absolute numbers and percentages. The Kruskal-Wallis ANOVA test was used to compare both continuous and categorical data.

Estimations of risk were performed using a Cox proportional hazards model. Only complete data were analyzed. All demographic; clinical; echocardiography; laboratory; medication; and Cp and NT-proBNP data, expressed as the top quartiles individually or as the combined top quartiles of Cp and NT-proBNP concentration, were included in a univariate Cox analysis. Variables with a value of $p \leq 0.05$ in the univariate analysis were included in the multivariate analysis. Two multivariate analysis models were built. The first model was based on the top Cp and NT-proBNP concentration quartiles separately and the second model was based on the combined top quartiles of Cp and NT-proBNP concentrations.

The results of the Cox analysis are presented as relative risks, with 95% confidence intervals (CIs). Cumulative survival curves for all-cause death or heart transplantation were constructed as the time to endpoint occurrence, using the Kaplan–Meier method. Survival curves were compared among groups according to quartiles of Cp, quartiles of NT-proBNP and between groups presented in Table 2, using the log-rank test, as appropriate.

The odds ratio (OR) of achieving the endpoint for the top quartiles of Cp and NT-proBNP concentrations were calculated. The same calculations were performed for the combined top quartiles of Cp and NT-proBNP concentrations. The predictive value of these parameters was then compared.

Statistical significance was set at $p < 0.05$. Statistical analyses were performed using STATISTICA 13.1 PL software (StatSoft, Cracow, Poland).

3. Results

3.1. Baseline Characteristics of the Entire Study Population and Subgroups in Relation to Ceruloplasmin Concentration

The study group included 741 systolic HF patients, with a median Cp concentration of 28.7 mg% (range, 23.7–35.8). The cohort was divided into quartiles of serum Cp concentration as follows: group I, 184 (24.8%) patients with a Cp concentration range of 8.0–23.6 mg/dL; group II, 184 (24.8%) patients with 23.7–28.6 mg/dL Cp; group III, 187 (25.2%) patients with 28.7–35.8 mg/dL Cp; and group IV, 186 (25.1%) patients with the highest Cp concentration quartile of 35.9–81.0 mg/dL. One hundred and twenty-eight (17.42%) patients reached the combined endpoint (101 deaths, 27 heart transplantations). The overall mortality rate during the 1-year follow-up period was 13.76% and the heart transplantation rate was 3.64%. The demographic, clinical, and laboratory parameters of all patient groups and subgroups, divided according to quartiles of serum Cp concentration, are presented in Table 1.

Table 1. Characteristic of the examined group with division according to ceruloplasmin concentration quartiles.

Ceruloplasmin Quartiles (mg/dL)	All Group	I Quartile 8.0–23.6	II Quartile 23.7–28.6	III Quartile 28.7–35.8	IV Quartile 35.9–81.0	
Number	N = 741	N = 184	N = 184	N = 187	N = 186	
Demographic and clinical parameters						ANOVA
Deaths (n)/HT (n) All n (%)	101/27 128 (17.27)	16/4 20 (10.87)	24/5 29 (15.76)	23/6 29 (15.51)	38/12 50 (26.88)	$p < 0.001$
Female n (%)	105 (14.17)	18 (9.78)	25 (13.59)	28 (14.97)	34 (18.28)	NS
Age (years)	54.00 (48.0–59.0)	54.00 (48.00–58.00)	55.00 (49.00–60.00)	54.00 (48.00–59.00)	55.00 (49.00–60.00)	NS
BMI (kg/m^2)	26.29 (23.50–29.32)	26.49 (24.04–29.06)	26.66 (23.58–29.70)	26.15 (23.36–29.69)	25.96 (22.50–28.89)	NS
Duration of symptoms before inclusion (months)	33.83 (13.07–69.67)	29.82 (13.40–58.47)	33.60 (12.80–69.02)	31.83 (12.90–68.70)	43.77 (14.13–79.93)	NS
Exercise, capacity, echocardiography						
NYHA class III–IV n (%)	417 (56.28)	77 (41.85)	99 (53.80)	119 (63.64)	122 (65.59)	$p < 0.001$
VO$_2$max (mL/min/kg b.w.)	14.35 (11.70–17.60)	15.30 (12.30–19.50)	14.70 (12.00–17.70)	14.20 (11.40–17.10)	13.40 (10.75–16.55)	$p < 0.001$
LVEF (%)	24.00 (20.00–30.00)	25.00 (20.50–32.50)	24.00 (20.00–30.00)	24.00 (22.00–28.00)	22.00 (19.00–28.00)	$p < 0.01$
Laboratory parameters						
NT-proBNP (pg/mL) /100	13.92 (6.44–31.55)	9.30 (5.00–20.09)	14.82 (6.64–34.77)	15.48 (6.55–31.95)	18.42 (8.97–37.96)	$p < 0.001$
Ceruloplasmin (mg/dL)	28.70 (23.70–35.80)	20.75 (18.20–22.40)	26.25 (24.90–27.50)	31.90 (30.00–33.50)	42.35 (38.10–49.30)	$p < 0.001$
Hemoglobin (g/dL)	14.02 (13.05–14.99)	14.02 (13.05–14.83)	14.02 (12.89–14.99)	14.02 (13.22–15.15)	14.18 (13.05–15.15)	NS
Leukocytes (10^9/L)	6.94 (5.82–8.27)	6.83 (5.53–8.26)	6.77 (5.55–8.27)	7.23 (5.88–8.65)	6.92 (6.07–7.84)	0.060
Blood platelets (10^9/L)	185.00 (152.00–223.00)	183.00 (148.00–218.50)	185.00 (156.50–220.50)	197.00 (160.00–238.00)	174.00 (150.00–218.00)	$p < 0.05$
Sodium (mmol/L)	136.00 (134.00–139.00)	137.00 (135.00–139.00)	137.00 (134.50–138.00)	135.00 (133.00–138.00)	136.00 (134.00–138.00)	$p < 0.001$
Creatinine clearance (mL/min)	95.11 (69.98–119.44)	101.49 (80.86–125.04)	93.51 (70.86–117.35)	88.85 (70.07–116.43)	93.27 (61.00–117.28)	$p < 0.01$
Uric acid (μmol/L)/10	40.90 (33.00–50.60)	37.85 (33.05–45.00)	41.10 (32.95–50.15)	41.50 (33.10–50.80)	43.25 (32.90–55.60)	$p < 0.001$

Table 1. Cont.

Ceruloplasmin Quartiles (mg/dL)	All Group	I Quartile 8.0–23.6	II Quartile 23.7–28.6	III Quartile 28.7–35.8	IV Quartile 35.9–81.0	
Number	N = 741	N = 184	N = 184	N = 187	N = 186	
Laboratory parameters						
Serum protein (g/L)	71.00 (67.00–75.00)	70.00 (66.00–73.50)	70.00 (66.00–74.00)	72.00 (67.00–76.00)	73.00 (69.00–77.00)	$p < 0.001$
Albumin (g/l)	42.00 (39.00–44.00)	42.00 (39.00–44.00)	41.00 (39.00–43.50)	41.00 (38.00–44.00)	43.00 (40.00–45.00)	$p < 0.05$
Fibrinogen (mg/dL)	397.00 (338.00–462.00)	367.00 (320.50–433.50)	395.50 (340.00–454.50)	425.00 (367.00–495.00)	409.50 (343.00–491.00)	$p < 0.001$
C-reactive protein (mg/dL)	2.94 (1.34–6.67)	1.97 (0.91–4.55)	2.65 (1.27–6.04)	4.11 (1.82–7.35)	3.83 (1.86–8.90)	$p < 0.001$
Iron concentration (μmol/L)	17.10 (12.00–22.20)	16.91 (13.00–20.25)	17.10 (11.14–21.40)	16.90 (11.80–22.40)	17.60 (12.00–23.92)	NS
Bilirubin (μmol/L)	13.70 (9.70–20.50)	12.00 (8.45–16.15)	13.65 (10.00–18.35)	14.70 (9.30–21.10)	16.55 (11.00–26.60)	$p < 0.001$
Aspartate transaminase (IU/L)	23.0 (19.0–30.9)	23.0 (18.0–29.0)	23 (19.0–28.6)	24 (18.0–310)	24 (20.0–33.0)	NS
Alanine transaminase (IU/L)	24 (17.0–36.0)	23 (17.5–35.5)	24 (17.0–36.0)	24 (17.0–34.0)	25 (18.0–38.0)	NS
γ-glutamyl transpeptidase (IU/L)	49 (27.0–100.0)	39 (24.5–75.5)	45.5 (27.0–79.0)	54 (27.0–112.0)	67.5 (33.0–152.0)	$p < 0.001$
Alkaline phosphatase (IU/L)	68.0 (56.0–90.0)	65.0 (52.0–80.4)	65.0 (54.0–84.0)	72.0 (58.0–94.0)	78.0 (61.0–108.0)	$p < 0.001$
Fasting glucose (mmol/L)	5.50 (5.00–6.20)	5.50 (5.00–6.20)	5.45 (4.85–6.20)	5.60 (5.10–6.70)	5.50 (4.90–6.10)	NS
Total Cholesterol (mmol/L)	4.29 (3.64–5.22)	4.30 (3.60–5.10)	4.25 (3.65–5.19)	4.25 (3.62–5.34)	4.41 (3.67–5.21)	NS
Triglycerides (mmol/L)	1.20 (0.89–1.73)	1.17 (0.83–1.73)	1.22 (0.89–1.93)	1.23 (0.97–1.69)	1.20 (0.85–1.74)	NS
Cholesterol HDL (mmol/L)	1.14 (0.94–1.40)	1.19 (0.98–1.43)	1.14 (0.92–1.39)	1.13 (0.94–1.32)	1.13 (0.88–1.42)	NS
Cholesterol LDL (mmol/L)	2.45 (1.90–3.16)	2.46 (1.89–3.08)	2.39 (1.88–3.20)	2.38 (1.85–3.25)	2.54 (2.00–3.16)	NS
Comorbidities						
Non ischemic DCM; n (%)	280 (37.79)	58 (31.52)	77 (41.85)	78 (41.71)	67 (36.02)	NS
Diabetes; n (%)	211 (28.48)	43 (23.37)	53 (28.80)	61 (32.62)	54 (29.03)	NS
Arterial hypertension; n (%)	408 (55.06)	100 (54.35)	104 (56.52)	91 (48.66)	113 (60.75)	NS
Permanent atrial fibrillation; n (%)	176 (23.75)	24 (13.04)	42 (22.83)	48 (25.67)	62 (33.33)	$p < 0.001$
ICD presence; n (%)	207 (27.94)	50 (27.17)	63 (34.24)	52 (27.81)	42 (22.58)	NS
Smoker; n (%)	257 (34.68)	64 (34.78)	78 (42.39)	72 (38.50)	43 (23.12)	$p < 0.001$
Pharmacotherapy						
Beta-blockers; n (%)	726 (97.98)	182 (98.91)	181 (98.37)	180 (96.26)	183 (98.39)	NS
ACE–inhibitors; n (%)	641 (86.50)	166 (90.22)	161 (87.50)	159 (85.03)	155 (83.33)	NS
Angiotensin-2 receptor blockers; n (%)	76 (10.26)	17 (9.24)	20 (10.87)	24 (12.83)	15 (8.06)	NS

Table 1. Cont.

Ceruloplasmin Quartiles (mg/dL)	All Group	I Quartile 8.0–23.6	II Quartile 23.7–28.6	III Quartile 28.7–35.8	IV Quartile 35.9–81.0	
Number	N = 741	N = 184	N = 184	N = 187	N = 186	
Pharmacotherapy						
ACE–inhibitor or/and * ARB; n (%)	693 (93.52)	178 (96.74)	174 (94,57)	174 (93,05)	167 (89,78)	$p < 0.05$
Loop diuretic; n (%)	647 (87.31)	145 (78.80)	168 (91.30)	169 (90.37)	165 (88.71)	$p < 0.001$
Thiazide diuretics; n (%)	93 (12.55)	14 (7.61)	19 (10.33)	34 (18.18)	26 (13.98)	$p < 0.05$
Aldosterone receptor antagonist; n (%)	683 (92.19)	163 (88.65)	171 (92.93)	177 (94.65)	172 (92.47)	NS
Statins; n (%)	487 (65.72)	128 (69.57)	127 (69.02)	124 (66.31)	108 (58.06)	NS
Digitalis; n (%)	339 (45.75)	57 (30.98)	82 (44.57)	102 (54.55)	98 (52.69)	$p < 0.001$

HT: Heart Transplantation; BMI: body mass index; NYHA: New York Heart Association functional class; VO$_2$max: maximum oxygen output; LVEF: left ventricle ejection fraction; NT-proBNP: N-terminal pro-B-type natriuretic peptide; HDL: high density lipoproteins; LDL: low density lipoproteins; ICD: Implantable Cardioverter Defibrillator; ACE-inhibitor: angiotensin-converting-enzyme inhibitor; ARB: angiotensin-2 receptor blockers; * (24 patients received ACE-I and ARB simultaneously).

Neither age, sex, BMI, nor duration of symptoms before enrollment differed between groups. LVEF was reduced to a greater extent in group IV. The percentage of patients with atrial fibrillation was higher in group IV, but the frequencies of coronary artery disease, hypertension, diabetes mellitus, and implantable cardioverter-defibrillators (ICDs) were similar between groups. Pharmacological treatments were comparable between groups in terms of the use of angiotensin-converting enzyme inhibitors (ACE-Is), angiotensin receptor blockers (ARBs), beta-blockers, mineralocorticoid receptor antagonists (MRAs), and statins, but loop and thiazide diuretics and digitalis were more frequently used by group III patients. If ACE-I or ARB treatment was analyzed, their use was the lowest in patients in the 4th Cp quartile.

The following laboratory parameters, assessed in serum samples, were different among groups: NT-proBNP, Cp, sodium, creatinine clearance, protein, fasting glucose, lipid parameters, uric acid, bilirubin, aspartate transaminase, alanine transaminase, alkaline phosphatase, and GGTP (Table 1). Characteristic of examined group with division according to ceruloplasmin and NT-proBNP concentration quartiles are presented in Table 2

Table 2. Characteristic of examined group with division according to ceruloplasmin and N-terminal pro-B-type natriuretic peptide (NT-proBNP) concentration quartiles.

Ceruloplasmin/NT-pro-BNP Quartiles (mg/dL)	I–III Quartile	IV–IV Quartiles	ANOVA
Number	N = 683	N = 58	
Demographic and clinical parameters			
Deaths (n)/HT (n) All n (%)	79/21 100 (14.64)	23/5 28 (48.28)	$p < 0.001$
Female n (%)	96 (14.06)	9 (15.52)	NS
Age (years)	54.00 (49.00–59.00)	56,50 (45,00–61,00)	NS
BMI (kg/m^2)	26.44 (23.74–29.41)	23.55 (19,86–26.76)	$p < 0.001$
Duration of symptoms before inclusion (months)	33.53 (12.93–68.70)	43.12 (14.3–92.20)	NS

Table 2. *Cont.*

Ceruloplasmin/NT-pro-BNP Quartiles (mg/dL)	I–III Quartile	IV–IV Quartiles	ANOVA
Number	N = 683	N = 58	
Exercise, capacity, echocardiography			
NYHA class III-IV n (%)	369 (54.03)	48 (82.76)	$p < 0.001$
VO$_2$max (mL/min/kg b.w.)	14.50 (11.70–18.00)	12.30 (9.20–14.50)	$p < 0.001$
LVEF (%)	24.00 (20.00-30.00)	20.00 (17.00-24.00)	$p < 0.001$
Laboratory parameters			
NT-proBNP (pg/mL) /100	12.78 (5.97–25.70)	52.34 (41.31–78.06)	$p < 0.001$
Ceruloplasmin (mg/dL)	28.00 (23.40–33.70)	46.30 (38.10–54.30)	$p < 0.001$
Hemoglobin (g/dL)	14.02 (13.05–14.99)	13.62 (12.73–15.15)	NS
Leukocytes (10^9/L)	6.94 (5.79–8.31)	7.01 (6.17–8.19)	NS
Blood platelets (10^9/L)	185.00 (152.00–224.00)	185.00 (152.00–219.00)	NS
Sodium (mmol/L)	137.00 (134.00–139.00)	134.00 (132.00–137.00)	$p < 0.001$
Creatinine clearance (mL/min)	96.93 (73.45–120.64)	66.41 (50.32–103.34)	$p < 0.001$
Uric acid (μmol/L)/10	40.80 (32.90–49.50)	44.40 (33.70–69.00)	$p < 0.01$
Serum protein (g/L)	71.00 (67.00–75.00)	71.50 (67.00–77.00)	NS
Albumin (g/L)	42.00 (39.00–44.00)	40.00 (38.00–44.00)	$p < 0.05$
Fibrinogen (ug/mL)	396.00 (337.00–458.00)	434.00 (360.00–536.00)	$p < 0.01$
C-reactive protein (mg/dL)	2.80 (1.27–6.12)	7.18 (2.67–14.75)	$p < 0.001$
Iron concentration (μmol/L)	17.20 (12.10–22.20)	16.15 (10.50–21.30)	NS
Bilirubin (μmol/L)	13.40 (9.50–19.30)	22.90 (13.80–32.50)	$p < 0.001$
Aspartate transaminase (IU/L)	23.00 (18.00–30.00)	27.00 (21.00–37.00)	$p < 0.01$
Alanine transaminase (IU/L)	24.00 (17.00–36.00)	25.00 (18.00–41.00)	NS
γ-glutamyl transpeptidase (IU/L)	47.00 (27.00–92.00)	133.50 (49.00–218.00)	$p < 0.001$
Alkaline phosphatase (IU/L)	67.00 (55.00–88.00)	99.50 (73.00–143.00)	$p < 0.001$
Fasting glucose (mmol/L)	5.50 (5.00–6.30)	5.20 (4.70–5.90)	$p < 0.05$
Total Cholesterol (mmol/L)	4.31 (3.66–5.27)	3.97 (3.33–3.86)	NS
Triglycerides (mmol/L)	1.22 (0.89–1.75)	1.07 (0.78–1.36)	$p < 0.05$
Cholesterol HDL (mmol/L)	1.15 (0.95–1.40)	1.05 (0.79–1.29)	$p < 0.05$
Cholesterol LDL (mmol/L)	2.46 (1.91–3.19)	2.29 (1.85–3.00)	NS

Table 2. Cont.

Ceruloplasmin/NT-pro-BNP Quartiles (mg/dL)	I–III Quartile	IV–IV Quartiles	ANOVA
Number	N = 683	N = 58	
Comorbidities			
Non ischemic DCM; n (%)	252 (36.90)	28 (48.27)	NS
Diabetes; n (%)	190 (27.82)	21 (36.21)	NS
Arterial hypertension; n (%)	382 (56.93)	20 (34.48)	$p < 0.01$
Permanent atrial fibrillation; n (%)	155 (22.69)	21 (36.21)	$p < 0.05$
ICD presence; n (%)	192 (28.11)	15 (25.86)	NS
Smoker; n (%)	241 (35.29)	16 (27.59)	NS
Pharmacotherapy			
Beta-blockers; n (%)	668 (97,80)	58 (100,00)	NS
ACE–inhibitors; n (%)	595 (87,12)	46 (79.310	NS
Angiotensin-2 receptor blockers; n (%)	71 (10,40)	5 (79,31)	NS
ACE–inhibitors or/and ARB; n (%)	643 (94.14)	50 (86,21)	$p < 0.05$
Loop diuretic; n (%)	590 (86.38)	57 (98.28)	$p < 0.05$
Thiazide diuretics; n (%)	79 (11.57)	14 (24.14)	$p < 05$
Aldosterone receptor antagonist; n (%)	628 (91,95)	54 (93,10)	NS
Statins; n (%)	457 (66.91)	30 (51.72)	$p < 0.05$
Digitalis; n (%)	305 (44.66)	34 (58.62)	NS

HT: Heart Transplantation; BMI: body mass index; NYHA: New York Heart Association functional class; VO$_2$max: maximum oxygen output; LVEF: left ventricle ejection fraction; NT-proBNP: N-terminal pro-B-type natriuretic peptide; HDL: high density lipoproteins; LDL: low density lipoproteins; ICD: Implantable Cardioverter Defibrillator; ACE-inhibitors: angiotensin-converting-enzyme inhibitor; ARB: angiotensin -2 receptor blockers.

3.2. Ceruloplasmin, NT-proBNP and Prognosis

3.2.1. Univariate Cox Regression Analysis

All demographic, clinical, exercise capacity, echocardiography, laboratory parameter, comorbidity, and pharmacotherapy data presented in Table 1 were assessed as risk factors for all-cause death or heart transplantation in a 1-year follow-up.

In univariate Cox regression analyses, among others, the top quartiles of NT-proBNP concentration (hazard ratio (HR) = 3.221, 95% CI (2.277–4.556)), Cp concentration (HR = 2.086, 95% CI (1.462–2.975)), and combined Cp and NT-proBNP concentration (HR = 4.253, 95% CI (2.795–6.471) were associated with a higher risk of death or heart transplantation.

All variables that reached $p < 0.05$ in a univariate Cox regression analysis are presented in Table 3.

3.2.2. Multivariate Cox Regression Analysis

In the first multivariate Cox regression model, after adjusting for other clinical and pharmacotherapeutic predictors, neither the top Cp concentration quartile nor the top NT-proBNP concentration quartile were significant predictors of unfavorable outcomes (Cp, HR = 1.511, 95% CI (0.980–2.330); NT-proBNP, HR = 1.287, 95% CI (0.815–2.033))

The results of the second multivariate Cox regression model, in which the top individual Cp and NT-proBNP concentration quartiles were replaced with the combined top quartiles of Cp and NT-proBNP concentrations, are presented in Table 3. In this model, an LVEF lower by 1 % (HR = 1.069, 95% CI (1.032–1.106)), a maximum measured VO_2 lower by 1 mL/min/kg b.m. (HR = 1.113, 95% CI (1.048–1.181)), absence of an ICD (HR = 7.575, 95% CI (3.278–17.502)), and lack of ACE-I and/or ARB therapy (HR = 2.195, 95% CI (1.234–3.906)) remained significant predictors of unfavorable outcomes. Among the laboratory parameters measured, only the combined top quartiles of Cp and NT-proBNP concentrations was associated with a higher risk of all-cause death and HT in a 1-year follow-up (HR = 2.120, 95% CI (1.233–3.646)).

Table 3. Predictors of death or heart transplantation in one-year follow-up. The results of uni- and multivariable Cox regression analysis, model-2.

	Univariable Cox Regression			Multivariable Cox Regression		
	HR	95%CI	P	HR	95%CI	P
General characteristics						
BMI ↑ (1 kg/m^2)	0.945	0.908–0.985	$p < 0.01$	0.966	0.912–1.022	NS
Duration of symptoms before inclusion ↑ (1month)	1.004	1.000–1.007	$p < 0.05$	1.000	0.996–1.004	NS
NYHA class ↑ (1 class)	2.936	2.280–3.779	$p < 0.001$	1.099	0.759–1.592	NS
VO_2max ↓ (1 mL/min/kg b.m.)	1.198	1.142–1.256	$p < 0.001$	1.113	1.048–1.181	$p < 0.001$
LVEF ↓ (1 %p)	1.091	1.059–1.122	$p < 0.001$	1.069	1.032–1.106	$p < 0.001$
Basic biochemistry						
Sodium ↓ (1 mmol/L)	1.111	1.070–1.155	$p < 0.001$	1.039	0.990–1.092	NS
Creatinine clearance ↓ (1 mL/min)	1.014	1.008–1.019	$p < 0.001$	1.001	0.993–1.008	NS
Albumin ↓ (1 g/L)	1.068	1.026–1.114	$p < 0.01$	1.023	0.966–1.083	NS
Cholesterol HDL ↓ (1 mmol/L)	1.805	1.121–2.907	$p < 0.05$	0.954	0.591–1.593	NS
Cp and NT-proBNP "both in top quartile" (yes/no)	4.253	2.795–6.471	$p < 0.001$	2.120	1.233–3.646	$p < 0.01$
Fibrinogen ↑ (1 mg/dL)	1.003	1.001–1.004	$p < 0.001$	1.001	1.000–1.003	NS
Uric acid ↑ (10 μmol/L)	1.030	1.018–1.041	$p < 0.001$	1.012	0.999–1.026	NS
Bilirubin ↑ (1 μmoL/L)	1.028	1.018–1.039	$p < 0.001$	0.994	0.976–1.012	NS
Alkaline phosphatase ↑ (1 U/L)	1.006	1.004–1.009	$p < 0.001$	1.000	0.995–1.006	NS
γ-Glutamyl trans peptidase ↑ (1 U/L)	1.001	1.000–1.002	$p < 0.05$	1.000	0.998–1.002	NS
Comorbidities						
Diabetes t.2 (yes/no)	1.604	1.123–2.291	$p < 0.01$	1.450	0.949–2.217	NS
ICD absence (yes/no)	9.929	3.922–20.000	$p < 0.001$	7.575	3.278–17.502	$p < 0.001$
Pharmacotherapy						
Lack of ACE - I or/and ARB (yes/no)	3.428	2.126–5.256	$p < 0.001$	2.195	1.234–3.906	$p < 0.01$
Loop diuretics (yes/no)	4.895	1.809–13.248	$p < 0.01$	1.735	0.525–5.730	NS
Thiazide diuretics (yes/no)	2.296	1.518–3.473	$p < 0.001$	1.317	0.781–2.221	NS
Statins (yes/no)	0.699	0.492–0.993	$p < 0.05$	1.294	0.825–2.032	NS
Digitalis (yes/no)	1.439	1.016–2.036	$p < 0.05$	0.833	0.547–1.267	NS

BMI: body mass index; NYHA: New York Heart Association functional class; VO_2max: maximum oxygen output; LVEF: left ventricle ejection fraction; NT-proBNP: N-terminal pro-B-type natriuretic peptide; Cp: ceruloplasmin, ICD: Implantable Cardioverter Defibrillator; ACE-I: angiotensin-converting-enzyme inhibitor; ARB: Angiotensin-2 receptor blocker.

3.2.3. Kaplan–Meier Survival Analysis and Endpoint Odds Ratios

There were 128 endpoints in groups I (20, 10.9%), II (29, 15.8%), III (29, 15.5%), and IV (50, 26.9%). Kaplan–Meier survival curves for the four groups according to Cp and NT-proBNP quartiles are presented in Figures 1 and 2. Patients with both Cp and NT-proBNP concentrations in the top quartile were compared with the remaining patients (quartile I–III of Cp or NT-proBNP concentration), as shown in Figure 3.

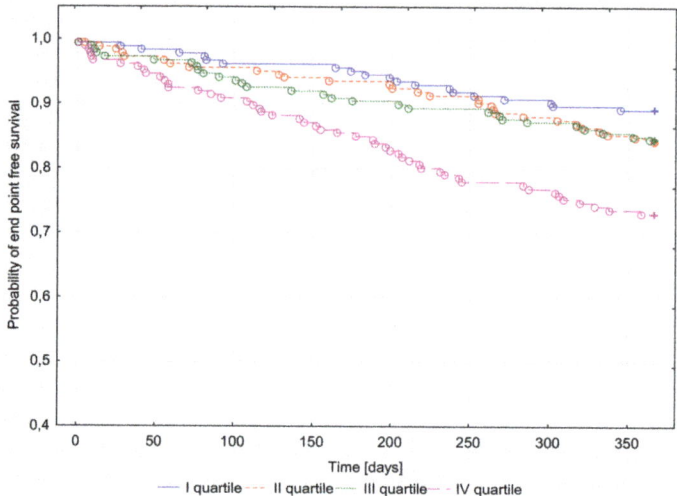

Figure 1. Probability of survival of time free of death or heart transplantation depending on quartiles of ceruloplasmin concentration in 1-year follow-up, $p < 0.001$.

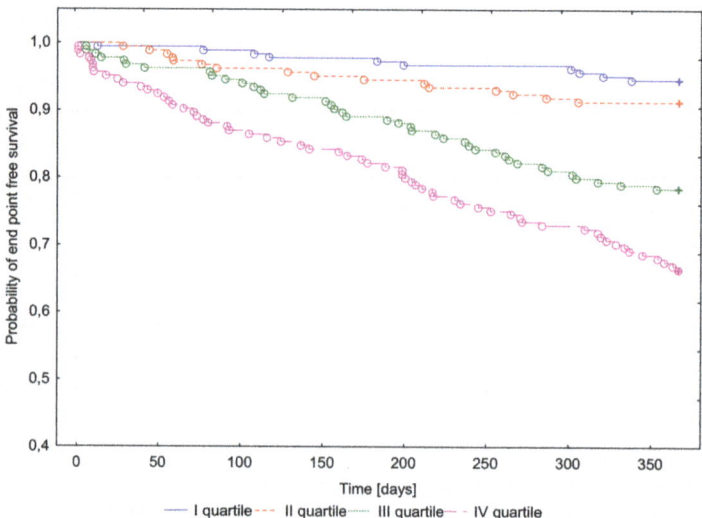

Figure 2. Probability of survival of time free of death or heart transplantation depending on quartiles of NT-proBNP concentrations in 1-year follow-up, $p < 0.001$.

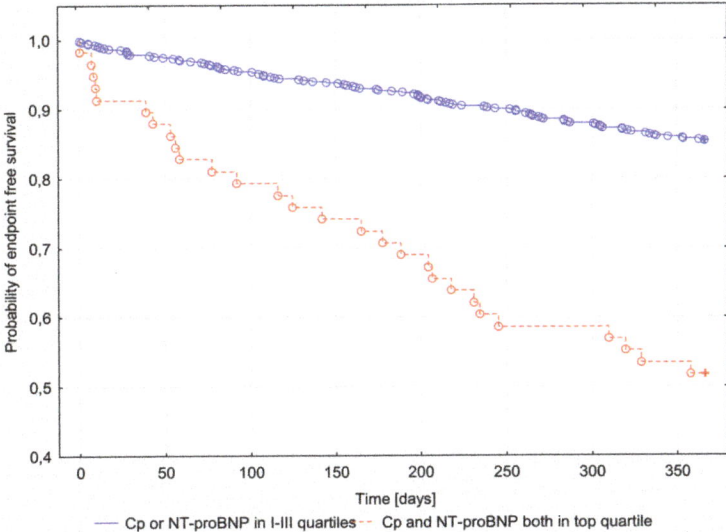

Figure 3. Probability of endpoint free survival in 1-year follow-up. Patients with Ceruloplasmin or NT-proBNP concentrations in I–III quartiles vs. both Cp and NT-proBNP in the top quartile, log rank $p < 0.001$.

A log-rank analysis revealed a significantly different probability of all-cause death or heart transplantation over time in patients stratified by quartiles of Cp or NT-proBNP concentration in the 1-year follow-up period ($p < 0.001$). After the stratification of patients based on the combination of CP and NT-proBNP concentration, patients with both Cp and NT-proBNP in the upper quartile had the highest probability of an endpoint occurrence (Table 4).

Table 4. Probability of death or heart transplantation occurrence in 1-year follow-up.

	I-III Quartiles of Cp (mg%) (8.0–35.8)	Top Quartile of Cp (mg%) (35.9–81.0)	I-III Quartiles of NT-proBNP (pg/mL) (122.9–3155.0)	Top Quartile of NTpro-BNP (pg/mL) (3156.0–22378.0)	I-III Quartiles of Cp or NT-proBNP	Cp and NT-proBNP Both in Top Quartile
End point (+) (n)	78	50	66	62	100	28
End point (−) (n)	477	136	490	123	583	30
Probability of end point (%) with confidence intervals	14.054 (11.159–16.941)	26.881 (20.508–33.251)	11.871 (9.182–14.558)	33.513 (26.708–40.312)	14.641 (11.989–17.291)	48.276 (35.416–61.136)
Odds ratio	2.248 95%CI (1.503–3.364) $p < 0.001$		3.742 95%CI (2.511–5.578) $p < 0.001$		5.441 95%CI (3.117–9.498) $p < 0.001$	
Sensitivity (%)	26.88		33.51		48.28	
Specificity (%)	77.81		79.93		95.10	

Cp—ceruloplasmin; NT-proBNP—N-terminal Type B pro peptide.

Detailed results for the top quartiles of Cp and NT-proBNP concentration, as well as the combination of the top quartiles of Cp and NT-proBNP concentrations, with the sensitivity and specificity of their predictive values, are presented in Table 4. For patients with a Cp concentration in the top quartile, the risk of death or heart transplantation was two-fold higher than in patients with Cp concentrations in quartiles I–III. Similarly, NT-proBNP concentration in the top quartile indicated approximately a 4-fold increase in the probability of an endpoint occurrence. The predictive values of Cp and NT-proBNP concentrations did not differ significantly (NT-proBNP vs. Cp, OR = 1.371, 95% CI (0.878–2.140)). The greatest prognostic value was seen for the combination of Cp and NT-proBNP concentrations in the top quartile, which was associated with more than a five-fold increased risk. Cp and NT-proBNP concentrations (both in the top quartile) showed a significantly higher predictive value than the top quartile of Cp (OR = 2.539; 95% CI (1.381–4.666)) or NT-proBNP (OR = 1.852; 95% CI (1.018–3.370)) concentrations individually (Table 4).

4. Discussion

There are many papers documenting the association between Cp and cardiovascular disease in clinical and experimental studies [20–22]. However, data confirming the effect of Cp concentration on prognosis in patients with HF are limited. This study intended to determine the clinical utility of a single baseline Cp measurement and other common risk factors as prognostic markers of all-cause mortality or heart transplantation in HF patients. We showed a significantly higher risk of all-cause death or heart transplantation in a 1-year follow-up of patients with Cp concentration in the top quartile. Similarly, patients with NT-proBNP concentration in the top quartile had a higher risk of endpoint occurrence. However, after adjustment for known clinical and laboratory parameters and treatments, neither NT-proBNP nor Cp remained significant predictors. Interestingly, the combination of elevated Cp and NT-proBNP concentrations (both in the top quartile) had greater specificity and sensitivity for endpoint prediction than CP or NT-proBNP concentrations alone. Other independent endpoint predictors were LVEF, peak VO_2, ACE-I/ARB therapy, and prior ICD implantation. Although clinical assessment had a strong prognostic role, it is worth highlighting that peak oxygen consumption (peak VO_2) rather than New York Heart Association class, should be used to estimate functional capacity. The utility of peak VO_2 and other parameters of the Heart Failure Survival Score (ischemic heart disease, mean blood pressure, LVEF, heart rate, serum sodium, intraventricular conduction defect) for predicting prognosis and assessing candidacy for heart transplantation, have been documented across races and genders [23].

Recently, Paolillo et al. showed that the cut-off values of peak VO_2 able to identify a 10% or 20% risk (in 10 years of follow-up) of unfavorable outcomes decreased over 20 years up to 2010, with similar cut-off values observed over this time period [24]. As a possible explanation, they suggested that the most effective treatment options were introduced to the guidelines by 2010, such that a similar risk level was observed in patients enrolled after 2010. In our study, patients were enrolled before 2010 and a decrease in peak VO_2 by 1 mL/min/kg was associated with an 11% increase in the risk of endpoints in a 1-year follow-up. Lower values of the main echocardiographic parameter, LVEF, were associated with increased mortality or heart transplantation rate.

On the contrary, Lai et al. showed that, at initial presentation, LVEF did not have outcome-predictive power Additionally, they showed that the 12-month mortality risk in patients with LVEF ≥ 50% was similar to those with LVEF < 40% [7]. However, in this study, patients were hospitalized with acute HF, and therefore, LVEF data may reflect exacerbated heart function, rather than a chronic stable status.

Referring to guideline-based therapy, patient treatment in our study was considered to be optimized by the physicians [25]. Although we did not analyze the reasons for not using this treatment, in most cases there were contraindications to the use of this therapy. Moreover, we did not analyze the ACE-I/ARB dose, since even low-dose ACE-I/ARB therapy is superior to no one treatment as it decreases 1-year mortality rates [26]. Patient treatment may be a limitation of the study (see study limitation section). Beta-blockers were used in the majority of patients (97%). Notably, the percentage of patients with ICDs in our study was rather low (approximately 27%). The lack of ICD implantation was an independent risk factor of all-cause mortality (not only sudden cardiac death) and heart transplantation. Improved survival of patients with implanted ICDs has previously been observed in clinical trials [27]. ICD implantation was different between groups according to Cp concentration quartiles. In the highest

Cp quartile the percentage of patients who did not receive ACE-I and /or ARB was the lowest. In our study, many of the analyzed laboratory parameters were risk factors of unfavorable outcomes only in univariable analyses. However, none of them were shown to affect mortality or heart transplantation after adjusting for other predictive factors. Only the combination of the top quartiles of NT-proBNP and Cp concentrations was useful for the prediction of unfavorable outcomes.

Previously, some investigations with various study designs have demonstrated the prognostic power of natriuretic peptide concentration [28–30]. Lai et al. reported that increased plasma NT-pro BNP level ($\geq$11755 ng/L) was an independent predictor of 1- and 3-month mortality, but not of mortality in more extended follow-up [7]. Bettencourt and colleagues showed that an NT-proBNP concentration > 6779 pg/mL at admission was a weaker predictor of readmission or death than a post-treatment NT-proBNP concentration of 4137 pg/mL, with an 8% increase in the probability of death or readmission over 6 months per 1000 pg/mL of NT-proBNP [31]. Finally, the current ACC/AHA/HFSA Guideline for the Management of Heart Failure recommends the assessment of natriuretic peptide biomarkers on admission in acutely decompensated HF patients and before discharge, to establish a prognosis [32].

We evaluated NT-proBNP concentrations in stable, nonhospitalized patients and found that an NT-proBNP concentration > 3155pg/mL (upper quartile) did not have significant predictive value in a multivariate analysis in a 1-year follow-up. A comparison of our results with other studies is difficult because of different follow-up periods, endpoint definitions, and types of cohorts. Bayes-Genis et al. performed a serial assessment of NT-proBNP concentration in an outpatient group (patient decompensated, but not requiring emergency hospital admission) with reduced LVEF (27 +/− 9%). The percentage reduction in NT-proBNP concentration in the first four weeks (not baseline concentration) was a predictor of death and hospitalization during three months of follow-up [33].

Multiple biomarker strategies, involving a combination of NPs with other biomarkers, have been proposed to create more accurate predictive scores in HF [34]. Multimarker approaches combining NT-pro-BNP and Cp have been used to assess the risk of HF incidence and mortality in patients in the Atherosclerosis Risk in Communities (ARIC) study. In this population, the strongest associations of Cp were observed with HF and all-cause mortality. These associations persisted after adjusting for biomarkers known to have a role in HF prediction, such as NT-proBNP, troponin, and CRP [35]. Engstrom et al. also reported Cp as a risk factor for HF incidence in Caucasian men with a high risk of cardiovascular disease [36].

Elevated Cp levels have been shown in many cardiovascular disorders, including coronary heart disease, myocardial infarction, and arteriosclerosis. The oxidative effects of Cp on serum lipids, in combination with decreased antioxidant protection, can predominate in CAD patients. Ceruloplasmin has diverse functions. It is involved in iron homeostasis and angiogenesis. It is the major source of serum ferroxidase activity and can act as a pro- or antioxidant molecule [37–39]. Many previous studies have reported an elevated Cp concentration during HF [40,41]. Some study demonstrated that the Cp can be a significant marker of heart failure in patients with ST segment elevated myocardial infarction [42]. A possible association between ceruloplasmin and progression of HF was study by Cabassi et al. [43].

To the best of our knowledge, only one previous study has evaluated the prognostic value of the simultaneous assessment of Cp and BNP in stable HF patients undergoing elective cardiac evaluation, including coronary angiography. In that study, Hammadah et al. reported that elevated Cp levels increase the risk of 5-year all-cause mortality. Even after adjusting for a large panel of other risk factors and medications, Cp concentration in the third or fourth quartile (> 25.6 mg/dL) remained a significant predictor of increased 5-year mortality. Further analysis, with additional adjustment for heart rate, QRS duration and ICD placement, revealed that a Cp concentration in the upper quartile (> 30.2 mg/dL) remained predictive. Additionally, within each group of defined BNP concentration range, higher Cp levels were associated with poorer outcomes. Similar to our study, the authors shown that the combined use of biomarkers can help identify patients with the highest probability of death [44].

The reasons for the increased Cp concentration in HF are not well understood, but it is possible that the measurement of Cp (in combination with NT-proBNP) can help identify patients with the highest long-term mortality risk.

5. Conclusions

The determination of Cp concentration is cost-effective and relatively easy. Data from the present study confirmed the association between Cp concentration and the severity of HF. The combined measurement of Cp and NT-proBNP concentrations has an advantage over measuring NT-proBNP concentration alone in selecting a group of high-risk HF patients in a 1-year follow-up.

Study Limitations

Our study has several limitations. Firstly, these results may not be applicable to the general population, since the age range of patients in this study was 48–59 years. Secondly, it was a single-center study of stable outpatients considered as potential recipients of the heart. Thirdly, ARNI and SGLT2 were not used, since patient enrollment occurred before 2010. Fourthly, low percentage of patients with implanted ICD.

Author Contributions: Conceptualization, E.R., C.W., and W.J.; Methodology, C.W., E.R., and W.J.; Software, W.J.; Validation, E.R., C.W., and W.J.; Formal Analysis, E.R., C.W., and W.J.; Investigation, E.R., C.W., and W.J.; Resources, M.G., E.Z., and P.R.; Data Curation, A.M., E.Z.; Writing—Original Draft Preparation, E.R., C.W., and W.J.; Writing—Review & Editing, E.R., C.W., and W.J.; Visualization, J.N., A.M., and W.J.; Supervision, M.G., P.R.; Project Administration, E.R., C.W., and W.J. All authors have read and agreed to the published version of the manuscript.

Funding: This work was founded by the Medical University of Silesia grant no. KNW-1/096/K/8/0, Poland.

Conflicts of Interest: The authors declare that there is no conflict of interest regarding the publication of this paper.

References

1. Seino, Y.; Ogawa, A.; Yamashita, T.; Fukushima, M.; Ogata, K.; Fukumoto, H.; Takan, T. Application of NT-proBNP and BNP measurements in cardiac care: A more discerning marker for the detection and evaluation of heart failure. *Eur. J. Heart Fail.* **2004**, *6*, 295–300. [CrossRef] [PubMed]
2. Anker, S.; Doehner, W.; Rauchhaus, M.; Sharma, R.; Francis, D.; Knosalla, C.; Davos, C.H.; Cicoira, M.; Shamim, W.; Kemp, M.; et al. Uric Acid and Survival in Chronic Heart Failure Validation and Application in Metabolic, Functional, and Hemodynamic Staging. *Circulation* **2003**, *107*, 1991–1997. [CrossRef] [PubMed]
3. Yin, W.H.; Chen, J.W.; Jen, L.H.; Chiang, M.C.; Huang, W.P.; Feng, A.N.; Young, M.S.; Lin, S.J. Independent prognostic value of elevated high-sensitivity C-reactive protein in chronic heart failure. *Am. Heart J.* **2004**, *147*, 931–938. [CrossRef] [PubMed]
4. Ponikowski, P.; Voors, A.A.; Anker, S.D.; Bueno, H.; Cleland, J.G.F.; Coats, A.J.S.; Falk, V.; González-Juanatey, J.R.; Harjola, V.P.; Jankowska, E.A.; et al. 2016 ESC Guidelines for the diagnosis and treatment of acute and chronic heart failure: The Task Force for the diagnosis and treatment of acute and chronic heart failure of the European Society of Cardiology (ESC). Developed with the special contribution of the Heart Failure Association (HFA) of the ESC. *Eur. Heart J.* **2016**, *37*, 2129–2200. [CrossRef]
5. Neuhold, S.; Huelsmann, M.; Strunk, G.; Stoiser, B.; Struck, J.; Morgenthaler, N.G.; Bergmann, A.; Moertl, D.; Berger, R.; Pacher, R. Comparison of copeptin, B-type natriuretic peptide, and amino-terminal pro-B-type natriuretic peptide in patients with chronic heart failure: Prediction of death at different stages of the disease. *J. Am. Coll. Cardiol.* **2008**, *52*, 266–272. [CrossRef]
6. Chow, S.L.; Chow, S.L.; Maisel, A.S.; Anand, I.; Bozkurt, B.; de Boer, R.A.; Felker, G.M.; Fonarow, G.C.; Greenberg, B.; Januzzi, J.L., Jr.; et al. Role of biomarkers for the prevention, assessment, and management of heart failure a scientific statement from the American Heart Association. *Circulation* **2017**, *135*, 1054–1091. [CrossRef]
7. Lai, M.Y.; Kan, W.C.; Huang, Y.T.; Chen, J.; Shiao, C.C. The Predictivity of N-Terminal Pro b-Type Natriuretic Peptide for All-Cause Mortality in Various Follow-Up Periods among Heart Failure Patients. *J. Clin. Med.* **2019**, *13*, 357. [CrossRef]

8. Januzzi, J.L.; Rehman, S.U.; Mohammed, A.A.; Bhardwaj, A.; Barajas, L.; Barajas, J.; Kim, H.N.; Baggish, A.L.; Weiner, R.B.; Chen-Tournoux, A.; et al. Use of amino-terminal pro-B type natriuretic peptide to guide outpatient therapy of patients with chronic left ventricular systolic dysfunction. *J. Am. Coll. Cardiol.* **2011**, *58*, 1881–1889. [CrossRef]
9. Floris, G.; Medda, R.; Padiglia, A.; Musci, G. The physiopathological significance of caeruloplasmin. *Biochem. Pharmacol.* **2000**, *60*, 1735–1741. [CrossRef]
10. Harris, E.D. A requirement for copper in angiogenesis. *Nutr. Rev.* **2004**, *62*, 60–64. [CrossRef]
11. Hannan, G.N.; McAuslen, B.R. Modulation of synthesis of specific proteins in endothelial cells by copper, cadmium, and disulfiram: An early response to an angiogenic inducer of cell migration. *J. Cell. Physiol.* **1982**, *111*, 207–212. [CrossRef] [PubMed]
12. Shukla, N.; Maher, J.; Masters, J.; Angelini, G.D.; Jeremy, J.Y. Does oxidative stress change ceruloplasmin from a protective to a vasculopathic factor. *Atherosclerosis* **2006**, *187*, 238–250. [CrossRef] [PubMed]
13. Shiva, S.; Wang, X.; Ringwood, L.A.; Xu, X.; Yuditskaya, S.; Annavajjhala, V.; Miyajima, H.; Hogg, N.; Harris, Z.L.; Gladwin, M.T. Ceruloplasmin is a NO oxidase and nitrite synthase that determines endocrine NO homeostasis. *Nat. Chem. Biol.* **2006**, *2*, 486–493. [CrossRef] [PubMed]
14. Xu, Y.; Lin, H.; Zhou, Y.; Cheng, G.; Xu, G. Ceruloplasmin and the extent of heart failure in ischemic and nonischemic cardiomyopathy patients. *Mediat. Inflamm.* **2013**, *2013*, 348145. [CrossRef] [PubMed]
15. Kaya, Z.; Kaya, B.; Sezen, H.; Bilinc, H.; Asoglu, R.; Yildiz, A.; Taskin, A.; Yalcin, S.; Sezen, Y.; Aksoy, N. Serum ceruloplasmin levels in acute decompensated heart failure. *Clin. Ter.* **2013**, *164*, 87–91.
16. Ahmed, M.S.; Jadhav, A.B.; Hassan, A.; Meng, Q.H. Acute Phase Reactants as Novel Predictors of Cardiovascular Disease. *ISRN Inflamm.* **2012**. [CrossRef]
17. Studies Investigating Co-Morbidities Aggravating Heart Failure (SICA-HF). 2016. Available online: https://clinicaltrials.gov/ (accessed on 18 November 2019).
18. Romuk, E.; Wojciechowska, C.; Jacheć, W.; Nowak, J.; Niedziela, J.; Malinowska-Borowska, J.; Głogowska-Gruszka, A.; Birkner, E.; Rozentryt, P. Comparison of Oxidative Stress Parameters in Heart Failure Patients Depending on Ischaemic or Nonischaemic Aetiology. *Oxid. Med. Cell. Longev.* **2019**, *2019*, 13. [CrossRef]
19. Richterich, R.; Gautier, E.; Stillharth, H.; Rossi, E. Serum ceruloplasmin concentration was determined spectrophotometrically according to Richterich reaction with p-phenyl-diamine. The heterogeneity of caeruloplasmin nd the enzymatic defect in Wilson's disease. *Helv. Paediatr. Acta* **1960**, *15*, 424–436.
20. Singh, T.K. Serum ceruloplasmin in acute myocardial infarction. *Acta Cardiol.* **1992**, *47*, 321–329.
21. Manttari, M.; Manninen, V.; Huttunen, J.K.; Palosuo, T.; Ehnholm, C.; Heinonen, O.P.; Frick, M.H. Serum ferritin and ceruloplasmin as coronary risk factors. *Eur. Heart J.* **1994**, *15*, 1599–1603. [CrossRef]
22. Atanasiu, R.; Dumoulin, M.J.; Chahine, R.; Mateescu, M.A.; Nadeau, R. Antiarrhythmic effects of ceruloplasmin during reperfusion in the ischemic isolated rat heart. *Can. J. Physiol. Pharmacol.* **1995**, *73*, 1253–1261. [CrossRef]
23. Goda, A.; Lund, L.H.; Mancini, D.M. Comparison across races of peak oxygen consumption and heart failure survival score for selection for cardiac transplantation. *Am. J. Cardiol.* **2010**, *15*, 1439–1444. [CrossRef]
24. Paolillo, S.; Veglia, F.; Salvioni, E.; Corrà, U.; Piepoli, M.; Lagioia, R.; Limongelli, G.; Sinagra, G.; Cattadori, G.; Scardovi, A.B.; et al. Heart failure prognosis over time: How the prognostic role of oxygen consumption and ventilatory efficiency during exercise has changed in the last 20 years. *Eur J. Heart Fail.* **2019**, *21*, 208–217. [CrossRef]
25. Tai, C.; Gan, T.; Zou, L.; Sun, Y.; Zhang, Y.; Chen, W.; Li, J.; Zhang, J.; Xu, Y.; Lu, H.; et al. Effect of angiotensin-converting enzyme inhibitors and angiotensin II receptor blockers on cardiovascular events in patients with heart failure: A meta-analysis of randomized controlled trials. *BMC Cardiovasc. Disord.* **2017**, *17*, 257. [CrossRef]
26. Rochon, P.A.; Sykora, K.; Bronskill, S.E.; Mamdani, M.; Anderson, G.M.; Gurwitz, J.H.; Gill, S.; Tu, J.V.; Laupacis, A. Use of angiotensin-converting enzyme inhibitor therapy and dose-related outcomes in older adults with new heart failure in the community. *J. Gen. Intern. Med.* **2004**, *19*, 676–683. [CrossRef]
27. Al-Khatib, S.M.; Hellkamp, A.; Bardy, G.H.; Hammill, S.; Hall, W.J.; Mark, D.B.; Anstrom, K.J.; Curtis, J.; Al-Khalidi, H.; Curtis, L.H.; et al. Survival of patients receiving a primary prevention implantable cardioverter-defibrillator in clinical practice vs clinical trials. *JAMA* **2013**, *309*, 55–62. [CrossRef]

28. Kociol, R.D.; Horton, J.R.; Fonarow, G.C.; Reyes, E.M.; Shaw, L.K.; O'Connor, C.M.; Felker, G.M.; Hernandez, A.F. Admission, discharge, or change in B-type natriuretic peptide and long-term outcomes: Data from Organized Program to Initiate Lifesaving Treatment in Hospitalized Patients with Heart Failure (OPTIMIZE-HF) linked to Medicare claims. *Circ. Heart Fail.* **2011**, *4*, 628–636. [CrossRef]
29. Khanam, S.S.; Son, J.W.; Lee, J.W.; Youn, Y.J.; Yoon, J.; Lee, S.H.; Kim, J.Y.; Ahn, S.G.; Ahn, M.S.; Yoo, B.S. Prognostic value of short-term follow-up BNP in hospitalized patients with heart failure. *BMC Cardiovasc. Disord.* **2017**, *17*, 215. [CrossRef]
30. Cheng, V.; Kazanagra, R.; Garcia, A.; Lenert, L.; Krishnaswamy, P.; Gardetto, N.; Clopton, P.; Maisel, A. A rapid bedside test for B-type peptide predicts treatment outcomes in patients admitted for decompensated heart failure: A pilot study. *J. Am. Coll. Cardiol.* **2001**, *37*, 386–391. [CrossRef]
31. Bettencourt, P.; Azevedo, A.; Pimenta, J.; Frioes, F.; Ferreira, S.; Ferreira, A. N-terminal-pro-brain natriuretic peptide predicts outcome after hospital discharge in heart failure patients. *Circulation* **2004**, *110*, 2168–2174. [CrossRef]
32. Yancy, C.W.; Jessup, M.; Bozkurt, B.; Butler, J.; Casey, D.E., Jr.; Colvin, M.M.; Drazner, M.H.; Filippatos, G.S.; Fonarow, G.C.; Givertz, M.M.; et al. 2017 ACC/AHA/HFSA Focused Update of the 2013 ACCF/AHA Guideline for the Management of Heart Failure. A Report of the American College of Cardiology/American Heart Association Task Force on Clinical Practice Guidelines and the Heart Failure Society of America. *Circulation* **2017**, *136*, 137–161. [CrossRef]
33. Bayes-Genis, A.; Pascual-Figal, D.; Fabregat, J.; Domingo, M.; Planas, F.; Casas, T.; Ordonez-Llanos, J.; Valdes, M.; Cinca, J. Serial NT-proBNP monitoring and outcomes in outpatients with decompensation of heart failure. *Int. J. Cardiol.* **2007**, *120*, 338–343. [CrossRef]
34. Bayes-Genis, A.; Ordonez-Llanos, J. Multiple biomarker strategies for risk stratification in heart failure. *Clin. Chim. Acta* **2015**, *443*, 120–125. [CrossRef]
35. Dadu, R.T.; Dodge, R.; Nambi, V.; Virani, S.S.; Hoogeveen, R.C.; Smith, N.L.; Chen, F.; Pankow, J.S.; Guild, C.; Tang, W.H.W.; et al. Ceruloplasmin and heart failure in the Atherosclerosis Risk in Communities study. *Circ. Heart Fail.* **2013**, *6*, 936–943. [CrossRef]
36. Engström, G.; Hedblad, B.; Tydén, P.; Lindgärde, F. Inflammation-sensitive plasma proteins are associated with increased incidence of heart failure: A population-based cohort study. *Atherosclerosis* **2009**, *202*, 617–622. [CrossRef]
37. Bustamante, J.B.; Mateo, M.C.; Fernandez, J.; de Quiros, B.; Manchado, O.O. Zinc, copper and ceruloplasmin in arteriosclerosis. *Biomed. Express* **1976**, *25*, 244–245.
38. Reunanen, A.; Knekt, P.; Aaran, R.K. Serumceruloplasmin level and the risk of myocardial infarction and stroke. *Am. J. Epidemiol.* **1992**, *136*, 1082–1090. [CrossRef]
39. Göçmen, A.Y.; Sahin, E.; Semiz, E.; Gümuşlü, S. Is elevated serum ceruloplasmin level associated with increased risk of coronary artery disease? *Can. J. Cardiol.* **2008**, *24*, 209–212. [CrossRef]
40. Sezen, H.; Sezen, Y. How to Change Ceruloplasmin Levels in Heart Disease? *Koşuyolu Heart J.* **2018**, *21*, 61–64. [CrossRef]
41. Cao, D.J.; Hill, J.A. Copper Futures: Ceruloplasmin and Heart Failure. *Circ. Res.* **2014**, *114*, 1678–1680. [CrossRef]
42. Correale, M.; Brunetti, M.D.; de Gennaro, L.; di Biase, M. Acute phase proteins in atherosclerosis*(Acute Coronary Syndrome). *Cardiovasc. Hematol. Agents Med. Chem.* **2008**, *6*, 272–277. [CrossRef]
43. Cabassi, A.; Binno, S.M.; Tedeschi, S.; Ruzicka, V.; Dancelli, S.; Rocco, R.; Vicini, V.; Coghi, P.; Regolisti, G.; Montanari, A.; et al. Low Serum Ferroxidase I Activity Is Associated With Mortality in Heart Failure and Related to Both Peroxynitrite-Induced Cysteine Oxidation and Tyrosine Nitration of Ceruloplasmin. *Circ. Res.* **2014**, *114*, 1723–1732. [CrossRef]
44. Hammadah, M.; Fan, Y.; Wu, Y.; Hazern, S.L.; Wilson Tang, W.H. Prognostic Value of Elevated Serum Ceruloplasmin Levels in Patients with Heart Failure. *J. Card. Fail.* **2014**, *20*, 946–952. [CrossRef]

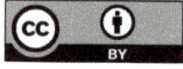

© 2020 by the authors. Licensee MDPI, Basel, Switzerland. This article is an open access article distributed under the terms and conditions of the Creative Commons Attribution (CC BY) license (http://creativecommons.org/licenses/by/4.0/).

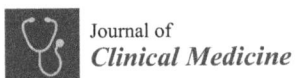
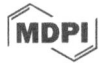

Article

Growth Differentiation Factor-8 (GDF8)/Myostatin Is a Predictor of Troponin I Peak and a Marker of Clinical Severity after Acute Myocardial Infarction

Alexandre Meloux [1,2], Luc Rochette [1], Maud Maza [1,2], Florence Bichat [1,2], Laura Tribouillard [2], Yves Cottin [1,2], Marianne Zeller [1] and Catherine Vergely [1,*]

1. Laboratoire Physiopathologie et Epidémiologie Cérébro-Cardiovasculaires (PEC2, EA 7460), Université de Bourgogne-Franche-Comté, UFR des Sciences de Santé; 7 Bd Jeanne d'Arc, 21000 Dijon, France; alexandre.meloux@u-bourgogne.fr (A.M.); luc.rochette@u-bourgogne.fr (L.R.); maud.maza@chu-dijon.fr (M.M.); florence.bichat@chu-dijon.fr (F.B.); yves.cottin@chu-dijon.fr (Y.C.); marianne.zeller@u-bourgogne.fr (M.Z.)
2. Department of Cardiology, University Hospital of Dijon, 21000 Dijon, France; laura.tribouillard@chu-dijon.fr
* Correspondence: cvergely@u-bourgogne.fr; Tel.: +33-3803-93292; Fax: +33-3803-93293

Received: 6 December 2019; Accepted: 20 December 2019; Published: 31 December 2019

Abstract: Objective: Growth differentiation factor-8 (GDF8), also known as myostatin, is a member of the transforming growth factor-β superfamily that inhibits skeletal muscle growth. We aimed to investigate the association between GDF8 and peak troponin I levels after acute myocardial infarction (AMI). Methods: All consecutive patients admitted from June 2016 to February 2018 for type 1 AMI in the Coronary Care Unit of University Hospital of Dijon Bourgogne (France) were included in our prospective study. Blood samples were harvested on admission, and serum levels of GDF8 were measured using a commercially available enzyme-linked immunosorbent assay kit. Results: Among the 296 patients with type 1 AMI, median age was 68 years and 27% were women. GDF8 levels (median (IQR) = 2375 ng/L) were negatively correlated with age, sex and diabetes ($p < 0.001$ for all). GDF8 levels were higher in patients with in-hospital ventricular tachycardia or fibrillation (VT/VF) than those without in-hospital VT/VF. GDF8 was positively correlated with troponin I peak (r = 0.247; $p < 0.001$). In multivariate linear regression analysis, log GDF8 (OR: 21.59; 95% CI 34.08–119.05; $p < 0.001$) was an independent predictor of troponin I peak. Conclusions: These results suggest that GDF8 levels could reflect the extent of myocardial damage during AMI, similar to peak troponin I, which is currently used to estimate infarct size. Further studies are needed to elucidate the underlying mechanisms linking the GDF8 cytokine with troponin I levels.

Keywords: GDF8; myostatin; AMI; troponin

1. Introduction

Patients with acute myocardial infarction (AMI) have a high rate of mortality, and the risk of fatal events is highest in the first hours following onset. The severity of AMI, which is usually determined early on with the measurement of circulating troponins, has a major impact on the development of late AMI consequences such as heart failure. Therefore, precise and rapid assessment of the severity of AMI critically affects treatment choices and patient prognoses. Recently, there has been interest in the potential role of new biomarkers for the assessment of severity in the early stages of AMI, with a particular focus on NT-pro-natriuretic peptide (NT-proBNP), heart-type fatty acid binding protein (hFABP) and circulating cytokines such as growth differentiation factor-15 [1].

Growth differentiation factor-8 (GDF8), also known as myostatin, is a member of the transforming growth factor-β (TGF-β) superfamily. GDF8 shares many structural similarities with other members such as growth differentiation factor-11 [2,3]. GDF8 is mainly expressed in skeletal muscles, particularly during the development period but also in adulthood, and is considered a negative regulator of muscle growth [4]. Genetic inhibition of myostatin leads to an increase in skeletal muscle mass and triggers a hyper-muscular phenotype in mammals [5,6]. In the heart muscle, GDF8 is expressed in fetal and adult myocardium [7], and its expression is increased in cardiac diseases such as advanced heart failure [8] or congenital heart disease [9]. Following experimental myocardial infarction, GDF8 is up-regulated in cardiomyocytes surrounding the infarcted area [7] and its concentration rapidly increases in the circulation [10]. However, the role of GDF8 during the acute phase of AMI in humans is poorly understood.

The aim of our study was to evaluate GDF8/myostatin levels in patients admitted for AMI, and to investigate the associations between GDF8 and markers of AMI severity such as troponin.

2. Methods

2.1. Patients

The methods and design of the French Regional Observatoire des Infarctus de Côte-d'Or (RICO) survey have been previously described [11]. From June 2016 to February 2018, all consecutive patients admitted to the coronary care unit of the Dijon University Hospital (France) for type 1 AMI were prospectively included. Type 1 MI is defined as an acute atherothrombotic coronary event resulting in the formation of an intra-luminal thrombus (plaque rupture, ulceration, erosion or coronary dissection) [12]. The present study is in agreement with the ethical guidelines of the Declaration of Helsinki. All of the participants provided consent prior to inclusion, and the Ethics Committee of the University Hospital of Dijon approved the protocol (BIOCARDIS-2016–9205AAO034S02117).

2.2. Data Collection

Patient characteristics were obtained at hospital admission. These included cardiovascular risk factors and history, and clinical and biological data. Risk scores were calculated (GRACE score and SYNTAX score). Blood samples were collected on admission to measure serum C-reactive protein (CRP), creatinine, creatine kinase peak, troponin Ic peak, NT-proBNP, blood lipids, glucose and hemoglobin. eGFR was calculated using Chronic Kidney Disease-EPIdemiology Collaboration formula (CKD-EPI). Echocardiographic data such as left ventricular ejection fraction (LVEF) were recorded. Finally, in-hospital events were documented, including death, cardiovascular death, re-infarction, stroke, development of heart failure and ventricular tachycardia or fibrillation (VT/VF).

2.3. Determination of Serum GDF8

Blood samples were collected on admission from a vein in the arm, centrifuged at 4 °C to isolate the serum, and samples were stored at −80 °C until use. Median (IQR) time from symptom onset to blood sampling was 16(8–30) hours. Serum GDF8 was measured in duplicate using a commercially available Quantitine kit (DGDF80, R&D systems, MN). The minimum detectable concentration was 2.25 ng/L, and the coefficient of variation between duplicates did not exceed 10%.

2.4. Statistical Analysis

Dichotomous variables are expressed as n (%) and continuous variables as mean ± SD or median (interquartile range). A Kolmogorov–Smirnov test was performed to test the normality of continuous variables. For non-normally distributed variables (i.e., NT-proBNP), they were log transformed. The Mann-Whitney test or Student's t test was used to compare continuous data, and the Chi 2 test or Fisher's test was used for dichotomous data, as appropriate.

Pearson correlation analyses (for normally distributed variables) or Spearman correlation analyses (one or two non-Gaussian variables) were performed. The threshold for significance was set at 5%.

Bivariate linear regression analyses were used to adjust GDF8 with age.

Multivariate logistic regression models were built to estimate in-hospital VT/VF and troponin Ic peak based on significant variables in univariate analysis. The inclusion threshold was set at 5%.

SPSS version 12.0.1 (IBM Inc, Armonk, NY, USA) was used for all of the statistical tests.

3. Results

The baseline characteristics of the study population are shown in Table 1. Predictors of GDF8 are shown in Table 2. GDF8 levels were significantly associated with age, sex and diabetes. Clinical data showed an association with systolic and diastolic blood pressure, STEMI, heart failure and GRACE risk score. Moreover, GDF8 was strongly correlated with CRP, creatine kinase peak, troponin Ic peak, NT-proBNP and LDL-cholesterol, as well as creatinine clearance and acute statin medication.

Table 1. Baseline characteristics.

	N (%) or Median (IQR) N = 296
Risk factors	
Age, y	68 (58–78)
Female	81 (27%)
BMI, kg/m^2	26 (24–30), n = 295
Hypertension	178 (60%)
Diabetes	75 (25%)
Hypercholesterolemia	117 (40%)
Family history of CAD	74 (25%)
Current smoking	85 (29%)
Cardiovascular history	
CAD	53 (18%)
Stroke	17 (6%)
Chronic kidney disease	16 (5%)
Clinical data	
LVEF, %	55 (50–60), n = 294
LVEF <40%	22 (7%)
HR, bpm	76 (64–87), n = 283
SBP, mmHg	142 (123–165), n = 275
DBP, mmHg	82 (70–94), n = 274
STEMI	143 (48%)
HF	56 (19%)
GRACE risk score	141 (116–170), n = 268
ICU length of stay, d	3 (3–4), n = 290
Coronary angiography	294 (99%)
SYNTAX score	12 (7–18), n = 284
Multivessel disease	184 (63%)
Percutaneous coronary intervention	252 (86%)
Biological data	
GDF8 relative expression	2375.0 (1640.0–3346.7)
CRP > 3 mg/L	158 (54%)
Creatinine, µmol/L	79 (68–95), n = 295
eGFR CKD, mL/min	82.7 (65.9–95.5), n = 295
eGFR CKD < 45 mL/min	34 (12%)
CK peak, UI/L	583 (195–1483), n = 291
Troponin Ic peak, ng/mL	15.00 (3.21–70.00), n = 295
Nt-ProBNP, pg/mL	394 (93–1588), n = 295
LDL cholesterol, g/L	1.24 (0.92–1.53), n = 293
HDL cholesterol, g/L	0.50 (0.40–0.60), n = 293
Total cholesterol, g/L	2.06 (1.70–2.35), n = 293
Triglycerides, g/L	1.21 (0.84–1.76), n = 293
Glycemia, mmol/L	6.80 (5.80–8.63), n = 295

Table 1. *Cont.*

	N (%) or Median (IQR) N = 296
In-hospital events	
Death	7 (2%)
Cardiovascular death	6 (2%)
Recurrent MI	7 (2%)
Stroke	2 (1%)
HF	75 (26%)
VT or VF	10 (3%)
Chronic medications	
Antiplatelet therapy	24 (8%)
Aspirin	72 (24%)
ARB	63 (21%)
ACE inhibitor	58 (20%)
Statin	92 (31%)
Beta blocker	83 (28%)
Diuretic	57 (19%)
Acute medications	
Antiplatelet therapy	283 (96%)
Aspirin	290 (98%)
ARB	36 (12%)
ACE inhibitor	179 (60%)
Statin	270 (91%)
Beta blocker	207 (70%)
Diuretic	65 (22%)

Data are expressed as n (%) or median (25th and 75th percentiles). n: number; GDF8: growth differentiation factor 8; BMI: body mass index; CAD: coronary artery disease; LVEF: left ventricular ejection fraction; HR: heart rate; HF: Heart failure; SBP: systolic blood pressure; DBP: diastolic blood pressure; STEMI: ST segment elevation myocardial infarction; GRACE: Global Registry of Acute Coronary Events; ICU: Intensive Care Unit; CRP: C-reactive protein; CK: creatine kinase; NT-proBNP: N-terminal pro-brain natriuretic peptide; LDL: low density lipoprotein; HDL: high density lipoprotein; ARB: angiotensin receptor blockers; ACE: angiotensin converting enzyme.

Table 2. Association between GDF8 levels and study variables ($n = 296$).

		Patients (n = 296)	GDF8 Relative Expression or r	*p* Value
CV risk factors				
Age (years)		68 (58–78)	−0.26	<0.001
Female	Yes	81 (27)	2002 (1284–2785)	<0.001
	No	215 (73)	2554.9 (1759–3489)	
BMI (kg/m^2)		26 (24–30)	0.08	0.191
Hypertension	Yes	178 (60)	2247 (1532–3321)	0.063
	No	118 (40)	2585 (1756–3381)	
Diabetes	Yes	75 (25)	1946 (1429–2621)	<0.001
	No	221 (75)	2574 (1751–3526)	
Hypercholesterolemia	Yes	117 (40)	2501 (1697–3397)	0.396
	No	179 (60)	2311 (1621–3304)	
Current smoking	Yes	85 (29)	2482 (1689–3396)	0.306
	No	211 (71)	2256 (1633–3320)	
Cardiovascular history				
CAD	Yes	53 (18)	2209 (1477–2991)	0.189
	No	243 (82)	2426 (1688–3381)	
Stroke	Yes	17 (6)	1742 (1070–2636)	0.062
	No	279 (94)	2431 (1679–3372)	
Chronic kidney disease	Yes	16 (5)	2712 (1315–3416)	0.885
	No	280 (95)	2368 (1663–3346)	
Clinical data				

Table 2. Cont.

		Patients (n = 296)	GDF8 Relative Expression or r	p Value
LVEF		55 (50–60)	−0.05	0.396
HR (bpm)		76 (64–87)	−0.06	0.304
SBP (mmHg)		142 (123–165)	0.14	0.022
DBP (mmHg)		82 (70–94)	0.22	<0.001
STEMI	Yes	143 (48)	2748 (1802–3445)	0.001
	No	153 (52)	2141 (1519–2973)	
Heart failure	Yes	56 (19)	2018 (1252–2775)	0.006
	No	238 (81)	2511 (1695–3413)	
GRACE risk score		141 (116–170)	−0.22	<0.001
ICU stay length (days)		3 (3–4)	−0.01	0.877
Biological data				
CRP ≥ 3 mg/L	Yes	158 (54)	2102 (1471–3197)	<0.001
	No	136 (46)	2722 (1957–3525)	
Creatinine clearance (CKD EPI) (mL/min)		83 (66–96)	0.15	0.010
CK peak (UI/L)		583 (195–1493)	0.26	<0.001
Peak troponin Ic (ng/mL)		15 (3–70)	0.25	<0.001
NT-proBNP (pg/mL)		394 (93–1588)	−0.27	<0.001
Glucose (mmol/L)		7 (6–9)	−0.02	0.684
LDL cholesterol (g/L)		1.2 (0.9–1.5)	0.25	<0.001
HDL cholesterol (g/L)		0.5 (0.4–0.6)	0.07	0.211
Triglycerides (g/L)		1.2 (0.8–1.8)	0.02	0.773

Data are expressed as n (%) or median (25th and 75th percentiles). n: number; r: correlation coefficient; GDF8: growth differentiation factor 8; BMI: body mass index; CAD: coronary artery disease; LVEF: left ventricular ejection fraction; HR: heart rate; SBP: systolic blood pressure; DBP: diastolic blood pressure; STEMI: ST segment elevation myocardial infarction; GRACE: Global Registry of Acute Coronary Events; ICU: Intensive Care Unit; CRP: C-reactive protein; CK: creatine kinase; NT-proBNP: N-terminal pro-brain natriuretic peptide; LDL: low density lipoprotein; HDL: high density lipoprotein; ARB: angiotensin II receptor blockers; ACE inhibitors: angiotensin converting enzyme inhibitors.

3.1. Baseline Characteristics

Among the 296 included patients, eighty-one (27%) were female. The median age was 68 years, 178 (60%) had hypertension, 117 (40%) had hypercholesterolemia, 75 (25%) had diabetes and 85 (29%) are active smokers. Median GDF8 was 2375 (1640–3347) ng/L.

3.2. Associations between GDF8 Levels and in-Hospital Development of Ventricular Tachycardia or Fibrillation

Ten patients (3%) developed VT/VF during their hospital stay. GDF8 levels were higher in these patients than in those who did not experience VT/VF (2565 ± 75 vs. 3852 ± 642 ng/L, $p = 0.034$, Figure 1). To assess VT/VF risk, a GDF8 cut-off value of 2878 ng/L was established with a receiver operating characteristic (ROC) curve analysis. The value was rounded to 2800 ng/L to improve clinical relevance. The area under the curve (AUC) was 0.697 ($p = 0.034$) and the sensitivity and specificity were good (70% and 66%, respectively). Among patients with GDF8 > 2800 ng/L (112/296), the risk of developing in-hospital VT/VF was higher than in patients with GDF8 < 2800 ng/L (184/296) ($p = 0.046$). The other relevant biomarkers (CK and peak troponin Ic) showed similar associations with the outcome (VT/VF): the respective AUC were 0.717 ($p = 0.027$) and 0.698 ($p = 0.034$), and the cut-off values were 400.5 UI/L and 7.6 ng/mL. Sensitivity and specificity were respectively 100% and 44% for CK and 100% and 43% for peak troponin IC. Both CK and troponin Ic were significantly associated with VT/VF in logistic regression analysis (CK peak: OR (95% CI): 6.034 (1.684–21.621) and troponin Ic peak: OR (95% CI): 2.751 (1.079–7.019)).

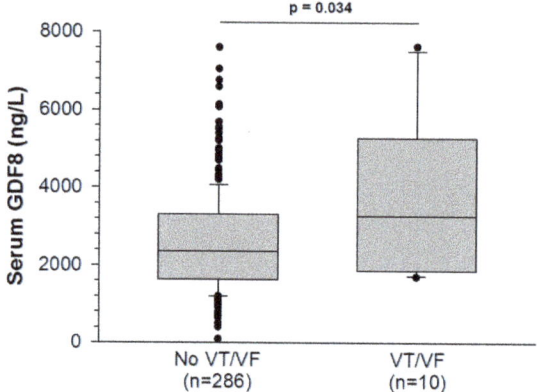

Figure 1. Serum growth differentiation factor-8 (GDF8) levels rise more in AMI patients with ventricular tachycardia or fibrillation (VT/VF) than AMI patients without VT/VF.

3.3. Associations between GDF8 Levels and Peak Troponin Ic

GDF8 was correlated with peak troponin Ic (r = 0.247; p <0.001). Patients with high (i.e., supramedian) GDF8 levels had a trend toward an increased risk of TV/FV compared with patients who had lower (i.e., inframedian) GDF8 levels (4.8% vs. 2%). Moreover, the troponin peak was much higher (X3) in patients with a supramedian GDF8 level, as shown in Table 3. In univariate analysis, diabetes (OR 11.82, 95% CI −3.49–43.03; p = 0.095), smoking (OR 11.34, 95% CI 0.78–45.40; p = 0.043), left ventricular ejection fraction <40% (OR 19.53, 95% CI 10.88–87.76; p = 0.012), GRACE risk score (OR 0.16, 95% CI 0.16–0.76; p = 0.003), and time to admission (OR 0.01, 95% CI −0.02–0.001; p = 0.065) and log GDF8 (OR 21.59, 95% CI 34.08–119.05; p <0.001) were associated with the prediction of troponin Ic peak. In multivariable analysis, log GDF8 remained associated to the prediction of troponin Ic peak, after adjustment for confounding factors (Table 4).

Table 3. Relevant outcomes according to high/low GDF8 levels (cutoff on median GDF8 value).

	GDF 8 ≤ 2400 ng/L N = 151	GDF 8 > 2400 ng/L N = 145	p Value
In-hospital VF/VT	3 (2.0%)	7 (4.8%)	0.211
Troponin Ic peak, ng/mL	8.30 (2.10–36.00)	29.50 (4.22–92.75)	<0.001
LVEF, %	56 (50–60)	55 (50–60)	0.498

Table 4. Logistic regression analysis for prediction of troponin I peak.

	Univariate			Multivariate		
	OR	95% CI	p Value	OR	95% CI	p Value
Diabetes	11.82	−3.49–43.03	0.095	12.98	7.86–59.00	0.011
Smoking	11.34	0.78–45.40	0.043	13.19	10.32–62.28	0.006
LVEF > 40%	19.53	10.88–87.76	0.012	22.23	6.75–94.34	0.024
GRACE risk score	0.15	0.16–0.76	0.003	0.168	0.39–1.05	<0.001
Time to admission, per min	0.01	−0.02–0.00	0.065	0.01	−0.02–0.01	0.233
Log GDF8, per unit	21.59	34.08–119.05	<0.001	26.68	67.05–172.17	<0.001

LVEF: left ventricular ejection fraction; GRACE: Global Registry of Acute Coronary Events; NT-proBNP: N-terminal pro-brain natriuretic peptide; GDF8: growth differentiation factor 8; OR: odds ratio; CI: confidence interval.

4. Discussion

In our study, GDF8 levels were shown to be negatively associated with older age, and positively with female sex; these results corroborate existing clinical data. For instance, previous studies have shown that GDF8 levels were highest in men in their 20s and statistically declined throughout subsequent decades [13]. Indeed, in men, serum GDF8 increases slightly with age until 57 years and then decreases [14]. In both the "Heart and Soul" and the HUNT3 cohorts, GDF11/8 levels were lower in older participants [15]. In patients aged 60 years and older, a recent study has shown that women had higher GDF8 plasma levels than men and that the circulating plasma GDF8 was negatively associated with muscle function [16].

In the present work, we also observed correlations between GDF8 levels and traditional cardiovascular risk factors such as diabetes, increased systolic and diastolic blood pressure, increased LDL cholesterol and CRP. The role of GDF8 in regulating tissue glucose uptake has been documented both in experimental [17] and clinical studies [18,19]. Blocked GDF8 expression in mice resulted in increased insulin signaling and better insulin sensitivity in skeletal muscle [20]. Therefore, in patients with insulin resistance, GDF8 inactivation is a potential target for the prevention of risk factors associated with the development of ischemic cardiovascular diseases. The clinical data are sparse for hypertension, cholesterol levels and CRP, but one experimental study has demonstrated that GDF8 deletion in a mouse model of metabolic syndrome resulted in increased muscle mass and prevented an increase in blood pressure [21]. Inactivation of GDF8 in in *Ldlr-/-* mice was shown to protect against the development of insulin resistance, proatherogenic dyslipidemia and aortic atherogenesis [22].

The main findings of the present study involve the association of GDF8 with the markers of AMI severity such as ST-elevation myocardial infarction (STEMI), occurrence of complicating heart failure, GRACE risk score, CK peak, NT-proBNP, and troponin levels. In multivariable analysis, log GDF8 was associated with the prediction of troponin I peak, even after adjustment for age. Moreover, among patients with the highest GDF8 levels (>2800 ng/L), the risk of developing in-hospital VT/VF was higher. To our knowledge, this is the first time that GDF8 has been associated with clinical severity in the acute phase of MI. Previous studies in sheep found that GDF8 was expressed in the fetal and adult heart and was localized in the cardiomyocytes and Purkinje fibers [7]. Furthermore, after experimental myocardial infarction, GDF8 expression was upregulated in the cardiomyocytes surrounding the infarcted zone. Studies performed in mice have shown that GDF8 was upregulated in the heart as early as 10 min after coronary artery ligation, reaching peak expression in tissue between 24 h and 1 month following the acute event. In the serum of the mice, GDF8 levels also promptly and steadily increased [10]. Indeed, elevated circulating levels of GDF8 have been observed in several types of serious myocardial diseases such as anthracycline-induced cardiotoxicity [23] and in experimental [24–26] and clinical heart failure [8,9,27]. In particular, serum GDF8 levels were shown to have predictive value for the severity of chronic heart failure and to be a predictor of adverse prognosis in these patients [27]. In myocardial infarction, both the destruction of the cardiac tissue and the up-regulation of its expression may account for the elevated levels found in serum. Consequently, it has been suggested that the heart could function as an endocrine organ promoting skeletal or myocardial muscle wasting, inducing cardiac muscle weakness [25]. In fact, the absence of GDF8 in GDF8-deficient mice subjected to myocardial infarction seemed to protect the heart, possibly by limiting the extent of fibrosis and improving survival [28]. We suggest here that during the course of AMI, GDF8 is produced and released by the cardiac tissue proportionally to the severity of the ischemia. GDF levels may therefore be strongly associated with peak troponin, but also with the occurrence of complications such as heart failure or ventricular arrhythmias. Of course, the estimation of myocardial damage is complex and might not be only reflected by one circulating factor such as GDF8 and/or troponin peak. Hemodynamic measurements, expansion index, and other exams as such as magnetic resonance imaging are necessary to quantify the extent of the infarct, the myocardial tissue loss and fibrosis after AMI [29,30]. Further studies should be conducted to evaluate whether GDF8 could be a predictor of poor outcomes after AMI, in particular those related to skeletal or myocardial muscle wasting.

5. Study Limitations

The first limitation of our study is the small number of patients who developed VT/VF ($n = 10$), limiting statistical power. The second limitation is the monocentric nature of the study with a subsequent selection bias. However, the strong association between GDF8 and the prediction of troponin I peak was supported by results of univariate regression analysis ($p < 0.001$) and the enduring significance after adjustment for determinants ($p < 0.001$). In future, these preliminary results need to be confirmed in larger studies.

6. Conclusions

To conclude, our original results suggest that GDF8 levels could reflect the extent of myocardial damage during AMI, similar to peak troponin I, which is currently used to estimate infarct size. Further studies are needed to elucidate the underlying mechanisms linking the GDF8 cytokine with troponin I levels.

Author Contributions: Conceptualization, C.V., L.R. and M.Z.; Methodology, C.V. and M.Z.; Validation, M.Z.; Formal analysis, A.M. and M.M.; Investigation, Y.C., A.M., F.B. and L.T.; Resources, L.T. and F.B.; Writing—original draft preparation, A.M., C.V., L.R. and M.Z.; writing—review and editing, C.V., L.R. and M.Z.; Supervision, C.V.; Project administration, C.V.; Funding acquisition, C.V., M.Z. and Y.C. All authors have read and agreed to the published version of the manuscript.

Funding: This work was supported by the Dijon University Hospital, the French Federation of Cardiology, the Association de Cardiology de Bourgogne, and by grants from the Agence Régionale de Santé (ARS) de Bourgogne-Franche-Comté and from the Regional Council of Burgundy-Franche-Comté.

Acknowledgments: The authors thank Suzanne Rankin for English revision of the manuscript, Ivan Porcherot and Morgane Laine for providing technical assistance.

Conflicts of Interest: The authors declare no conflict of interest.

References

1. Wollert, K.C.; Kempf, T.; Wallentin, L. Growth Differentiation Factor 15 as a Biomarker in Cardiovascular Disease. *Clin Chem.* **2017**, *63*, 140–151. [CrossRef] [PubMed]
2. Walker, R.G.; Poggioli, T.; Katsimpardi, L.; Buchanan, S.M.; Oh, J.; Wattrus, S.; Heidecker, B.; Fong, Y.W.; Rubin, L.L.; Ganz, P.; et al. Biochemistry and Biology of GDF11 and Myostatin: Similarities, Differences, and Questions for Future Investigation. *Circ. Res.* **2016**, *118*, 1125–1141. [CrossRef] [PubMed]
3. Rochette, L.; Zeller, M.; Cottin, Y.; Vergely, C. Growth and differentiation factor 11 (GDF11): Functions in the regulation of erythropoiesis and cardiac regeneration. *Pharmacol. Ther.* **2015**, *156*, 26–33. [CrossRef] [PubMed]
4. Argiles, J.M.; Orpi, M.; Busquets, S.; Lopez-Soriano, F.J. Myostatin: More than just a regulator of muscle mass. *Drug Discov. Today* **2012**, *17*, 702–709. [CrossRef]
5. McPherron, A.C.; Lee, S.J. Double muscling in cattle due to mutations in the myostatin gene. *Proc. Natl. Acad. Sci. USA* **1997**, *94*, 12457–12461. [CrossRef]
6. Mosher, D.S.; Quignon, P.; Bustamante, C.D.; Sutter, N.B.; Mellersh, C.S.; Parker, H.G.; Ostrander, E.A. A mutation in the myostatin gene increases muscle mass and enhances racing performance in heterozygote dogs. *PLoS Genet.* **2007**, *3*, e79. [CrossRef]
7. Sharma, M.; Kambadur, R.; Matthews, K.G.; Somers, W.G.; Devlin, G.P.; Conaglen, J.V.; Fowke, P.J.; Bass, J.J. Myostatin, a transforming growth factor-beta superfamily member, is expressed in heart muscle and is upregulated in cardiomyocytes after infarct. *J. Cell Physiol.* **1999**, *180*, 1–9. [CrossRef]
8. George, I.; Bish, L.T.; Kamalakkannan, G.; Petrilli, C.M.; Oz, M.C.; Naka, Y.; Lee Sweeney, H.; Maybaum, S. Myostatin activation in patients with advanced heart failure and after mechanical unloading. *Eur. J. Heart Fail.* **2010**, *12*, 444–453. [CrossRef]
9. Bish, L.T.; George, I.; Maybaum, S.; Yang, J.; Chen, J.M.; Sweeney, H.L. Myostatin is elevated in congenital heart disease and after mechanical unloading. *PLoS ONE* **2011**, *6*, e23818. [CrossRef]

10. Castillero, E.; Akashi, H.; Wang, C.; Najjar, M.; Ji, R.; Kennel, P.J.; Sweeney, H.L.; Schulze, P.C.; George, I. Cardiac myostatin upregulation occurs immediately after myocardial ischemia and is involved in skeletal muscle activation of atrophy. *Biochem. Biophys. Res. Commun.* **2015**, *457*, 106–111. [CrossRef]
11. Zeller, M.; Steg, P.G.; Ravisy, J.; Lorgis, L.; Laurent, Y.; Sicard, P.; Janin-Manificat, L.; Beer, J.C.; Makki, H.; Lagrost, A.C.; et al. Relation between body mass index, waist circumference, and death after acute myocardial infarction. *Circulation* **2008**, *118*, 482–490. [CrossRef] [PubMed]
12. Thygesen, K.; Alpert, J.S.; Jaffe, A.S.; Simoons, M.L.; Chaitman, B.R.; White, H.D. Third universal definition of myocardial infarction. *Circulation* **2012**, *126*, 2020–2035. [CrossRef] [PubMed]
13. Schafer, M.J.; Atkinson, E.J.; Vanderboom, P.M.; Kotajarvi, B.; White, T.A.; Moore, M.M.; Bruce, C.J.; Greason, K.L.; Suri, R.M.; Khosla, S.; et al. Quantification of GDF11 and Myostatin in Human Aging and Cardiovascular Disease. *Cell Metab.* **2016**, *23*, 1207–1215. [CrossRef] [PubMed]
14. Szulc, P.; Schoppet, M.; Goettsch, C.; Rauner, M.; Dschietzig, T.; Chapurlat, R.; Hofbauer, L.C. Endocrine and clinical correlates of myostatin serum concentration in men–the STRAMBO study. *J. Clin. Endocrinol. Metab.* **2012**, *97*, 3700–3708. [CrossRef]
15. Olson, K.A.; Beatty, A.L.; Heidecker, B.; Regan, M.C.; Brody, E.N.; Foreman, T.; Kato, S.; Mehler, R.E.; Singer, B.S.; Hveem, K.; et al. Association of growth differentiation factor 11/8, putative anti-ageing factor, with cardiovascular outcomes and overall mortality in humans: Analysis of the Heart and Soul and HUNT3 cohorts. *Eur. Heart J.* **2015**, *36*, 3426–3434. [CrossRef]
16. Fife, E.; Kostka, J.; Kroc, L.; Guligowska, A.; Piglowska, M.; Soltysik, B.; Kaufman-Szymczyk, A.; Fabianowska-Majewska, K.; Kostka, T. Relationship of muscle function to circulating myostatin, follistatin and GDF11 in older women and men. *BMC Geriatr.* **2018**, *18*, 200. [CrossRef]
17. Zhao, B.; Wall, R.J.; Yang, J. Transgenic expression of myostatin propeptide prevents diet-induced obesity and insulin resistance. *Biochem. Biophys. Res. Commun.* **2005**, *337*, 248–255. [CrossRef]
18. Brandt, C.; Nielsen, A.R.; Fischer, C.P.; Hansen, J.; Pedersen, B.K.; Plomgaard, P. Plasma and muscle myostatin in relation to type 2 diabetes. *PLoS ONE* **2012**, *7*, e37236. [CrossRef]
19. Hittel, D.S.; Berggren, J.R.; Shearer, J.; Boyle, K.; Houmard, J.A. Increased secretion and expression of myostatin in skeletal muscle from extremely obese women. *Diabetes* **2009**, *58*, 30–38. [CrossRef]
20. Zhang, C.; McFarlane, C.; Lokireddy, S.; Bonala, S.; Ge, X.; Masuda, S.; Gluckman, P.D.; Sharma, M.; Kambadur, R. Myostatin-deficient mice exhibit reduced insulin resistance through activating the AMP-activated protein kinase signalling pathway. *Diabetologia* **2011**, *54*, 1491–1501. [CrossRef]
21. Butcher, J.T.; Mintz, J.D.; Larion, S.; Qiu, S.; Ruan, L.; Fulton, D.J.; Stepp, D.W. Increased Muscle Mass Protects Against Hypertension and Renal Injury in Obesity. *J. Am. Heart Assoc.* **2018**, *7*, e009358. [CrossRef] [PubMed]
22. Tu, P.; Bhasin, S.; Hruz, P.W.; Herbst, K.L.; Castellani, L.W.; Hua, N.; Hamilton, J.A.; Guo, W. Genetic disruption of myostatin reduces the development of proatherogenic dyslipidemia and atherogenic lesions in Ldlr null mice. *Diabetes* **2009**, *58*, 1739–1748. [CrossRef] [PubMed]
23. Kesik, V.; Honca, T.; Gulgun, M.; Uysal, B.; Kurt, Y.G.; Cayci, T.; Babacan, O.; Gocgeldi, E.; Korkmazer, N. Myostatin as a Marker for Doxorubicin Induced Cardiac Damage. *Ann. Clin. Lab. Sci.* **2016**, *46*, 26–31. [PubMed]
24. Biesemann, N.; Mendler, L.; Wietelmann, A.; Hermann, S.; Schafers, M.; Kruger, M.; Boettger, T.; Borchardt, T.; Braun, T. Myostatin regulates energy homeostasis in the heart and prevents heart failure. *Circ. Res.* **2014**, *115*, 296–310. [CrossRef]
25. Heineke, J.; Auger-Messier, M.; Xu, J.; Sargent, M.; York, A.; Welle, S.; Molkentin, J.D. Genetic deletion of myostatin from the heart prevents skeletal muscle atrophy in heart failure. *Circulation* **2010**, *121*, 419–425. [CrossRef]
26. Damatto, R.L.; Lima, A.R.; Martinez, P.F.; Cezar, M.D.; Okoshi, K.; Okoshi, M.P. Myocardial myostatin in spontaneously hypertensive rats with heart failure. *Int. J. Cardiol.* **2016**, *215*, 384–387. [CrossRef]
27. Chen, P.; Liu, Z.; Luo, Y.; Chen, L.; Li, S.; Pan, Y.; Lei, X.; Wu, D.; Xu, D. Predictive value of serum myostatin for the severity and clinical outcome of heart failure. *Eur. J. Intern. Med.* **2019**, *64*, 33–40. [CrossRef]
28. Lim, S.; McMahon, C.D.; Matthews, K.G.; Devlin, G.P.; Elston, M.S.; Conaglen, J.V. Absence of Myostatin Improves Cardiac Function Following Myocardial Infarction. *Heart Lung Circ.* **2018**, *27*, 693–701. [CrossRef]

29. Flachskampf, F.A.; Schmid, M.; Rost, C.; Achenbach, S.; DeMaria, A.N.; Daniel, W.G. Cardiac imaging after myocardial infarction. *Eur. Heart J.* **2011**, *32*, 272–283. [CrossRef]
30. Ibanez, B.; James, S.; Agewall, S.; Antunes, M.J.; Bucciarelli-Ducci, C.; Bueno, H.; Caforio, A.L.P.; Crea, F.; Goudevenos, J.A.; Halvorsen, S.; et al. 2017 ESC Guidelines for the management of acute myocardial infarction in patients presenting with ST-segment elevation: The Task Force for the management of acute myocardial infarction in patients presenting with ST-segment elevation of the European Society of Cardiology (ESC). *Eur. Heart J.* **2018**, *39*, 119–177.

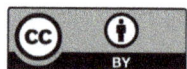

© 2019 by the authors. Licensee MDPI, Basel, Switzerland. This article is an open access article distributed under the terms and conditions of the Creative Commons Attribution (CC BY) license (http://creativecommons.org/licenses/by/4.0/).

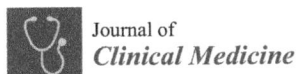 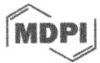

Article

New Imaging Markers of Clinical Outcome in Asymptomatic Patients with Severe Aortic Regurgitation

Radka Kočková [1,2,*], Hana Línková [3], Zuzana Hlubocká [4], Alena Pravečková [1], Andrea Polednová [1], Lucie Súkupová [1], Martin Bláha [1], Jiří Malý [5], Eva Honsová [6], David Sedmera [7] and Martin Pěnička [8]

1. Department of Cardiology, Institute for Clinical and Experimental Medicine, Prague 14021, Czech Republic; alena.praveckova@ikem.cz (A.P.); andrea.polednova@ikem.cz (A.P.); lucie.sukupova@gmail.com (L.S.); martin.blaha@ikem.cz (M.B.)
2. Faculty of Medicine in Hradec Králové, Charles University, Šimkova 870, Hradec Králové 500 03, Czech Republic
3. Department of Cardiology, Royal Vinohrady University Hospital, Prague 10034, Czech Republic; hana.linkova@fnkv.cz
4. Department of Cardiology, General University Hospital, Prague 12808, Czech Republic; zuzana.hlubocka@vfn.cz
5. Department of Cardiothoracic surgery, Institute for Clinical and Experimental Medicine, Prague 14021, Czech Republic; jiri.maly@ikem.cz
6. Institute for Clinical and Experimental Medicine, Clinical and Transplant Pathology Centre, Prague 14021, Czech Republic; eva.honsova@ikem.cz
7. First Faculty of Medicine, Institute of Anatomy, Charles University in Prague, Prague 12800, Czech Republic; david.sedmera@lf1.cuni.cz
8. Cardiovascular Center Aalst, OLV Clinic, 9300, Belgium; martin.penicka@olvz-aalst.be
* Correspondence: radka.kockova@ikem.cz; Tel.: +420-606-483-586

Received: 23 September 2019; Accepted: 6 October 2019; Published: 11 October 2019

Abstract: *Background:* Determining the value of new imaging markers to predict aortic valve (AV) surgery in asymptomatic patients with severe aortic regurgitation (AR) in a prospective, observational, multicenter study. *Methods:* Consecutive patients with chronic severe AR were enrolled between 2015–2018. Baseline examination included echocardiography (ECHO) with 2- and 3-dimensional (2D and 3D) vena contracta area (VCA), and magnetic resonance imaging (MRI) with regurgitant volume (RV) and fraction (RF) analyzed in CoreLab. *Results:* The mean follow-up was 587 days (interquartile range (IQR) 296–901) in a total of 104 patients. Twenty patients underwent AV surgery. Baseline clinical and laboratory data did not differ between surgically and medically treated patients. Surgically treated patients had larger left ventricular (LV) dimension, end-diastolic volume (all $p < 0.05$), and the LV ejection fraction was similar. The surgical group showed higher prevalence of severe AR (70% vs. 40%, $p = 0.02$). Out of all imaging markers 3D VCA, MRI-derived RV and RF were identified as the strongest independent predictors of AV surgery (all $p < 0.001$). *Conclusions:* Parameters related to LV morphology and function showed moderate accuracy to identify patients in need of early AV surgery at the early stage of the disease. 3D ECHO-derived VCA and MRI-derived RV and RF showed high accuracy and excellent sensitivity to identify patients in need of early surgery.

Keywords: aortic regurgitation; echocardiography; magnetic resonance imaging; vena contracta area; longitudinal strain; T1 mapping

1. Introduction

Chronic aortic regurgitation (AR) is the third most common valvular heart disease in Western countries, with a prevalence of 0.1% to 2.0%. Degenerative etiology on tricuspid or bicuspid aortic valves and annuloaortic ectasia are the most common causes of chronic AR. Rheumatic fever remains a frequent cause of chronic AR in developing countries [1–4]. In chronic AR, progressive left ventricular (LV) dilatation compensates for the increase of LV end-diastolic pressure. Left ventricular dilatation enables the preservation of cardiac output despite the large regurgitant volume of blood returning to the LV in diastole. Increased afterload in chronic AR is compensated by eccentric LV hypertrophy. This complex volume and pressure compensatory mechanisms explain the long asymptomatic course of the disease.

A combination of several clinical and imaging characteristics makes the timing of aortic valve (AV) intervention challenging. Patients with severe AR are often middle-aged males with a long asymptomatic course [1,2,5]. Furthermore, current indications for AV intervention (i.e., two-dimensional (2D) echocardiography (ECHO)-derived assessment of AR severity and left ventricular (LV) remodeling), appear to be rather specific but less sensitive [1,2,6–10]. This may lead to late AV intervention resulting in irreversible myocardial damage and impaired outcome [1–3,11,12]. Thus, a more a sensitive and accurate imaging marker to trigger early AV intervention may be of crucial importance.

Several promising imaging approaches to assess AR or its impact on LV structure and function have emerged recently [13–20]. For instance, three-dimensional (3D) ECHO- or magnetic resonance (MRI)-derived evaluation of AR severity may increase the accuracy of AR classification [16,19,20]. Assessment of LV myocardial fibrosis, strain or work may be more sensitive than LV diameters or ejection fraction (LVEF) to detect irreversible myocardial damage at an early stage [13–15,17,18,21]. Therefore, in a multicenter study, we thought to determine the value of new imaging markers to predict AV surgery in asymptomatic patients with severe AR and preserved LVEF. Imaging markers from all participating centers were analyzed centrally by a CoreLab.

2. Experimental Section

2.1. Design

A prospective, observational and multicenter study was conducted in three tertiary cardiology centers. All imaging markers were evaluated centrally in a CoreLab (Institute of Clinical and Experimental Medicine, Prague), which holds the European Association of Cardiovascular Imaging (EACVI) Laboratory accreditation and individual certification for both ECHO and MRI.

2.2. Patients

The study population consisted of all consecutive patients (age 44.4 ± 13.2 years, 85.4% males) with chronic severe AR and no indication for AV intervention who were referred to participating heart valve centers for AR assessment between March 2015 and September 2018. To be eligible for the study patients had to fulfil the following inclusion criteria: (1) severe AR defined by using the integrative 2D ECHO approach [10]; (2) absence of symptoms validated using bicycle ergometry; (3) preserved LVEF (>50%); (4) non-dilated LV end-diastolic diameter (≤70 mm) and LV end-systolic diameter index (≤25 mm/m^2); and (5) sinus rhythm. Patients with guideline indications for AV intervention, acute AR, aortic dissection, endocarditis, irregular heart rate, associated with more than mild valvular disease, complex congenital heart disease, intracardiac shunt, creatinine clearance <30 mL/min, pregnancy, or contra indication for MRI were excluded [1,2]. The study protocol and informed consent was approved by the ethics committees of all participating institutions. All patients had to sign informed consent prior to the enrollment. The study was registered in ClinicalTrials.gov under a unique identifier NCT02910349.

2.3. Protocol

An initial assessment was performed by specialized heart valve cardiologist in all participating centers. It included a history, clinical examination, Electrocardiography (ECG), bicycle ergometry, blood sampling, and comprehensive 2D and 3D ECHO. A cardiac MRI was performed in the center where the CoreLab was based for all participants. Patients from this particular center underwent MRI on the day of enrollment while patients from other two centers underwent an MRI within 2 weeks after the enrollment. Analysis of all ECHO- and MRI-derived markers were centralized in the CoreLab.

2.4. Follow-Up and Study Endpoints

After enrollment, patients were followed in participating heart valve centers every 6 months till 30 September 2018. The decision-making on conservative versus surgical treatment was left at the discretion of a particular heart valve team. In patients undergoing AV surgery, a perioperative biopsy was performed at the level of basal interventricular septum to assess the extent of myocardial fibrosis as previously described in our pilot study [14]. The follow-up data on AV interventions, mortality, and cardiac hospitalizations were obtained in all patients (100%) using population registry, medical files, and contact with referring physicians or family. Baseline clinical and imaging characteristics were analyzed to identify independent predictors of AV surgery. A prespecified study endpoint was cumulative of the indication for aortic valve intervention, ventricular arrhythmia occurrence (non-sustained or sustained ventricular tachycardia, ventricular ectopic beats >10%), hospitalization for heart failure, Brain natriuretic peptide (BNP) elevation >150 ng/L or cardiovascular death.

2.5. Doppler ECHO

A comprehensive 2D and 3D transthoracic ECHO was performed using a Vivid 7 and Vivid 9 (GE HealthCare, Horten, Norway) ultrasound system equipped with 4-dimensional active matrix 4-D volume phased array probe. Several 3D ECHO loops in each view were recorded using ECG-gated full-volume acquisition over four (LV function) to six (color Doppler) cardiac cycles during end-expiratory apnea. Images were optimized by adjusting the depth, sector size, gain, number of frames per second (FPS), the number of heart beats, and breath hold. All acquired images were digitally stored, anonymized, and analyzed using the commercially available software EchoPac BT 202, GE HealthCare. An average of at least 3 beats was taken for each measurement. Blood pressure and heart rate was recorded during each examination.

LV internal diameters were derived from an LV internal cavity using M-mode whenever possible. The biplane Simpson method was used to assess 2D LV volumes and Ejection fraction (EF) [21]. A semi-automatic contouring method with manual correction was used to measure 3D LV volumes and EF [21]. Global longitudinal strain (GLS) was assessed using a semi-automatic speckle tracking method with manual adjustment with frame rate of >60 FPS for 2D GLS (Figure 1B) and LV twist, and >25 FPS for 3D GLS [21]. Myocardial work was derived from 2D GLS, brachial blood pressure, and the timing of valvular events as described previously [18,22]. The severity of AR was assessed using the recommended approach integrating valve morphology, vena contracta width, the size of regurgitant jet in LV cavity and its width in LVOT, the jet pressure half time, the velocity of the diastolic flow reversal in the descending aorta, and the size of the proximal isovelocity surface area (PISA) [7,10]. Given the high prevalence of bicuspid valves in the study population and eccentric jets, the calculation of regurgitant volume (RV) using the PISA method was not consistently feasible. Therefore, the RV and regurgitant fraction (RF) of AR was assessed using the Doppler volumetric method, which uses the differences between the mitral and aortic stroke volumes (SV) to calculate RV and RF of AR [7,10]. Moderate-to-severe AR was defined by the presence of 2–3 specific criteria and RV of 45–59 mL or RF of 40%–49% [7,10]. Severe AR was defined by the presence of ≥4 specific criteria or by the presence of 2–3 specific criteria and RV ≥60 mL or RF ≥50% [10]. Moreover, 3D ECHO derived vena contracta area (VCA) was assessed in zoomed parasternal long-axis view (Figure 1A). In brief, the narrowest sector possible and multibeat acquisition was used to maximize the frame rate. To identify VCA, the 3D dataset was rotated to bisect the regurgitant color jet at the level of the leaflet coaptation zone perpendicularly to its long axis in 2 orthogonal planes. The image was cropped along the jet direction to visualize the cross-sectional area at the level of the vena contracta. Low velocity peripheral signals of the color spectrum were rejected. The VCA was defined as the high velocity core of the color spectrum [20].

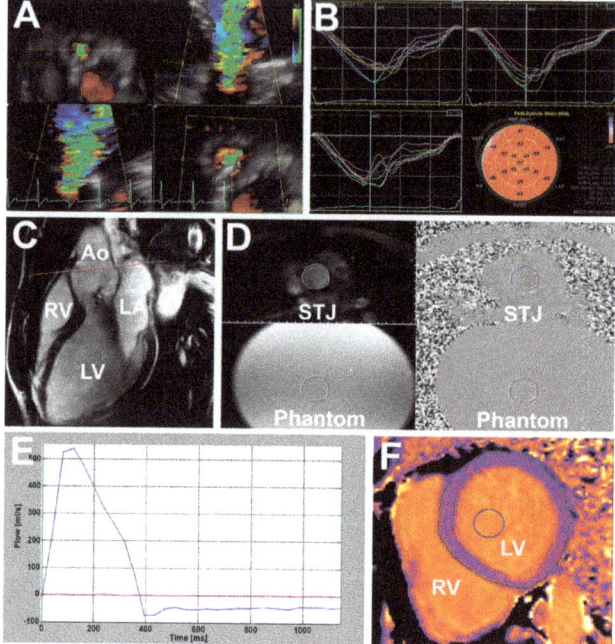

Figure 1. Imaging markers. (**A**) Echocardiography derived three-dimensional vena contracta area; (**B**) echocardiography two-dimensional global longitudinal strain; (**C**) magnetic resonance—the left ventricular outflow tract (cine), red line—through-plane flow sequence slice position displayed on, Ao—aorta, LA—left atrium, LV—left ventricle, RV—right ventricle; (**D**) through-plane flow sequence at sinotubular junction level (STJ) of the aorta (displayed on (**C**)), the blue circle is a manually drawn region of interest where the blood flow and regurgitant volume and fraction are calculated. The exact copy of the region interest is in all four images, phantom—stationary phantom used for flow measurement correction; (**E**) flow-time curve based on (**D**)—blue line shows blood flow at STJ and red line show flow in stationary phantom; (**F**) native T1 mapping from modified Look–Locker Inversion recovery sequence (MOLLI) sequence, blue circle—a semi-automatically drawn region of interest within the blood pool, blue ellipsoid—a manually drawn region of interest within the myocardium at the level of the interventricular septum utilized for myocardial fibrosis calculation.

2.6. Cardiac MRI

An examination was performed using a 1.5T scanner (Magnetom Avanto fit, Siemens, Munich, Germany). The protocol consisted of pilots, T2 weighted dark blood, cine with 2-, 4-, 3-chambers, and short axis (SA) images covering the entire end-diastolic ventricular length, through-plane phase-contrast velocity mapping at the level of the aortic root, contrast late gadolinium enhancement (LGE), and modified Look–Locker Inversion recovery sequence (MOLLI) [14,23]. Analysis was performed using a commercially available software (Segment CMR, Medviso AB 2018, Lund, Sweden). Blood pressure and heart rate was recorded during each examination.

LV volumes and LVEF were calculated using the steady state free precession cine imaging in short-axis stack (slice thickness 8 mm, slice spacing 0) with correction for the valve position in long-axis planes. LV radial, circumferential and longitudinal strain were assessed in the short axis and apical views. Native T1 relaxation time and extracellular volume fraction (ECV) were evaluated using the MOLLI sequence as previously described [14]. The T1 relaxation time measurement was performed in basal-to-mid short-axis slice 15 min pre and 15 min post contrast administration (Figure 1F). Parameters of the MOLLI sequence were as follows: field of view (FoV) 360 × 301 mm, matrix 118 × 256, slice thickness 8 mm, voxel size 1.4 mm × 1.4 mm × 8 mm, echo time 1.1 ms, repetition time 359 ms, flip angle 35°, bandwidth 1.085 Hz/Pixel.

Aortic forward and regurgitation flow were obtained by using the through-plane phase-contrast velocity mapping during breath-hold over 10–20 ms with retrospective ECG gating (Figure 1D). Parameters were as follows: temporal resolution 25–55 ms; echo time 2.7 ms; repetition time 46.8 ms, FoV 300 × 200 mm; matrix size 192 × 132; velocity window 1.5 to 4.0 m/s. Several image slices were prescribed at the level of the aortic root in end-diastole starting from 0.5 cm above AV annulus to 0.5 cm above the sinotubular junction (slice thickness 6 mm, spacing 0). Care was taken to align the slices perpendicularly to the direction of blood flow in two orthogonal imaging planes (Figure 1C). The lowest velocity encoding without flow aliasing was chosen for the analysis. Background velocity offset errors were corrected by using flow stationary phantom and post-processing correction. It has been shown previously that the ascending aorta slice location with the most accurate measurement of RV is between annulus and coronary ostia [24]. To reduce underestimation of RV and RF of AR, the closest slice to the AV without interference of turbulent flow was selected for the analysis [16,19]. Flow measurements from 3 acquisitions were averaged. Aortic forward volume (SV) and RV were derived by integration of the flow curve over 1 cardiac cycle. RF was calculated as RV/(SV * 100%) (Figure 1E).

2.7. New Imaging Markers

Apart from conventional clinical and imaging parameters, the value of the following new imaging markers to predict AV surgery was tested: 2D GLS, 2D myocardial work, 3D GLS, 3D VCA, MRI-derived native T1 relaxation time and ECV, MRI-derived GLS and circumferential strain, and MRI-derived RV and RF.

2.8. Statistical Analysis

Data are expressed as mean ± SD for continuous variables and as counts or percentages for categorical variables. Unpaired Student t-test, Pearson χ^2 or Fisher exact tests were used as appropriate. Receiver-operating characteristic curve analysis was used to identify imaging markers to predict future AV surgery. The optimal cutoff value for sensitivity and specificity was calculated according to the Youden's index and according to the clinical relevance. Several Cox proportional hazard models were used to identify independent predictors of aortic valve surgery (AVR). The selection of variables for the models was based on clinical relevance. Care was taken to avoid overfitting and to avoid combining mutually dependent variables in one analysis. Results were reported as hazard ratios (HRs) with the 95% of confidence interval (95% CI) of probability values. The Kaplan–Meier method and log-rank test was used for temporal analysis of differences in AV surgery between groups. For all tests, values of $p < 0.05$ were considered significant. Statistical analysis was performed using the SPSS version 20 (SPSS Inc, Chicago, IL, USA) and the GraphPad Prism version 6.0 (GraphPad Software, San Diego, CA, USA).

3. Results

3.1. Baseline Clinical and Imaging Characteristics

Tables 1 and 2 show baseline clinical and imaging characteristics, respectively. A two-dimensional ECHO study with satisfactory image quality was successfully completed in all patients. Feasibility of 3D ECHO was 99% for LV volumes, 89% for 3D GLS, and 100% for VCA. Three patients (3%) failed to complete the cardiac MRI because of claustrophobia ($n = 2$) or severe spine deformity ($n = 1$). Feasibility of MRI-derived T1 mapping and LV strain was 96% and 95%, respectively. Blood pressure and heart rate was similar during ECHO and MRI examination. The majority of patients were middle-aged males (86%) with bicuspid AV (76%). The most prevalent risk factor for coronary artery disease was hypertension (47%) with corresponding medication. Per study inclusion criteria, all patients were asymptomatic, in sinus rhythm, with normal LV dimensions, and LVEF. A total of 56 (54%) individuals had moderate-to-severe AR while the remaining 48 (46%) showed severe AR. During median follow-up of 587 days (interquartile range (IQR) 296–901 days), no patient died. A total of 20 (19%) individuals underwent AV surgery (surgical group) while the remaining patients were treated conservatively (conservative group). Median time to AV surgery was 236 days (IQR 125–460 days). Clinical characteristics, BNP, and creatinine values were similar between groups (Table 1).

Table 1. Baseline clinical characteristics.

	Total ($n = 104$)	Conservative ($n = 84$)	Surgical ($n = 20$)	p-Value
Age, years	44 ± 13	44 ± 13	45 ± 14	0.922
Male gender, N (%)	89 (86)	72 (86)	17 (85)	0.292
Hypertension, N (%)	50 (48)	40 (48)	10 (50)	0.801
Diabetes mellitus, N (%)	6 (6)	5 (6)	1 (5)	1.000
Hyperlipidemia, N (%)	29 (28)	24 (29)	5 (25)	0.773
Smoker, N (%)	14 (13)	11 (13)	3 (15)	1.000
Coronary artery disease, N (%)	4 (4)	3 (4)	1 (5)	0.542
Previous cardiac surgery, N (%)	4 (4)	3 (4)	1 (5)	1.000
Stroke, N (%)	1 (1)	0 (0)	1 (5)	0.175
Aspirin, N (%)	10 (10)	7 (8)	3 (15)	0.686
Oral anticoagulants, N (%)	5 (5)	3 (4)	2 (10)	0.542
ACEI/ARBs, N (%)	54 (52)	44 (52)	10 (50)	0.607
Beta-blockers, N (%)	25 (24)	21 (25)	4 (20)	0.231
Calcium channel blockers, N (%)	20 (19)	16 (19)	4 (20)	0.759
Diuretics, N (%)	15 (14)	9 (11)	6 (30)	0.261
Statins, N (%)	22 (21)	18 (21)	4 (20)	1.000
NYHA Class I, N (%)	104 (100)	84 (100)	20 (100)	1.000
Height, cm	180 ± 9	180 ± 9	181 ± 8	0.752
Weight, kg	85 ± 14	84 ± 14	86 ± 14	0.744
Systolic blood pressure, mmHg	136 ± 16	135 ± 16	139 ± 18	0.334
Diastolic blood pressure, mmHg	70 ± 12	71 ± 12	68 ± 12	0.292
Heart rate, beats per min	64 ± 10	63 ± 10	64 ± 13	0.965
Sinus rhythm, N (%)	104 (100)	84 (100)	20 (100)	1.000
B-natriuretic peptide, ng/L	27 (42)	24 (36)	34 (117)	0.054
Creatinine Clearance mL/min	118 ± 31	120 ± 32	107 ± 28	0.110
Aortic valve morphology				0.551
Trileaflet, N (%)	14 (13.6)	11 (12.9)	3 (16.7)	
Bicuspid, N (%)	79 (76.7)	65 (76)	14 (70)	
Unicuspid/quadricuspid, N (%)	4 (4)	4 (5)	0 (0)	
Unknown, N (%)	6 (6)	4 (5)	2 (10)	

Values are means ± standard deviations, median (interquartile range) or numbers (percentage). ACEI/ARB, angiotensin converting enzyme inhibitor/angiotensin receptor blocker; NYHA, New York Heart Association.

Table 2. Baseline imaging characteristics.

	Total (n = 104)	Medical (n = 84)	Surgical (n = 20)	p-Value
LV assessment				
2D ECHO end-diastolic diameter, mm	58 ± 6	58 ± 6	61 ± 4	0.031
2D ECHO end-systolic diameter, mm	37 ± 5	37 ± 5	40 ± 4	0.006
2D ECHO end-systolic diameter index, mm/m^2	18 ± 3	18 ± 3	20 ± 3	0.019
2D ECHO end-diastolic volume, mL	158 ± 68.0	156 ± 58	194 ± 60	0.008
2D ECHO end-diastolic volume index, mL/m^2	77 ± 31	76 ± 26	89 ± 32	0.019
2D ECHO end-systolic volume, mL	56 ± 32	56 ± 29	70 ± 39	0.069
2D ECHO end-systolic volume index, mL/m^2	28 ± 15.0	26 ± 14	33 ± 18	0.072
2D ECHO ejection fraction, %	64 ± 6	64 ± 6	64 ± 6	0.695
3D ECHO end-diastolic volume, mL	177 ± 51	175 ± 46	196 ± 68	0.125
3D ECHO end-diastolic volume index, mL/m^2	86 ± 23	85 ± 21	94.9 ± 28	0.108
3D ECHO end-systolic volume, mL	69 ± 24	68 ± 21	78 ± 34	0.12
3D ECHO end-systolic volume index, mL/m^2	33 ± 11	33 ± 10	38 ± 15	0.095
3D ECHO ejection fraction, %	62 ± 5	62 ± 5	61 ± 6	0.678
MRI end-diastolic volume, mL	234 ± 81	223 ± 80	293 ± 76	<0.001
MRI end-diastolic volume index, mL/m^2	118 ± 30	114 ± 27	142 ± 34	<0.001
MRI end-systolic volume, mL	88 ± 51	86 ± 41	124 ± 68	0.005
MRI end-systolic volume index, mL/m^2	43 ± 23	41 ± 20	60 ± 28	0.003
MRI ejection fraction, %	61 ± 6	61 ± 6	60 ± 5	0.248
MRI native T1 relaxation time, ms	1023 ± 30	1023 ± 30	1022 ± 29	0.934
MRI extracellular volume fraction, %	24 ± 3	24 ± 3	24 ± 2	0.819
2D ECHO global longitudinal strain, %	−18 ± 2	−19 ± 2	−17 ± 3	0.07
2D ECHO TWIST	14 ± 4	13 ± 4	14 ± 4	0.496
3D ECHO global longitudinal strain, %	−15 ± 4	−15 ± 4	−15 ± 4	0.518
MRI global longitudinal strain, %	−15 ± 2	−15 ± 2	−14 ± 3	0.62
MRI global circumferential strain, %	−22 ± 3	−22 ± 3	−21 ± 2	0.54
MRI global radial strain, %	31 ± 7	31 ± 7	31 ± 6	0.55
AR assessment				
Integrative approach				0.02
Moderate-to-severe AR, N (%)	56 (54)	50 (60)	6 (30)	
Severe AR, N (%)	48 (46)	34 (40)	14 (70)	
2D ECHO vena contracta width, mm	6.5 ± 1.5	6.3 ± 1.5	6.9 ± 1.6	0.118
Diastolic flow reversal velocity, cm/s	19.4 ± 4.3	18.8 ± 4.0	22.8 ± 4.0	<0.001
2D ECHO regurgitant volume, mL	52 ± 48	52 ± 47	69 ± 63	0.041
2D ECHO regurgitant fraction, %	36 ± 18	34 ± 18	45 ± 17	0.017
3D ECHO vena contracta area, mm^2	29 ± 13	26 ± 11	38 ± 15	<0.001
MRI regurgitation volume, mL	50 ± 28	44 ± 25	73 ± 30	<0.001
MRI regurgitation fraction, %	38 ± 17	36 ± 17	49 ± 11	0.001

Values are means ± standard deviations or numbers (percentage). 2D, two-dimensional; 3D, three dimensional; AR, aortic regurgitation; ECHO, echocardiography; MRI, magnetic resonance imaging; TWIST, left ventricular torsion.

3.2. Assessment of LV Morphology and Function

At 2D ECHO, patients who underwent AV surgery had significantly larger LV dimensions, end-diastolic volume (LVEDV) (all $p < 05$) and tended to have larger end-systolic volume (LVESV) than patients treated conservatively (Table 2). MRI-derived LV volumes showed a similar trend with significantly larger volumes in the surgical versus the conservative group (all $p < 0.01$). In contrast, LVEF derived by using whatever method was similar. Imaging markers of subtle myocardial damage (i.e., the MRI-derived T1 relaxation time or ECV, 2D-, 3D-, or MRI-derived LV strain), did not show statistically significant differences between groups, although 2D GLS tended to be lower in the surgical versus the conservative group ($p = 0.07$). Average myocardial fibrosis on perioperative myocardial biopsy ($n = 14$) was 15 ± 20%. The degree of myocardial fibrosis correlated significantly with MRI-derived LV mass (r = 0.66), native T1 relaxation time (r = 0.56), ECV (r = 0.31), and 2D ECHO-derived GLS (0.46).

3.3. Assessment of AR Severity

Using the integrative approach, the surgical group showed a significantly higher prevalence of severe AR than the conservative group (70% vs. 40%, $p = 0.02$). Accordingly, we observed significantly larger velocity of the diastolic flow reversal in the descending aorta, 2D ECHO RV and RF of AR, and 3D ECHO VCA in patients treated surgically versus conservatively (all $p < 0.05$) (Table 2). In contrast, 2D vena contracta width was similar between groups. MRI-derived RV and RF were significantly larger in patients undergoing surgery than in patients treated conservatively (both $p < 0.01$).

3.4. Prediction of AV Surgery

Table 3 and Figure 2 show accuracy of selected imaging markers to identify patients who underwent AV surgery. The integrative 2D ECHO approach had high negative predictive value (89%), but low positive predictive value (29%) to identify future AV surgery. All the ECHO- and MRI-derived indices of LV remodeling and function had an area under the curve (AUC) <0.7. Out of the ECHO-derived parameters, end-systolic diameter (LVESD), with an optimal cutoff value of >37 mm, its index (LVESDi), with an optimal cutoff value of >18 mm/m^2, had the largest AUC. Higher cutoff values of LVESD (>45 mm) or LVESDi (>22 mm/m^2), approaching the guideline recommendations, were highly specific (>90%) but lacked the sensitivity (<20%). The MRI-derived volumes and their indexed values were also rather specific than sensitive. Out of the ECHO-derived indices of AR severity, the largest AUC was observed for velocity of diastolic flow reversal in aorta descendens and 3D VCA. The optimal cutoff value of 3D VCA ≥30 mm^2 had a sensitivity of 80% and a specificity of 63% to identify future AV surgery (Figure 3A). A total of 31 patients treated conservatively had VCA ≥30 mm^2 (false positive). Combining VCA with LVESD or LVESDi increased the specificity up to 97% depending on the cutoff (Table 3). Out of all tested imaging markers, the MRI-derived RV, with a cutoff value ≥45 mL (Figure 3B), and the MRI-derived RF, with a cutoff value ≥34% (Figure 3C), showed the largest AUC (>0.75) with very high sensitivity (≥90%). A total of 33 out of 36 patients in the conservative group had RV ≥45 mL and RF ≥34%, respectively (false positive). Combining RV and RF with LV end-diastolic or end-systolic volume index increased the specificity up to 78% and 89%, respectively (Table 3). In Cox regression analysis, 3D VCA, MRI-derived RV and RF were identified as strongest independent predictors of AV surgery (Table 4). In contrast, LV strain, T1 time or ECV were not independent predictors.

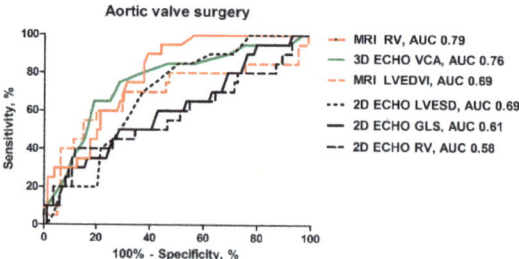

Figure 2. Receiver-operating characteristics curves of the MRI-derived: regurgitant volume (RV) and left ventricular end-diastolic volume index (LVEDVI); the 3D ECHO-derived: vena contracta area (VCA); 2D ECHO-derived: left ventricular end-systolic diameter (LVESD); RV and global longitudinal strain (GLS) to predict AV surgery.

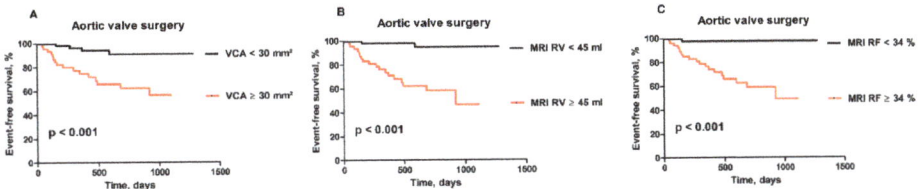

Figure 3. (**A**) Kaplan–Meier curves for aortic valve surgery (AVR) in patients with 3D ECHO-derived VCA ≥30 mm^2 vs. <30 mm^2, (**B**) MRI-derived RV ≥45 mL vs. <45 mL; and (**C**) MRI-derived RF ≥34% vs. <34%.

Table 3. Predictive accuracy of selected imaging markers to identify patients undergoing AV surgery.

	AUC (95% CI)	Cutoff Value	Sensitivity (%)	Specificity (%)
Markers of LV remodeling				
2D ECHO LVESD, mm	0.69 (0.57–0.80)	37	85	56
		40	55	69
		45	15	94
2D ECHO LVESDi, mm/m^2	0.66 (0.54–0.78)	18	80	53
		20	30	75
		22	15	90
MRI LVEDV, mL	0.68 (0.53–0.83)	281	50	84
MRI LVEDVi, mL/m^2	0.69 (0.54–0.84)	110	80	53
		124	70	70
		139	55	85
MRI LVESV, mL	0.64 (0.48–0.80)	121	50	84
MRI LVESVi, mL/m^2	0.65 (0.49–0.81)	42	70	53
		56	60	77
		58	50	81
2D ECHO GLS, %	0.61 (0.47–0.70)	−17.5	50	71
Markers of AR severity				
Diastolic flow reversal velocity, cm/s	0.72 (0.59–0.85)	22	65	78
2D ECHO RV, mL	0.58 (0.43–0.74)	93	40	88
2D ECHO RF, %	0.61 (0.47–0.76)	47	50	73
3D VCA (mm^2)	0.76 (0.64–0.88)	29	80	63
		31	75	71
		36	65	81
MRI RV, mL	0.79 (0.70–0.88)	41	95	56
		45	90	61
MRI RF, %	0.77 (0.68–0.86)	34	95	55
Integrative approach				
2D ECHO integrative approach	0.65 (0.52–0.78)	Severe AR	70	60
3D ECHO VCA ≥30 mm^2 and 2D ECHO LVESD or LVESDi	NA	LVESD >40 mm	80	71
		LVESD >45 mm	80	97
		LVESDi >20 mm/m^2	80	77
		LVESDi >22 mm/m^2	80	87
MRI regurgitant volume ≥45 mL and MRI LVEDVi or LVESVi	NA	LVEDVi >139 mL/m^2	90	78
		LVESVI >62 mL/m^2	90	78
MRI regurgitant fraction ≥34% and MRI LVEDVi or LVESVi	NA	LVEDVi >139 mL/m^2	95	89
		LVESVi >62 mL/m^2	95	89

2D, two-dimensional; 3D, three dimensional, AUC, area under curve; ECHO, echocardiography; GLS, global longitudinal strain; LV, left ventricle; LVEDV, left ventricular end-diastolic volume; LVEDVi, left ventricular end-diastolic volume index; LVESD, left ventricular end-systolic diameter; LVESDi, left ventricular end-systolic diameter index; LVESV, left ventricular end-systolic volume; LVESVi, left ventricular end-systolic volume index; MRI, magnetic resonance imaging; RF, regurgitant fraction; RV, regurgitant volume; VCA, vena contracta area.

Table 4. Independent predictors of aortic valve surgery.

	Univariable Analysis		Multivariable Analysis	
	HR (95% CI)	p-Value	HR (95% CI)	p-Value
2D ECHO LVEDD	1.08 (0.99–1.18)	0.084		
2D ECHO LVESD	1.12 (1.02–1.23)	0.014	1.12 (1.02–1.23)	0.018 *
2D ECHO LVESDi	1.18 (1.02–1.37)	0.031	1.18 (1.01–1.38)	0.042 *
MRI LVEDV	1.01 (1.00–1.02)	0.004	1.01 (1.00–1.01)	0.036 †
MRI LVEDVi	1.02 (1.00–1.03)	0.004	1.01 (1.00–1.03)	0.033 †
MRI LVESV	1.02 (1.00–1.03)	0.017		
MRI LVESVi	1.03 (1.01–1.06)	0.014		
2D ECHO RV	1.01 (1.00–1.02)	0.011	1.01 (1.00–1.02)	0.035 ‡
2D ECHO RF	1.03 (1.01–1.06)	0.018	1.03 (1.00–1.06)	0.020 ‡
3D VCA	1.07 (1.04–1.10)	<0.001	1.06 (1.03–1.10)	<0.001 ‡
MRI RV	1.03 (1.02–1.05)	<0.001	1.03 (1.01–1.04)	<0.001 §
MRI RF	1.05 (1.03–1.08)	<0.001	1.05 (1.02–1.08)	<0.001 §

CI, confidence interval; HR, hazard ratio; for other abbreviations see previous tables. * LVESD and LVESDi remained significant predictors of aortic valve (AV) surgery after adjustment for ECHO RV and ECHO RF but they lost predictive significance in combination with 3D VCA. † MRI LVEDV and LVEDVi showed borderline significance to predict AV surgery after adjustment with MRI RF but they lost predictive significance in combination with MRI RV. ‡ 2D ECHO RV, 2D ECHO RF and 3D VCA consistently retained their independent predictive value after adjustment for ECHO-derived LV diameters or their indices, 3D VCA was the strongest predictor. § MRI RV and RF were strong independent predictors after adjustment for MRI-derived LV volumes or their indices.

4. Discussion

The present study included asymptomatic patients with normal LVEF and non-dilated LV. Compared with the previous reports in asymptomatic AR patients, individuals included in the present study were younger, had less dilated LV, lower BNP, higher magnitude of GLS, and experienced less endpoints during follow-up [6,8,13,15,19,25]. This suggests the very early stage of AR disease. The findings of the present study can be summarized as follows: (1) AR severity seemed to be the major determinant of early disease progression while indices of LV morphology and function showed lower predictive accuracy; (2) new imaging markers of AR severity (i.e., 3D VCA, MRI-derived RV and RF), showed higher sensitivity than those derived using 2D Doppler ECHO; (3) integrating a sensitive with a specific parameter, for instance ECHO-derived VCA with LVESDi, or MRI-derived RV or RF with LVEDVi or LVESVi showed higher discriminative power than 2D ECHO integrative approach to identify patients undergoing early AV surgery.

4.1. LV Morphology and Function

Chronic AR leads to LV volume and pressure overload with subsequent hypertrophy, dilatation, systolic dysfunction, and heart failure. LV dimensions (LVESD >50 mm or LVESDi >25 mm/m^2), and LVEF (LVEF <50%) are currently used as indications for AV intervention [1]. Several recent studies demonstrated low sensitivity of these cutoffs by showing improved outcome in patients who had been operated on before the onset of these triggers [6,8]. In the present study, the optimal cutoff of LVEDSi (>18 mm/m^2), with acceptable sensitivity (80%), was lower than previously proposed [1,6,8]. Using higher cutoff of 20 or 22 mm/m^2 increased specificity (75%–93%) at the expense of unacceptably low sensitivity (15%–30%). MRI-derived volumes were rather specific but had lower sensitivity. It is of note, that a considerable proportion of patients (38%) showed increased LV volumes at MRI despite normal 2D ECHO dimensions. Nevertheless, the predictive accuracy of LV dimensions or volumes, derived by either technique, were moderate with an area under the curve <0.7 in all cases. Several new markers describing subtle myocardial damage or dysfunction have emerged recently [13–20]. MRI-derived native T1 mapping and ECV are accurate and validated markers of diffuse myocardial fibrosis [14,23,26]. ECHO-derived GLS has been introduced as a sensitive marker of early systolic dysfunction and potentially of clinical outcome in different valvular diseases [1,21]. Several studies reported independent association between speckle-tracking-derived GLS and the need for AV surgery [13,15,17]. In the present study, only 2D GLS tended to be lower in the surgical versus the conservative group while 3D GLS or MRI-derived strains, T1 relaxation time, and ECV were similar. The explanation of different findings can be that previous studies included more advanced disease as documented by a higher prevalence of endpoints, older age, more dilated LV or lower magnitude of GLS compared with our data [13,15]. Of interest, in the surgical group, we observed increased myocardial fibrosis (median 15%) at perioperative biopsy. These values are clearly elevated as a normal range between 1%–4.5% [27,28]. Both T1 relaxation time, ECV, and GLS showed significant correlation with the extent of fibrosis in histological samples. Moreover, T1 relaxation time was significantly longer (1022 ± 30 ms vs. 980 ± 22 ms, $p < 0.01$) and 2D GLS significantly lower (−18 ± 2% vs. −22.5 ± 2%, $p < 0.01$) compared with 30 healthy controls. Yet, these parameters failed to identify patients with early disease progression. This suggests that at the early stage of AR disease, the parameters reflecting subtle myocardial damage may not be accurate enough to predict early disease progression.

4.2. Assessment of AR Severity

The majority of recommended indices to assess AR are semiquantitative, lack the sensitivity or their accuracy is hampered by jet eccentricity [7,9,10]. Accordingly, in the present study with high prevalence bicuspid AV and eccentric jets, the consistent measurement of PISA-derived effective regurgitant orifice (ERO) and RV was not possible. It might have been for the same reasons that 2D vena contracta width did not show significant differences between groups. In contrast, 3D data can be rotated perpendicular to the jet direction in several planes to avoid the limitation introduced by jet eccentricity. The vena contracta area is a 3D-derived area of the vena contracta without any geometric assumption. VCA has been shown to be highly accurate, reproducible, and superior to the PISA method in different native valve regurgitations [20,29–31]. In the present study, 3D VCA had the highest accuracy out of all ECHO markers of AR severity to identify patients in need for early AV surgery. A combination of sensitive VCA with specific LVEDSi showed the optimal discriminative power. MRI-derived assessment of blood flow at the level of the aortic root is a highly reproducible and quantitative technique, which allows for direct assessment of RV of AR [16,19]. In the present study, MRI-derived RV and RF showed the largest accuracy out of all the imaging parameters to predict AV surgery. Our cutoff values of RV (≥45 mL) and RF (≥34%) were similar to values (RV >42 mL, RF >33%) published previously in more advanced AR disease [19]. In our study, both RV and RF were highly sensitive but less specific. In contrast, Myerson observed balanced high sensitivity (92%–85%) and specificity (85%–92%) for both indices [19]. This difference in specificity may be related to the very early stage of AR disease in our study while Myerson included older patients with more a dilated LV [19]. In the present study, combining sensitive RV or RF with specific LV volumes or their indices increased the specificity to identify future AV surgery. Of note, 2D ECHO integrative approach showed lower predictive accuracy. This suggests that, in asymptomatic patients with severe AR, both 3D ECHO-derived VCA and MRI-derived RV and RF may be clinically useful to increase sensitivity and accuracy of the recommended approach.

5. Conclusions

The present study assessed the clinical value of new imaging markers in asymptomatic patients with chronic severe AR at the early stage of the disease. Parameters related to LV morphology and function showed moderate accuracy to identify patients in need for early AV surgery. This suggests their limited accuracy at the early stage of AR disease while they may become useful later in the disease course with ongoing LV remodeling. In contrast, 3D ECHO-derived VCA and MRI-derived RV and RF showed the highest accuracy and excellent sensitivity to identify patients in need for early AV surgery. This suggests their clinical potential since the recommended integrative approach is rather specific than sensitive.

Author Contributions: Conceptualization, R.K. and M.P.; investigation, L.S., M.B., J.M., and E.H.; project administration, A.P. (Andrea Polednová); validation, H.L., Z.H. and A.P. (Alena Pravečková); writing—review and editing, D.S.

Funding: This study was supported by the Ministry of Health of the Czech Republic 17-28265A. No potential conflict of interest was reported by the authors.

Acknowledgments: We are grateful to Marek Maly at the National Institute of Public Health, Prague, Czech Republic, for his invaluable statistical analysis.

Conflicts of Interest: The authors declare no conflicts of interest.

References

1. Baumgartner, H.; Falk, V.; Bax, J.J.; Bonis, M.; Hamm, C.; Holm, P.J.; Iung, B.; Lancelloti, P.; Lansac, E.; Rodriguez Munoz, D.; et al. ESC Scientific Document Group. 2017 ESC/EACTS Guidelines for the management of valvular heart disease. *Eur. Heart J.* **2017**, *38*, 2739–2791. [CrossRef]
2. Nishimura, R.A.; Otto, C.M.; Bonow, R.O.; Carabello, B.A.; Erwin, J.P., 3rd; Fleisher, L.A.; Jneid, H.; Mack, M.J.; McLeod, C.J.; O'Gara, P.T.; et al. 2017 AHA/ACC Focused Update of the 2014 AHA/ACC Guideline for the Management of Patients with Valvular Heart Disease: A Report of the American College of Cardiology/American Heart Association Task Force on Clinical Practice Guidelines. *J. Am. Coll. Cardiol.* **2017**, *70*, 252–289. [CrossRef] [PubMed]
3. Iung, B.; Baron, G.; Butchart, E.G.; Delahaye, F.; Gohlke-Barwolf, C.; Levang, O.W.; Tornos, P.; Vanoverschelde, J.L.; Vermeer, F.; Boersma, E.; et al. A prospective survey of patients with valvular heart disease in Europe: The Euro Heart Survey on Valvular Heart Disease. *Eur. Heart J.* **2003**, *24*, 1231–1243. [CrossRef]
4. Nkomo, V.T.; Gardin, J.M.; Skelton, T.N.; Gottdiener, J.S.; Scott, C.G.; Enriquez-Sarano, M. Burden of valvular heart diseases: A population-based study. *Lancet* **2006**, *368*, 1005–1011. [CrossRef]
5. Klodas, E.; Enriquez-Sarano, M.; Tajik, A.J.; Mullany, C.J.; Bailey, K.R.; Seward, J.B. Surgery for aortic regurgitation in women. Contrasting indications and outcomes compared with men. *Circulation* **1996**, *94*, 2472–2478. [CrossRef] [PubMed]
6. de Meester, C.; Gerber, B.L.; Vancraeynest, D.; Pouleur, A.C.; Noirhomme, P.; Pasquet, A.; Gerber, B.L.; Vanoverschelde, J.L. Do Guideline-Based Indications Result in an Outcome Penalty for Patients with Severe Aortic Regurgitation? *JACC Cardiovasc. Imaging* **2019**, *12*, 2880. [CrossRef] [PubMed]
7. Lancellotti, P.; Tribouilloy, C.; Hagendorff, A.; Popescu, B.A.; Edvardsen, T.; Pierard, L.A.; Badano, L.; Zamorano, J.L.; Scientific Document Committee of the European Association of Cardiovascular Imaging. Recommendations for the echocardiographic assessment of native valvular regurgitation: an executive summary from the European Association of Cardiovascular Imaging. *Eur. Heart J. Cardiovasc. Imaging* **2013**, *14*, 611–644. [CrossRef] [PubMed]
8. Mentias, A.; Feng, K.; Alashi, A.; Rodriguez, L.L.; Gillinov, A.M.; Johnston, D.R.; Sabik, J.F.; Svensson, L.G.; Grimm, R.A.; Griffin, B.P.; et al. Long-Term Outcomes in Patients with Aortic Regurgitation and Preserved Left Ventricular Ejection Fraction. *J. Am. Coll. Cardiol.* **2016**, *68*, 2144–2153. [CrossRef] [PubMed]
9. Messika-Zeitoun, D.; Detaint, D.; Leye, M.; Tribouilloy, C.; Michelena, H.I.; Pislaru, S.; Brochet, E.; Iung, B.; Vahanian, A.; Enriquez-Sarano, M. Comparison of semiquantitative and quantitative assessment of severity of aortic regurgitation: clinical implications. *J. Am. Soc. Echocardiogr.* **2011**, *24*, 1246–1252. [CrossRef] [PubMed]
10. Zoghbi, W.A.; Adams, D.; Bonow, R.O.; Enriquez-Sarano, M.; Foster, E.; Grayburn, P.A.; Hahn, R.T.; Han, Y.; Hung, J.; Lang, R.M.; et al. Recommendations for Noninvasive Evaluation of Native Valvular Regurgitation: A Report from the American Society of Echocardiography Developed in Collaboration with the Society for Cardiovascular Magnetic Resonance. *J. Am. Soc. Echocardiog.* **2017**, *30*, 303–371. [CrossRef]
11. Krayenbuehl, H.P.; Hess, O.M.; Monrad, E.S.; Schneider, J.; Mall, G.; Turina, M. Left ventricular myocardial structure in aortic valve disease before, intermediate, and late after aortic valve replacement. *Circulation* **1989**, *79*, 744–755. [CrossRef] [PubMed]
12. Pizarro, R.; Bazzino, O.O.; Oberti, P.F.; Falconi, M.L.; Arias, A.M.; Krauss, J.G.; Cagide, A.M. Prospective validation of the prognostic usefulness of B-type natriuretic peptide in asymptomatic patients with chronic severe aortic regurgitation. *J. Am. Coll. Cardiol.* **2011**, *58*, 1705–1714. [CrossRef] [PubMed]

13. Ewe, S.H.; Haeck, M.L.; Ng, A.C.; Witkowski, T.G.; Auger, D.; Leong, D.P.; Abate, E.; Ajmone Marsan, N.; Holman, E.R.; Schalij, M.J.; et al. Detection of subtle left ventricular systolic dysfunction in patients with significant aortic regurgitation and preserved left ventricular ejection fraction: speckle tracking echocardiographic analysis. *Eur. Heart J. Cardiovasc. Imaging* **2015**, *16*, 992–999. [CrossRef] [PubMed]
14. Kockova, R.; Kacer, P.; Pirk, J.; Maly, J.; Sukupova, L.; Sikula, V.; Kotrc, M.; Barciakova, L.; Honsova, E.; Maly, M.; et al. Native T1 Relaxation Time and Extracellular Volume Fraction as Accurate Markers of Diffuse Myocardial Fibrosis in Heart Valve Disease- Comparison with Targeted Left Ventricular Myocardial Biopsy. *Circ. J.* **2016**, *80*, 1202–1209. [CrossRef] [PubMed]
15. Kusunose, K.; Agarwal, S.; Marwick, T.H.; Griffin, B.P.; Popovic, Z.B. Decision making in asymptomatic aortic regurgitation in the era of guidelines: incremental values of resting and exercise cardiac dysfunction. *Circ. Cardiovasc. Imaging* **2014**, *7*, 352–362. [CrossRef] [PubMed]
16. Lee, J.C.; Branch, K.R.; Hamilton-Craig, C.; Krieger, E.V. Evaluation of aortic regurgitation with cardiac magnetic resonance imaging: A systematic review. *Heart* **2018**, *104*, 103–110. [CrossRef]
17. Lee, J.K.T.; Franzone, A.; Lanz, J.; Siontis, G.C.M.; Stortecky, S.; Gräni, C.; Roost, E.; Windecker, S.; Pilgrim, T. Early Detection of Subclinical Myocardial Damage in Chronic Aortic Regurgitation and Strategies for Timely Treatment of Asymptomatic Patients. *Circulation* **2018**, *137*, 184–196. [CrossRef]
18. Manganaro, R.; Marchetta, S.; Dulgheru, R.; Ilardi, F.; Sugimoto, T.; Robinet, S.; Cimino, S.; Go, Y.Y.; Bernard, A.; Kacharava, G.; et al. Echocardiographic reference ranges for normal non-invasive myocardial work indices: Results from the EACVI NORRE study. *Eur. Heart J. Cardiovasc. Imaging* **2019**, *20*, 582–590. [CrossRef]
19. Myerson, S.G.; d'Arcy, J.; Mohiaddin, R.; Greenwood, J.P.; Karamitsos, T.D.; Francis, J.M.; Banning, A.P.; Christiansen, J.P.; Neubauer, S. Aortic regurgitation quantification using cardiovascular magnetic resonance: Association with clinical outcome. *Circulation* **2012**, *126*, 1452–1460. [CrossRef]
20. Vecera, J.; Bartunek, J.; Vanderheyden, M.; Kotrc, M.; Kockova, R.; Penicka, M. Three-dimensional echocardiography-derived vena contracta area at rest and its increase during exercise predicts clinical outcome in mild-moderate functional mitral regurgitation. *Circ. J.* **2014**, *78*, 2741–2749. [CrossRef]
21. Lang, R.M.; Badano, L.P.; Mor-Avi, V.; Afilalo, J.; Armstrong, A.; Emande, L.; Flachskampf, F.A.; Foster, E.; Goldstein, S.A.; Kuznetsova, T.; et al. Recommendations for cardiac chamber quantification by echocardiography in adults: An update from the American Society of Echocardiography and the European Association of Cardiovascular Imaging. *J. Am. Soc. Echocardiogr.* **2015**, *28*, 1–39. [CrossRef] [PubMed]
22. Russell, K.; Eriksen, M.; Aaberge, L.; Wilhelmsen, N.; Skulstad, H.; Remme, E.W.; Haugaa, K.H.; Opdahl, A.; Fjeld, J.G.; Gjesdal, O.; et al. A novel clinical method for quantification of regional left ventricular pressure-strain loop area: A non-invasive index of myocardial work. *Eur. Heart J.* **2012**, *33*, 724–733. [CrossRef] [PubMed]
23. Messroghli, D.R.; Radjenovic, A.; Kozerke, S.; Higgins, D.M.; Sivananthan, M.U.; Ridgway, J.P. Modified Look-Locker inversion recovery (MOLLI) for high-resolution T1 mapping of the heart. *Magn. Reson. Med.* **2004**, *52*, 141–146. [CrossRef] [PubMed]
24. Chatzimavroudis, G.P.; Walker, P.G.; Oshinski, J.N.; Franch, R.H.; Pettigrew, R.I.; Yoganathan, A.P. Slice location dependence of aortic regurgitation measurements with MR phase velocity mapping. *Magn. Reson. Med.* **1997**, *37*, 545–551. [CrossRef] [PubMed]
25. Detaint, D.; Messika-Zeitoun, D.; Maalouf, J.; Tribouilloy, C.; Mahoney, D.W.; Tajik, A.J.; Enriquez-Sarano, M. Quantitative echocardiographic determinants of clinical outcome in asymptomatic patients with aortic regurgitation: A prospective study. *JACC Cardiovasc. Imaging* **2008**, *1*, 1–11. [CrossRef] [PubMed]
26. Messroghli, D.R.; Moon, J.C.; Ferreira, V.M.; Frosse-Wortmann, L.; He, T.; Kellman, P.; Mascherbauer, J.; Nezafat, R.; Salerno, M.; Schelbert, E.B.; et al. Clinical recommendations for cardiovascular magnetic resonance mapping of T1, T2, T2* and extracellular volume: A consensus statement by the Society for Cardiovascular Magnetic Resonance (SCMR) endorsed by the European Association for Cardiovascular Imaging (EACVI). *J. Cardiovasc. Magn. Reson.* **2017**, *19*, 75. [CrossRef] [PubMed]
27. Meckel, C.R.; Wilson, J.E.; Sears, T.D.; Rogers, J.G.; Goaley, T.J.; McManus, B.M. Myocardial fibrosis in endomyocardial biopsy specimens: Do different bioptomes affect estimation? *Am. J. Cardiovasc. Pathol.* **1989**, *2*, 309–313. [PubMed]

28. Tanaka, M.; Fujiwara, H.; Onodera, T.; Wu, D.J.; Hamashima, Y.; Kawai, C. Quantitative analysis of myocardial fibrosis in normals, hypertensive hearts, and hypertrophic cardiomyopathy. *Br. Heart J.* **1986**, *55*, 575–581. [CrossRef]
29. Abudiab, M.M.; Chao, C.J.; Liu, S.; Naqvi, T.Z. Quantitation of valve regurgitation severity by three-dimensional vena contracta area is superior to flow convergence method of quantitation on transesophageal echocardiography. *Echocardiography* **2017**, *34*, 992–1001. [CrossRef]
30. Sato, H.; Ohta, T.; Hiroe, K.; Okada, S.; Shimizu, K.; Murakami, R.; Tanabe, K. Severity of aortic regurgitation assessed by area of vena contracta: A clinical two-dimensional and three-dimensional color Doppler imaging study. *Cardiovasc. Ultrasound.* **2015**, *5*, 13–24. [CrossRef]
31. Zeng, X.; Levine, R.A.; Hua, L.; Morris, E.L.; Kang, Y.; Flaherty, M.; Morgan, N.V.; Hung, J. Diagnostic value of vena contracta area in the quantification of mitral regurgitation severity by color Doppler 3D echocardiography. *Circ. Cardiovasc. Imaging* **2011**, *4*, 506–513. [CrossRef] [PubMed]

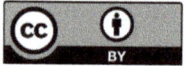

© 2019 by the authors. Licensee MDPI, Basel, Switzerland. This article is an open access article distributed under the terms and conditions of the Creative Commons Attribution (CC BY) license (http://creativecommons.org/licenses/by/4.0/).

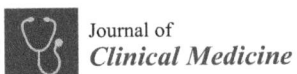

Article

Tissue-Specific miRNAs Regulate the Development of Thoracic Aortic Aneurysm: The Emerging Role of KLF4 Network

Stasė Gasiulė [1,†], Vaidotas Stankevičius [1,*,†], Vaiva Patamsytė [2], Raimundas Ražanskas [1], Giedrius Žukovas [3], Žana Kapustina [4], Diana Žaliaduonytė [5], Rimantas Benetis [2], Vaiva Lesauskaitė [2] and Giedrius Vilkaitis [1,*]

1. Institute of Biotechnology, Vilnius University, LT-10257 Vilnius, Lithuania; stase.gasiule@bti.vu.lt (S.G.); raimundas.razanskas@bti.vu.lt (R.R.)
2. Institute of Cardiology, Lithuanian University of Health Sciences, LT-50103 Kaunas, Lithuania; vaiva.patamsyte@lsmuni.lt (V.P.); rimantas.benetis@kaunoklinikos.lt (R.B.); vaiva.lesauskaite@lsmuni.lt (V.L.)
3. Department of Cardiac, Thoracic and Vascular Surgery, Lithuanian University of Health Sciences, LT-50103 Kaunas, Lithuania; giedrews@yahoo.com
4. Thermo Fisher Scientific Baltics, LT-02241 Vilnius, Lithuania; zana.kapustina@thermofisher.com
5. Department of Cardiology, Lithuanian University of Health Sciences, LT-50161 Kaunas, Lithuania; diana.zaliaduonyte@kaunoklinikos.lt
* Correspondence: vaidotas.stankevicius@gmc.vu.lt (V.S.); giedrius@ibt.lt (G.V.)
† These authors contributed equally to this manuscript.

Received: 5 August 2019; Accepted: 27 September 2019; Published: 3 October 2019

Abstract: MicroRNAs (miRNAs) are critical regulators of the functional pathways involved in the pathogenesis of cardiovascular diseases. Understanding of the disease-associated alterations in tissue and plasma will elucidate the roles of miRNA in modulation of gene expression throughout development of sporadic non-syndromic ascending thoracic aortic aneurysm (TAA). This will allow one to propose relevant biomarkers for diagnosis or new therapeutic targets for the treatment. The high-throughput sequencing revealed 20 and 17 TAA-specific miRNAs in tissue and plasma samples, respectively. qRT-PCR analysis in extended cohort revealed sex-related differences in miR-10a-5p, miR-126-3p, miR-155-5p and miR-148a-3p expression, which were the most significantly dysregulated in TAA tissues of male patients. Unexpectedly, the set of aneurysm-related miRNAs in TAA plasma did not resemble the tissue signature suggesting more complex organism response to the disease. Three of TAA-specific plasma miRNAs were found to be restored to normal level after aortic surgery, further signifying their relationship to the pathology. The panel of two plasma miRNAs, miR-122-3p, and miR-483-3p, could serve as a potential biomarker set (AUC = 0.84) for the ascending TAA. The miRNA-target enrichment analysis exposed TGF-β signaling pathway as sturdily affected by abnormally expressed miRNAs in the TAA tissue. Nearly half of TAA-specific miRNAs potentially regulate a key component in TGF-β signaling: TGF-β receptors, SMADs and KLF4. Indeed, using immunohistochemistry analysis we detected increased KLF4 expression in 27% of TAA cells compared to 10% of non-TAA cells. In addition, qRT-PCR demonstrated a significant upregulation of ALK1 mRNA expression in TAA tissues. Overall, these observations indicate that the alterations in miRNA expression are sex-dependent and play an essential role in TAA via TGF-β signaling.

Keywords: aortic disease; aneurysm; miRNA; TGF-β pathway; KLF4; synthetic phenotype

1. Introduction

Thoracic aortic aneurysms (TAAs) are usually silent and therefore deadly if not detected and repaired on time [1]. Most of them are affecting the root or ascending aorta [2]. TAA is categorized as syndromic (Marfan, Loyes-Dietz, Ehlers-Danlos, etc.), familial non-syndromic and sporadic [3]. The incidence of TAA is permanently increasing and remains much higher in males than females [4]. Similar trends are observed in hospital admissions for TAA [5]. The aortic diseases are more common in males but the outcome is worse in female patients, although reasons for sex differences are unknown [6]. Therefore, further investigation of molecular mechanisms for these differences are required as well [7]. Vascular smooth muscle cells (VSMC) have been shown to possess a natural plasticity to switch between contractile and synthetic phenotypes in order to repair small vascular injuries [8]. For the last few decades, VSMC dedifferentiation has been recognized as one of the key processes involved in arterial maintenance and development of vascular diseases [9]. This led to the identification of various regulators of VSMC phenotype including a transcription activator myocardin (*MyoCD*) [10], transcription factor Krüppel-like factor 4 (*KLF4*) [11], and components of a transforming growth factor beta (*TGF-β*) signalling pathway [12]. During the formation of TAA, VSMCs are thought to lose their contractile ability and start secretion of various extracellular matrix proteins and their inhibitors, but the mechanism of this phenotypic shift remains unknown.

Recent studies have focused on the emerging epigenetic regulation of gene expression and the short non-coding microRNAs (miRNAs) involved in post-transcriptional regulation of a target messenger RNA (mRNA) [13]. MiRNAs have been implicated in the pathogenesis of various cardiovascular diseases [14] and show the potential to be utilised as biomarkers in diagnosis, prognosis, and selection of treatment [15]. Over the last decade a variety of miRNAs have been identified in the regulation of VSMC phenotype [16–18] some of which have been associated with the formation of TAA [19,20]. The majority of miRNAs association studies were done using PCR or microarray techniques [21] and only a fraction of miRNAs have been validated in plasma samples [22]. However, to date, the global high-throughput miRNA sequencing data of TAA tissue is still missing. Furthermore, most of miRNA-related mechanistic insights of TAA development are made using cell cultures or knock-out animal models which only mildly represents human disease and could further lead to misinterpretation of biological processes occurring in human tissue *in vivo* [23].

A multidimensional approach is needed in order to uncover the complex mechanisms occurring in the human aortic wall during the formation of TAA and to evaluate the possibility of using circulating miRNAs as biomarkers for the development of the disease. In the present study, we aimed to profile miRNA changes in TAA tissue and blood plasma samples and to assess their role in the pathogenesis of the disease as well as to evaluate their potential to be used as biomarkers. Using high-throughput miRNA sequencing we identified 20 and 17 differentially expressed miRNAs in TAA tissue and TAA plasma samples compared to non-TAA specimens, respectively. Deregulation of selected miRNAs in TAA samples were further confirmed by qRT-PCR analysis, thus verifying reliability of miRNA-Seq results. A subsequent pathway enrichment analysis of miRNA target genes revealed significant relationship between nearly half of dysregulated miRNAs and TGF-β signalling pathway. Finally, we for the first time showed accumulation of KLF4, a master regulator of VSMC differentiation state, in TAA tissue obtained from patients. Altogether our results define potential candidates for TAA diagnostic biomarkers and provide new insights in regulatory miRNA-related mechanisms of TAA development.

2. Materials and Methods

2.1. Patient Samples

All experimental procedures using human tissue and plasma samples conform to the principles outlined in the Declaration of Helsinki and were approved by Kaunas Regional Biomedical Research Ethics Committee (Nr. P2-BE-2-12/2012).

The study included 40 patients with sporadic non-syndromic ascending thoracic aorta aneurysm (TAA group). Exclusion criteria were severe atherosclerosis showing calcified or ulcerating plaques of the ascending aorta, aortitis, phenotypic characteristics of the known genetic disorders such as Marfan, Ehlers Danlos and other syndromes. The diagnosis was confirmed by two-dimensional thoracic aorta echocardiography according to the 2014 ESC guidelines on the diagnosis and treatment of aortic diseases. Echocardiography was performed at the Department of Cardiology, Lithuanian University of Health Sciences (LUHS). TAA group included patients ($n = 23$) who underwent aortic reconstruction surgery at the Department of Cardiac, Thoracic and Vascular Surgery, LUHS and non-operated patients ($n = 17$) with ascending aorta aneurysm.

Study subjects without TAA (non-TAA group) included i) heart transplantation donors ($n = 6$), ii) patients who underwent isolated coronary artery bypass graft surgery (CABG) ($n = 72$) and iii) healthy volunteers ($n = 10$). All healthy volunteers were screened using two-dimensional transthoracic echocardiography to ensure the ascending aorta was not dilated. Detailed preparation of patients' tissue and plasma samples can be found in the Supplementary Methods.

2.2. Study Design

Study subjects ($n = 32$) selected for miRNA expression profiling in aortic tissue consisted of surgical TAA patients ($n = 8$), donors ($n = 4$) as well as CABG patients ($n = 2$). miRNA expression profiling in plasma was done in samples from surgical TAA patients ($n = 7$) before and 3 months after the aortic surgery (denoted as operated, $n = 4$), respectively. Seven volunteers without health complaints (n= 7) were used as non-TAA controls. Clinical and demographic characteristics of the groups are summarized in Table 1.

Table 1. Demographic and clinical characteristics of control and thoracic aortic aneurysm (TAA) patients selected for profiling of microRNA (miRNA) expression.

Variables	Tissue		Plasma		
	non-TAA ($n = 6$)	TAA ($n = 8$)	non-TAA ($n = 7$)	TAA ($n = 7$)	Operated ($n = 4$)
Age, years ± SD	47 ± 5	62 ± 10	54 ± 12	63 ± 11	64 ± 12
Sex, male (%)	4 (67 %)	6 (75 %)	4 (57 %)	5 (71 %)	3 (75 %)
Ascending aortic diameter, mm	36 ± 0.7 *	50 ± 3	35 ± 3	53 ± 5	52 ± 4
Aortic valve stenosis (%)	0 (0 %)	3 (38 %)	1 (14 %)	2 (29 %)	1 (25 %)
Bicuspid aortic valve (%)	0 (0 %)	5 (63 %)	0 (0 %)	4 (57 %)	2 (50 %)
Aortic valve insufficiency (%)	0 (0 %)	5 (63 %)	1 (14 %)	3 (43 %)	1 (25 %)
Hypertension (%)	2 (100 %) *	7 (88 %)	4 (57 %)	6 (86 %)	4 (100 %)
Smokers (%)	2 (100 %) *	1 (13 %)	1 (14 %)	1 (14 %)	0 (0 %)
Diabetes (%)	0 (0 %)	1 (13 %)	0 (0%)	3 (43 %)	1 (25 %)

Notes: * Data is missing from four aorta donors. Operated denotes patient samples collected after aortic surgery.

Validation group for miRNA expression in aortic tissue consisted of TAA surgical patients ($n = 17$), donors and CABG patients ($n = 35$). For the miRNA validation in plasma samples, we were able to collect larger TAA group ($n = 28$) and non-TAA group ($n = 34$) which consisted of healthy volunteers and CABG patients. Clinical and demographic characteristics of each validation group are presented in Supplementary Table S1. A significant difference in ascending aortic diameter ($p < 0.001$) was observed between TAA patients and non-TAA in both miRNA profiling groups supporting the selection criteria. Patients with bicuspid aortic valve were predominant in both TAA groups ($p < 0.001$) compared with non-TAA group.

Total RNA isolation, cDNA library sequencing, and miRNA-Seq differential and functional analysis are described in detail in Supplementary Methods. miRNA-Seq data are available at GEO database using accession number GSE122266. Validation of miRNA-Seq data was performed as described previously [24] and detailed qRT-PCR and immunohistochemistry analysis are depicted in Supplementary Methods.

3. Results

3.1. Differential miRNA Expression Analysis in TAA Tissue and Blood Plasma Samples

In order to determine miRNAs which expression levels are potentially deregulated in aorta tissue and blood plasma during the formation of TAA, in the present study we evaluated miRNA expression profiles in a learning set of patient tissue and plasma samples ($n = 32$) using Illumina high-throughput miRNA sequencing platform (Table 1; Figure 1A). The overview of miRNA-Seq experimental design and data quality is depicted in Supplementary Results. miRNA-Seq data analysis revealed a total of 20 differentially expressed miRNAs (selection criteria were fold change ≥ 1.5, p value < 0.05 and base mean higher than 10) in TAA tissue samples compared to non-TAA group (Table 2), among which the majority (15 of 20 miRNAs) were upregulated (Table 3). A detailed differential miRNA-Seq data evaluation of each sample assessed in the present study is depicted in Supplementary File 1 and Supplementary File 2. A heat map of expression signature for these dysregulated miRNAs in all 14 samples clearly clustered aorta tissues according to the presence or absence of aneurysm (Figure 1B).

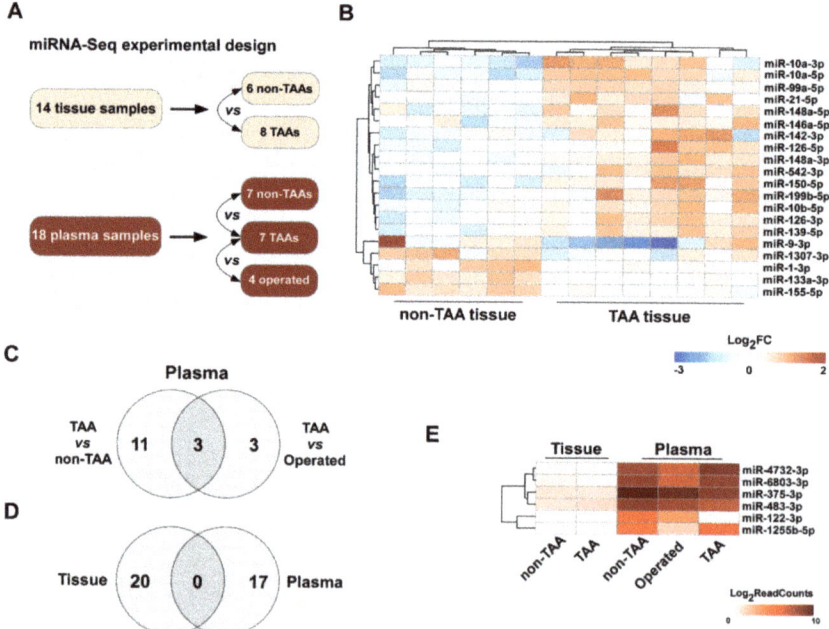

Figure 1. Differential miRNA expression analysis in TAA tissue and plasma samples using high-throughput RNA sequencing. (**A**) Schematic diagram of miRNA-Seq experiment. (**B**) Heat map showing a total of 20 miRNAs differentially expressed (fold change, FC > 1.5, p < 0.05, normalized read count average, RC > 10) in TAA tissue samples ($n = 8$) compared to normal aorta tissue ($n = 6$). Red color indicates upregulated log-transformed expression level ratios of corresponding miRNAs, blue – downregulated; (**C**) Venn's diagram showing the number of differentially expressed miRNAs (FC > 1.5, $p \leq 0.05$ and RC > 20) in TAA plasma samples ($n = 7$) compared to non-aneurysmal group ($n = 7$) and plasma samples obtained 3 months after aortic reconstructive surgery ($n = 4$); (**D**) Venn's diagram demonstrating the number of differentially expressed miRNAs in TAA tissue and plasma samples; (**E**) Heat map demonstrating the expression of six miRNAs, which were significantly deregulated in TAA plasma samples, but were almost absent in TAA tissue samples. Color intensity indicates log-transformed normalized read counts of corresponding miRNA.

Table 2. A number of miRNAs differentially expressed (fold change > 1.5) in TAA tissue and blood plasma samples compared to non-TAA controls.

Groups	Number of miRNAs	Upregulated	Downregulated
Tissue			
TAA vs. non-TAA	20	15	5
Plasma			
TAA vs. non-TAA	14	3	11
TAA v.s Op	6	4	2
TAA vs. non-TAA + Op	10	2	8

Notes: TAA—Thoracic Ascending Aneurysm; Op—Operated.

Table 3. List of differentially expressed miRNAs (selection criteria were fold change > 1.5, p value < 0.05 and base mean higher than 10) in TAA aortic tissue samples compared to miRNA expression levels in non-TAA controls.

No.	miRNAs	Fold Change	p Value
	Upregulated		
1	hsa-miR-10a-3p	2.69	2.05E−06
2	hsa-miR-10a-5p	2.45	8.63E−07
3	hsa-miR-150-5p	2.21	2.05E−05
4	hsa-miR-199b-5p	2.12	1.19E−04
5	hsa-miR-126-5p	1.89	7.95E−04
6	hsa-miR-126-3p	1,88	2.10E−05
7	hsa-miR-139-5p	1.74	7.22E−04
8	hsa-miR-148a-3p	1.71	3.44E−05
9	hsa-miR-10b-5p	1.70	7.78E−04
10	hsa-miR-148a-5p	1.70	0.0112
11	hsa-miR-99a-5p	1.68	1.76E−05
12	hsa-miR-21-5p	1.67	1.10E−03
13	hsa-miR-146a-5p	1.67	0.002
14	hsa-miR-142-3p	1.66	0.020
15	hsa-miR-542-3p	1.64	0.009
	Downregulated		
16	hsa-miR-1-3p	−1.59	0.001
17	hsa-miR-133a-3p	−1.64	2.96E−07
18	hsa-miR-1307-3p	−1.68	0.011
19	hsa-miR-9-3p	−1.79	0.021
20	hsa-miR-155-5p	−1.88	7.34E−08

Using the same workflow of miRNA-Seq analysis, we found 14 differentially expressed miRNAs in TAA patient plasma samples compared to non-TAA group. Out of these, 3 were upregulated and 11 were downregulated (Tables 2 and 4). Next, to determine alterations after the removal of aneurysm, we compared the miRNA expression levels between TAA plasma samples collected before and 3 months after aortic surgery. This analysis led to the detection of six differentially expressed miRNAs (Table 4; Supplementary Figure S1). Remarkably, the expression of three of TAA-specific plasma miRNAs, miR-1255b-5p, miR-122-3p and miR-23b-5p, returned to near non-TAA levels after the operation. Finally, to identify the most significantly dysregulated miRNAs in TAA plasma samples, we pooled data from both non-aneurysmal (non-TAA and TAA samples collected after the surgery) cohorts and compared to TAA group. The differential analysis determined ten differentially expressed miRNAs revealing the greatest fold change for miR-122-3p. Thus, the overall evaluation of miRNA expression changes in plasma samples discovered a total of 17 differentially expressed miRNAs in TAA samples compared to non-TAA samples, samples collected after aortic surgery or both groups of samples (Figure 1C).

Table 4. List of differentially expressed miRNAs (fold change > 1.5, p value ≤ 0.05-fold and base mean ≥ 20) in TAA patient blood plasma samples compared to miRNA expression levels in non-TAA controls.

Group	No.	miRNA	Regulation	Fold Change	p Value
TAA vs. non-TAA	1	hsa-miR-146b-3p	up	9.11	0.044
	2	hsa-miR-1255b-5p	up	8.87	0.015
	3	hsa-miR-889-3p	up	7.95	0.047
	4	hsa-miR-375-3p	down	−2.38	0.036
	5	hsa–miR-30a-5p	down	−2.54	0.033
	6	hsa-miR-483-3p	down	−2.68	0.015
	7	hsa-miR-23b-3p	down	−2.79	0.017
	8	hsa-miR-140-3p	down	−4.01	0.010
	9	hsa-miR-100-5p	down	−9.17	0.003
	10	hsa-miR-145-5p	down	−17.36	1.44E−04
	11	hsa-miR-143-3p	down	−17.74	3.27E−05
	12	hsa–miR-23b-5p	down	−24.93	0.013
	13	hsa-miR-122-3p	down	−69.32	3.31E−04
	14	hsa-miR-34a-5p	down	−71.95	4.01E−05
TAA vs. Operated	1	hsa-miR-1255b-5p	up	9.7203	0.045
	2	hsa-miR-4732-3p	up	3.9801	0.050
	3	hsa-miR-6803-3p	up	3.4495	0.011
	4	hsa-miR-22-3p	up	2.5198	0.029
	5	hsa-miR-122-3p	down	−18.4085	0.024
	6	hsa-miR-23b-5p	down	−44.7992	0.001
TAA vs. non-TAA & Operated	1	hsa-miR-1255b-5p	up	11.68	0.004
	2	hsa-miR-22-3p	up	1.73	0.034
	3	hsa-miR-375-3p	down	−2.12	0.049
	4	hsa-miR-483-3p	down	−2.29	0.035
	5	hsa-miR-23b-3p	down	−2.36	0.024
	6	hsa-miR-143-3p	down	−3.83	0.012
	7	hsa-miR-145-5p	down	−4.83	0.019
	8	hsa-miR-23b-5p	down	−29.67	0.003
	9	hsa-miR-34a-5p	down	−48.62	6.26E−05
	10	hsa-miR-122-3p	down	−53.67	2.31E−04

Surprisingly, a pattern of aneurysm-related alterations in plasma's miRNA profiles showed no resemblance to the tissue set. Indeed, none of the differentially expressed miRNAs overlapped in Venn's diagram (Figure 1D). Moreover, the expression levels of the six significantly deregulated miRNAs in TAA plasma samples, miR-4732-3p, miR-6803-3p, miR-375-3p, miR-483-3p, miR-122-3p and miR-1255b-5p, were negligible in aortic tissue samples (Figure 1E).

3.2. Validation of Selected miRNAs in TAA Tissue and Plasma Samples by qRT-PCR

In order to corroborate the RNA sequencing-based predictions, we performed qRT-PCR analysis to examine the abundance of five selected miRNAs (mir-10a-5p and miR-155-5p exhibited the greatest up/down fold changes; miR-126-3p, mir-133a-3p and miR-148a-3p were implicated in TGF-β signaling routes, see below) in the independent group of 37 samples containing 20 non-TAA and 17 thoracic aortic aneurysm tissues (Supplementary Table S1). Our analysis validated the up- and downregulated expression of miR-10a-5p, miR-126-3p, miR-133a-3p and miR-155-5p, respectively, in the sex-undivided set of TAA tissue samples compared to the non-TAA group (Figure 2A, Supplementary Figure S2). Whereas, the difference in miR-148a-3p expression levels was significant among the groups only when stratifying by sex ($p = 0.0203$ for a male patient set). Interestingly, a significantly greater differential expression of miR-126-3p ($p = 0.0062$ vs. $p = 0.0225$ for sex-undivided set), miR-155-5p ($p = 0.0003$ vs. $p = 0.0017$) and miR-10a-5p ($p = 0.0001$ vs. $p = 0.0002$), except miR-133a-3p ($p = 0.0068$ vs. $p = 0.0031$), also was observed between 13 TAA and 13 normal aorta tissue samples from male patients showing sex-related miRNA expression variances in the TAA tissue. Because of the scarce representation of female samples (7 non-TAA vs. 4 TAA) the extent of involvement of these miRNAs in the thoracic aneurysm formation in female patients requires further analysis.

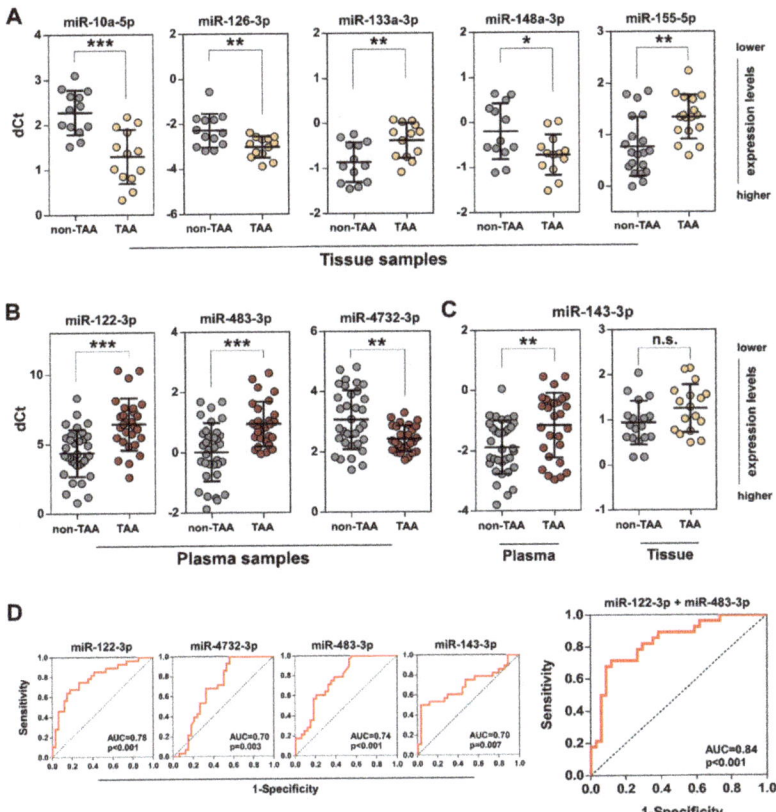

Figure 2. Validation of differentially expressed miRNAs in TAA tissue and plasma samples by qRT-PCR. qRT-PCR analysis was used for the comparison of relative miRNA expression levels between non-TAA and TAA groups in tissue (**A**) and plasma (**B**) both types (**C**) of samples. The cycle threshold (Ct) values of observed miRNAs were normalized to miR-152-3p and miR-185-5p for tissue and plasma samples, respectively, which were revealed as the most reliable endogenous controls according to miRNA-Seq data. Lines within boxes indicate relative miRNA expression median values; whiskers—5–95 percentile of the relative miRNA expression values. Significance between each group was evaluated using Student's t test and is shown as follows: n.s.—not significant; * $p < 0.05$; ** $p < 0.01$ and *** $p < 0.001$. (**D**) Diagnostic ROC curve analysis showing sensitivity and specificity of mir-122-3p, mir-483-3p, mir-4732-3p and mir-143-3p selected circulating miRNAs or the combination of mir-122-3p and mir-483-3p together. AUC denotes area under the ROC curve.

In contrast, the evaluation of the miRNA expression levels in 62 plasma samples (34 non-TAA vs. 28 TAA) demonstrated that all selected miRNAs, miR-4732-3p, miR-483-3p and miR-122-3p, exhibited statistically significant expression changes in TAA plasma samples compared to non-TAA group showing a good reliability of our miRNA-Seq data (Figure 2B). Of those, the difference of miR-122-3p expression levels was the most significant ($p < 0.0001$) between two plasma sample groups.

RNA-Seq analysis displayed that the difference of miR-143-3p expression was not statistically significant in TAA tissue samples compared to non-TAA. Consistently with this observation, a significant downregulation ($p = 0.0051$) was observed only in TAA plasma samples (Figure 2C) despite the decrement of miR-143-3p expression level in both TAA specimen groups compared to non-TAA group.

The diagnostic sensitivity and specificity of selected plasma circulating miRNAs which could serve as potential biomarkers of TAA was examined by ROC curve analysis (Figure 2D). The results demonstrated that miR-122-3p reached the most significant prognostic accuracy (AUC = 0.78, $p < 0.001$). Moreover, a combined analysis of miR-122-3p and miR-483-3p miRNAs showed even better diagnostic discrimination (AUC = 0.84, $p < 0.001$) indicating that these miRNAs could be applied as TAA biomarkers.

Finally, the statistical analysis showed no significant correlations between selected differential miRNAs, miR-10a-5p, miR-126-3p, mir-133a-3p miR-155-5p, miR-148a-3p, miR-122-3p, miR-483-3p, miR-4732-3p, miR-143-3p and chosen patient characteristics such as patients' age, aorta diameter, bicuspid (BAV)/tricuspid aortic valves (TAV)-associated aneurysms (data is not shown).

On the other hand, we revealed a significant moderate positive correlations between expression level of miR-126-3p and miR-148a-3p ($R = 0.67$) or miR-10a-5p ($R = 0.67$), miR-148a-3p and miR-10a-5p ($R = 0.49$), miR-133a-3p and miR-155-5p ($R = 0.67$) (Supplementary Table S2). Meanwhile, in plasma samples, the strongest correlation was observed between the expression of miR-122-3p and miR-483-3p ($R = 0.65$) (Supplementary Table S3).

3.3. Functional Analysis of miRNA Target Genes Involved in TAA Development

Next, we performed KEGG pathway enrichment analysis of dysregulated miRNA target genes to unravel the miRNA-mediated biological processes associated with TAA development. To provide the best set of relevant candidates for the bona fide miRNA-mRNA interactions, we evaluated combined scores from eight different miRNA target site prediction databases (see details in Methods). The examination identified 1133 target genes (exceeding combined score threshold value of 4) for group consisting of miRNAs which were differently expressed in TAA tissue (Supplementary File 3). The subsequent pathway enrichment analysis of the defined miRNA target sets revealed 48 KEGG categories significantly enriched in targeted genes (> 15 target genes in functional category, FDR < 0.05; Supplementary Table S4). In order to visualize the interconnection between signaling pathways regulated by miRNAs, we generated KEGG pathway network using Cytoscape plugin ClueGo. The network analysis clearly exposed three large functional clusters of KEGG categories closely related to immune response, cancer development and kinase signaling pathways, while any significant association of the remaining ten pathways to any other category was absent (Figure 3A, Supplementary Table S5). Transforming growth factor beta (*TGF-β*) signaling pathway, which plays a key role during aorta development and subsequent remodeling, was represented among these categories. To make a more detailed assessment of the miRNA-target interaction network, we additionally introduced target genes which were significantly related to differentially expressed miRNAs (target score > 4).

The expanded analysis revealed 17 target genes which could be potentially regulated by 9 out of 20 of miRNAs differentially expressed in TAA tissue (Figure 3B). Furthermore, our results defined two groups of genes sharing the similar functions which could be potentially affected by miRNAs - (i) *TGF-β* receptors and ligands and (ii) regulating *SMADs* (rSMADs) (Figure 3C, grey boxes). As shown above, the differential expression of two of them, miR-148a-3p and miR-155-5p, were additionally confirmed by qRT-PCR analysis. Moreover, miR-133a-3p, which was significantly downregulated in TAA tissue samples, has been previously described as a prominent indirect downregulator of Kruppel-like factor 4 (*KLF4*) [25]. According to these findings, we hypothesized that the miRNAs related to TAA could contribute significantly to critical changes in tissue remodeling in diseased aorta through of *TGF-β* signaling pathway: (i) leading to the functional dysregulation of the key regulators, *KLF4* and/or *MyoCD*, which determine the differentiation state of aorta smooth muscle cells (Figure 3C); (ii) the altered signaling balance between *TGF-β* receptors, ligands and rSMADs could provoke alternative *MyoCD*-independent *TGF-β* signaling routes which could boost TAA development.

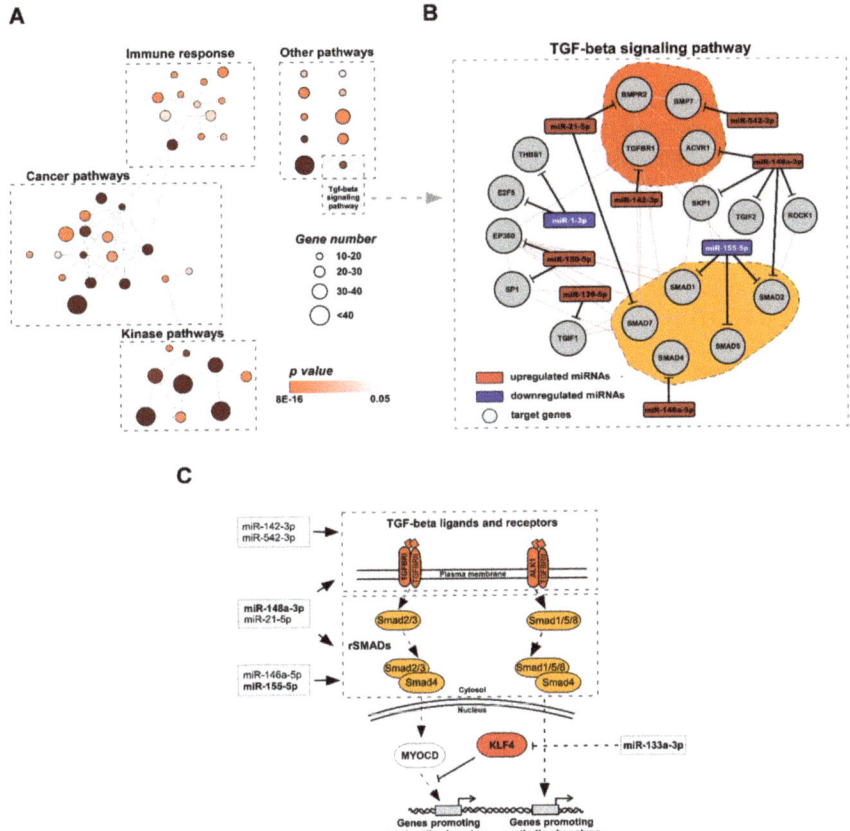

Figure 3. Functional analysis of target genes of miRNAs dysregulated in TAA. (**A**) Network analysis of 48 KEGG categories specified three clusters of closely related categories including immune response, cancer, kinase signaling pathways and ten separate groups that were not significantly associated with any other category. *TGF-β* signaling pathway is included in a grey box. The size of node represents gene number in particular, KEGG category, the node color – the significance level value of particular KEGG category. Edges indicate a statistically significant association between categories. (**B**) Expanded molecular network of miRNAs and their potential target genes involved in *TGF-β* signaling pathway. Grey nodes denote target genes, red and blue – upregulated and downregulated miRNAs, respectively. Dark orange area covers *TGF-β* ligands and receptors; light orange – regulatory *SMADs* (*rSMADs*). (**C**) Simplified hypothetical schema of *TGF-β* signal transduction in TAA tissue cells. miRNAs, which were differentially expressed in TAA tissue (grey boxes), could potentially disturb *TGF-β* signaling by targeting *TGF-β* ligands, receptors or rSMADs leading to dysregulation of *MyoCD–KLF4* transcription regulator axis and further TAA progression.

3.4. Number of VSMCs Expressing KLF4 Dramatically Increases during TAA Development

To further explore the compelling connection of the reprogramed miRNA network with *TGF-β* signaling pathway, we assessed the mRNA expression levels of *TGF-β* receptors, *TGFBR1* and *ALK1* (also known as *ACVRL1*), and transcription factors, *MyoCD* and *KLF4*, in non-TAA (n=21) and TAA ($n = 17$) tissue samples (Supplementary Figure S3A). We observed a relevant elevation of *ALK1* gene transcription in TAA tissues ($p = 0.0244$) compared to non-TAA group of normal aortas but found no significant difference in cellular mRNA levels of *TGFBR1*, *KLF4*, and *MyoCD*. It is noteworthy that we revealed a moderate positive correlation between the changes in expression of *ALK1*, miR-10a-5p, miR-126-3p and miR-148a-5p (Supplementary Table S6; Supplementary Figure S4) suggesting a putative biological relationship between these miRNAs and *TGF-β* signaling pathway. Thus, the obtained data pointed out to a weak regulation of studied genes, except *ALK1*, on transcription or mRNA decay level. However, it has been reported that many human miRNAs control post-transcriptional processes at the protein translation stage [26]. Therefore, we further evaluated the protein expression levels of the selected genes in non-TAA and TAA tissue samples using immunohistochemical analysis (IHC) (Figure 4; Supplementary Figure S3B). The IHC analysis revealed higher expression of *ALK1* both in normal and TAA tissues (IHC score median = 4), whereas the expression levels of *TGFBR1* remained lower in both aortic sample groups (IHC score median = 2). However, the difference of expression levels of both *TGF-β* receptors remained insignificant between TAA and non-TAA specimens (Supplementary Figure S3B). In contrast, although the overall expression levels of *KLF4* were low in both groups of aortic samples, we detected a significant three-fold accumulation ($p = 0.0037$) of *KLF4* positive cells in TAA tissues compared to non-TAA group (Figure 4). Meanwhile, IHC analysis strongly supported upregulated expression of osteopontin ($p = 0.0311$), which is indicating shift of vascular smooth muscles from contraction to synthetic phenotype and is a positive marker of aortic aneurysms [27,28]. Finally, despite IHC results displaying high levels of *MyoCD* in both groups of samples (IHC score median = 6), a significant expression difference was absent between groups (Figure 4, lower panel).

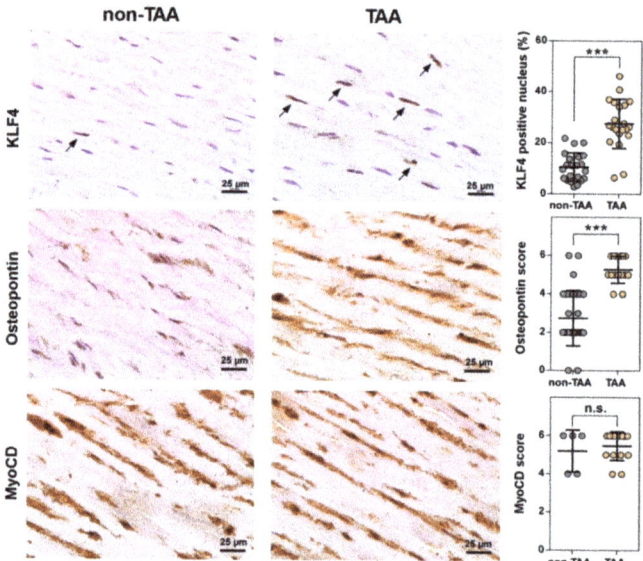

Figure 4. Immunohistochemical (IHC) analysis of KLF4, MyoCD, and osteopontin expression in non-TAA and TAA tissue samples. The abundance of proteins was examined by immunostaining and visualized with diaminobenzidine (brown). The sections were counterstained with hematoxylin (blue). Histological quantification of KLF4 was performed by counting KLF4 positive cell nucleus (black arrows; $n = 43$), whereas osteopontin ($n = 46$) and MyoCD ($n = 20$) by IHC score (graphs in right panel). Lines within boxes indicate KLF4 positive nucleus mean or MyoCD and osteopontin IHC score median values, whiskers – 5-95 percentile of KLF4 positive nucleus or MyoCD and osteopontin IHC score values. The histological data were assessed using Student's t test (for KLF4) or non-parametric Mann-Whitney U test (for MyoCD and osteopontin). The significance between each group is shown as follows: n.s.—not significant; * $p < 0.05$; ** $p < 0.01$, *** $p < 0.001$.

4. Discussion

Aneurysm is one of the most frequent diseases of the aorta [29]. The aortic aneurysms rarely cause any symptoms and thereby are commonly diagnosed incidentally. Consequently, the rupture or dissection of the aneurysm leads to lethal outcomes in over 15000 cases annually in the USA only [30]. Classification of aortic aneurysms is based on the anatomic location, with thoracic aortic aneurysms involving the ascending and descending aorta and abdominal aortic aneurysm [31]. The ascending aorta is derived from distinct embryonic origin defining some specific pathological aspects of aneurysms appearing in different locations [32]. The distinct disease entities at the molecular level may be regulated by specific, at least partially, miRNA networks. Previous studies have demonstrated that miRNAs play key roles during the formation of AAA by dysregulating VSMC homeostasis and extracellular matrix (ECM) composition or inducing vascular inflammatory response [33,34]. However, a global high-throughput miRNA-sequencing data of TAA tissue and plasma was still missing, despite some experimental data obtained by miRNA microarrays [19,20,35].

4.1. miRNA Expression Patterns in Tissues May Be Influenced by Aneurysmal Location and Sex

In the present study we determined a total of 20 miRNAs which were differentially expressed in ascending TAA tissues compared to non-aneurysmal group. A qRT-PCR testing further validated the differential expression of four selected miR-10a-5p, miR-133a-3p, miR-126-3p, miR-155-5p and miR-148a-3p in a larger set of independent samples supporting the reliability of miRNA-Seq results.

Despite a partial overlap (miR-126-3p, miR-155-5p and mir-133a-3p appeared to be involved in AAA [22,29,30]), our results confirmed previous assumptions indicating a quite distinct miRNA expression patterns between TAA and AAA tissues. This might be explained by different pathophysiological mechanism for ascending aneurysm development in comparison to AAA. The latter is most commonly caused by atherosclerosis [31]. In agreement with the present study, the dysregulated expression of miR-133a-3p, miR-126-3p and miR-155-5p has been previously associated with TAA [32]. However, the pathophysiological functions of selected miRNAs in TAA formation and how they modulate disease progression remain poorly understood. A significant upregulation of miR-155-5p was identified in various cardiovascular diseases including AAA and was linked to the inflammatory response in aortic wall. It was demonstrated that expression of miR-155 correlated with inflammatory macrophage response and extracellular matrix destruction in AAA model mice [33]. On the contrary, we identified miR-155-5p as the most strongly downregulated miRNA in TAA tissue. It might be explained by the absence of advanced atherosclerosis leading to inflammatory response in the studied ascending aorta samples obtained during aortic reconstruction. Meanwhile, vascular endothelium specific miR-126-3p is required for the maintenance of vascular integrity and endothelial cell homeostasis [34]. Reduced in proliferating VSMC miR-133a-3p switch on transcription factor *Sp1*, which activates *KLF4*, thus promoting synthetic phenotype [25,35]. miR-10a-5p, one of the most upregulated miRNAs in this study, and miR-148a-3p previously were not related to TAA. It was reported that increased miR-10a-5p expression leads to VSMC differentiation from embryonic stem cells through repression of histone deacetylase *HDAC4* [36]. Thus, we inferred that miR-10a-5p may be a potential modulator of VSMC phenotype as well.

We identified a positive correlation between expression levels of miR-126-3p and newly predicted TAA-related miR-10a-5p and miR-148a-3p (Supplementary Figure S4) indicating a possible functional or regulatory link between these miRNAs. Therefore, further studies of the molecular impact of miR-148a-3p and miR-10a-5p on TAA development is of interest.

An evaluation of sex-dependence revealed that miR-148a-3p varied significantly only in male TAA cohort (Supplementary Figure S1). Furthermore, miR-126-3p, miR-155-5p and miR-10a-5p expression changes were more statistically significant in male TAA patients. Notably, the incidence of TAA is more prevalent in males than females [4]. Moreover, previous reports emphasized relevant sex differences in the pathology of TAA, although underlying molecular mechanisms are unknown. Accordingly, aortic dilation rate was more than 3 times greater in women than in men [6]. This observation was associated with different levels of metalloproteinases *MMP2* and *MMP9*, inhibitory enzymes *TIMP1* and *TIMP2* and overall aortic stiffness highlighting a different ECM remodeling in female aortas [37]. Altogether, these findings suggest that sex-dependent physiological differences could be associated with different changes of miRNA levels in male aorta tissue during TAA development. Otherwise, a deregulation of miRNAs in sex-dependent manner could promote distinct pathways leading to different TAA progression and pathology rates in male patients.

4.2. Circulating miRNA Profile Does Not Match to Aneurysmal Signature of TAA Tissues

Herein we revealed 17 differentially expressed miRNAs in the TAA patients' plasma samples compared to the non-TAA group. The combination of two of them, miR-122-3p and miR-483-3p, allowed to distinguish TAA patients from non-TAA subjects suggesting a novel set of prognostic biomarkers for TAA non-invasive diagnostic. Notably, the majority of altered miRNAs were associated with TAA for the first time, and so far, have not been previously identified in AAA samples [22].

Suprisingly, the pattern of aneurysm-related alterations in TAA patients' plasma miRNA profile does not overlap with the tissue set (Figure 1D). Moreover, the expression of six miRNAs, which were among the most strongly deregulated in TAA plasma samples, was almost absent in TAA tissue. We can speculate that miRNA expression changes in TAA patient's plasma could be evoked by a complex physiological organismal response to the aortic aneurysm development passed by circulating miRNAs that are essential vehicles for organ-to-organ cross-talk between liver, pancreas, muscle, immune and endothelial cells [38]. For instance, miR-122, the most strongly downregulated miRNA in this study, is a key factor in liver development, homeostasis and metabolic functions [39]. The downregulation of miR-122 in the liver cells correlates with hepatic pathology [40], which could be further associated with metabolic syndrome and cardiovascular diseases [41]. In blood plasma, the downregulation of miR-122 was previously associated with other cardiovascular diseases including bicuspid aortic valve, myocardial infarction and cardiac arrest [42–44]. Thus, it seems that the dysregulation of circulating miR-122, highlighted in our study, is not TAA tissue-associated directly but rather is determined by response to the TAA. Meanwhile, an altered expression of mir-483-3p was associated with endothelial cell response to vascular injury [45].

4.3. miRNA Target Analysis Reveals KLF4 As a Key Factor for the TAA Development in vivo

Using bioinformatics approach, we exposed 48 KEGG pathways enriched in genes targeted by differentially expressed miRNAs in TAA tissue cells. Functional categories annotated by KEGG displayed overlapping among target genes which were mainly associated with the immune response, cancer, and kinase activity processes. We emphasized "TGF-β signaling pathway" as individual pathways of highest importance which could be involved in TAA development (Supplementary Table S5). Indeed, about half of differentially expressed miRNAs have predicted targets in 17 genes involved in *TGF-β* pathway. These miRNAs could interfere with the signal transduction by affecting two principal groups of target genes - *TGF-β* ligands/receptors and regulatory *SMAD*s (Figure 3C). Based on these findings, we hypothesized that the mis-expressed miRNAs could contribute significantly to critical changes in diseased aorta via alterations in components of *TGF-β* signaling pathway. It can lead to the functional dysregulation of the key downstream regulators, *KLF4* and/or *MyoCD*. On the other hand, the deregulated balance between *TGF-β* receptors, ligands and rSMADs might trigger alternative *MyoCD*-independent *TGF-β* signaling routes promoting further TAA development [46]. As shown in Figure 3, a group of *TGF-β* receptors/rSMADs-associated miRNAs was mis-regulated in TAA tissues. Previous reports revealed that deficiency of *SMAD4* and *TGFBR2* in VSMCs induced aortic dilation in TAA mice model indicating that the imbalance of TGF-β receptors and rSMADs could promote TAA progression [47,48]. On the other hand, the overexpression and over-activation of *SMAD2* was TGF-β signaling independent in TAA tissue samples suggesting a functional dissociation between the Smad2 activation and activity of the *TGF-β* receptors [47,49]. A signaling switch from canonical *TGFBRI/Smad2*-dependent to *ALK1/Smad1/5/8* signaling was shown to activate genes related to synthetic VSMC phenotype in mice model [50]. In addition, previous report indicated that the differentiation state of VSMCs is controlled by miR-26a via suppression of *TGF-β* signaling molecules [51] demonstrating a link between the dysregulated miRNA expression and aberrant *TGF-β* signaling during TAA development.

Herein we demonstrated a significant upregulation of *ALK1* mRNA expression in TAA tissue cells compared to non-TAA. The expression of *ALK1* positively correlated with the levels of miR-126-3p, mir-10a-5p and miR-148a-3p indicating a functional connection between these miRNAs and *TGF-β* signaling. A follow-up IHC analysis revealed no significant changes in *ALK1* protein level in TAA tissues. However, the discrepancy between mRNA and protein assessments could be related to insufficient sensitivity of the immunohistochemistry approach that hamper the quantification of the modest changes at the protein level. Nevertheless, the main advantage of IHC analysis compared to other methods evaluating total levels of gene expression is the feasibility to visualize precisely the protein localization in individual cells of tissue. Thereby, the number of cells strongly expressing *KLF4* factor in the nucleus was shown to be nearly three-fold higher in TAA tissues compared to non-TAA (27% vs. 10%). Meanwhile, myocardin expression level appeared to be similar, although the precise estimation of the nuclear protein is encumbered by rather high myocardin abundance in cytoplasm. Thus, our *in vivo* data indicate that upregulation of *KLF4* does not directly abrogate the myocardin expression but rather regulates VSMC phenotypic transition from more differentiated contractile to synthetic by competing with myocardin-*SRF* (serum responce factor) complex for the contractile gene promoters [52]. Thus, *KLF4* is an important player in aortic aneurysm morphogenesis by regulating VSMC phenotypic switching [53]. We suggest that a marked reduction of miR-133a-3p *in vivo* could be associated with upregulated *KLF4* expression in one third of smooth muscle cells in the TAA tissues (Figure 3C). This supposition is supported by previous *in vitro* studies in rodent cell cultures [25,35] showing that VSMC phenotype switch could be regulated by miR-133a-3p via indirect repression of *KLF4*.

This study has some potential limitations: i) In order to thoroughly examine a homogenous etiological category of aneurysms, we have limited our investigation to the sporadic non-syndromic TAA cases. The samples of patients with severe atherosclerosis (calcified or ulcerating plagues), aortitis or phenotypic characteristics of the known genetic syndromes (Marfan, Ehlers Danlos, and other) were excluded, because these features can lead to skewed results. As a consequence of the abovementioned restrictions the total number of samples used in the analysis was limited. ii) Female sample size was small. A larger cohort of female specimens needs to be examined in the future to reliably corroborate sex-specific variances of miRNA signatures in TAA tissues. iii) We profiled miRNA from TAA and non-TAA samples which differed by age. However, the sequencing data was then validated by qRT-PCR performed on larger TAA and non-TAA groups of comparable age. iv) The control group included heart transplant donors, patients who underwent CABG and healthy volunteers. To diminish the impact of such diversity on the outcome of the study, a strict clinical testing was performed on the control group to confirm the normal measurements of ascending aorta.

5. Conclusions

Taken together, these observations point to a critical role of aberrant miRNAs expression in promoting TAA via imbalanced repression of *TGF-β* signaling pathway components and following deregulation of *KLF4* transcription axis in vivo. The miRNA-mediated gene expression regulatory networks elucidated herein in clinical samples have paved the ways to further in vitro studies of the miRNAs functions in controlling of VSMC phenotype switch. Moreover, co-expression analysis of selected miRNAs, *KLF4* and VSMC markers inside the cells should be performed in the future to extend our understanding of the miRNA-modulated gene activation shift during TAA development.

Supplementary Materials: The following are available online at http://www.mdpi.com/2077-0383/8/10/1609/s1. Supplementary File 1. A detailed evaluation of differential miRNA-Seq data of each tissue sample assessed in the present study. Supplementary File 2. A detailed evaluation of differential miRNA-Seq data of each plasma sample assessed in the present study. Supplementary File 3. Dataset for miRNA target analysis. Supplementary Material. Supplementary methods, results, figures and tables.

Author Contributions: Conceptualization, S.G., V.S., G.V.; methodology, S.G., V.S., V.P., D.Z.; software, R.R.; validation, S.G. and V.S.; formal analysis, S.G. and V.S.; investigation, S.G., V.S., V.P., G.Z., Z.K., R.B.; data curation, S.G. and V.S.; writing—original draft preparation, V.S. and G.V; writing—review and editing, V.L.; visualization, V.S. and V.P.; supervision, V.L. and G.V.; project administration, S.G., V.P., V.L. and G.V.; funding acquisition V.L. and G.V.

Funding: This research was funded by a grant (No. SEN-05/2016) from the Research Council of Lithuania.

Acknowledgments: We thank Dovydas Gecys for technical assistance in preparing patients' aorta tissue and blood plasma samples.

Conflicts of Interest: The authors declare no conflict of interest. The funders had no role in the design of the study; in the collection, analyses, or interpretation of data; in the writing of the manuscript, or in the decision to publish the results.

References

1. Kuzmik, G.A.; Sang, A.X.; Elefteriades, J.A. Natural history of thoracic aortic aneurysms. *J. Vasc. Surg.* **2012**, *56*, 565–571. [CrossRef] [PubMed]
2. Elefteriades, J.A.; Farkas, E.A. Thoracic Aortic Aneurysm Clinically Pertinent Controversies and Uncertainties. *J. Am. Coll. Cardiol.* **2010**, *55*, 841–857. [CrossRef] [PubMed]
3. Quintana, R.A.; Taylor, W.R. Cellular Mechanisms of Aortic Aneurysm Formation. *Circ. Res.* **2019**, *124*, 607–618. [CrossRef] [PubMed]
4. Olsson, C.; Thelin, S.; Ståhle, E.; Ekbom, A.; Granath, F. Thoracic Aortic Aneurysm and Dissection. *Circulation* **2006**, *114*, 2611–2618. [CrossRef] [PubMed]
5. Von Allmen, R.S.; Anjum, A.; Powell, J.T. Incidence of Descending Aortic Pathology and Evaluation of the Impact of Thoracic Endovascular Aortic Repair: A Population-based Study in England and Wales from 1999 to 2010. *Eur. J. Vasc. Endovasc. Surg.* **2013**, *45*, 154–159. [CrossRef]
6. Cheung, K.; Boodhwani, M.; Chan, K.L.; Beauchesne, L.; Dick, A.; Coutinho, T. Thoracic Aortic Aneurysm Growth: Role of Sex and Aneurysm Etiology. *J. Am. Heart Assoc.* **2017**, *6*, e003792. [CrossRef]
7. Nicolini, F.; Vezzani, A.; Corradi, F.; Gherli, R.; Benassi, F.; Manca, T.; Gherli, T. Gender differences in outcomes after aortic aneurysm surgery should foster further research to improve screening and prevention programmes. *Eur. J. Prev. Cardiol.* **2018**, *25*, 32–41. [CrossRef]
8. Owens, G.K. Regulation of Differentiation of Vascular Smooth-Muscle Cells. *Physiol. Rev.* **1995**, *75*, 487–517. [CrossRef]
9. Owens, G.K.; Kumar, M.S.; Wamhoff, B.R. Molecular regulation of vascular smooth muscle cell differentiation in development and disease. *Physiol. Rev.* **2004**, *84*, 767–801. [CrossRef]
10. Wang, Z.G.; Wang, D.Z.; Pipes, G.C.T.; Olson, E.N. Myocardin is a master regulator of smooth muscle gene expression. *Proc. Natl. Acad. Sci. USA* **2003**, *100*, 7129–7134. [CrossRef]
11. Liu, Y.; Sinha, S.; McDonald, O.G.; Shang, Y.T.; Hoofnagle, M.H.; Owens, G.K. Kruppel-like factor 4 abrogates myocardin-induced activation of smooth muscle gene expression. *J. Biol. Chem.* **2005**, *280*, 9719–9727. [CrossRef] [PubMed]
12. Tang, Y.F.; Yang, X.H.; Friesel, R.E.; Vary, C.P.H.; Liaw, L. Mechanisms of TGF-beta-Induced Differentiation in Human Vascular Smooth Muscle Cells. *J. Vasc. Res.* **2011**, *48*, 485–494. [CrossRef] [PubMed]
13. Chuang, J.C.; Jones, P.A. Epigenetics and microRNAs. *Pediatr. Res.* **2007**, *61*, 24–29. [CrossRef] [PubMed]
14. Small, E.M.; Frost, R.J.A.; Olson, E.N. MicroRNAs Add a New Dimension to Cardiovascular Disease. *Circulation* **2010**, *121*, 1022–1032. [CrossRef]
15. Zhou, S.S.; Jin, J.P.; Wang, J.Q.; Zhang, Z.G.; Freedman, J.H.; Zheng, Y.; Cai, L. miRNAS in cardiovascular diseases: Potential biomarkers, therapeutic targets and challenges. *Acta Pharmacol. Sin.* **2018**, *39*, 1073–1084. [CrossRef] [PubMed]
16. Song, Z.F.; Li, G.H. Role of Specific MicroRNAs in Regulation of Vascular Smooth Muscle Cell Differentiation and the Response to Injury. *J. Cardiovasc. Transl. Res.* **2010**, *3*, 246–250. [CrossRef]

17. Merlet, E.; Atassi, F.; Motiani, R.K.; Mougenot, N.; Jacquet, A.; Nadaud, S.; Capiod, T.; Trebak, M.; Lompre, A.M.; Marchand, A. miR-424/322 regulates vascular smooth muscle cell phenotype and neointimal formation in the rat. *Cardiovasc. Res.* **2013**, *98*, 458–468. [CrossRef]
18. Dong, N.N.; Wang, W.; Tian, J.W.; Xie, Z.L.; Lv, B.; Dai, J.N.; Jiang, R.; Huang, D.; Fang, S.H.; Tian, J.T.; et al. MicroRNA-182 prevents vascular smooth muscle cell dedifferentiation via FGF9/PDGFR signaling. *Int. J. Mol. Med.* **2017**, *39*, 791–798. [CrossRef]
19. Jones, J.A.; Stroud, R.E.; O'Quinn, E.C.; Black, L.E.; Barth, J.L.; Elefteriades, J.A.; Bavaria, J.E.; Gorman, J.H.; Gorman, R.C.; Spinale, F.G.; et al. Selective MicroRNA Suppression in Human Thoracic Aneurysms Relationship of miR-29a to Aortic Size and Proteolytic Induction. *Circ-Cardiovasc. Genet.* **2011**, *4*, 605–613. [CrossRef]
20. Licholai, S.; Blaz, M.; Kapelak, B.; Sanak, M. Unbiased Profile of MicroRNA Expression in Ascending Aortic Aneurysm Tissue Appoints Molecular Pathways Contributing to the Pathology. *Ann. Thorac. Surg.* **2016**, *102*, 1245–1252. [CrossRef]
21. Boileau, A.; Lindsay, M.E.; Michel, J.B.; Devaux, Y. Epigenetics in Ascending Thoracic Aortic Aneurysm and Dissection. *Aorta* **2018**, *6*, 1–12. [CrossRef] [PubMed]
22. Moushi, A.; Michailidou, K.; Soteriou, M.; Cariolou, M.; Bashiardes, E. MicroRNAs as possible biomarkers for screening of aortic aneurysms: A systematic review and validation study. *Biomarkers* **2018**, *23*, 253–264. [CrossRef] [PubMed]
23. Raffort, J.; Lareyre, F.; Clement, M.; Mallat, Z. Micro-RNAs in abdominal aortic aneurysms: Insights from animal models and relevance to human disease. *Cardiovasc. Res.* **2016**, *110*, 165–177. [CrossRef]
24. Butkytė, S.; Čiupas, L.; Jakubauskienė, E.; Vilys, L.; Mocevicius, P.; Kanopka, A.; Vilkaitis, G. Splicing-dependent expression of microRNAs of mirtron origin in human digestive and excretory system cancer cells. *Clin. Epigenet.* **2016**, *8*, 33. [CrossRef] [PubMed]
25. Torella, D.; Iaconetti, C.; Catalucci, D.; Ellison Georgina, M.; Leone, A.; Waring Cheryl, D.; Bochicchio, A.; Vicinanza, C.; Aquila, I.; Curcio, A.; et al. MicroRNA-133 Controls Vascular Smooth Muscle Cell Phenotypic Switch In Vitro and Vascular Remodeling In Vivo. *Circ. Res.* **2011**, *109*, 880–893. [CrossRef] [PubMed]
26. Jonas, S.; Izaurralde, E. Towards a molecular understanding of microRNA-mediated gene silencing. *Nat. Rev. Genet.* **2015**, *16*, 421. [CrossRef] [PubMed]
27. Huusko, T.; Salonurmi, T.; Taskinen, P.; Liinamaa, J.; Juvonen, T.; Paakko, P.; Savolainen, M.; Kakko, S. Elevated messenger RNA expression and plasma protein levels of osteopontin and matrix metalloproteinase types 2 and 9 in patients with ascending aortic aneurysms. *J. Thorac. Cardiovasc. Surg.* **2013**, *145*, 1117–1123. [CrossRef]
28. Lesauskaite, V.; Tanganelli, P.; Sassi, C.; Neri, E.; Diciolla, F.; Ivanoviene, L.; Epistolato, M.C.; Lalinga, A.V.; Alessandrini, C.; Spina, D. Smooth muscle cells of the media in the dilatative pathology of ascending thoracic aorta: Morphology, immunoreactivity for osteopontin, matrix metalloproteinases, and their inhibitors. *Hum. Pathol.* **2001**, *32*, 1003–1011. [CrossRef]
29. Spin, J.M.; Li, D.Y.; Maegdefessel, L.; Tsao, P.S. Non-coding RNAs in aneurysmal aortopathy. *Vascul. Pharmacol.* **2018**, *114*, 110–121. [CrossRef]
30. Li, Y.H.; Maegdefessel, L. Non-coding RNA Contribution to Thoracic and Abdominal Aortic Aneurysm Disease Development and Progression. *Front. Physiol.* **2017**, *8*, 429. [CrossRef]
31. Ruddy, J.M.; Jones, J.A.; Spinale, F.G.; Ikonomidis, J.S. Regional heterogeneity within the aorta: Relevance to aneurysm disease. *J. Thorac. Cardiovasc. Surg.* **2008**, *136*, 1123–1130. [CrossRef] [PubMed]
32. Venkatesh, P.; Phillippi, J.; Chukkapalli, S.; Rivera-Kweh, M.; Velsko, I.; Gleason, T.; VanRyzin, P.; Aalaei-Andabili, S.H.; Ghanta, R.K.; Beaver, T.; et al. Aneurysm-Specific miR-221 and miR-146a Participates in Human Thoracic and Abdominal Aortic Aneurysms. *Int. J. Mol. Sci.* **2017**, *18*, 875. [CrossRef] [PubMed]
33. Zhang, Z.; Liang, K.; Zou, G.; Chen, X.; Shi, S.; Wang, G.; Zhang, K.; Li, K.; Zhai, S. Inhibition of miR-155 attenuates abdominal aortic aneurysm in mice by regulating macrophage-mediated inflammation. *Biosci. Rep.* **2018**, *38*. [CrossRef] [PubMed]
34. Welten, S.M.J.; Goossens, E.A.C.; Quax, P.H.A.; Nossent, A.Y. The multifactorial nature of microRNAs in vascular remodelling. *Cardiovasc. Res.* **2016**, *110*, 6–22. [CrossRef] [PubMed]
35. Deaton, R.A.; Gan, Q.; Owens, G.K. Sp1-dependent activation of KLF4 is required for PDGF-BB-induced phenotypic modulation of smooth muscle. *Am. J. Physiol. Heart Circ. Physiol.* **2009**, *296*, H1027–H1037. [CrossRef] [PubMed]

36. Huang, H.R.; Xie, C.Q.; Sun, X.; Ritchie, R.P.; Zhang, J.F.; Chen, Y.E. miR-10a Contributes to Retinoid Acid-induced Smooth Muscle Cell Differentiation. *J. Biol. Chem.* **2010**, *285*, 9383–9389. [CrossRef] [PubMed]
37. Sokolis, D.P.; Iliopoulos, D.C. Impaired mechanics and matrix metalloproteinases/inhibitors expression in female ascending thoracic aortic aneurysms. *J. Mech. Behav. Biomed.* **2014**, *34*, 154–164. [CrossRef]
38. Guay, C.; Regazzi, R. Exosomes as new players in metabolic organ cross-talk. *Diabetes Obes. Metab.* **2017**, *19*, 137–146. [CrossRef] [PubMed]
39. Hu, J.; Xu, Y.; Hao, J.; Wang, S.; Li, C.; Meng, S. MiR-122 in hepatic function and liver diseases. *Protein Cell* **2012**, *3*, 364–371. [CrossRef]
40. Bandiera, S.; Pfeffer, S.; Baumert, T.F.; Zeisel, M.B. miR-122–A key factor and therapeutic target in liver disease. *J. Hepatol.* **2015**, *62*, 448–457. [CrossRef]
41. Olijhoek, J.K.; van der Graaf, Y.; Banga, J.-D.; Algra, A.; Rabelink, T.J.; Visseren, F.L. The Metabolic Syndrome is associated with advanced vascular damage in patients with coronary heart disease, stroke, peripheral arterial disease or abdominal aortic aneurysm. *Eur. Heart J.* **2004**, *25*, 342–348. [CrossRef] [PubMed]
42. D'Alessandra, Y.; Devanna, P.; Limana, F.; Straino, S.; Di Carlo, A.; Brambilla, P.G.; Rubino, M.; Carena, M.C.; Spazzafumo, L.; De Simone, M.; et al. Circulating microRNAs are new and sensitive biomarkers of myocardial infarction. *Eur. Heart J.* **2010**, *31*, 2765–2773. [CrossRef] [PubMed]
43. Devaux, Y.; Salgado-Somoza, A.; Dankiewicz, J.; Boileau, A.; Stammet, P.; Schritz, A.; Zhang, L.; Vausort, M.; Gilje, P.; Erlinge, D.; et al. Incremental Value of Circulating MiR-122-5p to Predict Outcome after Out of Hospital Cardiac Arrest. *Theranostics* **2017**, *7*, 2555–2564. [CrossRef] [PubMed]
44. Martínez-Micaelo, N.; Beltrán-Debón, R.; Baiges, I.; Faiges, M.; Alegret, J.M. Specific circulating microRNA signature of bicuspid aortic valve disease. *J. Transl. Med.* **2017**, *15*, 76. [CrossRef] [PubMed]
45. Kraenkel, N.; Kuschnerus, K.; Briand, S.; Luescher, T.F.; Landmesser, U. miR-483 impairs endothelial homeostasis and response to vascular injury: Upregulation by high-glucose and in patients with type-2 diabetes. *Eur. Heart J.* **2013**, *34*, 762. [CrossRef]
46. Takeda, N.; Hara, H.; Fujiwara, T.; Kanaya, T.; Maemura, S.; Komuro, I. TGF-β Signaling-Related Genes and Thoracic Aortic Aneurysms and Dissections. *Int. J. Mol. Sci.* **2018**, *19*, 2125. [CrossRef]
47. Zhang, P.; Hou, S.Y.; Chen, J.C.; Zhang, J.S.; Lin, F.Y.; Ju, R.J.; Cheng, X.; Ma, X.W.; Song, Y.; Zhang, Y.Y.; et al. Smad4 Deficiency in Smooth Muscle Cells Initiates the Formation of Aortic Aneurysm. *Circ. Res.* **2016**, *118*, 388–399. [CrossRef] [PubMed]
48. Li, W.; Li, Q.L.; Jiao, Y.; Qin, L.F.; Ali, R.; Zhou, J.; Ferruzzi, J.; Kim, R.W.; Geirsson, A.; Dietz, H.C.; et al. Tgfbr2 disruption in postnatal smooth muscle impairs aortic wall homeostasis. *J. Clin. Investig.* **2014**, *124*, 755–767. [CrossRef]
49. Gomez, D.; Coyet, A.; Ollivier, V.; Jeunemaitre, X.; Jondeau, G.; Michel, J.B.; Vranckx, R. Epigenetic control of vascular smooth muscle cells in Marfan and non-Marfan thoracic aortic aneurysms. *Cardiovasc. Res.* **2011**, *89*, 446–456. [CrossRef]
50. Jones, J.A.; Barbour, J.R.; Stroud, R.E.; Bouges, S.; Stephens, S.L.; Spinale, F.G.; Ikonomidis, J.S. Altered Transforming Growth Factor-Beta Signaling in a Murine Model of Thoracic Aortic Aneurysm. *J. Vasc. Res.* **2008**, *45*, 457–468. [CrossRef]
51. Leeper, N.J.; Raiesdana, A.; Kojima, Y.; Chun, H.J.; Azuma, J.; Maegdefessel, L.; Kundu, R.K.; Quertermous, T.; Tsao, P.S.; Spin, J.M. MicroRNA-26a is a novel regulator of vascular smooth muscle cell function. *J. Cell. Physiol.* **2011**, *226*, 1035–1043. [CrossRef] [PubMed]
52. Frismantiene, A.; Philippova, M.; Erne, P.; Resink, T.J. Smooth muscle cell-driven vascular diseases and molecular mechanisms of VSMC plasticity. *Cell. Signal.* **2018**, *52*, 48–64. [CrossRef] [PubMed]
53. Salmon, M.; Johnston, W.F.; Woo, A.; Pope, N.H.; Su, G.; Upchurch, G.R.; Owens, G.K.; Ailawadi, G. KLF4 Regulates Abdominal Aortic Aneurysm Morphology and Deletion Attenuates Aneurysm Formation. *Circulation* **2013**, *128*, S163–S174. [CrossRef] [PubMed]

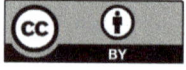

© 2019 by the authors. Licensee MDPI, Basel, Switzerland. This article is an open access article distributed under the terms and conditions of the Creative Commons Attribution (CC BY) license (http://creativecommons.org/licenses/by/4.0/).

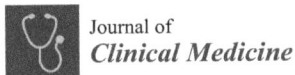

Article

Growth Differentiation Factor-15 (GDF-15) Is a Biomarker of Muscle Wasting and Renal Dysfunction in Preoperative Cardiovascular Surgery Patients

Toshiaki Nakajima [1,*], Ikuko Shibasaki [2], Tatsuya Sawaguchi [1], Akiko Haruyama [1], Hiroyuki Kaneda [1], Takafumi Nakajima [1], Takaaki Hasegawa [1], Takuo Arikawa [1], Syotaro Obi [1], Masashi Sakuma [1], Hironaga Ogawa [2], Shigeru Toyoda [1], Fumitaka Nakamura [3], Shichiro Abe [1], Hirotsugu Fukuda [2] and Teruo Inoue [1]

[1] Department of Cardiovascular Medicine, School of Medicine, Dokkyo Medical University, Shimotsuga-gun, Tochigi 321-0293, Japan; tswg0814@gmail.com (T.S.); hal@dokkyomed.ac.jp (A.H.); hirokane1010@gmail.com (H.K.); sho-taka.07@softbank.ne.jp (T.N.); thasegawa6134@gmail.com (T.H.); takuoari@dokkyomed.ac.jp (T.A.); syoutarouobi@yahoo.co.jp (S.O.); masakuma@dokkyomed.ac.jp (M.S.); s-toyoda@dokkyomed.ac.jp (S.T.); abenana@dokkyomed.ac.jp (S.A.); inouet@dokkyomed.ac.jp (T.I.)

[2] Department of Cardiovascular Surgery, School of Medicine, Dokkyo Medical University, Shimotsuga-gun, Tochigi 321-0293, Japan; sibasaki@dokkyomed.ac.jp (I.S.); hironaga_0722@yahoo.co.jp (H.O.); fukuda-h@dokkyomed.ac.jp (H.F.)

[3] Third Department of Internal Medicine, Teikyo University, Chiba Medical Center, Ichihara, Chiba 299-0111, Japan; fumitaka@med.teikyo-u.ac.jp

* Correspondence: nakat@dokkyomed.ac.jp

Received: 24 August 2019; Accepted: 25 September 2019; Published: 1 October 2019

Abstract: Frailty and sarcopenia increase the risk of complications and mortality when invasive treatment such as cardiac surgery is performed. Growth differentiation factor-15 (GDF-15) involves various pathophysiological conditions including renal dysfunction, heart failure and cachexia. We investigated the pathophysiological roles of preoperative GDF-15 levels in cardiovascular surgery patients. Preoperative skeletal muscle index (SMI) determined by bioelectrical impedance analysis, hand-grip strength, 4 m gait speed, and anterior thigh muscle thickness (TMth) measured by echocardiography were assessed in 72 patients (average age 69.9 years) who underwent cardiovascular surgery. The preoperative serum GDF-15 concentration was determined by enzyme-linked immunosorbent assay. Circulating GDF-15 level was correlated with age, brain natriuretic peptide, and estimated glomerular filtration rate (eGFR). It was also negatively correlated with SMI, hand-grip strength, and anterior TMth. In multivariate analysis, eGFR and anterior TMth were the independent determinants of GDF-15 concentration even after adjusting for age, sex, and body mass index. Alternatively, the GDF-15 level was an independent determinant of eGFR and anterior TMth. We concluded that preoperative GDF-15 levels reflect muscle wasting as well as renal dysfunction in preoperative cardiovascular surgery patients. GDF-15 may be a novel biomarker for identify high-risk patients with muscle wasting and renal dysfunction before cardiovascular surgery.

Keywords: GDF-15; cardiovascular surgery; operative risk; biomarkers; muscle wasting; sarcopenia; renal dysfunction; chronic kidney disease

1. Introduction

As life expectancy has increased, the number of older patients undergoing cardiovascular surgery has also increased, and many such patients have frailty. Frailty is a geriatric syndrome described as decreased reserves when confronted with stressors, which is associated with poor outcomes in both community cohorts and patients [1,2]. In cardiovascular surgery such as transcatheter valve implantation (TAVI), frailty is now identified as an important predictor of adverse outcomes in older patients [1,3,4]. Patients with higher frailty are at increased risk during the postoperative period, with long hospital stays, and postoperative complications such as stroke and death, compared to those with lower frailty [5]. Sarcopenia, the skeletal muscle loss associated with aging, also includes low physical function (hand-grip strength, walking speed) as a component of frailty [6,7]. It is frequently associated with chronic diseases including heart failure, chronic kidney disease (CKD), cancer, wasting, and cachexia [7]. Thus, it is generally accepted that frailty and sarcopenia, as well as physical function are predictors of survival in patients with cardiovascular diseases (CVD), and they increase the risk of complications and mortality when invasive treatments such as cardiovascular operations are performed. Therefore, it is quite important to identify high-risk patients with frailty and sarcopenia before cardiovascular surgery.

Growth differentiation fator-15 (GDF-15) is not highly expressed in most tissues under normal physiological conditions [8,9], but it increases under various pathophysiological conditions such as inflammation [10], oxidant stress [11], and ischemia/reperfusion [12]. Clinical trials reported that GDF-15 is a reliable biomarker of CVD [13–15], and heart failure [16], and it has independent prognostic value in patients with coronary artery bypass grafting (CABG) [17], acute coronary syndromes (ACS) [18,19], and heart failure (HF) [20]. In addition, it has been reported that GDF-15 is a novel serum biomarker of mortality in CKD, and can identify patients at high risk of developing CKD [21–23]. The preoperative GDF-15 level has been also reported to be a novel risk biomarker in association with the EuroSCORE for risk stratification independently of N-terminal pro-B-type natriuretic peptide (NTproBNP) and high-sensitive troponin T [24], and closely related to post-operative morbidity in cardiovascular surgery patients including those undergoing TAVI [25,26]. Furthermore, it has been reported to reflect post-operative acute kidney injury (AKI) in patients undergoing CABG [27] and myocardial injury in patients undergoing off-pump CABG [28]. Thus, GDF-15 appears to be a novel biomarker to identify surgical risk in patients undergoing cardiovascular surgery.

Circulating GDF-15 levels increase with age [20,22], and may partly reflect mitochondrial dysfunction in aging and age-related diseases [29]. Furthermore, several papers showed that GDF-15 may be involved in muscle wasting in a variety of patients including COPD [30], patients undergoing elective high-risk cardiothoracic surgery [31], intensive care unit (ICU) patients [32], and cancer patients [33]. Bloch et al. [31] showed that an elevation of postoperative GDF-15 levels is a potential factor associated with muscle atrophy in patients undergoing cardiovascular surgery. However, the physiological significance of the preoperative GDF-15 level in patients undergoing cardiovascular surgery still remains to be clarified.

Therefore, we investigated the pathophysiological roles of preoperative GDF-15 levels in cardiovascular surgery patients. We provided the first evidence that GDF-15 may be a novel biomarker for identifying high-risk patients with muscle wasting and renal dysfunction, compared with tumor necrosis factor α (TNFα) or insulin growth factor-1 (IGF-1) in cardiovascular surgery patients.

2. Methods

2.1. Participants

A total of 72 preoperative patients (42 males, 30 females) undergoing cardiovascular surgery at Dokkyo Medical Hospital were recruited in this study. The patient characteristics are summarized in Table 1. The mean age was 69.9 ± 13.1 years (23–89 years), and body mass index (BMI) was 24.3 ± 3.9 kg/m^2. Most of the patients had conventional risk factors such as hypertension (HT), diabetes (DM), hyperlipidemia (HL), current smoking, and hemodialysis (HD) as shown in Table 1. The average preoperative New York Heart Association (NYHA) classification was 2.2 ± 1.0. Table 1 also shows the number of patients classified by surgical procedures for cardiovascular disease. The study was approved by the Ethics Committee of the Dokkyo Medical University (No. 27077), and informed consents were obtained from all participants.

Table 1. Patient Characteristics.

Number	72
Male, Female	42, 30
Age, y	69.9 ± 13.1
BMI, kg/m²	24.3 ± 3.9
Risk factors (percentage)	
Hypertension	75
Diabetes	35
Dyslipidemia	46
Smoking	11
Hemodialysis	8
NYHA classification	2.2 ± 1.0
Coronary artery disease (percentage)	
0-vessel disease	53
1-vessel disease	11
2-vessel disease	6
3-vessel disease	30
Cardiovascular surgery (percentage)	
CABG	26
AVR	21
Other valve replacement/repair (MVR, MVP, TAP, TAR, LAAAC)	17
CABG combined with valve replacement/repair (AVR, MVP, TAP)	8
AVR combined with other valve (MVP, TAP, LAAC) or aortic diseases (TAR)	11
Aortic disease (TAR, TEVAR, et al.)	7
Others	10
Drugs (percentage)	
β-blockers	49
Ca-blockers	38
ACE-I/ARB	58
Diuretics	49
Statins	53
Oral antidiabetic drugs	31
Insulin	8

The mean ± SD values are shown. BMI, body mass index; NYHA, New York Heart Association; CABG, coronary artery bypass grafting; AVR, aortic valve replacement; MVR, mitral valve replacement; MVP, mitral valve plasty; TAP, tricuspid annuloplasty; LAAC, left atrial appendage closure; TAR, total arch replacement; TEVAR, thoracic endovascular aortic repair; ACE-I, angiotensin converting enzyme inhibitors; ARB, angiotensin II receptor blockers; Oral anti-diabetic drugs included α-glucosidase inhibitors, sulfonylurea, biguanide, dipeptidyl peptidase-4 inhibitors, and sodium glucose cotransporter 2 inhibitors.

The biochemical data were analyzed using routine chemical methods in Dokkyo Medical University Hospital clinical laboratory. Hemoglobin A1c (HbA1c), brain natriuretic peptide (BNP), and estimated glomerular filtration rate (eGFR) were measured before the operation. The eGFR was calculated by the following equations:

$$\text{Males: eGFR (mL/min/1.73m}^2) = 194 \, (\text{creatinine}^{-1.094}) \, (\text{age}^{-0.287})$$

$$\text{Females: eGFR (mL/min/1.73m}^2) = 0.739 \, \{194(\text{creatinine}^{-1.094}) \, (\text{age}^{-0.287})\}$$

The high-sensitivity C-reactive protein (hsCRP) was measured by a latex-enhanced nephelometric immunoassay (N Latex CRP II and N Latex SAA, Dade Behring Ltd., Tokyo, Japan). The homeo-static model assessment of insulin resistance (HOMA-IR), which indicates an index of insulin resistance, was calculated from the fasting blood insulin (immunoreactive insulin (IRI)) concentration and the fasting blood glucose (FBS) level early in the morning, based on the following equation.

$$\text{HOMA-IR} = (\text{IRI}) \, (\text{FBS})/405$$

To measure fasting serum GDF-15, TNFα, and IGF-1 levels, peripheral venous blood was drawn into pyrogen-free tubes with and without EDTA on the morning of cardiovascular surgery. Plasma and serum were stored in aliquots at −80 °C for all enzyme linked immunosorbent assay (ELISA).

2.2. Enzyme Linked Immunosorbent Assay (ELISA)

Serum GDF-15 level was measured by a Human Quantikine ELISA Kit (DGD150 for GDF-15, R&D Systems, Minneapolis, MN, USA). Samples, reagents, and buffers were prepared according to the manufacturers' manuals. The detection threshold of GDF-15 was 2.0 pg/mL. The serum concentrations of TNFα were measured by a Human Quantikine HS ELISA Kit (HSTA00E, R&D Systems, Minneapolis, MN, USA), and the detection threshold was 0.022 pg/mL. The serum IGF-1 concentration was measured by a Human Quantikine ELISA Kit (DG100, R&D Systems), and the detection threshold was 0.026 ng/mL.

2.3. Measurement of Gait Speed, Hand-Grip Strength, and Voluntary Isometric Contraction

Maximum voluntary isometric contraction (MVIC) of the hand-grip was measured by using a factory-calibrated hand dynamometer (TKK 5401, TAKEI Scientific Instruments Co., Ltd., Tokyo, Japan). Each patient performed two trials, and the highest value was adopted for analysis. The gait speed was measured as the time needed to walk 4 m at an ordinary pace. MVIC of the knee extensors was measured by using a digital handheld dynamometer (μTas MT-1, ANIMA Co., Ltd., Tokyo, Japan) as described previously [34]. Each subject performed two trials, and the highest score was adopted for analysis.

2.4. Measurements with the Bioelectrical Impedance Analyzer (BIA)

A multi-frequency bioelectrical impedance analyzer (BIA), InBody S10 Biospace device (Biospacte Co, Ltd., Korea/Model JMW140) was used to measure muscle and fat volume as described in detail previously [34]. Thirty impedance measurements were performed using 6 different frequencies (1, 5, 50, 250, 500, and 1000 kHz) at the five segments of the body (right arm, left arm, trunk, right leg, and left leg). The measurements were performed while the subjects rested in the supine position, with their elbows extended and relaxed along their trunk. Body fat volume, body fat percentage, and skeletal muscle volume were measured. Skeletal muscle mass index (SMI; appendicular skeletal muscle mass/height^2, kg/m^2) was also calculated as the sum of lean soft tissue of the two upper limbs and two lower limbs. In this study, sarcopenia was defined according to the Asian Working Group for Sarcopenia (AWGS) [7] criteria (age ≥ 65 years; handgrip < 26 kg or gait speed ≤ 0.8 m/s, and SMI < 7.0 kg/m^2 for males; handgrip < 18 kg or gait speed ≤ 0.8 m/s, and SMI < 5.7 kg/m^2 for females.

2.5. Measurement of Muscle Thickness by Ultrasound

The anterior mid-thigh muscle thickness was measured on the right leg using a real-time linear electronic scanner with a 10.0-MHz scanning head and Ultrasound Probe (L4–12t-RS Probe, GE Healthcare Japan, Tokyo, Japan) and LOGIQ e ultrasound (GE Healthcare Japan), as previously described [34]. From the ultrasonic image, the subcutaneous adipose tissue-muscle interface and the muscle-bone interface were identified. The perpendicular distance from the adipose tissue-muscle interface to the muscle-bone interface was considered to represent the anterior thigh muscle thickness (TMth). The measurement was performed twice in both the supine and standing positions, and the average value was adopted for analysis.

2.6. Statistical Analysis

Data are presented as mean value ± SD. After testing for normality (Kolmogorov-Smirnov), the comparison of means between groups was analyzed by a two-sided, unpaired Student's *t*-test in the case of normally distributed parameters or by the Mann-Whitney-U-Test in the case of non-normally distributed parameters. Associations among parameters were evaluated using Pearson or Spearman correlation coefficients. Multiple linear regression analysis with log (serum GDF-15 concentration), eGFR, or anterior TMth as the dependent variable was performed to identify the independent factors (clinical laboratory data, or physical data) that influenced these dependent variables. Age, sex, and BMI were employed as covariates. When the independent data were not normally distributed, the data were logarithmically transformed to achieve a normal distribution. Receiver operating characteristic (ROC) curves were plotted to identify an optimal cut-off level of the serum concentration of GDF-15 for detecting impaired eGFR. All analyses were performed using SPSS version 24 for Windows (IBM Corp., New York, NY, USA). A p value less than 0.05 was regarded as significant.

3. Results

3.1. Patient Characteristics

All patients had medical treatment including β-blocking agents (49%), calcium-channel blockers (38%), angiotensin receptor blockers (ARB)-/-angiotensin converting enzyme inhibitors (ACEI) (58%), diuretics (49%), statins (53%), and anti-diabetic drugs (31%) (Table 1).

The sex differences of the study patients are shown in Table 2. The mean age of females was significantly higher than that of males ($p < 0.05$). The BMI value was not different between males and females, but body fat percentage (%) in females was significantly higher, compared with that in men ($p < 0.05$).

Table 2. Sex differences in various parameters.

	Total ($n = 72$)	Male ($n = 42$)	Female ($n = 30$)
Age, years	69.9 (13.1)	66.9 (14.4)	73.7 (10.0) *
BMI, kg/m^2	24.3 (3.9)	24.9 (4.5)	24.7 (5.5)
NYHA classification	2.2 (1.0)	2.3 (1.1)	2.1 (0.9)
Gait speed, m/s	0.93 (0.32)	0.99 (0.34)	0.86 (0.28)
Hand-grip strength, kgf	22.8 (8.5)	27.1 (7.9)	16.5 (4.6) ***
Knee extension strength, kgf	20.8 (9.5)	24.4 (9.3)	15.6 (7.1) ***
Body fat percentage, %	32.3 (9.3)	28.4 (7.8)	37.6 (8.7) ***
Skeletal muscle mass index (SMI), kg/m^2	6.5 (1.4)	7.2 (1.3)	5.4 (0.9) ***
Anterior thigh muscle thickness (TMth) (supine), cm	2.28 (0.75)	2.41 (0.80)	2.1 (0.6)
Anterior thigh muscle thickness (TMth) (standing), cm	3.47 (0.95)	3.68 (0.97)	3.2 (0.9) *
HbA1c, %	6.2 (0.9)	6.3 (1.0)	6.0 (0.8)
BNP, pg/mL	355 (570)	399 (673)	268 (345)
eGFR, ml/min/1.73 m^2	58.2 (24.0)	55.7 (26.6)	63.4 (19.3)
Hb, g/dL	12.2 (1.8)	12.3 (1.9)	11.9 (1.7)
HOMA-IR	2.75 (4.20)	3.46 (5.29)	1.64 (1.29)
hsCRP, mg/L	5.9 (12)	7.4 (13.8)	3.3 (7.9)
GDF-15, pg/mL	1676 (1465)	1928 (1655)	1325 (1078)
TNFα, pg/mL	3.5 (2.8)	4.1 (2.9)	2.6 (1.9) *
IGF-1, ng/mL	74.4 (33.4)	77.3 (36.5)	70.4 (28.5)

* $p < 0.05$. *** $p < 0.001$. Males vs. Females hsCRP, high sensitivity C-reactive protein; BNP, brain natriuretic peptide; eGFR, estimate glomerular filtration rate; HOMA-IR, Homeostasis model assessment of insulin resistance; GDF-15, growth differentiation factor-15; TNFα, tissue necrosis factor α; IGF-1, insulin growth factor-1.

The hand-grip strength, knee extension strength, and SMI in females were significantly lower than those in males. The anterior TMth (standing) in males was significantly higher, compared with that in females ($p < 0.05$). The BNP level was not different between males and females (399 ± 673 pg/mL vs. 268 ± 345 pg/mL). The mean eGFR of all the patients was 58.2 ± 24.0 mL/min/1.73 m^2. Furthermore, patients were classified into five groups based on the eGFR levels: normal (eGFR ≥ 90 mL/min/1.73 m^2), low (eGFR 60–89 mL/min/1.73 m^2), moderate (eGFR 30–59 mL/min/1.73 m^2), severe (eGFR 15–29 mL/min/1.73 m^2), and kidney failure (eGFR < 15 mL/min/1.73 m^2). Among total 72 patients, there were 3 patients (normal), 36 patients (low),

25 patients (moderate), 2 patients (severe), and 6 patients (kidney failure). Therefore, the overall prevalence of CKD (eGFR < 60 mL/min/1.73 m^2) was 33 patients out of 72 (44%). The serum TNFα level was 3.5 ± 2.8 pg/mL in all of the patients. It was higher in males than in females (males, 4.1 ± 2.9 pg/mL; females, 2.6 ± 1.9 pg/mL, p < 0.05). The serum GDF-15 level did not significantly differ between males and females (males, 1928 ± 1655 pg/mL; females, 1325 ± 1078 pg/mL). The serum IGF-1 concentration also did not significantly differ between males and females (males, 77.3 ± 36.5 ng/mL; females, 70.4 ± 28.5 pg/mL).

3.2. Correlation between Various Parameters and Serum GDF-15, TNFα, and IGF-1 Concentration

The correlations between serum GDF-15, TNFα, and IGF-1 concentrations and the clinical data are shown in Table 3 and Figure 1. Table 3 shows the data obtained from males and females separately, and Figure 1 shows the correlations in all of the patients. The serum GDF-15 level was positively correlated with age in all of the patients (r = 0.438, p < 0.001, Figure 1Aa), but not TNFα (r = 0.192, p = 0.105, Figure 1Ba), and serum IGF-1 concentration declined with age (r = −0.346, p = 0.003, Figure 1Ca). In addition, the serum GDF-15 level was positively correlated with age in both males and females (males, r = 0.436, p = 0.004; females, r = 0.637, p < 0.001). The concentration of GDF-15 was positively correlated with BNP in both sexes (males, r = 0.427, p = 0.005; females, r = 0.480, p = 0.007), but the serum TNFα level was positively correlated with BNP only in men (r = 0.465, p = 0.002). The concentration of GDF-15 and TNFα (Figure 1Ab, Figure 1Bb), but not IGF-1 (Figure 1Cb), was negatively correlated with eGFR (Figure 1Ab, GDF-15, r = −0.768, p < 0.001; Figure 1Bb, TNFα, r = −0.551, p < 0.001) in all of the patients and both sexes (Table 2). Both GDF-15 and TNFα were negatively correlated with hemoglobin (Hb) in males (GDF-15, r = −0.560, p < 0.001; TNFα, r = −0.566, p < 0.001).

Table 3. Correlation matrix between various parameters and serum GDF-15, and TNFα, IGF-1 concentration.

	GDF-15 Males/Females	TNFα Males/Females	IGF-1 Males/Females
Age	0.436 (0.004) **/0.637 (<0.001) ***	0.244 (0.120)/0.261 (0.164)	−0.319 (0.036) */−0.339 (0.066)
BMI	−0.143 (0.367)/−0.062 (0.745)	−0.263 (0.092)/−0.055 (0.772)	0.047 (0.769)/0.194 (0.303)
HbA1C	−0.155 (0.340)/−0.229 (0.223)	−0.154 (0.342)/−0.127 (0.503)	0.261 (0.104)/0.344 (0.063)
BNP	0.427 (0.005) **/0.480 (0.007) **	0.465 (0.002) **/0.214 (0.257)	−0.059 (0.710)/−0.353 (0.055)
eGFR	−0.792 (<0.001) ***/−0.726 (<0.001) ***	−0.642 (<0.001) ***/−0.394 (0.031) *	0.144 (0.363)/0.301 (0.106)
Hb	−0.560 (<0.001) ***/−0.370 (0.044) *	−0.566 (<0.001) ***/−0.065 (0.732)	0.079 (0.617)/−0.006 (0.977)
Body fat percentage	−0.140 (0.403)/0.300 (0.128)	−0.146 (0.382)/0.135 (0.502)	−0.119 (0.479)/0.197 (0.326)
SMI	−0.392 (0.014) */−0.529 (0.005) **	−0.368 (0.021) */−0.189 (0.346)	0.313 (0.053)/0.153 (0.446)
Hand-grip	−0.456 (0.002) **/−0.656 (<0.001) ***	−0.393 (0.010) */−0.298 (0.117)	0.240 (0.126)/0.244 (0.202)
Knee extension	−0.222 (0.169)/−0.541 (0.003) **	−0.431 (0.005) **/−0.192 (0.329)	0.140 (0.390)/0.061 (0.758)
Gait speed	−0.218 (0.165)/−0.558 (0.002) **	−0.190 (0.229)/−0.336 (0.074)	0.256 (0.102)/0.253 (0.186)
Anterior TMth (supine)	−0.636 (<0.001) ***/−0.391 (0.044) *	−0.509 (0.001) **/−0.200 (0.316)	0.429 (0.005) **/0.057 (0.779)
Anterior TMth (standing)	−0.600 (<0.001) ***/−0.557 (0.003) **	−0.434 (0.005) **/−0.267 (0.178)	0.366 (0.020) */0.301 (0.127)
GDF-15	-/-	0.657 (<0.001) **/0.434 (0.017) *	−0.203 (0.198)/−0.553 (0.002) **
TNFα	0.657 (<0.001) ***/0.434 (0.017) *	-/-	−0.233 (0.137)/−0.479 (0.007) **

* p < 0.05 ** p < 0.01 *** p < 0.001. SMI, skeletal muscle mass index; TMth, thigh muscle thickness.

Table 3 also shows the relationships between serum GDF-15, TNFα, IGF-1 concentrations and the physical data. Figure 2 shows the correlations between serum GDF-15, TNFα, IGF-1 concentrations and the physical data in men. The serum GDF-15 level was negatively correlated with hand-grip strength, SMI, anterior TMth (supine, and standing) in both males and females, as shown in Table 3. As shown in Figure 2, there was a negative correlation between the serum GDF-15 level and both anterior TMth (supine) (r = −0.636, p < 0.001, Figure 2Aa), and hand-grip strength (r = −0.456, p = 0.002, Figure 2Ab) in men. Similar results were obtained in females as shown in Table 3. On the other hand, a negative correlation was observed between the serum TNFα level and grip strength, knee extension strength, SMI, and anterior TMth (supine, standing) in males, but not in females (Table 3). A negative correlation between the serum TNFα level and both anterior TMth (supine) (r = −0.509, p = 0.001, Figure 2Ba), and grip strength (r = −0.393, p = 0.010, Figure 2Bb) was observed in men. On the other hand, a positive correlation was observed between the serum IGF-1 level and anterior TMth (supine) in men (r = 0.429,

$p = 0.005$, Figure 2Ca, Table 3), but not hand-grip strength ($r = 0.240$, $p = 0.126$, Figure 2Cb, Table 3). Furthermore, there were no correlations between the serum IGF-1 level and anterior TMth (supine, and standing) in females.

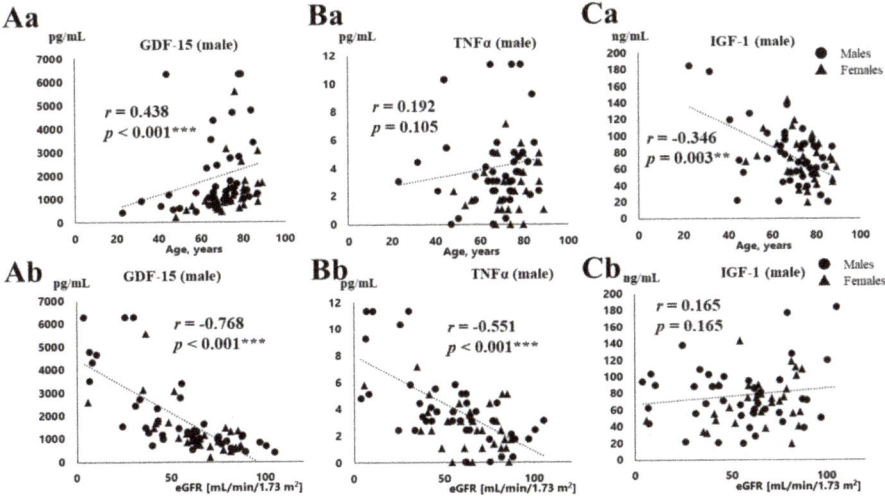

Figure 1. Correlations between clinical data (age, eGFR) and serum concentrations of GDF-15, TNF-α, and IGF-1. Relationships between laboratory data (age (**a**), eGFR (**b**)) and serum concentrations of GDF-15 (**Aa,Ab**), TNF-α (**Ba,Bb**) and IGF-1 (**Ca,Cb**) in males and females. ** $p < 0.01$, *** $p < 0.001$.

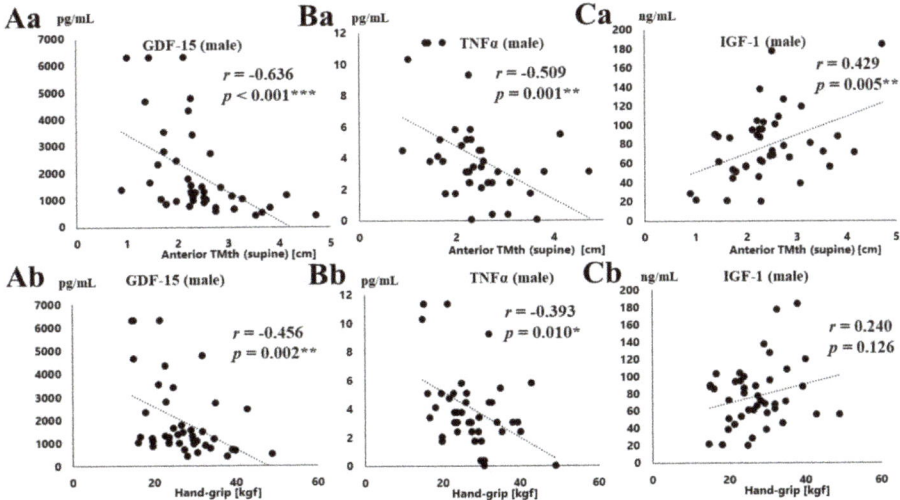

Figure 2. Correlations between the physical data (anterior thigh muscle thickness, grip strength) and serum concentrations of GDF-15, TNF-α, and IGF-1. Relationships between the laboratory data (anterior thigh muscle thickness (TMth, supine) (**a**), grip strength (**b**) and serum concentrations of GDF-15 (**Aa,Ab**), TNF-α (**Ba,Bb**) and IGF-1 (**Ca,Cb**) in males * $p < 0.05$, ** $p < 0.01$, *** $p < 0.001$.

3.3. Relationships among Serum GDF-15, TNFα, and IGF-1 Concentration

Table 3 shows the relationships among the serum GDF-15, TNFα, and IGF-1 concentrations. The serum level of GDF-15 was positively correlated with that of TNFα in both sexes (males, r = 0.657,

$p < 0.001$; females, $r = 0.434$, $p = 0.017$). A negative correlation was observed between the serum IGF-1 concentration and GDF-15 ($r = -0.553$, $p = 0.002$) and TNFα ($r = -0.479$, $p = 0.007$) in females, but not males.

3.4. Multiple Regression Analysis of Serum GDF-15 Levels and the Clinical Parameters

The linear regression analysis with serum GDF-15 levels as the dependent variable and clinical data (eGFR, BNP, Hb, SMI, hand-grip strength and anterior TMth (supine) as independent variable were investigated in all of the patients as shown in Table 4A. Univariate regression analysis (Table 4A) showed that eGFR (β = −0.650, $p < 0.001$), and anterior TMth (supine) (β = −0.358, $p = 0.001$) were independent variable to predict serum GDF-15 levels. Multiple regression analysis also showed that eGFR (β = −0.597, $p < 0.001$) and anterior TMth (supine) (β = −0.272, $p = 0.019$) were the independent determinants of GDF-15 concentration after adjusting for age, sex, and body mass index.

Table 4. Multiple linear regression analysis between serum GDF-15 levels and the clinical parameters.

A: Multiple linear regression analysis of GDF15 and the clinical data				
	Dependent variable: log (GDF−15)			
	Model 1	Model 2	Model 3	Model 4
Independent variable.	β-value (p)	β-value (p)	β-value (p)	β-value (p)
eGFR	−0.650 (<0.001) ***	−0.655 (<0.001) ***	−0.613 (<0.001) ***	−0.597 (<0.001) ***
BNP (log)	−0.009 (0.929)	−0.011 (0.912)	−0.042 (0.649)	−0.040 (0.663)
Hb	−0.106 (0.257)	−0.110 (0.253)	−0.079 (0.372)	−0.084 (0.343)
SMI	0.036 (0.722)	0.031 (0.771)	−0.171 (0.139)	−0.196 (0.098)
Hand−grip strength	0.106 (0.312)	0.323 (0.104)	−0.105 (0.367)	−0.059 (0.632)
Anterior TMth (supine)	−0.358 (0.001) **	−0.362 (0.001) **	−0.233 (0.033) *	−0.272 (0.019) *
B: Multiple linear regression analysis of anterior thigh muscle thickness (supine) and serum markers				
	Dependent variable: anterior thigh muscle thickness (supine)			
	Model 1	Model 2	Model 3	Model 4
Independent variable	β-value (p)	β-value (p)	β-value (p)	β-value (p)
GDF−15 (log)	−0.401 (0.005) **	−0.311 (0.024) *	−0.384 (0.007) **	−0.390 (0.004) **
TNFα (log)	−0.007 (0.955)	−0.054 (0.671)	−0.068 (0.584)	−0.054 (0.644)
IGF−1	0.256 (0.031) *	0.094 (0.456)	0.071 (0.656)	0.078 (0.506)
C: Multiple linear regression analysis of eGFR and the clinical data				
	Dependent variable: eGFR			
	Model 1	Model 2	Model 3	Model 4
Independent variable	β-value (p)	β-value (p)	β-value (p)	β-value (p)
BNP (log)	−0.164 (0.070)	−0.149 (0.106)	−0.149 (0.113)	−0.170 (0.070)
hsCRP (log)	−0.070 (0.377)	−0.094 (0.262)	−0.097 (0.257)	−0.085 (0.999)
Hb	0.035 (0.685)	0.005 (0.958)	0.002 (0.984)	0.011 (0.657)
GDF−15 (log)	−0.583 (<0.001) ***	−0.571 (<0.001) ***	−0.577 (<0.001) ***	−0.565 (<0.001) ***
TNFα (log)	−0.177 (0.069)	−0.196 (0.050)	−0.198 (0.050)	−0.197 (0.050)

Model 1, unadjusted; Model 2, adjusted by age; Model 3, adjusted by age and sex; Model 4, adjusted by age, sex, and BMI.

Alternatively, multiple regression analysis showed that GDF-15 (β = −0.390, $p = 0.004$) was the independent determinant of anterior TMth (supine), even adjusting for age, sex, and BMI (Table 4B).

The regression analysis between eGFR and the clinical data (BNP, CRP, Hb, GDF-15, and TNFα) were performed as shown in Table 4C. Multiple regression analysis showed that GDF-15 (β = −0.565, $p < 0.001$) and TNFα (β = −0.197, $p = 0.050$) were the independent variable to predict eGFR after adjusting for age, sex, and BMI. These results suggest that the serum GDF-15 concentration is a predictor for low eGFR. The ROC curves were plotted to identify the optimal cut-off levels of GDF-15, TNFα, and Hb for detecting eGFR lower than 60 mL/min/1.73 m^2, which was approximately the same value as the mean eGFR (58.2 mL/min/1.73 m^2). To construct the ROC curves, different cut-off values of GDF-15, TNFα, and Hb were used to predict eGFR lower than 60 mL/min/1.73 m^2, with true positives plotted on the vertical axis (sensitivity) and false-positives (1-specificity) plotted on the horizontal axis. The area under the curves (AUCs) for GDF-15, TNFα, and Hb were 92.1%, 78.6%, and 67.5%, respectively. Sensitivity and specificity were 88.2% and 82.9% for GDF-15, 81.8% and 61.5% for TNFα, and 45% and 83% for Hb, respectively. The optimal cut-off value of GDF-15 was 1154 pg/mL as shown in Figure 3.

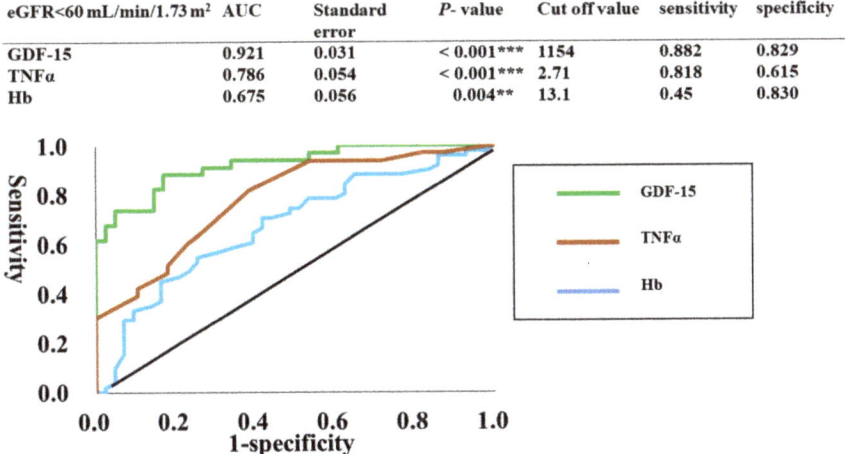

Figure 3. ROC curves to identify the optimal cut-off level of GDF-15, TNFα, and Hb for detecting eGFR < 60. In the ROC curves shown, different cut-off values of GDF-15, and TNFα, and Hb were used to predict eGFR < 60, with true positives plotted on the vertical axis (sensitivity) and Figure 1. plotted on the horizontal axis.

3.5. Relationships between Sarcopenia and Serum Concentration of GDF-15, TNFα and IGF-1

Sarcopenia was identified in 24 (36%) of a total of 66 patients evaluated based on the sarcopenia criteria. Serum GDF-15, TNFα and IGF-1 levels were compared in patients with and without sarcopenia (Table 5). Patients with sarcopenia had significantly higher age and BNP levels in both males and females, compared to those without sarcopenia (Table 5). On the other hand, they had significant lower gait speed, hand-grip strength, extension strength, SMI, and anterior TMth (supine, standing). Furthermore, both males and females with sarcopenia had significantly higher GDF-15 levels, compared to those without sarcopenia (males, 1483 ± 1125 pg/mL vs. 3053 ± 2346 pg/m, $p < 0.05$; females, 891 ± 700 pg/mL vs. 1625 ± 1302 pg/mL, $p < 0.05$). The TNFα concentration was significantly higher in males with than without sarcopenia (3.06 ± 1.95 pg/mL vs. 6.07 ± 3.27 pg/mL, $p < 0.01$). IGF-1 levels did not significantly differ between patients with and without sarcopenia in both males and females.

Table 5. Differences in clinical data between the patients with and without sarcopenia.

	Male		Female	
	Sarcopenia (−)	Sarcopenia (+)	Sarcopenia (−)	Sarcopenia (+)
Number	28	11	14	13
Age (years)	63.4 (14.2)	75.6 (10.8) ***	68.9 (10.5)	76.2 (7.3) *
BMI (kg/m^2)	26.0 (4.8)	22.6 (3.0) *	24.9 (3.1)	25.9 (7.3)
Physical capacity				
Gait speed (m/s)	1.08 (0.34)	0.77 (0.28) *	1.01 (0.17)	0.73 (0.32) *
Grip strength (kgf)	30.0 (7.4)	20.2 (4.4) ***	20.1 (3.1)	13.9 (3.5) ***
Knee extension (kgf)	26.9 (8.4)	17.5 (7.3) **	19.2 (7.5)	13.6 (4.8)*
BIA findings				
Body fat percentage (%)	28.8 (7.4)	27.9 (8.9)	35.7 (6.6)	39.8 (10.3)
Skeletal muscle mass index (SMI) (kg/m^2)	7.68 (1.15)	5.90 (0.53) ***	6.05 (0.53)	4.74 (0.63) ***
Muscle thickness				
Anterior TMth (supine) (cm)	2.64 (0.68)	1.65 (0.53) ***	2.45 (0.68)	1.89 (0.48) *
Anterior TMth (standing) (cm)	3.98 (0.88)	2.78 (0.46) ***	3.70 (0.74)	2.77 (0.79) **
HbA1c, %	6.3 (0.9)	6.4 (1.3)	6.12 (0.98)	5.97 (0.60)
BNP, pg/mL	209 (285)	646 (722) **	162 (250)	366 (427) *
eGFR, ml/min/1.73 m^2	59.7 (26.4)	47.9 (26.1)	70.6 (14.4)	56.1 (22.1)
Hb, g/dL	13.0 (1.6)	11.0 (1.7)	12.5 (1.7)	11.5 (1.6)
hsCRP, mg/L	7.1 (12.7)	9.9 (18.5)	4.5 (11.3)	2.0 (2.3)
GDF-15, pg/mL	1483 (1125)	3053 (2346) *	891 (700)	1625 (1302) *
TNFα, pg/mL	3.06 (1.95)	6.07 (3.27) **	2.23 (2.10)	2.92 (1.66)
IGF-1, ng/mL	84.1 (40.0)	62.7 (25.6)	74.7 (23.6)	70.6 (34.6)

* $p < 0.05$. ** $p < 0.01$***. $p < 0.001$. Males vs. Females.

4. Discussion

The major findings of the present study are as follows: (1) In preoperative cardiovascular surgery patients, the circulating GDF-15 level was correlated with age, BNP, and eGFR. It also had a negative correlation with SMI, hand-grip strength, and anterior TMth. The GDF-15 levels were significantly higher in sarcopenia patients. (2) In multivariate analysis, eGFR and anterior TMth were independent determinants of GDF-15 concentration after adjusting for age, sex, and BMI. Furthermore, the GDF-15 level was an independent determinant of eGFR and anterior TMth. These results suggests that an increased GDF-15 level reflects muscle wasting as well as renal dysfunction in preoperative cardiovascular surgery patients. Thus, GDF-15 may be a novel biomarker for identifying high-risk patients with muscle wasting and renal dysfunction in cardiovascular surgery patients.

4.1. Association of Serum GDF-15 Levels with eGFR

The present study showed that the preoperative GDF-15 level in patients undergoing cardiovascular surgery including CABG and AVR was positively associated with age, eGFR, and BNP. This is compatible with the previous paper showing that preoperative GDF-15 levels in patients undergoing CABG were positively associated with age, chronic renal failure, and high NT-proBNP [25]. Clinical studies have also shown that the GDF-15 concentration correlated strongly with age in healthy elderly individuals and patients with coronary artery diseases [20,28]. GDF-15 is expressed in various tissue types such as kidneys, macrophages, cardiomyocytes, and endothelial cells. The expression occurs in response to various stimuli including oxidative and metabolic stress, tissue injury, and inflammation [10–12]. It has been reported that an increase in GDF-15 levels in community-based patients is associated with endothelial dysfunction and subclinical cardiovascular disease [35].

Moreover, clinical trials have shown that GDF-15 can be regarded as a reliable biomarker of CVD [13–15], and chronic heart failure [16]. In addition, GDF-15 is a novel serum biomarker of mortality in CKD and can identify patients at high risk of developing CKD [21,22]. The presence and progression of CVD are often intimately associated with CKD [36,37]. Valvular heart disease, specifically aortic stenosis, is also a well-known complication of renal dysfunction [38,39]. Gibson et al. [40] utilized eGFR in the analysis of outcomes after valve replacement. They showed that a decrease in eGFR of 10 mL/min/1.73 m^2 corresponded to a 31% increase in the risk of postoperative death, and eGFR less than 60 mL/min/1.73 m^2 was the most useful variable in predicting 30 day and midterm mortality. The postoperative GDF-15 value has also been reported to reflect post-operative acute kidney injury (AKI) in CABG patients [27]. In our study, using multivariate analysis, eGFR was an independent determinant of the preoperative GDF-15 level, even after adjusting for age, sex, and BMI. In addition, the GDF-15 level, was an independent determinant of eGFR. In ROC curve analysis, different cut-off levels of GDF-15 were used to predict eGFR lower than 60 mL/min/1.73 m^2, and the AUCs was 92.1% with an optimal cut-off value of 1154 pg/mL. Given that the normal range for human serum GDF-15 level has been reported to be 150-1150 pg/mL [41], and 733-999 pg/mL [42], the cut-off value of 1154 pg/mL shown in our study appears to be a reasonable value for detecting CKD in patients hospitalized for cardiovascular surgery. Thus, GDF-15 appears to be a novel biomarker for identifying surgical risk in patients undergoing cardiovascular surgery. However, further studies using postoperative follow-up are needed to clarify whether the preoperative GDF-15 level can be used as a novel biomarker to identify surgical risk in patients undergoing cardiovascular surgery.

4.2. Association of Serum GDF-15 Levels with Muscle Loss

In cardiac surgery such as TAVI, frailty is identified as a major predictor of adverse outcomes in older surgical patients [1,3–5]. Sarcopenia, the skeletal muscle loss associated with aging, also includes low physical function (grip strength, walking speed) as a component of frailty [6,7]. Sarcopenia is frequently associated with chronic diseases including heart failure, COPD, CKD, cancer, wasting, and cachexia [7]. Thus, frailty and sarcopenia increase the risk of complications and mortality when cardiovascular surgery is performed. We have previously shown that the prevalence of sarcopenia including sarcopenic obesity in CVD patients was 47.5% in males and 60.2% in females [34]. In the present study using preoperative cardiovascular surgery patients, sarcopenia was identified in 36%. In these cardiovascular surgery patients, we found that the circulating GDF-15 level had a negative correlation with SMI, hand-grip strength, and anterior TMth. In multivariate analysis, the GDF-15 level was an independent determinant of anterior TMth, even after correction for age, gender, and BMI. In addition, preoperative GDF-15 levels were significantly higher in those with than without sarcopenia. The results were consistent with previous reports showing that the circulating GDF-15 concentration was negatively correlated with the cross-sectional area of rectus femoris in COPD [30], ICU [32], and cancer patients [33]. Bloch et al. [31] showed that patients who show wasting of the rectus femoris following cardiac surgery are exposed to a more sustained elevation of GDF-15 than those without muscle wasting. Moreover, several recent papers reported the relationships between GDF-15 levels and physical function such as gait speed, and hand-grip strength in community-dwelling older adults [43,44]. In the present study, a significant relationship between hand-grip strength/knee extension and the GDF-15 level was observed in preoperative cardiovascular surgery patients. From these results, it is very likely that circulating preoperative GDF-15 level may be a biomarker for identifying muscle wasting and sarcopenia in cardiovascular surgery patients.

Several mechanisms underlying GDF-15-induced muscle wasting have been proposed. First, an increase of GDF-15 may cause appetite loss, anorexia, and cachexia as shown in patients with cancer [41,45]. Animal studies also showed that GDF15 causes anorexia/cachexia, and then weight loss through a direct effect on the hypothalamus [46,47]. On the other hand, animal studies showed that local over-expression of GDF-15 in mice causes wasting of the tibialis anterior muscle directly [30], and the in vitro studies using C2C12 myotubes showed that GDF-15 treatment elevates expression of muscle atrophy-related genes, and causes muscle wasting, possibly by a direct effect of GDF-15 on skeletal muscle [32]. Further studies are required to clarify the mechanisms of action of GDF-15 on muscle wasting in patients with CVD including cardiovascular surgery.

4.3. Relationships between GDF-15 and TNFα, IGF-1 Concentration

It has been reported that several pro-inflammatory cytokines including TNFα are associated with cachexia and anorexia in both humans and rodents [48,49]. Higher concentrations of TNFα are also associated with a decline in muscle mass and grip strength in older persons [50]. In addition, systemic inflammation and increased circulating TNFα levels have been implicated in various conditions accompanied by muscle atrophy [51]. GDF-15 has been reported to be induced by inflammatory cytokines such as TNFα [10]. In our study, the serum GDF-15 level was positively correlated with the TNFα level, and a correlation was observed between TNFα and muscle mass and grip strength in men. However, multivariate regression analysis showed that that GDF-15, but not TNFα, was the independent determinant of anterior TMth (supine), even adjusting for age, sex, and BMI. These results suggest that GDF-15 is an independent marker of muscle mass, irrespective of TNF-α. Moreover, IGF-1 levels decrease with age and are regarded as a potential mediator of sarcopenia or frailty [52]. Wang et al. [53] showed that GDF-15 inhibits the release of IGF-1 from the liver in children with concomitant disease and failure. In our study, a negative correlation between GDF-15 and IGF-1 concentrations was observed only in females, but not in males. The reason of this sex discrepancy remains unknown. However, whereas the present study showed that IGF-1 was correlated negatively with age and positively with muscle mass, and anterior TMth, there were no significant differences in IGF-1 levels between patients with and without sarcopenia. Furthermore, we found no relationships between IGF-1 levels and hand-grip/extension strength. Thus, the contribution of serum IGF-1 levels to sarcopenia and muscle wasting remains unclear in our cardiovascular surgery patients.

4.4. Limitations

This study has several limitations. First, the results do not imply causality, because it was a cross-sectional study. Second, the study had a small number of cardiovascular surgery patients, especially females, and the patients underwent different types of cardiovascular surgery. Therefore, our findings are not necessarily applicable to the general population of cardiovascular surgery patients. Furthermore, most of the subjects had medical treatment. The use of drugs such as β-blockers, ACE-I, and ARB might have affected serum cytokine level. Therefore, the further studies using a large number of patients are required to clarify the pathophysiological roles of GDF-15 in preoperative cardiovascular surgery patients.

5. Conclusions

An elevated GDF-15 level reflects muscle wasting as well as renal dysfunction in preoperative cardiovascular surgery patients. Thus, serum GDF-15 concentration may be a novel biomarker for identifying high-risk patients with muscle wasting and renal dysfunction in cardiovascular surgery patients.

Author Contributions: Conceptualization, T.N. (Toshiaki Nakajima); methodology, A.H.; Resources, T.N. (Toshiaki Nakajima); formal analysis, T.S., T.N. (Toshiaki Nakajima); investigation, H.K., T.N. (Takafumi Nakajima), T.H.; T.A., S.O., S.A., M.S., S.T.; data curation, I.S., H.O.; supervision, F.N., H.F., T.I.; Funding acquisition, T.N. (Toshiaki Nakajima).

Funding: This study was supported in part by JSPS KAKENHI Grant Number 19H03981, 19H03981 (to T.N.).

Conflicts of Interest: The authors declare no conflict of interest.

Abbreviations

CVD	cardiovascular disease
CABG	coronary artery bypass graft
AVR	aortic valve replacement
MVR	mitral valve replacement
MVP	mitral valve plasty
TVP	tricuspid valve plasty
TAVI	transcatheter valve implantation procedure
TVR	tricuspid valve replacement
TAR	total arch replacement
EVAR	endovascular aneurysm repair
BMI	body mass index
NYHA	New York Heart Association
TNFα	tumor necrosis factor α
GDF-15	growth differentiation factor-15
IGF-1	insulin growth factor 1
TGF-β;	transforming growth factor β
SMI	skeletal muscle mass index
BNP	brain natriuretic peptide
eGFR	estimated glomerular filtration rate
hsCRP	high-sensitivity C-reactive protein
ROC	receiver operating characteristic
AUC	area under the curve
TMth	thigh muscle thickness
COPD	chronic obstructive pulmonary disease
HbA1c	hemoglobin A1c
MVIC	maximum voluntary isometric contraction
ELISA	enzyme-linked immunosorbent assay
ICU	intensive care unit
ACS	acute coronary syndrome
AKI	acute kidney disease
BIA	bioelectric impedance analyzer
HF	heart failure
HT	hypertension
HD	hemodialysis
CKD	chronic kidney disease

References

1. Partridge, J.S.; Harari, D.; Dhesi, J.K. Frailty in the older surgical patient: A review. *Age Ageing* **2012**, *41*, 142–147. [CrossRef] [PubMed]
2. Clegg, A.; Young, J.; Iliffe, S.; Rikkert, M.O.; Rockwood, K. Frailty in elderly people. *Lancet* **2013**, *381*, 752–762. [CrossRef]
3. Makary, M.A.; Segev, D.L.; Pronovost, P.J.; Syin, D.; Bandeen-Roche, K.; Patel, P.; Takenaga, R.; Devgan, L.; Holzmueller, C.G.; Tian, J.; et al. Frailty as a predictor of surgical outcomes in older patients. *J. Am. Coll. Surg.* **2010**, *210*, 901–908. [CrossRef] [PubMed]
4. Shimura, T.; Yamamoto, M.; Kano, S.; Kagase, A.; Kodama, A.; Koyama, Y.; Tsuchikane, E.; Suzuki, T.; Otsuka, T.; Kohsaka, S.; et al. OCEAN-TAVI Investigators. Impact of the Clinical Frailty Scale on Outcomes After Transcatheter Aortic Valve Replacement. *Circulation* **2017**, *135*, 2013–2024. [CrossRef] [PubMed]
5. Afilalo, J.; Alexander, K.P.; Mack, M.J.; Maurer, M.S.; Green, P.; Allen, L.A. Frailty assessment in the cardiovascular care of older adults. *J. Am. Coll. Cardiol.* **2014**, *63*, 747–762. [CrossRef]
6. Rosenberg, I.H. Sarcopenia: Origins and clinical relevance. *J. Nutr.* **1997**, *127* (Suppl. 5), 990S–991S. [CrossRef]

7. Chen, L.K.; Liu, L.K.; Woo, J.; Assantachai, P.; Auyeung, T.W.; Bahyah, K.S.; Chou, M.Y.; Chen, L.Y.; Hsu, P.S.; Krairit, O.; et al. Sarcopenia in Asia: Consensus report of the Asian Working Group for Sarcopenia. *J. Am. Med. Dir. Assoc.* **2014**, *15*, 95–101. [CrossRef]
8. Mimeault, M.; Batra, S.K. Divergent molecular mechanisms underlying the pleiotropic functions of macrophage inhibitory cytokine-1 in cancer. *J. Cell. Physiol.* **2010**, *224*, 626–635. [CrossRef]
9. Shi, Y.; Massagué, J. Mechanisms of TGF-beta signaling from cell membrane to the nucleus. *Cell* **2003**, *113*, 685–700. [CrossRef]
10. Bootcov, M.R.; Bauskin, A.R.; Valenzuela, S.M.; Moore, A.G.; Bansal, M.; He, X.Y.; Zhang, H.P.; Donnellan, M.; Mahler, S.; Pryor, K.; et al. MIC-1, a novel macrophage inhibitory cytokine, is a divergent member of the TGF-beta superfamily. *Proc. Natl. Acad. Sci. USA* **1997**, *94*, 11514–11519. [CrossRef]
11. Dandrea, T.; Hellmold, H.; Jonsson, C.; Zhivotovsky, B.; Hofer, T.; Wärngård, L.; Cotgreave, I. The transcriptosomal response of human A549 lung cells to a hydrogen peroxide-generating system: Relationship to DNA damage, cell cycle arrest, and caspase activation. *Free Radic. Biol. Med.* **2004**, *36*, 881–896. [CrossRef] [PubMed]
12. Kempf, T.; Eden, M.; Strelau, J.; Naguib, M.; Willenbockel, C.; Tongers, J.; Heineke, J.; Kotlarz, D.; Xu, J.; Molkentin, J.D.; et al. The transforming growth factor-beta superfamily member growth-differentiation factor-15 protects the heart from ischemia/reperfusion injury. *Circ. Res.* **2006**, *98*, 351–360. [CrossRef] [PubMed]
13. Lind, L.; Wallentin, L.; Kempf, T.; Tapken, H.; Quint, A.; Lindahl, B.; Olofsson, S.; Venge, P.; Larsson, A.; Hulthe, J.; et al. Growth-differentiation factor-15 is an independent marker of cardiovascular dysfunction and disease in the elderly: Results from the Prospective Investigation of the Vasculature in Uppsala Seniors (PIVUS) Study. *Eur. Heart J.* **2009**, *30*, 2346–2353. [CrossRef] [PubMed]
14. Eggers, K.M.; Kempf, T.; Wallentin, L.; Wollert, K.C.; Lind, L. Change in growth differentiation factor 15 concentrations over time independently predicts mortality in community-dwelling elderly individuals. *Clin. Chem.* **2013**, *59*, 1091–1098. [CrossRef] [PubMed]
15. Wollert, K.C.; Kempf, T.; Wallentin, L. Growth Differentiation Factor 15 as a Biomarker in Cardiovascular Disease. *Clin. Chem.* **2017**, *63*, 140–151. [CrossRef] [PubMed]
16. George, M.; Jena, A.; Srivatsan, V.; Muthukumar, R.; Dhandapani, V.E. GDF 15-A Novel Biomarker in the Offing for Heart Failure. *Curr. Cardiol. Rev.* **2016**, *12*, 37–46. [CrossRef] [PubMed]
17. Preeshagul, I.; Gharbaran, R.; Jeong, K.H.; Abdel-Razek, A.; Lee, L.Y.; Elman, E.; Suh, K.S. Potential biomarkers for predicting outcomes in CABG cardiothoracic surgeries. *J. Cardiothorac. Surg.* **2013**, *8*, 176. [CrossRef]
18. Wollert, K.C.; Kempf, T.; Lagerqvist, B.; Lindahl, B.; Olofsson, S.; Allhoff, T.; Peter, T.; Siegbahn, A.; Venge, P.; Drexler, H.; et al. Growth differentiation factor 15 for risk stratification and selection of an invasive treatment strategy in non ST-elevation acute coronary syndrome. *Circulation* **2007**, *116*, 1540–1548. [CrossRef]
19. Khan, S.Q.; Ng, K.; Dhillon, O.; Kelly, D.; Quinn, P.; Squire, I.B.; Davies, J.E.; Ng, L.L. Growth differentiation factor-15 as a prognostic marker in patients with acute myocardial infarction. *Eur. Heart J.* **2009**, *30*, 1057–1065. [CrossRef]
20. Kempf, T.; von Haehling, S.; Peter, T.; Allhoff, T.; Cicoira, M.; Doehner, W.; Ponikowski, P.; Filippatos, G.S.; Rozentryt, P.; Drexler, H.; et al. Prognostic utility of growth differentiation factor-15 in patients with chronic heart failure. *J. Am. Coll. Cardiol.* **2007**, *50*, 1054–1060. [CrossRef]
21. Breit, S.N.; Carrero, J.J.; Tsai, V.W.; Yagoutifam, N.; Luo, W.; Kuffner, T.; Bauskin, A.R.; Wu, L.; Jiang, L.; Barany, P.; et al. Macrophage inhibitory cytokine-1 (MIC-1/GDF15) and mortality in end-stage renal disease. *Nephrol. Dial. Transplant.* **2012**, *27*, 70–75. [CrossRef] [PubMed]
22. Ho, J.E.; Hwang, S.J.; Wollert, K.C.; Larson, M.G.; Cheng, S.; Kempf, T.; Vasan, R.S.; Januzzi, J.L.; Wang, T.J.; Fox, C.S. Biomarkers of cardiovascular stress and incident chronic kidney disease. *Clin. Chem.* **2013**, *59*, 1613–1620. [CrossRef] [PubMed]
23. Nair, V.; Robinson-Cohen, C.; Smith, M.R.; Bellovich, K.A.; Bhat, Z.Y.; Bobadilla, M.; Brosius, F.; de Boer, I.H.; Essioux, L.; Formentini, I.; et al. Growth Differentiation Factor-15 and Risk of CKD Progression. *J. Am. Soc. Nephrol.* **2017**, *28*, 2233–2240. [CrossRef] [PubMed]
24. Heringlake, M.; Charitos, E.I.; Gatz, N.; Käbler, J.H.; Beilharz, A.; Holz, D.; Schön, J.; Paarmann, H.; Petersen, M.; Hanke, T. Growth differentiation factor 15: A novel risk marker adjunct to the EuroSCORE for risk stratification in cardiac surgery patients. *J. Am. Coll. Cardiol.* **2013**, *66*, 672–681. [CrossRef] [PubMed]

25. Kahli, A.; Guenancia, C.; Zeller, M.; Grosjean, S.; Stamboul, K.; Rochette, L.; Girard, C.; Vergely, C. Growth differentiation factor-15 (GDF-15) levels are associated with cardiac and renal injury in patients undergoing coronary artery bypass grafting with cardiopulmonary bypass. *PLoS ONE* **2014**, *9*, e105759. [CrossRef] [PubMed]
26. Krau, N.C.; Lünstedt, N.S.; Freitag-Wolf, S.; Brehm, D.; Petzina, R.; Lutter, G.; Bramlage, P.; Dempfle, A.; Frey, N.; Frank, D. Elevated growth differentiation factor 15 levels predict outcome in patients undergoing transcatheter aortic valve implantation. *Eur. J. Heart Fail.* **2015**, *17*, 945–955. [CrossRef] [PubMed]
27. Guenancia, C.; Kahli, A.; Laurent, G.; Hachet, O.; Malapert, G.; Grosjean, S.; Girard, C.; Vergely, C.; Bouchot, O. Pre-operative growth differentiation factor 15 as a novel biomarker of acute kidney injury after cardiac bypass surgery. *Int. J. Cardiol.* **2015**, *197*, 66–71. [CrossRef] [PubMed]
28. Yuan, Z.; Li, H.; Qi, Q.; Gong, W.; Qian, C.; Dong, R.; Zang, Y.; Li, J.; Zhou, M.; Cai, J.; et al. Plasma levels of growth differentiation factor-15 are associated with myocardial injury in patients undergoing off-pump coronary artery bypass grafting. *Sci. Rep.* **2016**, *6*, 28221. [CrossRef]
29. Fujita, Y.; Taniguchi, Y.; Shinkai, S.; Tanaka, M.; Ito, M. Secreted growth differentiation factor 15 as a potential biomarker for mitochondrial dysfunctions in aging and age-related disorders. *Geriatr. Gerontol. Int.* **2016**, *16* (Suppl. 1), 17–29. [CrossRef]
30. Patel, M.S.; Lee, J.; Baz, M.; Wells, C.E.; Bloch, S.; Lewis, A.; Donaldson, A.V.; Garfield, B.E.; Hopkinson, N.S.; Natanek, A.; et al. Growth differentiation factor-15 is associated with muscle mass in chronic obstructive pulmonary disease and promotes muscle wasting in vivo. *J. Cachexia Sarcopenia Muscle* **2016**, *7*, 436–448. [CrossRef]
31. Bloch, S.A.; Lee, J.Y.; Wort, S.J.; Polkey, M.I.; Kemp, P.R.; Griffiths, M.J. Sustained elevation of circulating growth and differentiation factor-15 and a dynamic imbalance in mediators of muscle homeostasis are associated with the development of acute muscle wasting following cardiac surgery. *Crit. Care Med.* **2013**, *41*, 982–989. [CrossRef] [PubMed]
32. Bloch, S.A.; Lee, J.Y.; Syburra, T.; Rosendahl, U.; Griffiths, M.J.; Kemp, P.R.; Polkey, M.I. Increased expression of GDF-15 may mediate ICU-acquired weakness by down-regulating muscle microRNAs. *Thorax* **2015**, *70*, 219–228. [CrossRef] [PubMed]
33. Lerner, L.; Hayes, T.G.; Tao, N.; Krieger, B.; Feng, B.; Wu, Z.; Nicoletti, R.; Chiu, M.I.; Gyuris, J.; Garcia, J.M. Plasma growth differentiation factor 15 is associated with weight loss and mortality in cancer patients. *J. Cachexia Sarcopenia Muscle* **2015**, *6*, 317–324. [CrossRef] [PubMed]
34. Yasuda, T.; Nakajima, T.; Sawaguchi, T.; Nozawa, N.; Arakawa, T.; Takahashi, R.; Mizushima, Y.; Katayanagi, S.; Matsumoto, K.; Toyoda, S.; et al. Short Physical Performance Battery for cardiovascular disease inpatients: Implications for critical factors and sarcopenia. *Sci. Rep.* **2017**, *7*, 17425. [CrossRef] [PubMed]
35. Wang, T.J.; Gona, P.; Larson, M.G.; Tofler, G.H.; Levy, D.; Newton-Cheh, C.; Jacques, P.F.; Rifai, N.; Selhub, J.; Robins, S.J.; et al. Multiple biomarkers for the prediction of first major cardiovascular events and death. *N. Engl. J. Med.* **2006**, *355*, 2631–2639. [CrossRef]
36. Sarnak, M.J.; Levey, A.S.; Schoolwerth, A.C.; Coresh, J.; Culleton, B.; Hamm, L.L.; McCullough, P.A.; Kasiske, B.L.; Kelepouris, E.; Klag, M.J.; et al. American Heart Association Councils on Kidney in Cardiovascular Disease, High Blood Pressure Research, Clinical Cardiology, and Epidemiology and Prevention. Kidney disease as a risk factor for development of cardiovascular disease: A statement from the American Heart Association Councils on Kidney in Cardiovascular Disease, High Blood Pressure Research, Clinical Cardiology, and Epidemiology and Prevention. *Circulation* **2003**, *108*, 2154–2169. [PubMed]
37. Wali, R.K.; Henrich, W.L. Chronic kidney disease: A risk factor for cardiovascular disease. *Cardiol. Clin.* **2005**, *23*, 343–362. [CrossRef]
38. Ibáñez, J.; Riera, M.; Saez de Ibarra, J.I.; Carrillo, A.; Fernández, R.; Herrero, J.; Fiol, M.; Bonnin, O. Effect of preoperative mild renal dysfunction on mortality and morbidity following valve cardiac surgery. *Interact. Cardiovasc. Thorac. Surg.* **2007**, *6*, 748–752. [CrossRef] [PubMed]
39. Thourani, V.; Keeling, W.B.; Sarin, E.L.; Guyton, R.A.; Kilgo, P.D.; Dara, A.B.; Puskas, J.D.; Chen, E.P.; Cooper, W.A.; Vega, J.D.; et al. Impact of preoperative renal dysfunction on long-term survival for patients undergoing aortic valve replacement. *Ann. Thorac. Surg.* **2011**, *91*, 1798–1806. [CrossRef]
40. Gibson, P.H.; Croal, B.L.; Cuthbertson, B.H.; Chiwara, M.; Scott, A.E.; Buchan, K.G.; El-Shafei, H.; Gibson, G.; Jeffrey, R.R.; Hillis, G.S. The relationship between renal function and outcome from heart valve surgery. *Am. Heart J.* **2008**, *156*, 893–899. [CrossRef]

41. Bauskin, A.R.; Brown, D.A.; Kuffner, T.; Johnen, H.; Luo, X.W.; Hunter, M.; Breit, S.N. Role of macrophage inhibitory cytokine-1 in tumorigenesis and diagnosis of cancer. *Cancer Res.* **2006**, *66*, 4983–4986. [CrossRef]
42. Krintus, M.; Braga, F.; Kozinski, M.; Borille, S.; Kubica, J.; Sypniewska, G.; Panteghini, M. A study of biological and lifestyle factors, including within-subject variation, affecting concentrations of growth differentiation factor 15 in serum. *Clin. Chem. Lab. Med.* **2019**, *57*, 1035–1043. [CrossRef] [PubMed]
43. Rothenbacher, D.; Dallmeier, D.; Christow, H.; Koenig, W.; Denkinger, M.; Klenk, J.; ActiFE study group. Association of growth differentiation factor 15 with other key biomarkers, functional parameters and mortality in community-dwelling older adults. *Age Ageing* **2019**, *48*, 541–546. [CrossRef] [PubMed]
44. Semba, R.D.; Gonzalez-Freire, M.; Tanaka, T.; Biancotto, A.; Zhang, P.; Shardell, M.; Moaddel, R.; Ferrucci, L.; CHI Consortium. Elevated Plasma Growth and Differentiation Factor-15 is Associated with Slower Gait Speed and Lower Physical Performance in Healthy Community-Dwelling Adults. *J. Gerontol. A Biol. Sci. Med. Sci.* **2019**. [CrossRef]
45. Welsh, J.B.; Sapinoso, L.M.; Kern, S.G.; Brown, D.A.; Liu, T.; Bauskin, A.R.; Ward, R.L.; Hawkins, N.J.; Quinn, D.I.; Russell, P.J.; et al. Large-scale delineation of secreted protein biomarkers overexpressed in cancer tissue and serum. *Proc. Natl. Acad. Sci. USA* **2003**, *100*, 3410–3415. [CrossRef]
46. Johnen, H.; Lin, S.; Kuffner, T.; Brown, D.A.; Tsai, V.W.; Bauskin, A.R.; Wu, L.; Pankhurst, G.; Jiang, L.; Junankar, S.; et al. Tumor-induced anorexia and weight loss are mediated by the TGF-beta superfamily cytokine MIC-1. *Nat. Med.* **2007**, *13*, 1333–1340. [CrossRef] [PubMed]
47. Tsai, V.W.; Macia, L.; Johnen, H.; Kuffner, T.; Manadhar, R.; Jørgensen, S.B.; Lee-Ng, K.K.; Zhang, H.P.; Wu, L.; Marquis, C.P.; et al. TGF-b superfamily cytokine MIC-1/GDF15 is a physiological appetite and body weight regulator. *PLoS ONE* **2013**, *8*, e55174. [CrossRef]
48. Hubbard, R.E.; O'Mahony, M.S.; Savva, G.M.; Calver, B.L.; Woodhouse, K.W. Inflammation and frailty measures in older people. *J. Cell. Mol. Med.* **2009**, *13*, 3103–3109. [CrossRef] [PubMed]
49. Utech, A.E.; Tadros, E.M.; Hayes, T.G.; Garcia, J.M. Predicting survival in cancer patients: The role of cachexia and hormonal, nutritional and inflammatory markers. *J. Cachexia Sarcopenia Muscle* **2012**, *3*, 245–251. [CrossRef]
50. Schaap, L.A.; Pluijm, S.M.; Deeg, D.J.; Harris, T.B.; Kritchevsky, S.B.; Newman, A.B.; Colbert, L.H.; Pahor, M.; Rubin, S.M.; Tylavsky, F.A.; et al. Health ABC Study. Higher inflammatory marker levels in older persons: Associations with 5-year change in muscle mass and muscle strength. *J. Gerontol. A Biol. Sci. Med. Sci.* **2009**, *64*, 1183–1189. [CrossRef] [PubMed]
51. von Haehling, S.; Steinbeck, L.; Doehner, W.; Springer, J.; Anker, S.D. Muscle wasting in heart failure: An overview. *Int. J. Biochem. Cell Biol.* **2013**, *45*, 2257–2265. [CrossRef] [PubMed]
52. Leng, S.X.; Cappola, A.R.; Andersen, R.E.; Blackman, M.R.; Koenig, K.; Blair, M.; Walston, J.D. Serum levels of insulin-like growth factor-I (IGF-I) and dehydroepiandrosterone sulfate (DHEA-S), and their relationships with serum interleukin-6, in the geriatric syndrome of frailty. *Aging Clin. Exp. Res.* **2004**, *16*, 153–157. [CrossRef] [PubMed]
53. Wang, T.; Liu, J.; McDonald, C.; Lupino, K.; Zhai, X.; Wilkins, B.J.; Hakonarson, H.; Pei, L. GDF15 is a heart-derived hormone that regulates body growth. *EMBO. Mol. Med.* **2017**, *9*, 1150–1164. [CrossRef] [PubMed]

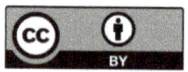

© 2019 by the authors. Licensee MDPI, Basel, Switzerland. This article is an open access article distributed under the terms and conditions of the Creative Commons Attribution (CC BY) license (http://creativecommons.org/licenses/by/4.0/).

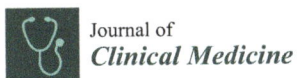 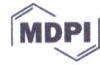

Article

Catestatin in Acutely Decompensated Heart Failure Patients: Insights from the CATSTAT-HF Study

Josip A. Borovac [1,2,3], Duska Glavas [3,4], Zora Susilovic Grabovac [3], Daniela Supe Domic [5,6], Domenico D'Amario [7] and Josko Bozic [1,*]

1. Department of Pathophysiology, University of Split School of Medicine, Soltanska 2, 21000 Split, Croatia
2. Institute of Emergency Medicine of Split-Dalmatia County (ZHM SDZ), Spinciceva 1, 21000 Split, Croatia
3. Clinic for Cardiovascular Diseases, University Hospital of Split, Spinciceva 1, 21000 Split, Croatia
4. Department of Internal Medicine, University of Split School of Medicine, Soltanska 2, 21000 Split, Croatia
5. Department of Medical Laboratory Diagnostics, University Hospital of Split, Spinciceva 1, 21000 Split, Croatia
6. Department of Health Studies, University of Split, Rudjera Boskovica 35, P.P. 464, 21000 Split, Croatia
7. Department of Cardiovascular and Thoracic Sciences, IRCCS Fondazione Policlinico A. Gemelli, Università Cattolica Sacro Cuore, Largo Francesco Vito 1, 00168 Rome, Italy
* Correspondence: josko.bozic@mefst.hr; Tel.: +385-21-557-871

Received: 24 June 2019; Accepted: 29 July 2019; Published: 30 July 2019

Abstract: The role of catestatin (CST) in acutely decompensated heart failure (ADHF) and myocardial infarction (MI) is poorly elucidated. Due to the implicated role of CST in the regulation of neurohumoral activity, the goals of the study were to determine CST serum levels among ninety consecutively enrolled ADHF patients, with respect to the MI history and left ventricular ejection fraction (LVEF) and to examine its association with clinical, echocardiographic, and laboratory parameters. CST levels were higher among ADHF patients with MI history, compared to those without (8.94 ± 6.39 vs. 4.90 ± 2.74 ng/mL, $p = 0.001$). CST serum levels did not differ among patients with reduced, midrange, and preserved LVEF (7.74 ± 5.64 vs. 5.75 ± 4.19 vs. 5.35 ± 2.77 ng/mL, $p = 0.143$, respectively). In the multivariable linear regression analysis, CST independently correlated with the NYHA class ($\beta = 0.491$, $p < 0.001$), waist-to-hip ratio (WHR) ($\beta = -0.237$, $p = 0.026$), HbA1c ($\beta = -0.235$, $p = 0.027$), LDL ($\beta = -0.231$, $p = 0.029$), non-HDL cholesterol ($\beta = -0.237$, $p = 0.026$), hs-cTnI ($\beta = -0.221$, $p = 0.030$), and the admission and resting heart rate ($\beta = -0.201$, $p = 0.036$ and $\beta = -0.242$, $p = 0.030$), and was in positive association with most echocardiographic parameters. In conclusion, CST levels were increased in ADHF patients with MI and were overall associated with a favorable cardiometabolic profile but at the same time reflected advanced symptomatic burden (CATSTAT-HF ClinicalTrials.gov number, NCT03389386).

Keywords: acute myocardial infarction; biomarkers; catestatin; coronary artery disease; heart failure; heart failure decompensation; left ventricular ejection fraction; troponin; NT-proBNP; NYHA functional class

1. Introduction

Acute decompensated heart failure (ADHF) is a complex clinical syndrome associated with high morbidity, mortality, and healthcare expenditures [1–3]. During the acute decompensation event, a cascade of multiple cellular pathways is activated and this activity can be quantified by measuring levels of circulating biomarkers [4]. Decades ago, Viquerat et al. showed that levels of endogenous norepinephrine and dopamine are elevated in patients with congestive heart failure (HF), compared to the healthy controls, thus, reflecting an increased sympathetic nervous system (SNS) activity [5]. Importantly, among patients with established HF, activation of the SNS, renin-angiotensin-aldosterone system (RAAS), and T-cell-mediated immune response is higher among those with ischemic etiology of the disease compared to non-ischemic idiopathic dilated cardiomyopathy [6]. Finally, patients with the ischemic HF also exhibit a higher resting muscle sympathetic nerve activity than patients with non-ischemic HF [7]. On the other hand, catestatin (CST) is a pleiotropic cardioprotective peptide that counterbalances the negative effects of SNS by promoting vasodilation [8] and by inhibiting catecholamine secretion [9,10]. Previous studies have demonstrated that high levels of CST might reflect increased sympathoadrenal activity [11–13], are associated with increased mortality in HF [14,15], and are a marker of poor ventricular remodeling after myocardial infarction (MI) [16]. Furthermore, CST levels were associated with disease severity in HF [17,18] and were similar between patients with preserved (HFpEF) and reduced (HFrEF) left ventricular ejection fraction (LVEF) phenotypes [17].

Due to the compensatory actions of CST with respect to adverse neurohumoral activation that is particularly pronounced in ischemic disease, we hypothesized that circulating CST levels would likely be higher in ADHF patients with a previous MI, compared to those without MI. Moreover, since CST reflects increased SNS activity, we further hypothesized that CST levels might be higher in ADHF patients with more reduced LVEF, thus, we expected to see a positive correlation of CST levels with the functional burden of the disease, as assessed by the New York Heart Association (NYHA) classification. Finally, since associations of CST with relevant biochemical and echocardiographic markers in ADHF population are poorly elucidated, our secondary objectives were to investigate the relationship of CST serum levels with echocardiographic parameters of the left ventricle/left atrium and laboratory biomarkers that are commonly used in the workup of ADHF patients. While this part of the study was exploratory in nature, we expected to generally observe beneficial associations of CST with these parameters, based on the corroborations from previous preclinical/mechanistic studies.

For reasons stated above, we sought to determine and compare the CST serum levels between patients, with and without, the previous history of MI and across the whole LVEF phenotype spectrum (HFrEF, HFmrEF, and HFpEF). Secondly, we aimed to investigate the relationship of CST serum levels with the NYHA functional class, echocardiographic indices of the left ventricle/left atrium, and select laboratory biomarkers.

2. Materials and Methods

2.1. Study Population

This was a non-randomized clinical cross-sectional study with a prospective follow-up planned in future analyses. Between January 2018 and February 2019, a total of 118 consecutive patients presenting with signs and symptoms of heart failure at the emergency department (ED) were considered eligible for the study inclusion and were hospitalized at the Department of Cardiology.

In this study, we consecutively enrolled HF patients (of both sexes) with the New York Heart Association (NYHA) functional class II–IV and with a positive history of admission due to HF, who agreed to participate in the study and signed the informed written consent. The clinical and physical examination of the patients was undertaken according to the Framingham criteria for HF [19]. Diagnosis of the acute event due to heart failure was mandatorily confirmed as per the current European Society of Cardiology (ESC) guidelines, for the diagnosis and treatment of acute and chronic heart failure with the final diagnosis adjudicated and verified by the ESC-certified HF specialist who was on-site investigator for the study [20]. All patients received standard-of-care HF-directed treatment, according to their individual clinical status. In order to obtain a well-selected population with clear and undisputable cardiac etiology of dyspnea, a rigorous exclusion criteria were employed, which included adults <35 years and >90 years of age, patients with documented or newly-established severe valvular or pericardial disease, infiltrative or hypertrophic cardiomyopathy, cor pulmonale, primary pulmonary disease, diabetes mellitus type I, primary renal or hepatic disease, active malignant or infectious disease, systemic autoimmune disease, hemorrhagic diathesis or significant coagulopathy, systemic immunological, or an immunosuppressive disorder, or a positive recent history of immunosuppressive/cancer chemotherapeutic drug use, positive history of acute coronary syndrome or stroke within 3 months prior to study enrolment, positive history of excessive alcohol, drug, narcotics or sedative consumption, and significantly debilitating psychiatric or neurological condition (Figure 1). Additionally, patients not included in the analysis were those that, at the ED or in-ward admission, had NT-proBNP levels <300 pg/mL as a "rule-out" strategy, while age-adjusted NT-proBNP cut-off values for the "rule-in" of heart failure diagnosis were applied as following—450 pg/mL for age <50 years, 900 pg/mL for 50–75 years, and 1,800 pg/mL for ≥75 years, based on the data from PRIDE [21] and International Collaborative of NT-proBNP [22] studies, later validated in the ICON-Reloaded study [23].

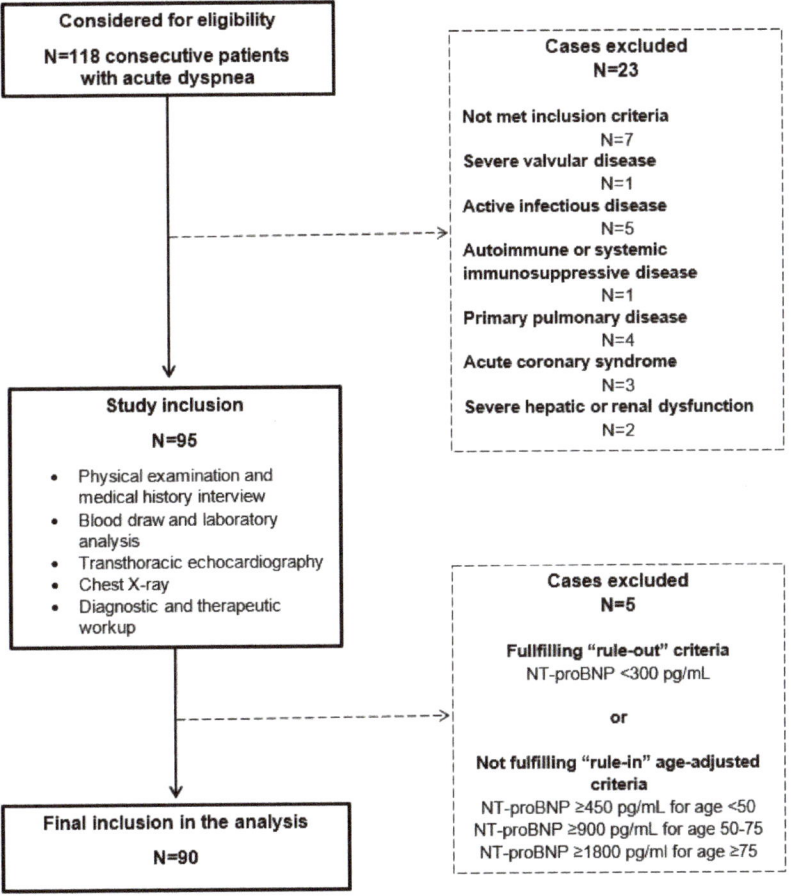

Figure 1. Flowchart of the CATSTAT-HF study.

The study protocol was approved by the Ethics Committee of the University Hospital of Split (approval no. 2181-147-01/06/M.S.-17-2) and University of Split School of Medicine Ethics Committee. All medical procedures were undertaken as in accordance with the Declaration of Helsinki and its latest revision in 2013. A study was registered on 3 January 2018 at ClinicalTrials.gov registry before the enrolment of the first patient (Serum Catestatin Expression and Cardiometabolic Parameters in Patients with Congestive Heart Failure (CATSTAT-HF); ClinicalTrials.gov number NCT03389386).

2.2. Data Measurement

All patients were evaluated in the first 24 h of admission and this evaluation consisted of physical examination, medical history interview (via custom checklist questionnaire), antecubital venous blood sampling for laboratory analyses, peripheral arterial blood gas sampling, transthoracic echocardiography (TTE), chest X-ray imaging, and a standard 12-lead electrocardiography (ECG) recording. All patients were assessed for the medical history, demographic data (age and sex), body weight and height, body mass index (BMI), body surface area (BSA), waist-to-hip ratio (WHR) and pharmacotherapy use. Patients were specially assessed for the documented previous history of myocardial infarction (defined as non-ST segment myocardial infarction-NSTEMI or ST-elevation myocardial infarction-STEMI and verified by the medical records). For the body weight (kg) and height (cm) measurements we used a calibrated scale (Seca, Birmingham, UK) and the BMI was calculated by the body weight (kg) being divided by height-squared (m^2). BSA was calculated using the Mosteller formula [24]. Waist circumference (cm) was measured while standing at the mid-point between the inferior tip of the ribcage and the superior aspect of the iliac crest, while hip circumference (cm) was measured at the point providing maximum circumference over the buttocks, using a tape measure. WHR was calculated by dividing the waist by the hip circumference. Heart rate (HR) at admission was recorded at the first medical contact in hospital by using a 12-lead ECG machine, while resting HR was recorded at the bedside when the patients were stable, by using the AliveCor®Kardia mobile device system (AliveCor Inc., Mountain View, CA, USA) attached to an Apple iPhone (Apple Inc., Cupertino, CA, USA).

2.3. Definitions

Patients with systolic blood pressure >140 mmHg or diastolic blood pressure >90 mmHg or those taking antihypertensive medications were considered to have arterial hypertension [25]. Dyslipidemia was defined as total cholesterol (TC) ≥5.0 mmol/L or low-density lipoprotein cholesterol (LDL-c) ≥3.0 mmol/L serum levels or current treatment with lipid-lowering agents. Non-high-density lipoprotein (HDL) cholesterol fraction was calculated by the formula = (total cholesterol − HDL cholesterol). Chronic kidney disease (CKD) was defined as an estimated glomerular filtration rate (eGFR) <60 mL/min/1.73 m^2, calculated by the Chronic Kidney Disease Epidemiology Collaboration (CKD-EPI) formula [26]. Hyperuricemia was defined as uric acid plasma levels >337 μmol/L for women and >403 μmol/L for men, as per our institutional laboratory cutoffs. Diabetes mellitus was defined as plasma glycated hemoglobin (HbA1c) ≥6.5% or fasting plasma glucose ≥7.0 mmol/L, according to the American Diabetes Association (ADA) guidelines or current treatment with oral hypoglycemic and/or insulin agents [27]. Obesity was determined by the BMI ≥30 kg/m^2 as defined by the World Health Organization (WHO) criteria. Patients with admission hemoglobin count <119 g/L for women and <138 g/L for men were considered to have anemia. Smoking was defined as current or former/past smoking. Left bundle branch block (LBBB) was defined based on the analysis of the available in-hospital ECG tracings, according to established recommendations [28]. For the evaluation of HF-related symptom burden, we used a New York Heart Association (NYHA) functional classification of heart failure, adjudicated by the same on-site principal investigator in collaboration with the HF-certified cardiology specialist.

2.4. Echocardiography

A transthoracic echocardiography (TTE) examination was performed on the same day as blood samples were collected. All measurements were taken while patients were at rest and in the left lateral decubitus position and by following recommendations for cardiac chamber quantification by echocardiography in adults endorsed by the American Society of Echocardiography (ASE) and the European Association of Cardiovascular Imaging (EACVI) [29]. A single on-site cardiology consultant with an expertise in ultrasonography performed all echocardiographic examinations. Measurements included quantification of left ventricle (LV) internal dimensions in diastole (LVEDd, mm), systole (LVESd, mm) in parasternal long-axis view, and M-mode tracing while LV volumes were measured in the apical four- and two-chamber views. LV ejection fraction (LVEF) was measured several times by the 2D biplane method, according to the modified Simpson's rule and the average value was recorded [30]. Fractional shortening (FS, %) was derived from linear measurements obtained from 2D images. Posterior left ventricular wall thickness (LVPWd, mm) and interventricular septal thickness (IVSd, mm) were measured by the linear method. LV mass was calculated by the linear method and the Cube formula—LV Mass (g) = $0.8 \times 1.04 \times [(LVEDd + IVSd + LVPWd)^3 - LVEDd^3] + 0.6$. Left ventricular mass index (LVMI) was calculated by dividing LV mass with body surface area (BSA) and expressed in g/m^2. Left-ventricular remodeling was assessed by calculating relative wall thickness (RWT) that allowed for the further classification of the LV mass increase as either concentric hypertrophy (RWT > 0.42) or eccentric hypertrophy (RWT ≤ 0.42), while RWT was calculated by the formula RWT = $(2 \times LVPWd)/LVEDd$. Left atrium (LA, mm) size quantification was performed in the parasternal long-axis view, perpendicular to the aortic root long axis at the end of the LV systole, while aortic root (Ao, mm) measurements were obtained in the parasternal long-axis view. LA/Ao represents the ratio of LA internal diameter and diameter of Ao. Echocardiographic parameters were used to aid in the diagnosis of HFpEF and to be considered for the HFpEF diagnosis, patients had to have symptoms and signs of HF, LVEF ≥50% and elevated natriuretic peptides further accompanied with relevant structural or functional heart alterations, as assessed by echocardiography. Structural abnormalities included left-ventricular hypertrophy, left atrial enlargement, or left ventricular mass index (LVMI) ≥115 g/m^2 for men and ≥95 g/m^2 for women. Significant functional alterations were considered if the ratio of the peak early mitral inflow velocity over the early diastolic mitral annular velocity (E/e') ≥13 cm/s and mean early diastolic myocardial relaxation velocities (e' septal and lateral wall) were <9 cm/s. Doppler estimation of pulmonary artery systolic pressure (PASP) >35 mmHg was also used to aid in the diagnosis. Where necessary, to unmask diastolic dysfunction and alter pseudonormal filling into impaired relaxation, a Valsalva maneuver was performed in patients.

All images were acquired using the Vivid 9 ultrasound system (GE Medical Systems, Milwaukee, WI, USA) and stored/analyzed on the Echo PAC workstation (EchoPac PC, version 112; GE Medical Systems, Milwaukee, WI, USA).

2.5. Laboratory Analyses

Blood was drawn after patients fasted from the antecubital vein by using a polyethylene butterfly needle and was stored into two vials, one with a clot activator (BD Vacutainer®CAT-Clot Activator Tube, 2.0 mL) and other containing anticoagulant K3 EDTA (BD Vacutainer®K3E 3.5 mg, 2.0 mL). These samples were then immediately transferred to the Department of Medical Laboratory Diagnostics, where they were further processed according to good laboratory practice. From one of the vials, blood was centrifuged (20 min at 2,000 rpm at 4 °C) and the obtained sera were divided into two aliquots and stored at a temperature of −80 °C, until analysis. All blood samples were analyzed in the same certified institutional biochemical laboratory, by using the standard laboratory procedures.

Catestatin levels in serum were determined by an enzyme-linked immunosorbent assay (ELISA), by using a commercially-available diagnostic kit (EK-053-27CE, EIA kit, Phoenix Pharmaceuticals Inc., Burlingame, CA, USA). According to the manufacturer's instruction, the kit measurement range was 0–100 ng/mL. Reported sensitivity for catestatin was 0.05 ng/mL with a linear range of 0.05–0.92 ng/mL. Cross-reactivity with endogenous human catestatin peptide for this assay kit was 100% with the intra-assay and inter-assay coefficient of variability being <10% and <15%, respectively. High-sensitivity cardiac troponin I (hs-cTnI) concentrations were determined by using Abbot Diagnostics hs-cTnI assay (Abbott ARCHITECT ci16200 analyzer, Abbott, Chicago, IL, USA) with the upper limit of 99th percentile being 34.2 ng/L for men and 15.6 ng/L for women. The N-terminal (1–76) pro brain natriuretic peptide (NT-proBNP) concentrations were determined using Eclesys®Cobas e601 NT-proBNP assay via the electrochemiluminescense (ECLIA) method (Roche Diagnostics, Manheim, Germany). Hemoglobin

A1c (HbA1c) levels were measured by using high-performance liquid chromatography (HPLC) (Tosoh G8, Tosoh Bioscience, Tokyo, Japan). Electrolyte levels were determined by the potentiometric method, while C-reactive protein (CRP) was determined by the immunoturbidimetric method on the Architect c16200 system (Abbott, Chicago, IL, USA). Complete blood count and differential blood count were determined by using standard flow-cytometry-based hematologic analyses (ADVIA 2120i, Siemens Healthcare, Erlangen, Germany). Fasting glucose, total cholesterol, high-density lipoprotein cholesterol (HDL-c), low-density lipoprotein cholesterol (LDL-c), triglycerides, blood urea nitrogen (BUN), creatinine, D-dimer, and uric acid concentrations were analyzed through the standard laboratory methods (ARCHITECT ci16200, Abbott, Chicago, IL, USA).

2.6. Statistical Analysis

Data were analyzed using SPSS Statistics for Windows®(version 25.0, IBM, Armonk, NY, USA) and Prism 6 for Windows®(version 6.01, GraphPad, La Jolla, CA, USA). Data were presented as mean ± standard deviation (SD) or median (interquartile range) based on the variable distribution normality or number (N) with percentage (%), within the particular category of interest. Normality of distribution for continuous variables was assessed with the Kolmogorov-Smirnov test. For differences between groups, an independent samples t-test was used for continuous variables with normal distribution, while the Mann–Whitney U test was used for continuous variables with non-normal distribution. The chi-squared (χ^2) test was used to determine differences between groups in terms of categorical variables, while the Fisher Exact test was employed in cases where a group of interest had <5 cases. For comparisons of continuous variables among >2 groups of interest, a one-way ANOVA was used with a post-hoc Tukey test. Finally, a multivariable linear regression analysis with forward algorithm was applied to determine significant and independent correlates of the catestatin serum level, which was defined as a dependent continuous variable. This linear regression model was weighted by sex, previous history of MI, and covariate-adjusted for age, BMI, eGFR, arterial systolic blood pressure, and LVEF. To further minimize the chance of overfitting, separate multivariable linear regression analyses were undertaken for each variable of interest. In these analyses, univariate beta coefficient and its respective significance value was reported for every evaluated variable, while the unstandardized coefficient (B) with standard error (SE), standardized coefficient (β), t-statistics, and their associated *p*-value were reported only for those variables that retained significance in the multivariable model. A two-tailed *p*-value <0.05 was considered to be statistically significant.

3. Results

3.1. Patients' Baseline Characteristics

Out of 118 consecutive patients that presented with acute dyspnea, a total of 90 patients were included in the final analysis, after applying the study exclusion criteria (Figure 1).

There was equal representation of sexes, with a slight predominance of women (N = 47, 52.2%) and the mean age of the population being 70.3 ± 10.2 years. The majority of patients were in the NYHA III functional class (62.2%), followed by NYHA IV (21.1%), while 15 (16.7%) were in the NYHA II class. Less than half of the patients (N = 40, 44.4%) had suffered MI in the past, 37 (41.1%) were diabetics, 34 (37.8%) were present or former smokers, while 84 (93.3%) had arterial hypertension. Atrial fibrillation was documented in 55.6% of patients, while more than half of the patients (51.1%) were in the CKD stage 3 or higher. Furthermore, 36 (40%) patients had at least one HF-related hospitalization during the previous year. Most of the patients had HFrEF phenotype (N = 39, 43.4%), followed by HFpEF (N = 31, 34.4%), while 20 (22.2%) had a midrange LVEF. Baseline characteristics of the patient cohort are available in Table 1.

Table 1. Baseline data and pharmacotherapy of the enrolled cohort stratified by the positive history of myocardial infarction.

VARIABLE	Total Cohort N = 90	ADHF without MI N = 50	ADHF with MI N = 40	p-Value *
Demographics and clinical profile				
Age, years	70.3 ± 10.2	69.8 ± 10.8	70.9 ± 9.6	0.610
Female sex	47 (52.2)	33 (66.0)	14 (35.0)	**0.003**
Body mass index, kg/m^2	30.2 ± 4.2	30.8 ± 4.4	29.6 ± 3.9	0.182
Body surface area, m^2	2.02 ± 0.18	2.02 ± 0.19	2.03 ± 0.17	0.792
Waist-to-hip ratio	0.98 ± 0.08	0.97 ± 0.09	0.99 ± 0.06	0.095
Systolic blood pressure, mmHg	137 ± 28	134 ± 23	140 ± 32	0.285
Diastolic blood pressure, mmHg	80 ± 13	79 ± 12	82 ± 14	0.279
Heart rate at admission, beats/min	95 ± 31	94 ± 28	96 ± 35	0.726
Heart rate at rest, beats/min	88 ± 26	90 ± 28	84 ± 22	0.300
HF-related hospitalization event in a previous year	36 (40.0)	15 (30.0)	21 (52.5)	**0.030**
Pacemaker/ICD/CRT device	13 (14.4)	3 (6.0)	10 (25.0)	**0.011**
Left bundle branch block	35 (38.9)	19 (38.0)	16 (40.0)	0.847
NYHA functional class	3.0 ± 0.62	2.9 ± 0.53	3.2 ± 0.69	**0.031**
CKD stage	2.6 ± 0.9	2.3 ± 1.0	2.9 ± 0.8	**0.004**
LVEF ≤35%, biplane Simpson	37 (41.1)	16 (32.0)	20 (50.0)	0.083
SaO_2 <90% at admission	34 (37.8)	18 (36.0)	10 (40.0)	0.777
Comorbidities and concomitant clinical conditions				
Diabetes mellitus	37 (41.1)	17 (34.0)	20 (50.0)	0.125
Anemia	36 (40.0)	12 (24.0)	14 (35.0)	0.253
Obesity	38 (42.2)	25 (55.6)	13 (35.1)	0.065
Hyperuricemia	75 (83.3)	40 (83.3)	35 (87.5)	0.193
Dyslipidemia	60 (66.6)	33 (66.6)	27 (67.5)	0.743
Chronic obstructive pulmonary disease	21 (23.3)	14 (28.0)	7 (17.5)	0.242
Chronic kidney disease	46 (51.1)	21 (42.0)	25 (62.5)	0.053
Arterial hypertension	84 (93.3)	45 (90.0)	39 (97.5)	0.156
Atrial fibrillation	50 (55.6)	28 (56.0)	22 (55.0)	0.924
Peripheral artery disease	19 (21.1)	9 (18.0)	10 (25.0)	0.419
Smoker, present or former	34 (37.8)	14 (28.0)	20 (50.0)	**0.032**
History of stroke or transient ischemic attack	7 (7.8)	4 (8.0)	3 (7.5)	0.930
Pharmacotherapy				
ACE inhibitor or ARB	70 (77.8)	41 (82.0)	29 (72.5)	0.245
Sacubitril-valsartan	24 (26.7)	11 (22.0)	13 (32.5)	0.154
β-blocker	81 (90.0)	43 (86.0)	38 (95.0)	0.235
Ca^{2+} channel blocker	13 (14.4)	9 (18.0)	4 (10.0)	0.305
MRA	42 (46.7)	24 (48.0)	18 (45.0)	0.953
Diuretics	82 (91.1)	45 (90.0)	37 (92.5)	0.274
Digoxin	18 (20.0)	9 (18.0)	9 (22.5)	0.554
Aspirin	35 (38.9)	13 (26.0)	22 (55.0)	**0.005**
Warfarin	23 (25.6)	14 (28.0)	9 (22.5)	0.617
NOAC	22 (24.4)	13 (26.0)	9 (22.5)	0.821
Statin	33 (36.7)	14 (28.0)	19 (47.5)	**0.035**

Values are mean ± SD or N (%); * an independent samples t-test or Chi-squared test or Fisher Exact test were used for comparisons between two groups of interest, as appropriate. Abbreviations: ACE—angiotensin-converting enzyme; ARB—angiotensin receptor blocker; CKD—chronic kidney disease; CRT—cardiac resynchronization therapy; HF—heart failure; ICD—implantable cardioverter defibrillator; LVEF—left ventricular ejection fraction; MI—myocardial infarction; MRA—mineralocorticoid receptor antagonist; NOAC—novel oral anticoagulant; NYHA—New York Heart Association; SaO_2—peripheral arterial oxygen saturation. Bold: statistical significance <0.05.

3.2. ADHF Patients with a History of MI and Those Without

Patients with a history of MI (MI+) tended to be males and smokers; they had more advanced kidney diseases and functional disease burden (as assessed by the NYHA classification), more HF-related hospitalizations in the previous year and more pacemaker/ICD/resynchronization devices implanted, compared to patients without any history of MI (MI−) (Table 1).

Regarding pharmacotherapy use prior to hospital discharge, a higher use of aspirin and statins was recorded among MI+ patients, compared to those without a history of MI. Among all patients, the coverage of guideline-directed medical therapy was 77.8% for angiotensin-converting enzyme (ACE) inhibitors or angiotensin receptor blockers (ARBs), 90% for beta-blockers, 26.7% for sacubitril-valsartan, while mineralocorticoid receptor antagonists were used in 46.7% of all patients. Diuretics were used by the vast majority of patients (91.1%), whereas half of the patients were on anticoagulation medications (Table 1).

In terms of laboratory data, MI+ patients had higher serum creatinine (139.8 ± 70.4 vs. 99.9 ± 42.0 mmol/L, $p = 0.001$) and lower eGFR (49.2 ± 21.7 vs. 63.8 ± 25.7 mL/min/1.73 m^2, $p = 0.005$) values, compared to the MI– group. Biomarker values of NT-proBNP and hs-cTnI were significantly higher among MI+ than MI– patients (5,227 (3,079–12,004) versus 2,286 (1,110–5,976) pg/mL, $p = 0.008$ and 35.8 (19.3–84.2) versus 16.0 (10.0–27.3) ng/L, $p = 0.001$, respectively). Furthermore, the average glycated hemoglobin value was significantly higher among MI+ compared to MI– patients (6.97 ± 1.50 vs. 6.33 ± 0.94%, $p = 0.017$, respectively). Finally, MI+ patients had lower concentrations of total cholesterol (4.1 ± 1.3 vs. 4.7 ± 1.3 mmol/L, $p = 0.030$) and its HDL and LDL fractions [0.9 (0.8–1.1) versus 1.0 (0.9–1.2) mmol/L, $p = 0.023$ and 2.4 ±1.1 vs. 2.9 ± 1.1 mmol/L, $p = 0.029$, respectively) compared to the MI– patients (Table 2).

Table 2. Laboratory data of the enrolled cohort stratified by the history of myocardial infarction.

Variable	Total Cohort N = 90	ADHF without Prior MI N = 50	ADHF with Prior MI N = 40	p-Value *
Laboratory values				
Sodium, mmol/L	138.9 ± 3.7	139.0 ± 4.1	138.7 ± 3.2	0.725
Potassium, mmol/L	4.2 ± 0.4	4.1 ± 0.4	4.2 ± 0.5	0.252
Creatinine, μmol/L	117.6 ± 59.5	99.9 ± 42.0	139.8 ± 70.4	**0.001**
BUN, mmol/L	4.9 ± 2.6	4.5 ± 2.5	5.4 ± 2.8	0.132
eGFR, mL/min/1.73 m^2	57.3 ± 24.9	63.8 ± 25.7	49.2 ± 21.7	**0.005**
Uric acid, μmol/L	535 ± 165	511 ± 179	565 ± 143	0.130
Albumin, g/L	38.7 ± 4.1	38.6 ± 4.1	38.8 ± 4.2	0.849
Total proteins, g/L	68.2 ± 7.2	67.5 ± 7.8	69.0 ± 6.3	0.314
Hemoglobin, g/L	133.4 ± 19.2	134.1 ± 18.7	132.6 ± 19.9	0.706
WBC count, ×10^9/L	8.08 ± 2.59	7.73 ± 2.49	8.51 ± 2.66	0.156
Erythrocytes, ×10^{12}/L	4.48 ± 0.69	4.46 ± 0.69	4.51 ± 0.71	0.775
Thrombocytes, ×10^9/L	214 ± 60	217 ± 61	209 ± 58	0.522
Lymphocytes, ×10^9/L	1.50 ± 1.35	1.49 ± 0.70	1.50 ± 0.68	0.970
Neutrophils, ×10^9/L	5.64 ± 2.18	5.41 ± 2.11	5.92 ± 2.24	0.278
Fasting glucose, mmol/L	8.2 ± 3.0	7.7 ± 2.6	8.8 ± 3.4	0.091
HbA1c, %	6.61 ± 1.26	6.33 ± 0.94	6.97 ± 1.50	**0.017**
NT-proBNP, pg/mL	3586 (1361–7787)	2286 (1110–5976)	5277 (3079–12004)	**0.008**
hs-cTnI, ng/L	22.9 (11.6–49.0)	16.0 (10.0–27.3)	35.8 (19.3–84.2)	**0.001**
CRP, mg/L	8.4 (4.9–20.5)	7.9 (4.7–17.7)	11.5 (6.6–30.6)	0.110
D-dimer, mg/L	1.62 ± 1.35	1.55 ± 1.33	1.72 ± 1.40	0.718
Triglycerides, mmol/L	1.56 ± 0.64	1.51 ± 0.64	1.61 ± 0.65	0.471
Total cholesterol, mmol/L	4.4 ± 1.3	4.7 ± 1.3	4.1 ± 1.3	**0.030**
HDL cholesterol, mmol/L	1.0 (0.8–1.2)	1.0 (0.9–1.2)	0.9 (0.8–1.1)	**0.023**
LDL cholesterol, mmol/L	2.7 ± 1.1	2.9 ± 1.1	2.4 ± 1.1	**0.029**

Values are mean ± SD or median (interquartile range); * Based on the variable distribution, an independent samples t-test or Mann–Whitney U test were used for the group comparisons, as appropriate. Abbreviations: BUN–blood urea nitrogen; CRP–C-reactive protein; eGFR–estimated glomerular filtration rate by chronic kidney disease epidemiology collaboration (CKD–EPI) formula; HDL–high-density lipoprotein; HbA1c–glycated hemoglobin; hs-cTnI–high sensitivity cardiac troponin I; LDL–low-density lipoprotein; NTproBNP—N-terminal pro B-type natriuretic peptide; WBC–white blood cells count. Bold: statistical significance <0.05.

No significant differences between two groups stratified by MI history were observed with regards to the echocardiographic parameters, while the mean LVEF in the total ADHF sample was 43.4 ± 16.4 percent (Table 3).

Table 3. Echocardiographic parameters of the total cohort and data stratified by the history of myocardial infarction.

Variable	Total Cohort N = 90	ADHF without Prior MI N = 50	ADHF with Prior MI N = 40	p-Value *
LVEF, biplane Simpson, %	43.4 ± 16.4	46.3 ± 15.8	39.9 ± 16.6	0.066
LV mass, g	254.4 ± 95.7	250.2 ± 93.9	258.5 ± 97.5	0.686
LVMI, g/m^2	119.0 ± 47.3	117.3 ± 46.5	120.7 ± 48.1	0.744
LV EDd, mm	57.9 ± 9.4	56.9 ± 8.5	58.9 ± 10.4	0.322
LV ESd, mm	42.6 ± 12.1	40.9 ± 11.3	44.6 ± 12.9	0.152
IVSd, mm	11 (10–13)	11 (10–13.5)	11 (10–12)	0.405
LV PWd, mm	10.9 ± 2.0	11.0 ± 1.9	10.9 ± 2.1	0.734
FS, %	27.3 ± 11.5	28.4 ± 11.4	25.9 ± 11.6	0.326
LV EDV, mL/m^2 **	85.2 ± 32.3	80.4 ± 26.4	91.1 ± 38.0	0.142
LV ESV, mL/m^2 **	45.0 ± 29.7	40.0 ± 25.4	51.3 ± 33.6	0.096
LA diameter, mm	49.9 ± 8.9	49.5 ± 9.7	50.3 ± 7.7	0.685
Aortic root diameter, mm	33.8 ± 5.1	33.3 ± 5.3	34.5 ± 4.9	0.295
LA/Ao ratio	1.49 ± 0.28	1.49 ± 0.31	1.48 ± 0.24	0.757

Values are mean ± SD or median (interquartile range); * Based on variable distribution, an independent samples t-test or the Mann–Whitney U test were used for group comparisons, as appropriate; ** Indexed to body surface area. Abbreviations: Ao—aortic root diameter; BSA—body surface area; EDd—end-diastolic diameter; EDV—end-diastolic volume; ESd—end-systolic diameter; ESV—end-systolic volume; FS—fractional shortening; IVSd—interventricular septum diameter; LA—left atrium; LV—left ventricle; LVEF—left ventricular ejection fraction; LVMI—left ventricular mass index; PWd—posterior wall diameter.

3.3. CST Serum Levels Stratified by the History of MI and Across Different LVEF Phenotypes

When stratified by the history of myocardial infarction, MI+ patients had two-fold higher serum CST levels compared to MI− patients (8.94 ± 6.39 vs. 4.90 ± 2.74 ng/mL, $p = 0.001$) (Figure 2).

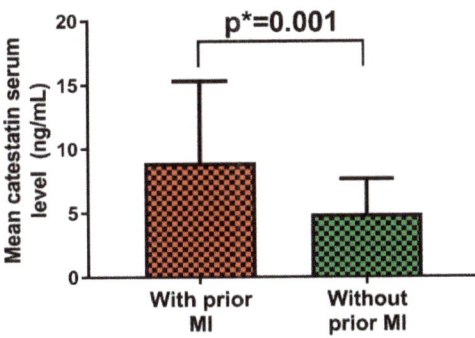

Figure 2. Catestatin (CST) serum levels in acutely decompensated heart failure patients stratified by the previous history of acute myocardial infarction.

CST serum levels did not significantly differ between the three LVEF phenotypes ($p = 0.143$). Patients in the HFrEF group exhibited the highest catestatin levels (7.74 ± 5.64 ng/mL), followed by the HFmrEF (5.75 ± 4.19 ng/mL) and HFpEF (5.35 ± 2.77 ng/mL) groups (Figure 3).

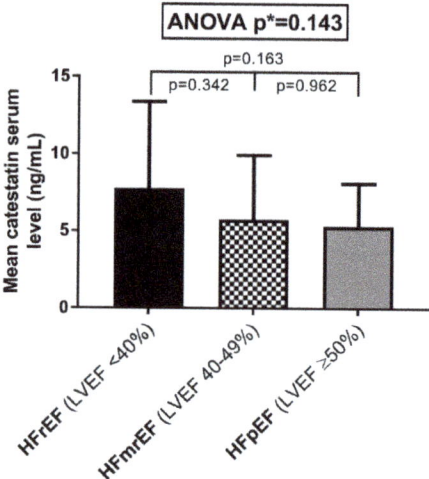

Figure 3. CST serum levels according to the left ventricular ejection fraction, stratified into three groups—heart failure with reduced ejection fraction (HFrEF), heart failure with midrange ejection fraction (HFmrEF), and heart failure with preserved ejection fraction (HFpEF).

3.4. Associations of Serum CST Levels with Clinical and Laboratory Parameters

In multivariable linear regression analysis performed among the total patient sample, CST serum levels positively correlated with the NYHA functional class ($\beta = 0.491$, $p < 0.001$). Furthermore, CST levels were in inverse correlation with WHR ($\beta = -0.237$, $p = 0.026$), HbA1c ($\beta = -0.235$, $p = 0.027$), LDL ($\beta = -0.231$, $p = 0.029$), non-HDL cholesterol ($\beta = -0.237$, $p = 0.026$), and hs-cTnI ($\beta = -0.221$, $p = 0.030$) concentrations. Finally, heart rate, both at admission and measured at rest, negatively correlated with the CST serum level ($\beta = -0.201$, $p = 0.036$ and $\beta = -0.242$, $p = 0.030$, respectively) (Table 4). Each variable was tested in a multivariable linear regression model adjusted for covariates, with following univariate β estimates and p-values—age ($\beta = -0.122$, $p = 0.320$), BMI ($\beta = -0.098$, $p = 0.801$), eGFR ($\beta = -0.109$, $p = 0.374$), systolic blood pressure ($\beta = 0.162$, $p = 0.412$), LVEF ($\beta = 0.311$, $p = 0.015$), female sex ($\beta = 0.249$, $p = 0.039$), and previous history of MI ($\beta = 0.378$, $p < 0.001$).

Table 4. Univariate beta estimates and results from multivariable linear regression showing associations of serum CST levels (ng/mL) with the clinical and laboratory parameters of interest.

Variable	Univariate β	p-Value *	B	SE	β	t	p-Value **
NYHA class	0.533	<0.001	0.361	0.082	0.491	4.257	<0.001
WHR	−0.335	0.012	−1.360	0.615	−0.237	−2.231	0.026
Heart rate at admission, bpm	−0.164	0.125	−0.933	0.418	−0.201	−1.960	0.036
Heart rate at rest, bpm	−0.189	0.098	−0.951	0.451	−0.242	−2.177	0.030
Total cholesterol, mmol/L	−0.108	0.268					
Triglycerides, mmol/L	−0.201	0.101					
HDL-c, mmol/L	−0.082	0.508					
LDL-c, mmol/L	−0.272	0.019	−0.089	0.040	−0.231	−2.123	0.029
Non-HDL cholesterol, mmol/L	−0.281	0.014	−0.094	0.045	−0.237	−2.298	0.026
NT-proBNP, pg/mL	−0.193	0.074					
hs-cTnI, ng/L	−0.260	0.015	−0.080	0.111	−0.221	−0.799	0.030
CRP, mg/L	0.147	0.490					
D-dimer, mg/L	−0.094	0.770					
Glucose, fasting, mmol/L	−0.165	0.159					
HbA1c, %	−0.264	0.023	−0.085	0.039	−0.235	−1.248	0.027

* Statistical significance for univariate beta estimate; ** Multivariable linear regression model when testing each variable was separately adjusted for age, body mass index, estimated glomerular filtration rate, systolic blood pressure, left ventricular ejection fraction, and weighted by sex and the history of myocardial infarction. Abbreviations: CRP-C—reactive protein; HDL—high-density lipoprotein; HbA1c—glycated hemoglobin; hs-cTnI—high sensitivity cardiac troponin I; LDL—low-density lipoprotein; NT-proBNP—N-terminal pro B-type natriuretic peptide; NYHA—New York Heart Association; WHR—Waist-to-Hip Ratio. Bold: statistical significance <0.05.

3.5. Associations of Serum CST Levels with Echocardiographic Parameters

CST serum levels were in positive correlation with LVEF (β = 0.271, p = 0.022) and fractional shortening (β = 0.255, p = 0.029), while an inverse relationship was observed with respect to the left ventricular mass (β = −0.249, p = 0.031), left ventricular mass index (β = −0.237, p = 0.015), left ventricular end-diastolic (β = −0.341, p = 0.001) and end-systolic (β = −0.311, p = 0.005) diameters. Furthermore, left ventricular end-diastolic and end-systolic volumes, indexed to BSA, were in a negative correlation with the CST serum levels (β = −0.324, p = 0.002 and β = −0.328, p = 0.002, respectively). Finally, diameter of the left atrium inversely correlated with the CST serum levels (β = −0.255, p = 0.021) (Table 5).

Table 5. Univariate beta estimates and results from multivariable linear regression showing associations of serum CST levels (ng/mL), with echocardiographic parameters.

Variable	Univariate β	p-Value *	B	SE	β	t	p-Value **
LVEF, %	0.323	0.010	0.700	0.299	0.271	2.350	0.022
LV mass, g	−0.312	0.019	−0.001	0.001	−0.249	−2.185	0.031
LVMI, g/m^2	−0.301	0.022	−0.002	0.001	−0.237	−2.488	0.015
LV EDd, mm	−0.463	<0.001	−0.020	0.005	−0.341	−3.203	0.001
LV ESd, mm	−0.411	<0.001	−0.013	0.004	−0.311	−2.762	0.005
IVSd, mm	0.181	0.139					
LV PWd, mm	−0.165	0.180					
LV EDV, indexed to BSA, mL/m^2	−0.375	<0.001	−0.002	0.001	−0.324	−3.211	0.002
LV ESV, indexed to BSA, mL/m^2	−0.349	<0.001	−0.003	0.001	−0.328	−3.157	0.002
LA diameter, mm	−0.297	0.010	−0.012	0.005	−0.262	−2.415	0.019
Aortic root diameter, mm	−0.070	0.574					
LA/Ao ratio	−0.032	0.795					
LAEDV, mL	−0.171	0.251					
LAVI, mL/m^2	−0.233	0.101					
Fractional shortening, %	0.292	0.021	0.011	0.003	0.255	2.198	0.029

* Statistical significance for univariate beta estimate; ** Multivariable linear regression model when testing each variable separately was adjusted for age, body mass index, estimated glomerular filtration rate, systolic blood pressure, and weighted by sex and the history of myocardial infarction; Abbreviations: Ao—aortic root diameter; BSA—body surface area; EDd—end-diastolic diameter; EDV—end-diastolic volume; ESd—end-systolic diameter; ESV—end-systolic volume; IVSd—interventricular septum diameter; LA—left atrium; LV—left ventricle; LVEF—left ventricular ejection fraction; LVMI—left ventricular mass index; PWd—posterior wall diameter. Bold: statistical significance <0.05.

Finally, in terms of LV remodeling assessed by the value of relative wall thickness (RWT) derived from echocardiographic measurements, more than half of the patients (N = 47, 52.2%) had eccentric hypertrophy while one-quarter (N = 23, 25.8%) had concentric hypertrophy. Less than one-quarter of patients had normal left ventricular geometry (N = 20, 22.4%) (Figure 4).

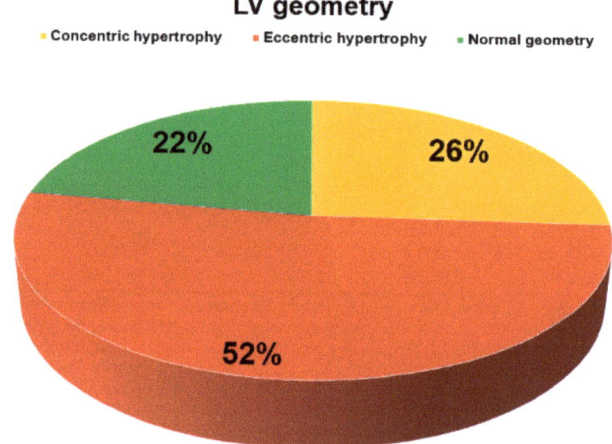

Figure 4. The distribution of left ventricular (LV) geometries as estimated by the relative wall thickness.

4. Discussion

We report that, among ADHF patients, serum catestatin levels were higher by two-fold among individuals that previously had AMI, while no significant differences in catestatin serum levels were observed among the different HF phenotypes stratified by LVEF (HFrEF versus HFmrEF versus HFpEF). Furthermore, the catestatin serum levels positively correlated with the NYHA functional class, independent of other covariates, while they were in negative correlation with WHR, LDL, and non-HDL cholesterol, hs-cTnI, glycated hemoglobin, and heart rate (both at admission and at rest). Finally, the catestatin serum levels correlated favorably with most of the relevant structural and functional echocardiographic parameters of the left ventricle (LV), such as LVEF, fractional shortening, LV volumes and diameters, LV mass and mass index, as well as the size of the left atrium.

We hypothesized that, due to the elevated neurohumoral and SNS activation in patients with heart failure and ischemic heart disease [5–7,31], serum CST levels would likely be higher among patients that previously suffered AMI, compared to those that did not. Importantly, circulating CST levels closely paralleled norepinephrine levels in different myocardial ischemia states, among patients with CAD [32]. Furthermore, since catecholamines are co-stored and co-released with a group of acidic secretory proteins (such as ChgA), from the storage vesicles in adrenal chromaffin cells and adrenergic neurons [33,34], it is plausible that CST levels might closely relate to the catecholaminergic "milieu" in the HF setting. As we hypothesized, our HF AMI+ cohort had more than two-fold higher levels of circulating catestatin, compared to the AMI– patients. This finding is comparable to another study of Liu et al. showing that plasma CST concentrations were significantly higher among HF patients with ischemic versus non-ischemic etiology of the disease, however, this finding was limited to patients in the NYHA III or IV class, and only HFpEF and HFrEF patients without a frank definition of ischemic disease [17].

Catestatin is a part of a complex neurohumoral feedback system and is most likely secreted peripherally as a counter-regulatory peptide attenuating excess catecholamine and SNS activity. Thus, higher levels of this peptide in peripheral blood might indirectly reflect increased neurohumoral burden and dysfunctional baroreflex control. However, precise pathophysiologic significance of the elevated CST levels in HF remains unknown [17,35]. Interestingly, this difference in catestatin serum levels between the AMI+ and AMI− cohort was persistent in our study, regardless of the baseline systolic blood pressure and guideline-directed pharmacotherapy targeting neurohumoral activation pathways, since both groups were similar in that regard. By measuring the circulating catestatin among similar HF patient groups (in terms of baseline characteristics and medication intake), it might be possible to quantify any "residual" neurohumoral activity that could be additionally targeted by uptitration or introduction of additional neurohumoral disease-modifying drugs that might be used in HF. This could be relevant for hard clinical outcomes, since high circulating catestatin levels measured during index admission of CHF patients, independently predicted post-discharge all-cause death (HR 1.84, 95% CI 1.02–3.32) and cardiac death (OR 2.41 95% CI 1.26–4.62), while these effects were even stronger if the natriuretic peptide levels were high [14]. However, this finding must be cautiously interpreted, as it was based on a single-center study that enrolled 200 patients, thus, signaling that more studies with larger enrollment are required in order to further determine the prognostic value of CST as a biomarker implicated in HF.

Even more, CST measurement in combination with other disease biomarkers such as NT-proBNP might give additional prognostic information in the HF population [14]. Interestingly, in a study by Liu et al., plasma CST levels did not significantly decrease and remained high after treatment and alleviation of the HF-related symptoms, while BNP plasma levels were significantly reduced [17]. This finding might suggest that residual catecholaminergic and SNS activity is preserved in these patients, despite therapeutic intervention and subsequent short-term improvement of symptoms and reduction of the circulating natriuretic peptides. It might also suggest that CST is a chronic, rather than acute-response biomarker of neurohumoral activity in HF. Finally, multimarker strategies accumulating independent information from a battery of biomarkers in terms of risk stratification in ADHF and CHF are recommended nowadays, since each biomarker provides insight into different aspects of the HF pathophysiology [36,37].

In the present study, ADHF patients within the whole spectrum of LVEF were included and, to our knowledge, this is the first study that reported on CST levels in patients with "midrange" LVEF. Although CST levels did not significantly differ between the three LVEF phenotypes, there is a clear trend towards HFrEF patients having higher CST levels, while statistical significance was not reached most likely due to the limited sample size. Additionally, circulating CST levels were highest in the NYHA IV, followed by NYHA III, and were lowest in the NYHA II subgroup. This finding was supported by a study of Liu et al. showing that plasma CST concentrations gradually increased among CHF patients from NYHA I to IV class and no difference in CST concentrations was observed between the HFrEF and HFpEF patients [17]. However, one study showed that the catestatin levels decreased gradually from stage A to C of HF, when using the American Heart Association (AHA) and American College of Cardiology (ACC) classification of HF [18]. In accordance with the previous study by Liu et al, our findings might suggest that CST is a marker of advanced HF and its circulating levels are dependent on a constellation of factors beyond the ejection fraction. Since the NYHA class is consistently associated with hospitalizations and mortality in HF [38–40], our finding is of further relevance because higher plasma CST levels measured at index hospitalization were independently associated to increased risk of all-cause and cardiac death among CHF patients, during the median follow-up of 52.5 months [14].

Importantly, our study showed that serum CST levels positively correlated with LVEF and fraction shortening. Higher catestatin levels were associated with smaller LV volumes and dimensions, as well as decreased LV mass and LA size. These are novel findings suggesting the cardioprotective association of catestatin with structural and functional properties of left ventricle and dimensions of the left atrium. Previous studies in which similar positive associations were observed were only reported in the rat model of AMI [41] and in patients with AMI [16], but not in the ADHF setting. One study conducted in the setting of AMI failed to demonstrate the relationship between catestatin and LVEF [42]. Furthermore, patients with essential hypertension and left ventricular hypertrophy, as determined by echocardiography, had a significantly lower catestatin-to-norepinephrine ratio [43], while mice with ablated ChgA gene showed increased LV mass and LV cavity dimensions. This suggests that deficiency of the prohormone ChgA and its downstream products such as catestatin are responsible for the loss of endogenous "brake" on adrenergic activity and mediation of pathologic LV remodeling [44]. Unlike our findings, Liu et al. did not find LVEF as an independent correlate of plasma CST levels in their CHF cohort but rather reported the NYHA class, ischemic etiology of the cardiomyopathy, and eGFR as independent predictors of CST levels [17].

We further expanded on these findings since our multivariable regression analysis showed that independent negative predictors of CST serum levels were HbA1c, LDL and non-HDL cholesterol fractions, hs-cTnI, WHR, and HR (both at admission and at rest). These are novel findings in the context of HF and can be related to some reports on the role of CST in other diseases. Of note, catestatin suppressed hepatic glucose production and was associated with improved insulin sensitivity in mice with diet-induced obesity [45], while it also induced glucose uptake and GLUT4 trafficking in adult rat cardiomyocytes, thus, likely improving cardiac energetics [46]. One study performed among obese children and adolescents found that catestatin negatively correlated with the homeostatic model assessment of insulin resistance (HOMA-IR) and its levels were significantly reduced in obese subjects, compared to the control group [47]. CST also improved peripheral leptin sensitivity and promoted lipolysis and fatty acid oxidation in a preclinical model [48], thus, confirming its antiobesic effect [49]. These data altogether suggest that CST is associated with improved systemic glycemia and metabolic profile and these inferences are concordant to our findings in the ADHF population, since we observed negative associations of glycated hemoglobin and WHR with serum CST concentrations.

In terms of catestatin and lipid metabolism, no comparable data are available for the HF population. In a study among untreated hypertensive patients, catestatin levels correlated positively with HDL-cholesterol levels but no associations were observed with respect to the total cholesterol or other cholesterol fractions [50], while CST correlated negatively with HDL cholesterol among obstructive sleep apnea patients [11]. Similarly, catestatin significantly retarded aortic atherosclerotic lesions with declined lipoprotein-induced foam cell formation in a preclinical experiment [51], while its levels were inversely associated with the severity of atherosclerosis, among patients with CAD [52]. These data suggest that CST is associated with an improved lipid profile and likely exerts antiatherosclerotic effects, thus, partially explaining the negative associations of LDL and non-HDL cholesterol fractions with the CST levels, as observed in this study.

Relationship of CST with cardiac troponin, a hallmark biomarker of myocardial injury, has not been previously described, especially not in the HF setting. Our study revealed a weak but significant and independent inverse association of hs-cTnI concentrations with CST. Increased troponin levels in HF are common and can occur due to many mechanisms other than myocardial ischemia, such as elevated filling pressures, increased wall stress, tachycardias, arrhythmias, anemia, hypotension, and increased cardiomyocyte membrane permeability, causing a leak of cardiac troponin from the cytosolic pool into circulation [53]. Furthermore, pathologic processes in HF that occur on a cellular level, such as cardiomyocyte apoptosis, dysfunctional autophagy, and chronic breakdown of contractile apparatus, can result in a rise of circulating troponin levels, particularly those detected with high-sensitivity assays [53,54]. Since CST was associated with improved structural and functional echocardiographic parameters and lower left ventricular mass in our study, it is plausible that these effects might attenuate the extent of myocardial injury during the acute HF decompensation. However, it remains unknown whether this relationship is of chronic or acute nature and what are the dynamics of circulating troponin and CST during the natural course of HF.

Finally, CST serum levels were independently and inversely related to HR, both at admission and bedside rest. Previously, CST was characterized as an endocrine modulator of cardiac inotropism and lusitropism, by exhibiting cardiosuppressive effects on basal cardiac function and antagonistic action on beta-adrenergic positive inotropism and endothelin-1-mediated vasoconstriction, especially under stressed conditions [55–57]. Likewise, a study performed in mice showed that CST has a profound effect on autonomic function as its administration improved HR variability and decreased tachycardia by 10% in a ChgA knockout mice model, while wildtype mice had significantly lower HR at baseline compared to a ChgA knockout [58]. Our findings seem to support these preclinical observations, since patients with higher CST levels were more likely to have a generally lower HR.

There are several limitations to this study. This is a single-center clinical report with the cross-sectional design and no follow-up, therefore, we lack data on CST dynamics at various time-points and no causal inferences could be made due to the possibility of interference of non-measured confounders. Thus, enrolment of a larger number of patients might be required to generalize these results and to ascertain the potential relationship of CST with other relevant parameters of interest. Due to the lack of mechanistic insights, associations of CST with the measured parameters cannot be verified through a direct pathophysiological link, thereby, requiring further elucidation in future mechanistic preclinical and translational studies. Furthermore, direct measurements of circulating or urinary catecholamines or SNS activity parameters have not been performed in this study, therefore, we could not quantify catecholamine burden or sympathetic "excess" in our ADHF cohort. Finally, we lack data on specific pulmonary function parameters and lifestyle-related parameters as these were not prespecified and measured in our study design.

5. Conclusions

Results of this study are novel for this population and suggest that the role of CST in HF is complex and multidimensional. On the one hand, higher CST levels are associated with beneficial metabolic and cardioprotective effects and, on the other, high CST levels reflect higher disease severity and most likely parallel increased neurohumoral activity that might translate to adverse outcomes during the natural course of disease. These findings could have clinical impact in the sense that CST could serve as a chronic marker of increased or residual sympathetic activation and could potentially be measured alongside established HF biomarkers, such as natriuretic peptides in the identification of HF patients with advanced disease burden and an increased risk of post-discharge mortality. Furthermore, future treatments developed to target neurohumoral pathways and to attenuate sympathetic nervous system activity in HF might translate to changes in circulating CST levels, thus, making them appropriate for the measurement of response to HF-directed therapy. Finally, further mechanistic studies and larger clinical studies with follow-up powered for relevant clinical endpoints are required to confirm the findings obtained in this study.

Author Contributions: Conceptualization, J.A.B. and J.B.; Data curation, J.A.B. and D.S.D.; Formal analysis, J.A.B., Z.S.G., D.D., and J.B.; Funding acquisition, J.B.; Investigation, J.A.B., D.G., Z.S.G., and D.S.D.; Methodology, J.A.B., D.S.D., and J.B.; Project administration, J.A.B., D.G., and J.B.; Resources, D.G., Z.S.G., D.S.D., D.D., and J.B.; Supervision, J.A.B. and D.S.D.; Visualization, J.A.B., Z.S.G., and D.D.; Writing—original draft, J.A.B.; Writing—review & editing, J.A.B., D.G., Z.S.G., D.S.D., D.D., and J.B.

Acknowledgments: The summary figures for this article has been designed by using some illustration elements that were kindly provided by Servier. Servier Medical Art is licensed under a Creative Commons Attribution V.3.0 Unported License.

Conflicts of Interest: The authors declare no conflict of interest.

References

1. Kurmani, S.; Squire, I. Acute heart failure: Definition, classification and epidemiology. *Curr. Heart Fail. Rep.* **2017**, *14*, 385–392. [CrossRef] [PubMed]
2. Roger, V.L. Epidemiology of heart failure. *Circ. Res.* **2013**, *113*, 646–659. [CrossRef] [PubMed]
3. Savarese, G.; Lund, L.H. Global public health burden of heart failure. *Card. Fail. Rev.* **2017**, *3*, 7–11. [CrossRef]
4. Ibrahim, N.E.; Januzzi, J.L. Established and emerging roles of biomarkers in heart failure. *Circ. Res.* **2018**, *123*, 614–629. [CrossRef] [PubMed]
5. Viquerat, C.E.; Daly, P.; Swedberg, K.; Evers, C.; Curran, D.; Parmley, W.W.; Chatterjee, K. Endogenous catecholamine levels in chronic heart failure. Relation to the severity of hemodynamic abnormalities. *Am. J. Med.* **1985**, *78*, 455–460. [CrossRef]

6. Deng, M.C.; Brisse, B.; Erren, M.; Khurana, C.; Breithardt, G.; Scheld, H.H. Ischemic versus idiopathic cardiomyopathy: Differing neurohumoral profiles despite comparable peak oxygen uptake. *Int. J. Cardiol.* **1997**, *61*, 261–268. [CrossRef]
7. Notarius, C.F.; Spaak, J.; Morris, B.L.; Floras, J.S. Comparison of muscle sympathetic activity in ischemic and nonischemic heart failure. *J. Card. Fail.* **2007**, *13*, 470–475. [CrossRef]
8. Fung, M.M.; Salem, R.M.; Mehtani, P.; Thomas, B.; Lu, C.F.; Perez, B.; Rao, F.; Stridsberg, M.; Ziegler, M.G.; Mahata, S.K.; et al. Direct vasoactive effects of the chromogranin A (CHGA) peptide catestatin in humans in vivo. *Clin. Exp. Hypertens.* **2010**, *32*, 278–287. [CrossRef]
9. Mahata, S.K.; O'Connor, D.T.; Mahata, M.; Yoo, S.H.; Taupenot, L.; Wu, H.; Gill, B.M.; Parmer, R.J. Novel autocrine feedback control of catecholamine release. A discrete chromogranin a fragment is a noncompetitive nicotinic cholinergic antagonist. *J. Clin. Invest.* **1997**, *100*, 1623–1633. [CrossRef]
10. Mahata, S.K.; Kiranmayi, M.; Mahapatra, N.R. Catestatin: A Master regulator of cardiovascular functions. *Curr. Med. Chem.* **2018**, *25*, 1352–1374. [CrossRef]
11. Borovac, J.A.; Dogas, Z.; Supe-Domic, D.; Galic, T.; Bozic, J. Catestatin serum levels are increased in male patients with obstructive sleep apnea. *Sleep Breath* **2019**, *23*, 473–481. [CrossRef] [PubMed]
12. Gaede, A.H.; Pilowsky, P.M. Catestatin, a chromogranin A-derived peptide, is sympathoinhibitory and attenuates sympathetic barosensitivity and the chemoreflex in rat CVLM. *Am. J. Physiol. Regul. Integr. Comp. Physiol.* **2012**, *302*, R365–R372. [CrossRef] [PubMed]
13. Wang, X.; Xu, S.; Liang, Y.; Zhu, D.; Mi, L.; Wang, G.; Gao, W. Dramatic changes in catestatin are associated with hemodynamics in acute myocardial infarction. *Biomarkers* **2011**, *16*, 372–377. [CrossRef] [PubMed]
14. Peng, F.; Chu, S.; Ding, W.; Liu, L.; Zhao, J.; Cui, X.; Li, R.; Wang, J. The predictive value of plasma catestatin for all-cause and cardiac deaths in chronic heart failure patients. *Peptides* **2016**, *86*, 112–117. [CrossRef] [PubMed]
15. Ottesen, A.H.; Carlson, C.R.; Louch, W.E.; Dahl, M.B.; Sandbu, R.A.; Johansen, R.F.; Jarstadmarken, H.; Bjoras, M.; Hoiseth, A.D.; Brynildsen, J.; et al. Glycosylated chromogranin A in heart failure: Implications for processing and cardiomyocyte calcium homeostasis. *Circ. Heart Fail.* **2017**, *10*, e003675. [CrossRef] [PubMed]
16. Meng, L.; Wang, J.; Ding, W.H.; Han, P.; Yang, Y.; Qi, L.T.; Zhang, B.W. Plasma catestatin level in patients with acute myocardial infarction and its correlation with ventricular remodelling. *Postgrad. Med. J.* **2013**, *89*, 193–196. [CrossRef] [PubMed]
17. Liu, L.; Ding, W.; Li, R.; Ye, X.; Zhao, J.; Jiang, J.; Meng, L.; Wang, J.; Chu, S.; Han, X.; et al. Plasma levels and diagnostic value of catestatin in patients with heart failure. *Peptides* **2013**, *46*, 20–25. [CrossRef] [PubMed]
18. Zhu, D.; Wang, F.; Yu, H.; Mi, L.; Gao, W. Catestatin is useful in detecting patients with stage B heart failure. *Biomarkers* **2011**, *16*, 691–697. [CrossRef]
19. McKee, P.A.; Castelli, W.P.; McNamara, P.M.; Kannel, W.B. The natural history of congestive heart failure: The Framingham study. *N. Engl. J. Med.* **1971**, *285*, 1441–1446. [CrossRef]
20. Ponikowski, P.; Voors, A.A.; Anker, S.D.; Bueno, H.; Cleland, J.G.; Coats, A.J.; Falk, V.; Gonzalez-Juanatey, J.R.; Harjola, V.P.; Jankowska, E.A.; et al. 2016 ESC Guidelines for the diagnosis and treatment of acute and chronic heart failure: The task force for the diagnosis and treatment of acute and chronic heart failure of the European society of cardiology (ESC). Developed with the special contribution of the heart failure association (HFA) of the ESC. *Eur. J. Heart Fail.* **2016**, *18*, 891–975.
21. Januzzi, J.L.; van Kimmenade, R.; Lainchbury, J.; Bayes-Genis, A.; Ordonez-Llanos, J.; Santalo-Bel, M.; Pinto, Y.M.; Richards, M. NT-proBNP testing for diagnosis and short-term prognosis in acute destabilized heart failure: An international pooled analysis of 1256 patients: The international collaborative of NT-proBNP study. *Eur. Heart J.* **2006**, *27*, 330–337. [CrossRef]
22. Januzzi, J.L., Jr.; Camargo, C.A.; Anwaruddin, S.; Baggish, A.L.; Chen, A.A.; Krauser, D.G.; Tung, R.; Cameron, R.; Nagurney, J.T.; Chae, C.U.; et al. The N-terminal Pro-BNP investigation of dyspnea in the emergency department (PRIDE) study. *Am. J. Cardiol.* **2005**, *95*, 948–954. [CrossRef]
23. Januzzi, J.L.; Chen-Tournoux, A.A.; Christenson, R.H.; Doros, G.; Hollander, J.E.; Levy, P.D.; Nagurney, J.T.; Nowak, R.M.; Pang, P.S.; Patel, D.; et al. N-terminal pro–B-type natriuretic peptide in the emergency department: The ICON-RELOADED study. *J. Am. Coll. Cardiol.* **2018**, *71*, 1191–1200. [CrossRef]
24. Mosteller, R.D. Simplified calculation of body-surface area. *N. Engl. J. Med.* **1987**, *317*, 1098.

25. Williams, B.; Mancia, G.; Spiering, W.; Agabiti Rosei, E.; Azizi, M.; Burnier, M.; Clement, D.L.; Coca, A.; de Simone, G.; Dominiczak, A.; et al. 2018 ESC/ESH Guidelines for the management of arterial hypertension. *Eur. Heart J.* **2018**, *39*, 3021–3104. [CrossRef]
26. Levey, A.S.; Stevens, L.A.; Schmid, C.H.; Zhang, Y.L.; Castro, A.F., 3rd; Feldman, H.I.; Kusek, J.W.; Eggers, P.; Van Lente, F.; Greene, T.; et al. A new equation to estimate glomerular filtration rate. *Ann. Intern. Med.* **2009**, *150*, 604–612. [CrossRef]
27. American Diabetes Association. (2) Classification and diagnosis of diabetes. *Diabetes Care* **2015**, *38*, S8–S16.
28. Surawicz, B.; Childers, R.; Deal Barbara, J.; Gettes Leonard, S. AHA/ACCF/HRS Recommendations for the Standardization and interpretation of the electrocardiogram. *Circulation* **2009**, *119*, e235–e240. [CrossRef]
29. Lang, R.M.; Badano, L.P.; Mor-Avi, V.; Afilalo, J.; Armstrong, A.; Ernande, L.; Flachskampf, F.A.; Foster, E.; Goldstein, S.A.; Kuznetsova, T.; et al. Recommendations for cardiac chamber quantification by echocardiography in adults: An update from the American Society of Echocardiography and the European Association of Cardiovascular Imaging. *Eur. Heart J. Cardiovasc. Imaging* **2015**, *16*, 233–270. [CrossRef]
30. Folland, E.D.; Parisi, A.F.; Moynihan, P.F.; Jones, D.R.; Feldman, C.L.; Tow, D.E. Assessment of left ventricular ejection fraction and volumes by real-time, two-dimensional echocardiography. A comparison of cineangiographic and radionuclide techniques. *Circulation* **1979**, *60*, 760–766. [CrossRef]
31. Remme, W.J. The sympathetic nervous system and ischaemic heart disease. *Eur. Heart J.* **1998**, *19*, F62–F71.
32. Liu, L.; Ding, W.; Zhao, F.; Shi, L.; Pang, Y.; Tang, C. Plasma levels and potential roles of catestatin in patients with coronary heart disease. *Scand. Cardiovasc. J.* **2013**, *47*, 217–224. [CrossRef]
33. Taupenot, L.; Harper, K.L.; O'Connor, D.T. The chromogranin-secretogranin family. *N. Engl. J. Med.* **2003**, *348*, 1134–1149. [CrossRef]
34. Helle, K.B. The granin family of uniquely acidic proteins of the diffuse neuroendocrine system: Comparative and functional aspects. *Biol. Rev. Camb. Philos. Soc.* **2004**, *79*, 769–794. [CrossRef]
35. Gayen, J.R.; Gu, Y.; O'Connor, D.T.; Mahata, S.K. Global disturbances in autonomic function yield cardiovascular instability and hypertension in the chromogranin a null mouse. *Endocrinology* **2009**, *150*, 5027–5035. [CrossRef]
36. Pascual-Figal, D.A.; Manzano-Fernandez, S.; Boronat, M.; Casas, T.; Garrido, I.P.; Bonaque, J.C.; Pastor-Perez, F.; Valdes, M.; Januzzi, J.L. Soluble ST2, high-sensitivity troponin T-and N-terminal pro-B-type natriuretic peptide: Complementary role for risk stratification in acutely decompensated heart failure. *Eur. J. Heart Fail.* **2011**, *13*, 718–725. [CrossRef]
37. Aimo, A.; Januzzi, J.L., Jr.; Vergaro, G.; Ripoli, A.; Latini, R.; Masson, S.; Magnoli, M.; Anand, I.S.; Cohn, J.N.; Tavazzi, L.; et al. High-sensitivity troponin T, NT-proBNP and glomerular filtration rate: A multimarker strategy for risk stratification in chronic heart failure. *Int. J. Cardiol.* **2019**, *277*, 166–172. [CrossRef]
38. Ahmed, A. A propensity matched study of New York Heart Association class and natural history end points in heart failure. *Am. J. Cardiol.* **2007**, *99*, 549–553. [CrossRef]
39. Ahmed, A.; Aronow, W.S.; Fleg, J.L. Higher New York Heart Association classes and increased mortality and hospitalization in patients with heart failure and preserved left ventricular function. *Am. Heart J.* **2006**, *151*, 444–450. [CrossRef]
40. Muntwyler, J.; Abetel, G.; Gruner, C.; Follath, F. One-year mortality among unselected outpatients with heart failure. *Eur. Heart J.* **2002**, *23*, 1861–1866. [CrossRef]
41. Wang, D.; Liu, T.; Shi, S.; Li, R.; Shan, Y.; Huang, Y.; Hu, D.; Huang, C. Chronic administration of catestatin improves autonomic function and exerts cardioprotective effects in myocardial infarction rats. *J. Cardiovasc. Pharmacol. Ther.* **2016**, *21*, 526–535. [CrossRef]
42. Zhu, D.; Xie, H.; Wang, X.; Liang, Y.; Yu, H.; Gao, W. Correlation of plasma catestatin level and the prognosis of patients with acute myocardial infarction. *PLoS ONE* **2015**, *10*, e0122993. [CrossRef]
43. Meng, L.; Ye, X.J.; Ding, W.H.; Yang, Y.; Di, B.B.; Liu, L.; Huo, Y. Plasma catecholamine release-inhibitory peptide catestatin in patients with essential hypertension. *J. Cardiovasc. Med.* **2011**, *12*, 643–647. [CrossRef]
44. Mahapatra, N.R.; O'Connor, D.T.; Vaingankar, S.M.; Hikim, A.P.; Mahata, M.; Ray, S.; Staite, E.; Wu, H.; Gu, Y.; Dalton, N.; et al. Hypertension from targeted ablation of chromogranin A can be rescued by the human ortholog. *J. Clin. Invest.* **2005**, *115*, 1942–1952. [CrossRef]

45. Ying, W.; Mahata, S.; Bandyopadhyay, G.K.; Zhou, Z.; Wollam, J.; Vu, J.; Mayoral, R.; Chi, N.W.; Webster, N.J.G.; Corti, A.; et al. Catestatin inhibits obesity-induced macrophage infiltration and inflammation in the liver and suppresses hepatic glucose production, leading to improved insulin sensitivity. *Diabetes* **2018**, *67*, 841–848. [CrossRef]
46. Gallo, M.P.; Femmino, S.; Antoniotti, S.; Querio, G.; Alloatti, G.; Levi, R. Catestatin induces glucose uptake and GLUT4 trafficking in adult rat cardiomyocytes. *Biomed. Res. Int.* **2018**, *2018*, 2086109. [CrossRef]
47. Simunovic, M.; Supe-Domic, D.; Karin, Z.; Degoricija, M.; Paradzik, M.; Bozic, J.; Unic, I.; Skrabic, V. Serum catestatin concentrations are decreased in obese children and adolescents. *Pediatr. Diabetes* **2019**. Epub ahead of print. [CrossRef]
48. Bandyopadhyay, G.K.; Vu, C.U.; Gentile, S.; Lee, H.; Biswas, N.; Chi, N.W.; O'Connor, D.T.; Mahata, S.K. Catestatin (chromogranin A (352–372)) and novel effects on mobilization of fat from adipose tissue through regulation of adrenergic and leptin signaling. *J. Biol. Chem.* **2012**, *287*, 23141–23151. [CrossRef]
49. Bandyopadhyay, G.K.; Mahata, S.K. Chromogranin A regulation of obesity and peripheral insulin sensitivity. *Front. Endocrinol.* **2017**, *8*, 20. [CrossRef]
50. Durakoglugil, M.E.; Ayaz, T.; Kocaman, S.A.; Kirbas, A.; Durakoglugil, T.; Erdogan, T.; Cetin, M.; Sahin, O.Z.; Cicek, Y. The relationship of plasma catestatin concentrations with metabolic and vascular parameters in untreated hypertensive patients: Influence on high-density lipoprotein cholesterol. *Anatol. J. Cardiol.* **2015**, *15*, 577–585. [CrossRef]
51. Kojima, M.; Ozawa, N.; Mori, Y.; Takahashi, Y.; Watanabe-Kominato, K.; Shirai, R.; Watanabe, R.; Sato, K.; Matsuyama, T.A.; Ishibashi-Ueda, H.; et al. Catestatin prevents macrophage-driven atherosclerosis but not arterial injury-induced neointimal hyperplasia. *Thromb. Haemost.* **2018**, *118*, 182–194. [CrossRef]
52. Chen, Y.; Wang, X.; Yang, C.; Su, X.; Yang, W.; Dai, Y.; Han, H.; Jiang, J.; Lu, L.; Wang, H.; et al. Decreased circulating catestatin levels are associated with coronary artery disease: The emerging anti-inflammatory role. *Atherosclerosis* **2019**, *281*, 78–88. [CrossRef]
53. Wettersten, N.; Maisel, A. Role of cardiac troponin levels in acute heart failure. *Card. Fail. Rev.* **2015**, *1*, 102–106. [CrossRef]
54. Januzzi, J.L., Jr.; Filippatos, G.; Nieminen, M.; Gheorghiade, M. Troponin elevation in patients with heart failure: On behalf of the third Universal definition of myocardial infarction global task force: Heart failure section. *Eur. Heart J.* **2012**, *33*, 2265–2271. [CrossRef]
55. Angelone, T.; Quintieri, A.M.; Brar, B.K.; Limchaiyawat, P.T.; Tota, B.; Mahata, S.K.; Cerra, M.C. The antihypertensive chromogranin a peptide catestatin acts as a novel endocrine/paracrine modulator of cardiac inotropism and lusitropism. *Endocrinology* **2008**, *149*, 4780–4793. [CrossRef]
56. Imbrogno, S.; Garofalo, F.; Cerra, M.C.; Mahata, S.K.; Tota, B. The catecholamine release-inhibitory peptide catestatin (chromogranin A344-363) modulates myocardial function in fish. *J. Exp. Biol.* **2010**, *213*, 3636–3643. [CrossRef]
57. Mazza, R.; Gattuso, A.; Mannarino, C.; Brar, B.K.; Barbieri, S.F.; Tota, B.; Mahata, S.K. Catestatin (chromogranin A344–364) is a novel cardiosuppressive agent: Inhibition of isoproterenol and endothelin signaling in the frog heart. *Am. J. Physiol. Heart Circ. Physiol.* **2008**, *295*, H113–122. [CrossRef]
58. Dev, N.B.; Gayen, J.R.; O'Connor, D.T.; Mahata, S.K. Chromogranin a and the autonomic system: Decomposition of heart rate variability and rescue by its catestatin fragment. *Endocrinology* **2010**, *151*, 2760–2768. [CrossRef]

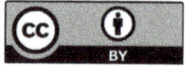

© 2019 by the authors. Licensee MDPI, Basel, Switzerland. This article is an open access article distributed under the terms and conditions of the Creative Commons Attribution (CC BY) license (http://creativecommons.org/licenses/by/4.0/).

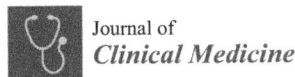

Article
New Cardiovascular Biomarkers in Ischemic Heart Disease—GDF-15, A Probable Predictor for Ejection Fraction

Daniel Dalos [1], Georg Spinka [1], Matthias Schneider [1], Bernhard Wernly [2], Vera Paar [2], Uta Hoppe [2], Brigitte Litschauer [3], Jeanette Strametz-Juranek [1] and Michael Sponder [1,*]

1. Division of Cardiology, Medical University of Vienna, 1090 Vienna, Austria
2. Division of Cardiology, Paracelsus Medical University of Salzburg, 5020 Salzburg, Austria
3. Department of Pharmacology, Medical University of Vienna, 1090 Vienna, Austria
* Correspondence: michael.sponder@meduniwien.ac.at; Tel.: +43-1-40-400-46140; Fax: +43-1-40-400-42160

Received: 12 June 2019; Accepted: 24 June 2019; Published: 27 June 2019

Abstract: Background: Various biomarkers have been associated with coronary artery disease (CAD) and ischemic heart failure. The aim of this study was to investigate the correlation of serum levels of soluble urokinase-type plasminogen activator receptor (suPAR), growth differentiation factor 15 (GDF-15), heart-type fatty acid-binding protein (H-FABP), and soluble suppression of tumorigenicity 2 (sST2) with left ventricular ejection fraction (EF) in CAD patients and controls. Methods and Results: CAD patients were divided into three groups according to their EF as measured by the biplane Simpson method (53–84%, 31–52%, ≤30%). Overall, 361 subjects were analyzed. In total, 155 CAD patients had an EF of 53–84%, 71 patients had an EF of 31–52%, and 23 patients had an EF of ≤30% as compared to 112 healthy controls (age 51.3 ± 9.0 years, 44.6% female). Mean ages according to EF were 62.1 ± 10.9, 65.2 ± 10.1, and 66.6 ± 8.2 years, respectively, with females representing 29.0, 29.6, and 13.0%. suPAR, GDF-15, H-FABP, and sST2 values were significantly higher in CAD patients and showed an exponential increase with decreasing EF. In a multiple logistic regression model, GDF-15 ($p = 0.009$), and NT-brain natriuretic peptide ($p = 0.003$) were independently associated with EF. Conclusion: Biomarkers such as suPAR, GDF-15, H-FABP, and sST2 are increased in CAD patients, especially in highly impaired EF. Besides NT-proBNP as a well-known marker for risk prediction, GDF-15 may be an additional tool for diagnosis and clinical follow-up.

Keywords: heart failure; ejection fraction; soluble urokinase-type plasminogen activator receptor (suPAR); growth differentiation factor 15 (GDF-15); heart-type fatty acid-binding protein (H-FABP); soluble suppression of tumorigenicity 2 (sST2)

1. Introduction

Coronary artery disease (CAD) resulting in chronic heart failure (CHF) is still one of the most important topics in socio-economic fields despite various advancements in treatment options over the last decades.

Several pathophysiological processes such as inflammation or myocardial stress have to be considered to understand the complexity of CAD and the ventricular remodeling mechanisms leading to CHF. During the last years, cardiovascular biomarkers reflecting these sequences have raised the attention of many research groups in order to identify patients at risk at an early timepoint, as well as to optimize their treatment strategies.

Elevated levels of soluble urokinase-type plasminogen activator receptor (suPAR), a membrane-bound receptor, have been associated with coronary calcification [1], systemic inflammation [2], and CHF [3].

Growth differentiation factor 15 (GDF-15) is a transforming growth-factor beta cytokine that is mainly expressed in inflammatory settings [4,5], and its prognostic utility has been previously described in cardiovascular disease [6], especially in CHF [7].

Heart-type fatty acid-binding protein (H-FABP) represents a protein in cardiomyocyte cytoplasm and can be found in skeletal muscle [8], cardiac microvasculature, and endothelial cells as well [9]. H-FABP in cardiomyocytes is indispensable to ensure a high flux of long-chain fatty acids and therefore plays an important role in the energy supply.

Suppression of tumorigenicity (ST) 2 is an interleukin (IL)-1 receptor, which can occur as transmembrane receptor and a soluble form (sST2). The natural ligand of ST2 is IL-33, which acts as a traditional cytokine and as a transcription factor [10] binding to circulating sST2. Soluble ST2 serves as a decoy receptor inhibiting the IL-33/ST2-ligand (ST2L) complex resulting in an attenuation of IL-33-mediated inflammation [11], and consequently limits the cardioprotective effect of IL-33/ST2L activation. Increased levels of sST2 have been described in acute coronary syndromes [12], CHF [13], chronic obstructive pulmonary disease, and sepsis [14].

Although there is quite a wide range of studies depicting the impact of aforesaid biomarkers on poor clinical outcome in CHF [7,15–20], their detailed course of plasma levels in decreasing left ventricular ejection fraction (EF) has not yet been investigated. The aim of this analysis was to determine suPAR, GDF-15, H-FABP, and sST2 levels in CHF patients and, furthermore, to investigate their association with EF in comparison to the well-established biomarker N-terminal pro brain natriuretic peptide (NT-proBNP).

2. Methods

The clinical trials registration number was NCT02097199 (IPHAAB-study)/NCT02159235, under the title "Heavy Metals, Angiogenesis Factors and Osteopontin in Coronary Artery Disease".

2.1. Subjects and Patient Population

Between October 2011 and December 2017, 249 patients with recently angiographically proven CAD were recruited in course of their inpatient stay at the Medical University of Vienna, Austria, in the Department of Internal Medicine II/Cardiology. Patients were included if coronary angiography revealed any atherosclerotic alteration in at least one coronary artery, regardless of any criteria necessitating coronary intervention. Patients were also included if any coronary intervention had been performed ≤7 days prior to enrolment. This cohort was further subdivided into three subgroups depending on left ventricular ejection fraction (EF): (1) 53–84%, (2) 31–52%, and (3) ≤30%. This classification was done in adherence to the current recommendations of the American Society of Echocardiography and the European Association of Cardiovascular Imaging [21] without any gender-specific analysis.

As a control group (to obtain reference values for the mentioned biomarkers) we recruited 112 subjects without angiographically proven CAD. In this group we performed a bicycle stress test (Ergometer eBike comfort, GE Medical Systems, Freiburg, Germany). Only subjects without corresponding anamnesis, typical symptoms, and/or ischemia-related ECG-abnormalities at rest or exhaustion were included in the control group.

In both groups detailed anthropometric and anamnestic data as well as routine laboratory parameters were assessed.

The study was carried out in adherence to the Declaration of Helsinki and its later amendments. The protocol has been approved by the Ethics Committee of the Medical University of Vienna and informed consent was obtained from all participating subjects prior to any study-related procedure.

2.2. Echocardiographic Analysis

Echocardiographic data was obtained with the use of the commercially available ultrasound systems (GE Medical Systems Vivid 7 Dimensions, Horton, Norway). All measurements were performed by experienced board-certified physicians according to the recommendations of the American Society of Echocardiography and the European Association of Cardiovascular Imaging [21]. The examiners were blinded to the levels of suPAR, GDF-15, H-FABP, and sST2. EF was calculated using the biplane method of disks with the following formula: (end-diastolic volume minus end-systolic volume) divided by end-diastolic volume (biplane Simpson method).

2.3. Laboratory Analysis

Blood samples were taken from an arm vein after 10 minutes in a lying position with a tube/adapter system. Samples were then placed in a standard centrifuge (Rotanta 460, Hettich GmbH & Co. KG, Tuttlingen, Germany) and were processed with 2500 rpm for 10 min.

Serum levels of suPAR, GDF-15, H-FABP, and sST2 were analyzed by utilizing enzyme-linked immunosorbent assay (ELISA) kits that are commercially available (Duoset DY206, DY1678, DY807, DY957; R&D Systems, Minneapolis, MN, USA). Preparation of all necessary reagents and measurements were performed according to the instructions supplied by the manufacturer. In short, patient serum samples and standard protein were added to the wells of the ELISA plates (Nunc MaxiSorp flat-bottom 96-well plates, VWR International GmbH, Vienna, Austria) and were incubated for two hours. ELISA plates were then washed using a Tween 20/PBS solution (Sigma Aldrich, St. Louis, MO, USA). In the next step, a biotin-labelled antibody was added and plates were incubated for another two hours. Plates were then washed once more and a streptavidin-horseradish-peroxidase solution was added to the wells. By adding tetramethylbenzidine (TMB; Sigma Aldrich, St. Louis, MO, USA) a color reaction was generated. Optical density (OD) values were measured at 450 nm on an ELISA plate-reader (iMark Microplate Absorbance Reader, Bio-Rad Laboratories, Vienna, Austria).

The analysis was performed according to the manufacturer's instructions. The coefficients of variation (CV) were for suPAR: 2.1–2.7% (intra-assay) and 5.1–5.9% (inter-assay); for H-FABP: 0.3–4.7% (intra-assay) and 1.3–17.4% (inter-assay); for sST2: 4.4–5.6% (intra-assay) and 5.4–7.1% (inter-assay); and for GDF-15: 4.7–5.9% (intra-assay) and 1.8–2.8% (inter-assay).

2.4. Statistical Analysis

Statistical analysis was done with SPSS 20.0 (IBM, Armonk, NY, USA). Dichotomous variables are expressed as frequencies or percentages. Continuous and normally distributed data is described by means ± standard deviation (SD), not normally distributed data as median/25th quartile/75th quartile. Comparisons between groups were made using the Chi-square or Fisher's exact test for categorical variables, and the Student t-test or Mann–Whitney U test for continuous variables, as appropriate. Correlations between continuous parameters were calculated using the Spearman coefficient.

The influence of relevant parameters on EF was investigated first by univariate logistic regression. To identify the most relevant predictors a multiple regression model was selected from the scope of variables that reached statistical significance in univariate analysis by a backward procedure. The significance limit for a predictor to enter the model was 0.05. All tests were two-sided and p-values ≤ 0.05 were considered significant.

3. Results

3.1. Baseline Characteristics

Out of 249 CAD patients, 155 had an EF of 53–84%, 71 had 31–52%, and 23 patients had a severely impaired EF ($\leq$30%). Patients were 62.1 ± 10.9, 65.2 ± 10.1 and 66.6 ± 8.2 years old, and were female in 29.0%, 29.6%, and 13.0% of cases, respectively. The control group consisted of 112 healthy adults with a mean age of 51.3 ± 9.0 years and with a higher proportion of women (44.6%). The detailed baseline characteristics concerning cardiovascular risk factors and routine laboratory assessment according to the four different groups are depicted in Table 1.

Table 1. Baseline characteristics.

	Control (n = 112)	EF 53–84% (n = 155)	EF 31–52% (n = 71)	EF ≤ 30% (n = 23)	p-Value
Age (years)	51.3 ± 9.0	62.1 ± 10.9	65.2 ± 10.1	66.6 ± 8.2	<0.001
Female sex (%)	44.6	29.0	29.6	13.0	0.006
Hypertension (%)	38.4	92.9	93.0	95.7	<0.001
Family history of CAD (%)	42.0	59.4	56.3	52.2	0.040
Diabetes (%)	5.4	21.9	25.2	34.8	<0.001
Dyslipidemia (%)	34.8	92.3	91.5	73.9	<0.001
BMI (kg/m^2)	27.4 ± 4.2	27.8 ± 4.8	28.6 ± 5.7	29.5 ± 6.4	0.226
SBP (mmHg)	138 ± 16	131 ± 16	128 ± 16	129 ± 19	0.004
DBP (mmHg)	84 ± 12	76 ± 10	74 ± 10	79 ± 17	<0.001
HR (bpm)	67 ± 9	68 ± 12	71 ± 15	77 ± 13	0.003
Cholesterol (mg/dL)	200 ± 40	180 ± 52	164 ± 41	163 ± 56	<0.001
Triglycerides (mg/dL)	129 ± 78	153 ± 88	149 ± 83	148 ± 72	0.605
LDL (mg/dL)	117 ± 35	107 ± 40	94 ± 41	96 ± 35	0.495
HDL (mg/dL)	58 ± 18	48 ± 14	43 ± 12	37 ± 10	0.005
Creatinine (mg/dL)	0.9 ± 0.2	1.1 ± 0.8	1.2 ± 0.4	1.4 ± 0.5	0.003
ASAT (U/L)	26 ± 13	52 ± 61	52 ± 78	35 ± 25	0.311
ALAT (U/L)	27 ± 15	37 ± 27	43 ± 12	31 ± 25	0.569
Gamma GT (U/L)	30 ± 40	56 ± 100	89 ± 133	78 ± 88	0.076
HbA$_{1c}$ (rel%)	5.4 ± 0.6	6.0 ± 0.9	6.6 ± 1.7	7.1 ± 2.4	<0.001
Erythrocytes (T/L)	4.7 ± 0.5	4.5 ± 0.6	4.4 ± 0.6	4.6 ± 0.7	0.028
Hemoglobin (g/dL)	13.8 ± 1.4	13.3 ± 1.8	12.8 ± 1.8	12.8 ± 2.4	0.012
Hematocrit (%)	40 ± 3	39 ± 5	39 ± 5	39 ± 7	0.392
Platelet count (G/L)	243 ± 56	236 ± 74	250 ± 101	217 ± 89	0.040
Leukocytes (G/L)	6.6 ± 1.7	12.7 ± 2.0	8.0 ± 2.5	7.2 ± 2.1	0.494

Continuous variables are shown as mean ± standard deviation; ALAT: alanine aminotransferase; ASAT: aspartate aminotransferase; BMI: body mass index; CAD: coronary artery disease; DBP: diastolic blood pressure; EF: ejection fraction; GT: glutamyltransferase; HDL: high-density lipoprotein; HR: heart rate; LDL: low-density lipoprotein; SBP: systolic blood pressure.

3.2. Biomarkers

Every investigated biomarker showed a constant increase with decreasing EF. suPAR levels from controls were 1852 ± 759 pg/mL compared to 3181 ± 1387 in the worst EF group ($p < 0.001$). There was a slight trend between the control cohort and CAD patients with normal EF (1852 ± 759 vs. 2178 ± 1108 pg/mL, $p = 0.087$), whereas there was a steep increase between normal EF and EF 31–52% (2178 ± 1108 vs. 2851 ± 1260 pg/mL, $p < 0.001$) (Figure 1).

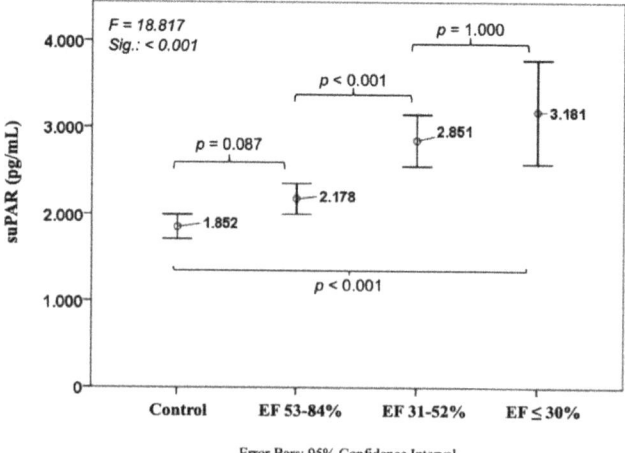

Figure 1. Course of soluble urokinase-type plasminogen activator receptor in ischemic heart disease. EF: ejection fraction; suPAR: soluble urokinase-type plasminogen activator receptor; EF: ejection fraction.

Levels of GDF-15 were 699 ± 554 pg/mL in the control cohort with a significant difference to the group with EF ≤ 30% (3173 ± 3008, $p < 0.001$). We also observed a relevant distinction between controls and normal EF patients (1500 ± 1337, $p < 0.001$) and a slight trend between normal and mid-range EF (1975 ± 1405, $p = 0.086$) (Figure 2).

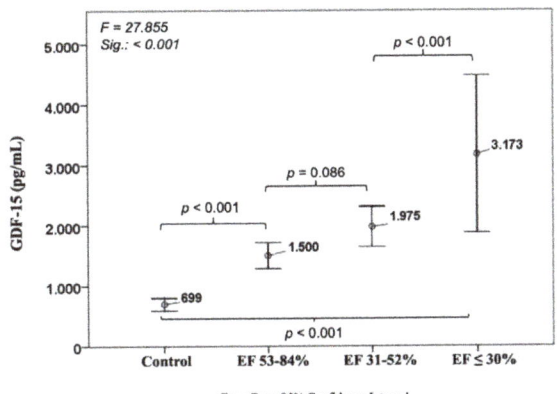

Figure 2. Course of growth differentiation factor 15 in ischemic heart disease. GDF-15: Growth differentiation factor 15.

Such as suPAR and GDF-15, H-FABP showed an increase with decreasing EF, but in contrast to the mentioned markers, this difference did neither show significant differences between controls 2.54 ± 4.16 ng/mL and EF ≤ 30% (5.92 ± 4.48 ng/mL, $p = 0.114$), nor in between the three EF groups (Figure 3).

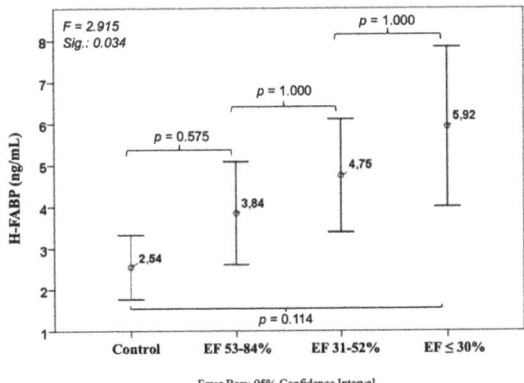

Figure 3. Course of heart-type fatty acid-binding protein in ischemic heart disease. H-FABP: heart-type fatty acid-binding protein.

Soluble ST2 levels were 6476 ± 2916 pg/mL in patients without CAD and CHF with a considerable increase compared to the worst CHF patients (9632 ± 6346 pg/mL, $p = 0.038$). No differences were observed amongst the other cohorts (Figure 4).

Concerning the well-established NT-proBNP we found the expected values of 58 ± 103 ng/L in controls, with a significant rise in CHF patients with poor EF (7041 ± 8791 ng/L, $p < 0.001$). There was a trend between the control cohort and CAD patients with normal EF (1239 ± 3298 ng/L, $p = 0.077$), whereas there was a significant increase between normal and mid-range EF patients (2843 ± 4306 ng/L, $p = 0.017$) as well as between mid-range and poor EF ($p < 0.001$) (Figure 5).

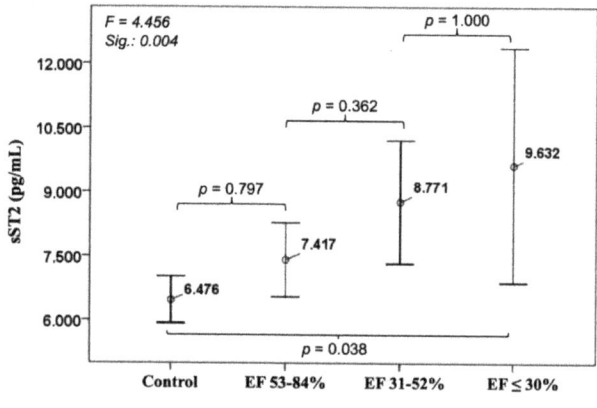

Figure 4. Course of soluble suppression of tumorigenicity 2 (sST2) in ischemic heart disease.

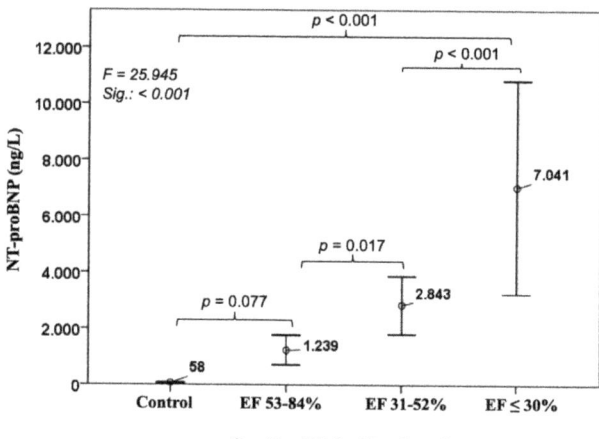

Figure 5. Course of N-terminal pro brain natriuretic peptide in ischemic heart disease. NT-proBNP: N-terminal pro brain natriuretic peptide.

In a multiple, backward logistic regression analysis, positive predictors for EF were age ($p < 0.001$), sex ($p < 0.001$), body mass index ($p = 0.010$), GDF-15 ($p = 0.009$) and NT-proBNP ($p = 0.003$, Table 2).

Table 2. Multiple logistic regression analysis for ejection fraction.

Parameters	Regression Coefficient B	Standard Error	Beta	T	p-Value
Constant	−2.056	0.334		−6.149	<0.001
Age (years)	0.029	0.004	0.379	7888	<0.001
Sex	0.351	0.083	0.188	2.614	<0.001
BMI (kg/m^2)	0.020	0.008	0.115	2.584	0.010
GDF-15 (pg/mL)	9.177×10^{-5}	0.001	0.158	2.614	0.009
NT-proBNP (pg/mL)	3.702×10^{-5}	0.001	0.172	2.983	0.003
$F = 38.0; p < 0.001; r^2_{adj}:0.346$					

BMI: body mass index; GDF-15: growth differentiation factor 15; NT-proBNP: N-terminal pro brain natriuretic peptide.

4. Discussion

In this analysis, we were able to confirm the diagnostic power of the biomarkers suPAR, GDF-15, H-FABP, sST2, and NT-proBNP in CHF patients compared to healthy adults. In addition, to the best of our knowledge, this is the first study to describe the detailed course of these biomarkers by means of left ventricular EF. Furthermore, we were able to show a significant association of GDF-15 with EF besides the well-established NT-proBNP in this specific patient population.

Circulating H-FABP levels increase during myocardial ischemia caused by pathological events, such as myocardial infarction, by leaking into the extracellular space [22]. However, in some cases myocardial damage due to acute physical activity might also increase its levels but they return to baseline within a few hours [23] and long-term physical training has been shown to lead to a significant decrease in H-FABP levels [24]. It can be assumed that high H-FABP levels in patients with low EF might be a sign of chronically impaired myocardial perfusion resulting in myocardial damage.

One could speculate that an increase in sST2 serum levels might be due to the chronic inflammatory state as it has been previously described in CHF patients [25]. As sST2 acts as a decoy receptor for IL-33, an upregulation might buffer an exuberant inflammation response.

Similar to sST2, suPAR (the soluble form of uPAR which is measurable after cleavage and release of membrane-bound uPAR) is involved in inflammation processes caused by numerous diseases, inter alia coronary calcification [1] and heart failure [3], and has been identified as marker for an unfavorable clinical outcome including mortality [26]. In our cohort we were able to confirm these findings as we found increasing suPAR levels dependent on the severity of CHF.

Interestingly, we observed an upregulation of GDF-15 with worsening EF as well as their independent association, together with NT-proBNP. GDF-15 is mainly secreted as a response to inflammation and hypoxemia. Due to the interaction with p53, it is released in sporadic severe stress situations, but also responds to low-level stressors during daily life activities [27,28]. These changes are reflected by circulating levels of GDF-15 that have been assigned protective effects regarding cell apoptosis [29] and myocardial hypertrophy [30,31].

While GDF-15 is expressed in visceral and subcutaneous adipose tissue in obese patients [32], it may also be released in atherosclerotic plaques in coronary arteries [33], in the myocardium in the course of acute cellular damages [5], as well as in peripheral tissue [34]. Due to its induction in different clinical scenarios, the use of GDF-15 as a diagnostic marker in acute cardiovascular care settings (e.g., chest pain, dyspnea) is limited.

In CAD, levels of GDF-15 are independently correlated with age, diabetes, high-sensitive C-reactive protein (hs-CRP), and natriuretic peptides in the AtheroGene study [35], which is in line with our finding of a significant correlation between GDF-15 and NT-proBNP in our CAD cohort ($r = 0.727$, $p < 0.001$). Furthermore, in the AtheroGene study, where 1352 patients with stable CAD were investigated, GDF-15 levels were independently associated with cardiac mortality. Schopfer et al. were able to depict the prognostic importance of GDF-15 concerning all-cause mortality in the Heart and Soul Study with 984 patients [36]. Circulating GDF-15 remains relatively stable after acute coronary syndromes without signs of HF, compared to other biomarkers such as cardiac troponin or hs-CRP showing a curve-shaped course [37,38], suggesting that GDF-15 reflects chronic disease burden.

In CHF with reduced EF, GDF-15 concentrations are elevated and their constant increase in relation to HF severity, as reflected by New York Heart Association functional class and NT-proBNP, has already been described [7,39]. This can be confirmed by our analysis with the additional input of a better characterized cohort by means of EF. Recently, the group of Li et al. investigated fewer patients with a much smaller control cohort than in our study and found similar results. The combination of GDF-15 and NT-proBNP significantly improved the accuracy of diagnosing HF [18]. Remarkably, circulating GDF-15 is also increased in HF patients with preserved ejection fraction (HFpEF) which is in line with the theory of Paulus and Tschöpe regarding a continuous inflammatory state as the central pathomechanism in HFpEF [40,41].

In severely impaired CHF patients that underwent implantation of left ventricular assist devices, the mechanical support has led to a significant decrease of measurable GDF-15, showing the reversibility of even highly increased levels [42]. How this reduction may affect the protective effects of GDF-15 remains a matter of debate, especially concerning potential therapeutic interventions targeting GDF-15 with unknown effects on clinical outcome.

In summary, elevated values of GDF-15 need to be interpreted with respect to other comorbidities, clinical symptoms and laboratory values. Likewise, with NT-proBNP values that may be adulterated by renal insufficiency or significant valvular disease, GDF-15 has to be evaluated simultaneously with other inflammatory parameters in order to rule out significant infections or even septic conditions.

5. Conclusions

Levels of the cardiovascular biomarkers suPAR, GDF-15, H-FABP, and sST2 constantly increase when left ventricular EF decreases in CHF patients, which is comparable to the course of the well-established NT-proBNP. However, only GDF-15 is significantly associated with EF in a multivariate model and therefore may expand the spectrum of biomarkers in identifying these patients without further needs of cost-intensive diagnostic modalities.

6. Limitations

Due to the single-center design of this study, a center-specific bias cannot be excluded and due to a small proportion of female patients we could not perform a sex-specific analysis. Additionally, unknown or un-controlled circumstances might have influenced the investigated parameters. Finally, although alterations in GDF-15 were shown in Caucasian and Asian tumor patients [43], there is little evidence regarding racial diversification in CAD and HF [44]. Our analysis was performed in Caucasian patients only; therefore, the results have to be interpreted cautiously with regard to other ethnicities.

Author Contributions: D.D.: recruitment, manuscript preparation, statistical analysis; M.S.: echocardiographic analysis, manuscript preparation; G.S.: echocardiographic analysis; B.W.: laboratory analysis; V.P.: laboratory analysis; U.H.: manuscript preparation; B.L.: statistical analysis; J.S.-J.: study design, manuscript preparation; M.S.: study design, recruitment, manuscript preparation, statistical analysis.

Funding: This study was funded by means of the Medical University of Vienna, Austria and the Paracelsus Medical University of Salzburg, Austria.

Acknowledgments: The authors would like to thank Markus Vertesich for his technical support.

Conflicts of Interest: The authors declare no conflict of interest.

References

1. Sorensen, M.H.; Gerke, O.; Eugen-Olsen, J.; Munkholm, H.; Lambrechtsen, J.; Sand, N.P.; Mickley, H.; Rasmussen, L.M.; Olsen, M.H.; Diederichsen, A. Soluble urokinase plasminogen activator receptor is in contrast to high-sensitive C-reactive-protein associated with coronary artery calcifications in healthy middle-aged subjects. *Atherosclerosis* **2014**, *237*, 60–66. [CrossRef] [PubMed]
2. Lyngbaek, S.; Marott, J.L.; Sehestedt, T.; Hansen, T.W.; Olsen, M.H.; Andersen, O.; Linneberg, A.; Haugaard, S.B.; Eugen-Olsen, J.; Hansen, P.R.; et al. Cardiovascular risk prediction in the general population with use of suPAR, CRP, and Framingham Risk Score. *Int. J. Cardiol.* **2013**, *167*, 2904–2911. [CrossRef] [PubMed]
3. Borne, Y.; Persson, M.; Melander, O.; Smith, J.G.; Engstrom, G. Increased plasma level of soluble urokinase plasminogen activator receptor is associated with incidence of heart failure but not atrial fibrillation. *Eur. J. Heart Fail.* **2014**, *16*, 377–383. [CrossRef] [PubMed]
4. Bootcov, M.R.; Bauskin, A.R.; Valenzuela, S.M.; Moore, A.G.; Bansal, M.; He, X.Y.; Zhang, H.P.; Donnellan, M.; Mahler, S.; Pryor, K.; et al. MIC-1, a novel macrophage inhibitory cytokine, is a divergent member of the TGF-beta superfamily. *Proc. Natl. Acad. Sci. USA* **1997**, *94*, 11514–11519. [CrossRef] [PubMed]

5. Kempf, T.; Eden, M.; Strelau, J.; Naguib, M.; Willenbockel, C.; Tongers, J.; Heineke, J.; Kotlarz, D.; Xu, J.; Molkentin, J.D.; et al. The transforming growth factor-beta superfamily member growth-differentiation factor-15 protects the heart from ischemia/reperfusion injury. *Circ. Res.* **2006**, *98*, 351–360. [CrossRef] [PubMed]
6. Wollert, K.C.; Kempf, T.; Wallentin, L. Growth differentiation factor 15 as a biomarker in cardiovascular disease. *Clin. Chem.* **2017**, *63*, 140–151. [CrossRef]
7. Kempf, T.; von Haehling, S.; Peter, T.; Allhoff, T.; Cicoira, M.; Doehner, W.; Ponikowski, P.; Filippatos, G.S.; Rozentryt, P.; Drexler, H.; et al. Prognostic utility of growth differentiation factor-15 in patients with chronic heart failure. *J. Am. Coll. Cardiol.* **2007**, *50*, 1054–1060. [CrossRef]
8. Zschiesche, W.; Kleine, A.H.; Spitzer, E.; Veerkamp, J.H.; Glatz, J.F. Histochemical localization of heart-type fatty-acid binding protein in human and murine tissues. *Histochem. Cell Biol.* **1995**, *103*, 147–156. [CrossRef]
9. Bathia, D.P.; Carless, D.R.; Viswanathan, K.; Hall, A.S.; Barth, J.H. Serum 99th centile values for two heart-type fatty acid binding protein assays. *Ann. Clin. Biochem.* **2009**, *46*, 464–467. [CrossRef]
10. Martin, N.T.; Martin, M.U. Interleukin 33 is a guardian of barriers and a local alarmin. *Nat. Immunol.* **2016**, *17*, 122–131. [CrossRef]
11. Lassus, J.; Gayat, E.; Mueller, C.; Peacock, W.F.; Spinar, J.; Harjola, V.P.; van Kimmenade, R.; Pathak, A.; Mueller, T.; Disomma, S.; et al. Incremental value of biomarkers to clinical variables for mortality prediction in acutely decompensated heart failure: The Multinational Observational Cohort on Acute Heart Failure (MOCA) study. *Int. J. Cardiol.* **2013**, *168*, 2186–2194. [CrossRef] [PubMed]
12. Kohli, P.; Bonaca, M.P.; Kakkar, R.; Kudinova, A.Y.; Scirica, B.M.; Sabatine, M.S.; Murphy, S.A.; Braunwald, E.; Lee, R.T.; Morrow, D.A. Role of ST2 in non-ST-elevation acute coronary syndrome in the MERLIN-TIMI 36 trial. *Clin. Chem.* **2012**, *58*, 257–266. [CrossRef] [PubMed]
13. Anand, I.S.; Rector, T.S.; Kuskowski, M.; Snider, J.; Cohn, J.N. Prognostic value of soluble ST2 in the Valsartan Heart Failure Trial. *Circ. Heart Fail.* **2014**, *7*, 418–426. [CrossRef] [PubMed]
14. Dieplinger, B.; Januzzi, J.L., Jr.; Steinmair, M.; Gabriel, C.; Poelz, W.; Haltmayer, M.; Mueller, T. Analytical and clinical evaluation of a novel high-sensitivity assay for measurement of soluble ST2 in human plasma—The presage ST2 assay. *Clin. Chim. Acta* **2009**, *409*, 33–40. [CrossRef] [PubMed]
15. Ho, J.E.; Lyass, A.; Courchesne, P.; Chen, G.; Liu, C.; Yin, X.; Hwang, S.J.; Massaro, J.M.; Larson, M.G.; Levy, D. Protein biomarkers of cardiovascular disease and mortality in the community. *J. Am. Heart Assoc.* **2018**, *7*. [CrossRef] [PubMed]
16. Kazimierczyk, E.; Kazimierczyk, R.; Harasim-Symbor, E.; Kaminski, K.; Sobkowicz, B.; Chabowski, A.; Tycinska, A. Persistently elevated plasma heart-type fatty acid binding protein concentration is related with poor outcome in acute decompensated heart failure patients. *Clin. Chim. Acta* **2018**, *487*, 48–53. [CrossRef] [PubMed]
17. Koller, L.; Stojkovic, S.; Richter, B.; Sulzgruber, P.; Potolidis, C.; Liebhart, F.; Mortl, D.; Berger, R.; Goliasch, G.; Wojta, J.; et al. Soluble urokinase-type plasminogen activator receptor improves risk prediction in patients with chronic heart failure. *JACC Heart Fail.* **2017**, *5*, 268–277. [CrossRef]
18. Li, J.; Cui, Y.; Huang, A.; Li, Q.; Jia, W.; Liu, K.; Qi, X. Additional diagnostic value of growth differentiation factor-15 (GDF-15) to N-Terminal B-type natriuretic peptide (NT-proBNP) in patients with different stages of heart failure. *Med. Sci. Monit.* **2018**, *24*, 4992–4999. [CrossRef]
19. Vorovich, E.; French, B.; Ky, B.; Goldberg, L.; Fang, J.C.; Sweitzer, N.K.; Cappola, T.P. Biomarker predictors of cardiac hospitalization in chronic heart failure: A recurrent event analysis. *J. Card. Fail.* **2014**, *20*, 569–576. [CrossRef]
20. Weinberg, E.O.; Shimpo, M.; Hurwitz, S.; Tominaga, S.; Rouleau, J.L.; Lee, R.T. Identification of serum soluble ST2 receptor as a novel heart failure biomarker. *Circulation* **2003**, *107*, 721–726. [CrossRef]
21. Lang, R.M.; Badano, L.P.; Mor-Avi, V.; Afilalo, J.; Armstrong, A.; Ernande, L.; Flachskampf, F.A.; Foster, E.; Goldstein, S.A.; Kuznetsova, T.; et al. Recommendations for cardiac chamber quantification by echocardiography in adults: An update from the American Society of Echocardiography and the European Association of Cardiovascular Imaging. *Eur. Heart J. Cardiovasc. Imaging.* **2015**, *16*, 233–270. [CrossRef] [PubMed]
22. Viswanathan, K.; Hall, A.S.; Barth, J.H. An evidence-based approach to the assessment of heart-type Fatty Acid binding protein in acute coronary syndrome. *Clin. Biochem. Rev.* **2012**, *33*, 3–11. [PubMed]

23. Lippi, G.; Schena, F.; Montagnana, M.; Salvagno, G.L.; Guidi, G.C. Influence of acute physical exercise on emerging muscular biomarkers. *Clin. Chem. Lab. Med.* **2008**, *46*, 1313–1318. [CrossRef] [PubMed]
24. Sponder, M.; Lichtenauer, M.; Wernly, B.; Paar, V.; Hoppe, U.; Emich, M.; Fritzer-Szekeres, M.; Litschauer, B.; Strametz-Juranek, J. Serum heart-type fatty acid-binding protein decreases and soluble isoform of suppression of tumorigenicity 2 increases significantly by long-term physical activity. *J. Investig. Med.* **2018**. [CrossRef] [PubMed]
25. Shirazi, L.F.; Bissett, J.; Romeo, F.; Mehta, J.L. Role of inflammation in heart failure. *Curr. Atheroscler. Rep.* **2017**, *19*, 27. [CrossRef] [PubMed]
26. Rasmussen, L.J.; Ladelund, S.; Haupt, T.H.; Ellekilde, G.; Poulsen, J.H.; Iversen, K.; Eugen-Olsen, J.; Andersen, O. Soluble urokinase plasminogen activator receptor (suPAR) in acute care: A strong marker of disease presence and severity, readmission and mortality. A retrospective cohort study. *Emerg. Med. J.* **2016**, *33*, 769–775. [CrossRef] [PubMed]
27. Yang, H.; Filipovic, Z.; Brown, D.; Breit, S.N.; Vassilev, L.T. Macrophage inhibitory cytokine-1: A novel biomarker for p53 pathway activation. *Mol. Cancer Ther.* **2003**, *2*, 1023–1029.
28. Vousden, K.H.; Lane, D.P. p53 in health and disease. *Nat. Rev. Mol. Cell Biol.* **2007**, *8*, 275–283. [CrossRef]
29. Li, J.; Yang, L.; Qin, W.; Zhang, G.; Yuan, J.; Wang, F. Adaptive induction of growth differentiation factor 15 attenuates endothelial cell apoptosis in response to high glucose stimulus. *PLoS ONE* **2013**, *8*, e65549. [CrossRef]
30. Schillaci, G.; Verdecchia, P.; Porcellati, C.; Cuccurullo, O.; Cosco, C.; Perticone, F. Continuous relation between left ventricular mass and cardiovascular risk in essential hypertension. *Hypertension* **2000**, *35*, 580–586. [CrossRef]
31. Xu, X.Y.; Nie, Y.; Wang, F.F.; Bai, Y.; Lv, Z.Z.; Zhang, Y.Y.; Li, Z.J.; Gao, W. Growth differentiation factor (GDF)-15 blocks norepinephrine-induced myocardial hypertrophy via a novel pathway involving inhibition of epidermal growth factor receptor transactivation. *J. Biol. Chem.* **2014**, *289*, 10084–10094. [CrossRef] [PubMed]
32. Ding, Q.; Mracek, T.; Gonzalez-Muniesa, P.; Kos, K.; Wilding, J.; Trayhurn, P.; Bing, C. Identification of macrophage inhibitory cytokine-1 in adipose tissue and its secretion as an adipokine by human adipocytes. *Endocrinology* **2009**, *150*, 1688–1696. [CrossRef] [PubMed]
33. Schlittenhardt, D.; Schober, A.; Strelau, J.; Bonaterra, G.A.; Schmiedt, W.; Unsicker, K.; Metz, J.; Kinscherf, R. Involvement of growth differentiation factor-15/macrophage inhibitory cytokine-1 (GDF-15/MIC-1) in oxLDL-induced apoptosis of human macrophages in vitro and in arteriosclerotic lesions. *Cell Tissue Res.* **2004**, *318*, 325–333. [CrossRef] [PubMed]
34. Lok, S.I.; Winkens, B.; Goldschmeding, R.; van Geffen, A.J.; Nous, F.M.; van Kuik, J.; van der Weide, P.; Klopping, C.; Kirkels, J.H.; Lahpor, J.R.; et al. Circulating growth differentiation factor-15 correlates with myocardial fibrosis in patients with non-ischaemic dilated cardiomyopathy and decreases rapidly after left ventricular assist device support. *Eur. J. Heart Fail.* **2012**, *14*, 1249–1256. [CrossRef] [PubMed]
35. Kempf, T.; Sinning, J.M.; Quint, A.; Bickel, C.; Sinning, C.; Wild, P.S.; Schnabel, R.; Lubos, E.; Rupprecht, H.J.; Munzel, T.; et al. Growth-differentiation factor-15 for risk stratification in patients with stable and unstable coronary heart disease: Results from the AtheroGene study. *Circ. Cardiovasc. Genet.* **2009**, *2*, 286–292. [CrossRef] [PubMed]
36. Schopfer, D.W.; Ku, I.A.; Regan, M.; Whooley, M.A. Growth differentiation factor 15 and cardiovascular events in patients with stable ischemic heart disease (The Heart and Soul Study). *Am. Heart J.* **2014**, *167*, 186–192. [CrossRef]
37. Bonaca, M.P.; Morrow, D.A.; Braunwald, E.; Cannon, C.P.; Jiang, S.; Breher, S.; Sabatine, M.S.; Kempf, T.; Wallentin, L.; Wollert, K.C. Growth differentiation factor-15 and risk of recurrent events in patients stabilized after acute coronary syndrome: Observations from PROVE IT-TIMI 22. *Arterioscler. Thromb. Vasc. Biol.* **2011**, *31*, 203–210. [CrossRef] [PubMed]
38. Eggers, K.M.; Kempf, T.; Lagerqvist, B.; Lindahl, B.; Olofsson, S.; Jantzen, F.; Peter, T.; Allhoff, T.; Siegbahn, A.; Venge, P.; et al. Growth-differentiation factor-15 for long-term risk prediction in patients stabilized after an episode of non-ST-segment-elevation acute coronary syndrome. *Circ. Cardiovasc. Genet.* **2010**, *3*, 88–96. [CrossRef]

39. Anand, I.S.; Kempf, T.; Rector, T.S.; Tapken, H.; Allhoff, T.; Jantzen, F.; Kuskowski, M.; Cohn, J.N.; Drexler, H.; Wollert, K.C. Serial measurement of growth-differentiation factor-15 in heart failure: Relation to disease severity and prognosis in the Valsartan Heart Failure Trial. *Circulation* **2010**, *122*, 1387–1395. [CrossRef]
40. Chan, M.M.; Santhanakrishnan, R.; Chong, J.P.; Chen, Z.; Tai, B.C.; Liew, O.W.; Ng, T.P.; Ling, L.H.; Sim, D.; Leong, K.T.; et al. Growth differentiation factor 15 in heart failure with preserved vs. reduced ejection fraction. *Eur. J. Heart Fail.* **2016**, *18*, 81–88. [CrossRef]
41. Paulus, W.J.; Tschope, C. A novel paradigm for heart failure with preserved ejection fraction: Comorbidities drive myocardial dysfunction and remodeling through coronary microvascular endothelial inflammation. *J. Am. Coll. Cardiol.* **2013**, *62*, 263–271. [CrossRef] [PubMed]
42. Ahmad, T.; Wang, T.; O'Brien, E.C.; Samsky, M.D.; Pura, J.A.; Lokhnygina, Y.; Rogers, J.G.; Hernandez, A.F.; Craig, D.; Bowles, D.E.; et al. Effects of left ventricular assist device support on biomarkers of cardiovascular stress, fibrosis, fluid homeostasis, inflammation, and renal injury. *JACC Heart Fail.* **2015**, *3*, 30–39. [CrossRef] [PubMed]
43. Wang, Y.; Jiang, T.; Jiang, M.; Gu, S. Appraising growth differentiation factor 15 as a promising biomarker in digestive system tumors: A meta-analysis. *BMC Cancer* **2019**, *19*, 177. [CrossRef] [PubMed]
44. Hsu, L.A.; Wu, S.; Juang, J.J.; Chiang, F.T.; Teng, M.S.; Lin, J.F.; Huang, H.L.; Ko, Y.L. Growth differentiation factor 15 may predict mortality of peripheral and coronary artery diseases and correlate with their risk factors. *Mediators Inflamm.* **2017**, *2017*, 9398401. [CrossRef] [PubMed]

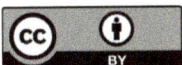 © 2019 by the authors. Licensee MDPI, Basel, Switzerland. This article is an open access article distributed under the terms and conditions of the Creative Commons Attribution (CC BY) license (http://creativecommons.org/licenses/by/4.0/).

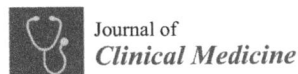 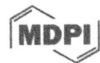

Article

Very Low-Density Lipoproteins of Metabolic Syndrome Modulates STIM1, Suppresses Store-Operated Calcium Entry, and Deranges Myofilament Proteins in Atrial Myocytes

Yi-Lin Shiou [1,2,3], Hsin-Ting Lin [1], Liang-Yin Ke [1,2], Bin-Nan Wu [4], Shyi-Jang Shin [5], Chu-Huang Chen [1,2], Wei-Chung Tsai [3,5], Chih-Sheng Chu [1,3,5] and Hsiang-Chun Lee *[,1,2,3,5,6]

1. Center for Lipid Biosciences, Kaohsiung Medical University Hospital, Kaohsiung 807, Taiwan; irpu10.yls@gmail.com (Y.-L.S.); hsintinglin2007@gmail.com (H.-T.L.); thwangg@gmail.com (L.-Y.K.); cchen@heart.thi.tmc.edu (C.-H.C.); jujuson993@gmail.com (C.-S.C.)
2. Lipid Science and Aging Research Center, Kaohsiung Medical University, Kaohsiung 807, Taiwan
3. Division of Cardiology, Department of Internal Medicine, Kaohsiung Medical University Hospital, Kaohsiung Medical University, Kaohsiung 807, Taiwan; azygo91@gmail.com
4. Department of Pharmacology, College of Medicine, Kaohsiung Medical University, Kaohsiung 807, Taiwan; binnan@gap.kmu.edu.tw
5. Department of Internal Medicine, Faculty of Medicine, College of Medicine, Kaohsiung Medical University, Kaohsiung 807, Taiwan; sjshin@kmu.edu.tw
6. Institute/Center of Medical Science and Technology, National Sun Yat-sen University, Kaohsiung 807, Taiwan
* Correspondence: hclee@kmu.edu.tw

Received: 31 May 2019; Accepted: 15 June 2019; Published: 20 June 2019

Abstract: Individuals with metabolic syndrome (MetS) are at high risk for atrial myopathy and atrial fibrillation. Very low-density lipoproteins (VLDLs) of MetS (MetS-VLDLs) are cytotoxic to atrial myocytes in vivo and in vitro. The calcineurin–nuclear factor of activated T-cells (NFAT) pathway, which is regulated by stromal interaction molecule 1 (STIM1)/ calcium release-activated calcium channel protein 1 (Orai1)–mediated store-operated Ca^{2+} entry (SOCE), is a pivotal mediator of adaptive cardiac hypertrophy. We hypothesized that MetS-VLDLs could affect SOCE and the calcineurin–NFAT pathway. Normal-VLDL and MetS-VLDL samples were isolated from the peripheral blood of healthy volunteers and individuals with MetS. VLDLs were applied to HL-1 atrial myocytes for 18 h and were also injected into wild-type C57BL/6 male mouse tails three times per week for six weeks. After the sarcoplasmic reticulum (SR) Ca^{2+} store was depleted, SOCE was triggered upon reperfusion with 1.8 mM of Ca^{2+}. SOCE was attenuated by MetS-VLDLs, along with reduced transcriptional and membranous expression of STIM1 ($P = 0.025$), and enhanced modification of O-GlcNAcylation on STIM1 protein, while Orai1 was unaltered. The nuclear translocation and activity of calcineurin were both reduced ($P < 0.05$), along with the alteration of myofilament proteins in atrial tissues. These changes were absent in normal-VLDL-treated cells. Our results demonstrated that MetS-VLDLs suppressed SOCE by modulating STIM1 at the transcriptional, translational, and post-translational levels, resulting in the inhibition of the calcineurin–NFAT pathway, which resulted in the alteration of myofilament protein expression and sarcomere derangement in atrial tissues. These findings may help explain atrial myopathy in MetS. We suggest a therapeutic target on VLDLs to prevent atrial fibrillation, especially for individuals with MetS.

Keywords: very low-density lipoprotein; metabolic syndrome; STIM1; SOCE; atrial myopathy; atrial fibrillation

1. Introduction

Despite advances in current therapy, the prevention of atrial fibrillation remains a challenge. Changes in Ca^{2+} regulation and related processes are important mechanisms leading to the initiation and maintenance of atrial fibrillation [1]. The pathogenesis of early atrial myopathy remains unclear. Intracellular Ca^{2+} homeostasis is critical for normal cellular function, particularly for cardiomyocytes, and may be dysregulated in early atrial myopathy.

Store-operated Ca^{2+} entry (SOCE) is recognized to coexist with voltage-gated Ca^{2+} channels in cardiomyocytes and, though this is debated, is suggested to contribute to basal Ca^{2+} homeostasis [2]. A general function of SOCE is to replenish depleted sarcoplasmic reticulum (SR) Ca^{2+} stores [3]. It is commonly thought that beat-to-beat Ca^{2+} handling is mediated by excitation–contraction coupling. Nevertheless, upon facing different cardiac stressors, a sustained increase in intracellular Ca^{2+} takes place upon SOCE, which in turn activates the calcineurin–NFAT pathway, which is responsible for cardiac hypertrophy as an adaptive response [4]. Several studies have identified the essential role of SOCE in mediating NFAT nuclear translocation to develop cardiac hypertrophy induced either by IP3-generating agonists or by following pressure overload [2,5–7].

Stromal interaction molecule 1 (STIM1), a Ca^{2+}-binding protein and a Ca^{2+} sensor in the SR, is capable of triggering SOCE by interacting with Ca^{2+} inward channels on the plasma membrane [8,9]. Stress-triggered STIM1 re-expression and consequent SOCE enhancement are critical upstream elements that facilitate an essential increase in cytosolic Ca^{2+} levels to control cardiac hypertrophy [4]. A hypothetical model of STIM1 activation is that STIM1 couples with calcium release-activated calcium channel protein 1, Orai1, the Ca^{2+} inward channel located in the plasma membrane, and forms an SR/plasma membrane junction as they mediate crucial Ca^{2+} communication between the SR lumen, the cytoplasm, and the extracellular space [9,10].

O-GlcNAcylation is a post-translational modification of protein in serine and threonine residues that occurs in the cytoplasm and nucleus. The addition and removal of O-GlcNAc is catalyzed by O-GlcNAc transferase and neutral β-*N*-acetylglucosaminidase, respectively [11]. There is compelling evidence for a pivotal role of O-GlcNAcylation in the regulation of Ca^{2+} signaling [12]. STIM1 is a target of O-GlcNAcylation, and increased O-GlcNAcylation modification of STIM1 has been shown to attenuate SOCE in cardiomyocytes [13,14]. O-GlcNAcylation is also important in the development of diabetic cardiomyopathy and hyperglycemia-induced arrhythmias [15,16]. Additionally, O-GlcNAcylation may integrate environmental and genetic information in disease pathologies such as metabolic syndrome (MetS) [17], with a potential mechanism linking the metabolic and calcium signaling pathways. Although it has been reported that O-GlcNAcylation is involved in cardiomyopathy correlated with insulin resistance [12,15,18], there have only been a few studies related to the role of O-GlcNAcylation of STIM1 and SOCE in atrial myopathy.

Our previous study demonstrated that very low-density lipoproteins (VLDLs) isolated from individuals with MetS (MetS-VLDLs) exert cardiac lipotoxicity and induce atrial remodeling and vulnerability to atrial fibrillation [19]. MetS-VLDLs are suggested to play a pivotal role in early atrial myopathy [19]. In addition, MetS-VLDLs induce O-GlcNAcylation on gap junction proteins and as a result causing intracardiac conduction delay [20]. We further hypothesized that STIM1-regulated SOCE and O-GlcNAcylation are involved in the pathophysiology of atrial myopathy for individuals with MetS. Therefore, the objective of this study was to assess how VLDLs affect STIM1 and SOCE in atrial myocytes. HL-1 cells derived from murine atrial myocytes have essential SOCE machinery with expression of STIM1 and channel Orai1 and are therefore useful for investigating SOCE in the atrium [21]. This study used HL-1 cells to assess the effects of MetS-VLDLs on STIM1 expression, the O-GlcNAcylation modification of STIM1, the regulation of SOCE and subsequent calcineurin–NFAT signaling, and myofilament protein expression.

2. Materials and Methods

2.1. VLDL Isolation

This study followed Helsinki Declaration principles, and the study was approved by the Kaohsiung Medical University Hospital Ethics Review Board. Blood was obtained from individuals who either met the criteria for MetS or were otherwise healthy and gave informed consent. Blood samples from five male MetS patients (55.0 ± 15.5 years old, all with type 2 diabetes mellitus, elevated triglyceride levels, and hypertension) and three healthy individuals (non-MetS subjects, 34.3 ± 9.3 years old) were used in this study. Normal-VLDLs (VLDL from non-MetS subjects) and MetS-VLDLs (d = 0.930–1.006 g/mL) were isolated by sequential ultracentrifugation as previously described [19,22,23]. Pooled VLDL samples were applied for subsequent experiments.

2.2. HL-1 Atrial Myocyte Culture and Incubation with Isolated VLDLs

Murine HL-1 atrial myocyte cells were maintained with fresh Claycomb medium in precoated culture flasks at 37 °C in a humidified atmosphere containing 5% CO_2. Culture medium was supplemented with 87% Claycomb medium, 2 mM/L L-glutamine, 10% fetal bovine serum, 100 U/mL penicillin, 100 µg/mL streptomycin, and 0.1 mM/L norepinephrine, which is necessary for maintaining a differentiated cardiac phenotype in HL-1 culture [24]. The HL-1 cells were treated with 25 µg/mL specific VLDLs for 18 h. For experiments on testing the effects of the modulation of O-GlcNAcylation on STIM1 expression (see below), the inhibitor 6-Diazo-5-oxo-L-norleucine (5 µM/L) (DON, Sigma-Aldrich, St Louis, MO, USA) and the enhancer Thiamet G (10 µM/L) (Thm-G, Sigma-Aldrich, St Louis, MO, USA) were used.

2.3. Quantitative Real-Time Reverse Transcriptase PCR

Total RNA of HL-1 cells was prepared using TRI Reagent (Sigma-Aldrich, St Louis, MO, USA) and was then reverse-transcribed (Invitrogen, Carlsbad, CA, USA). Quantitative real-time RT-PCR was performed using an ABI 7500 real-time system (Applied Biosystems, Foster City, CA, USA) and TaqMan Universal Master Mix II (Applied Biosystems, Foster City, CA, USA) with TaqMan probe STIM1 (Mm01158413_m1; Thermo Fisher Scientific, Waltham, MA, USA) and Rn18S (Mm03928890_g1; Thermo Fisher Scientific, Waltham, MA, USA).

2.4. Isolation of Nuclear, Cytoplasmic, and Membrane Proteins from HL-1 Cells

The HL-1 cells were resuspended in 500 µL of ice-cold hypotonic buffer (10 mM HEPES, 0.5 mM dithiothreitol, 0.5 mM phenylmethylsulfonyl fluoride, and protease inhibitor (Sigma-Aldrich Corp., St. Louis, MO, USA), pH 7.9) and disrupted with 30 strokes of a tight-fitting Dounce homogenizer. The homogenate was centrifuged to remove the nuclei and mitochondria at 8000 rpm for 15 min. Afterward, the supernatant was centrifuged at 24,000 rpm for 30 min to remove cytoplasmic proteins. The membrane fraction was obtained as the pellet. The pellet underwent hypotonic buffer wash and was dissolved in 200 µL of hypotonic buffer. Membrane proteins were released through treatment with 0.25% Triton X-100 for 1 h.

2.5. Western Blot

Protein samples were separated using SDS-polyacrylamide gel and transferred to nitrocellulose membranes. Blots were incubated with 1:1000 anti-STIM1 (Cell Signaling, #4916, Danvers, MA, USA), 1:1000 anticalcineurin (Cell Signaling, #2641, Danvers, MA, USA), 1:500 anti-Orai1 (Santa Cruz, sc-68895, Dallas, TX, USA), 1:1000 anti-NFATc3 (Santa Cruz, sc-8321, Dallas, TX, USA), and 1:500 antiphosphorylated NFATc3 (Santa Cruz, sc-365785, Dallas, TX, USA). The membranes were then incubated with horseradish peroxidase-linked secondary antibody. The immunoblots were identified with SuperSignal West Picochemiluminescent substrate (Thermo Fisher Scientific, Waltham, MA, USA).

Band intensity was calculated using ImageJ (National Institutes of Health), and intensity data from cytoplasmic, membranous, and nuclear proteins of interest were normalized to 1:1000 α-tubulin (Santa Cruz, sc-23948, Dallas, TX, USA), 1:1000 pan-cadherin (Sigma-Aldrich, C1821, St. Louis, MO, USA), and 1:500 lamin B (Santa Cruz, sc-6216, Dallas, TX, USA), respectively. Antidesmin (1:500, Upstate, Cat. #04-585, Lake Placid, NY, USA) was used for immunoblotting atrial tissue proteins.

2.6. Detection of O-GlcNAcylation STIM1 by Immunoprecipitation

Protein extract was isolated from HL-1 cells using lysis buffer: 1 mg of protein was mixed with 1:1000 anti-STIM1 (Cell Signaling, #4916, Danvers, MA, USA) at 4 °C for 1 h and then incubated with Pierce™ protein A/G magnetic beads (Thermo Fisher Scientific, St. Peters, MO, USA) overnight at 4 °C. The immunoprecipitation matrix was washed twice with PBS containing 1% NP-40. The matrix-bound protein was eluted in sample buffer and then separated by 10% SDS-PAGE electrophoresis. The magnetic beads were saturated to capture all STIM1 proteins in the cell lysate. The immunoblot was done with 1:1000 anti-O-GlcNAc (MA1-076, Thermo Fisher Scientific, St Peters, MO, USA) and 1:1000 anti-STIM1 incubation overnight at 4 °C, and signals were detected by secondary antibodies with chemiluminescent visualization.

2.7. Measurement of Calcineurin Activity

The intracellular calcineurin activity of HL-1 cells was measured using an in vitro calcineurin phosphatase activity assay kit (Abcam, cat no. ab139461) according to the instruction protocols. The HL-1 cells were seeded to the 96-well plate, and the VLDLs were treated for 18 h. Whole-cell protein of HL-1 cells was determined and controlled for the activity assay. Calcineurin activity was calculated as the ratio of the phosphate release amount that was reflected as optical density, which was read on a microplate reader (Epoch Microplate Spectrophotometer, BioTek, Winooski, VT, USA) at wavelength of 620 nm.

2.8. Measurement of SR Calcium Load and SOCE

Prior to experiments (48–72 h), HL-1 cells (5.0×10^3) were washed twice with PBS and plated on 35-mm optical dishes. For imaging, HL-1 cells were incubated with a Ca^{2+} indicator dye, fura-2-AM (Invitrogen, Waltham, MA), for 30 min. Furo-2-AM stock solution was made up in DMSO (1 mM/mL). For a working concentration of 2 μM/mL, 2 μL of stock was added to 1 mL of calcium-free Hank's balanced salt solution (HBSS, Thermo Fisher Scientific, St Peters, MO, USA). Calcium imaging capture was performed on attached HL-1 cells on an Olympus Cell R system. To measure SOCE, dishes were perfused with 10 μM thapsigargin (TG) (Sigma-Aldrich, St Louis, MO, USA) in calcium-free HBSS (Thermo Fisher Scientific, St Peters, MO, USA) (0 mM Ca^{2+}) to trigger SR Ca^{2+} release. At the peak of the TG response, dishes were perfused with 10 mM of caffeine (Caff) in HBSS (0 mM Ca^{2+}) to test if the SR Ca^{2+} pool was depleted. The peak TG/Caff responses reflected the SR load. After the Ca^{2+} signals returned to a stable baseline, cells were reperfused with calcium content solution HBSS (1.8 mM Ca^{2+}). SOCE was triggered upon reperfusion with 1.8 mM Ca^{2+} solution, and the peak response was measured. After SOCE declined, myocytes were tested for viability at the end with potassium chloride (KCl) (80 mM). Data were eliminated if the KCl response was less than a 100% increase above the baseline fluorescence. The data for each experiment were the average of 8 to 11 cells' ratiometric changes in the same dish. Each group had five dishes. For the positive control groups, the STIM1 inhibitor SKF 96365 (Santa Cruz, Dallas, TX, USA) was applied (10 μM incubated for 48 h and 5 μM incubated for 72 h) before the SOCE measurement. The prolonged inhibition of STIM1 was chosen to be consistent with the experiments demonstrating the subsequent myofilament protein changes (shown below).

2.9. Tissue Protein Isolation from Mice Atrial Tissue

MetS-VLDLs or normal-VLDLs were administered by intravenous injection in 9-month-old wild-type C57BL/6 mice tail veins at a dose of 15 μg/g three times per week for 6 consecutive weeks, as in our previous study [19]. After anesthetization with 50–90 mg/kg of pentobarbital injected intraperitoneally, the mice chests were opened, their hearts were excised, and the atrial tissues were snap frozen in liquid nitrogen and stored in a freezer at −80 °C before use. Frozen tissue samples ($n = 3$ per group) were thawed for protein extraction. Mice atrial tissue samples were disrupted with 30 strokes of tissue grinder, and tissue protein extraction was isolated through incubation with 200 μL of lysis buffer on ice for 1 h. The homogenate was centrifuged at 12,000 rpm for 20 min. The protein concentration was calibrated with a Pierce™ BCA Protein Assay Kit (Thermo Fisher Scientific, St. Peters, MO, USA) at 37 °C for 30 min and was determined at 570 nm by an ELISA reader. All applicable institutional and governmental regulations concerning the ethical use of animals were conformed to, including the National Institutes of Health (NIH) guidelines being followed, and all animal procedures were approved by the Institutional Animal Care and Use Committee of Kaohsiung Medical University.

2.10. Myofilament and Contractile Protein Expression and Phosphorylation Analysis in VLDL-Treated HL-1 Cells and Atrial Tissues of VLDL-Injected Mice

Proteins were separated by electrophoresis on 1D-PAGE 15% polyacrylamide gels. Gels were loaded with an equal volume on each lane. Phosphorylated proteins were detected by Pro-Q® Diamond stain following the manufacturer's protocol (Invitrogen, Waltham, MA, USA). In short, the gels were fixed in 5% acetic acid and 50% methanol and incubated with Pro-Q® Diamond stock solution in 25 mL of staining buffer for 1.5 h. The gel was scanned using a Typhoon 9400 (GE Healthcare, Chicago, IL, USA). Subsequently, total proteins were detected by SYPRO® Ruby stain. The gels were fixed with 50% methanol and 7% acetic acid and stained with SYPRO® Ruby stain overnight. Phospho-bands were identified according to the molecular weight, normalized to the total lane individually, and then averaged ($n = 5$ per group). For positive control groups, the STIM1 inhibitor SKF 96365 (Santa Cruz, Dallas, TX, USA) was applied (5 μM) for 72 h, and the calcineurin inhibitor FK506 (Sigma-Aldrich, St. Louis, MO, USA) was applied (30 μM) for 24 h. The same Pro-Q method was applied to the mice atrial tissue ($n = 3$ per group).

2.11. Transmission Electron Microscopy (TEM)

After rinsing with phosphate-buffered saline, small pieces of atrial tissue were immediately fixed in 2.5% glutaraldehyde in 0.1 M of Sørensen's buffer at 4 °C. Following dehydration, samples were post-fixed in 1% osmium tetroxide (OsO4) and embedded in EPON 812 (Electron Microscopy Sciences, Hatfield, PA, USA). Ultrathin sections (60 nm) were stained with uranyl acetate and lead citrate. Images were captured on a Transmission Electron Microscope HT7700 (HITACHI, Tokyo, Japan).

2.12. Data Analysis and Statistics

Data are expressed as means ± SD unless indicated otherwise, and n indicates the number of cell samples. One-way ANOVA and Tukey's multiple comparisons test were used to compare values between groups. For the experiments with small n numbers, nonparametric tests were also performed to confirm the statistical significance (Prism; GraphPad, San Diego, CA, USA). Statistical significance was considered to be a P-value ≤ 0.05.

3. Results

3.1. MetS-VLDLs, but Not Normal-VLDLs, Induced the Downregulation of STIM1 at the Transcriptional and Translational Levels in HL-1 Cells

First, the expression of two key components of SOCE in HL-1 cells and the effects of two different VLDLs on their expression were examined (Figure 1a–d). The effects of VLDLs on STIM1 expression were investigated by quantitative RT-PCR and western blot. Only MetS-VLDLs significantly reduced STIM1 in HL-1 cells, and the reduction was at both the transcriptional (0.81 ± 0.02-fold versus control, Figure 1a) and the translational levels (0.33 ± 0.03-fold versus control, Figure 1c). The protein expression of STIM1 was analyzed specifically in the membrane fraction. The degree of STIM1 reduction in membrane proteins and in RNA expression was different. Nevertheless, the expression of Orai1, which was only analyzed on the protein level, remained unchanged (normal-VLDLs 0.94 ± 0.17-fold versus control and MetS-VLDLs 0.95 ± 0.06-fold versus control, Figure 1d). The effect of MetS-VLDLs on O-GlcNAcylation in the whole cell was examined using whole-cell immunoblot (Figure 1g). The results showed that MetS-VLDLs enhanced O-GlcNAcylation in proteins extracted from compartments of the nucleus, cytosol, and membrane. To further determine whether enhanced O-GlcNAcylation alone could cause any change in STIM1 expression, the HL-1 cells were treated with a specific inhibitor (deoxynorleucine) and an enhancer (Thiamet G) of O-GlcNAcylation for 24 h (Figure 1g,h). The manipulation of O-GlcNAcylation did not change STIM1 expression. The results suggested that the MetS-VLDL-induced STIM1 reduction did not result from its effect on the modulation of O-GlcNAcylation.

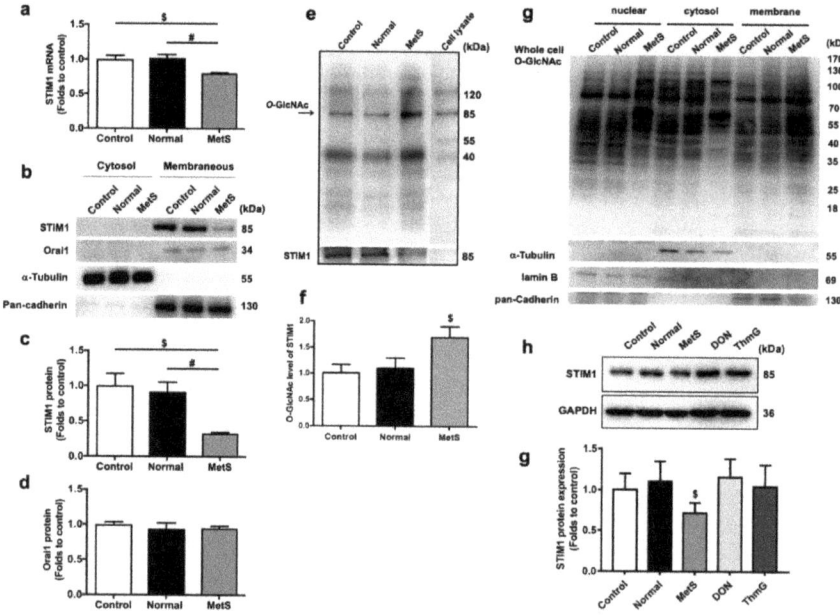

Figure 1. Effects of metabolic syndrome (MetS)-very low-density lipoproteins (VLDLs) on the expression of stromal interaction molecule 1 (STIM1) and calcium release-activated calcium channel protein 1 (Orai1) and the O-GlcNAcylation of STIM1. (**a**) Quantitative RT-PCR of STIM1 ($n = 4$ for each group). Reduced STIM1 mRNA in the MetS-VLDL-treated group (MetS) ($^\$ P = 0.012$, $^\# P = 0.005$). (**b**) Representative bands of western blots for STIM1 and Orai1 channel proteins. (**c**) Reduced STIM1 membrane protein expression in the MetS-VLDL group ($n = 4$ for each group; $^\$ P = 0.025$, $^\# P = 0.021$). (**d**) Orai1 channel membrane protein expression among groups ($n = 4$ for each group; $P = 0.5223$). (**e,f**) Representative immunoblots and densitometry analysis ($n = 4$ for each group). Although STIM1 protein expression was reduced, the O-GlcNAcylation (85 kDa, indicated by the arrow) was larger in the MetS group. $^\$ P = 0.038$ for the MetS group versus the control. All of the changes in the MetS group were absent in the normal-VLDL group (Normal). (**g**) Whole-cell O-GlcNAcylation immunoblotting showed enhanced O-GlcNAcylation of the nuclear, cytosol, and membranous protein fractions in the MetS groups. (**g,h**) The inhibition (with 5 μM deoxynorleucine (DON)) and enhancement (with 10 nM Thiamet G (ThmG)) of O-GlcNAcylation did not affect the expression of STIM1.

3.2. MetS-VLDLs Enhanced the O-GlcNAcylation of STIM1 Proteins

Since it is known that O-GlcNAcylated STIM1 exerts less activation, we therefore assessed if MetS-VLDLs enhanced the O-GlcNAcylation of STIM1 proteins. The immunoprecipitation results (Figure 1e,f) showed enhanced O-GlcNAcylation in the MetS-VLDL group (1.70 ± 0.41-fold versus control), with no change in the normal-VLDL group (1.10 ± 0.44-fold versus control, $P = 0.731$). The O-GlcNAcylation blots revealed another strong band at 120 kDa that also changed in the MetS-VLDL group (Figure 1e). Since STIM1 and Orai1 can undergo unimolecular coupling [25], the 120-kDa band very likely represents the unimolecular coupling of STIM1 and Orai1.

3.3. MetS-VLDLs Suppressed SOCE in HL-1 Cells

To determine if SOCE can be suppressed by MetS-VLDLs along with the modulation of STIM1, the Ca^{2+} response was assessed in fluorescent Ca^{2+}-labeled HL-1 cells (Figure 2). First, the SR store was assessed by the response of HL-1 upon administration of TG and caffeine to deplete the Ca^{2+} store in the SR. This response was demonstrated as an up-and-down wave using ratiometric tracing (Figure 2a–e). The peak of the TG/caffeine response was smaller in the MetS-VLDL group compared to the controls (Figure 2f). After the SR Ca^{2+} store was depleted, cells were perfused with 1.8 mM of Ca^{2+} solution. The SOCE was demonstrated as another up-and-down wave in ratiometric tracing. The peak was measured, and the average of 8–11 cells was obtained for each dish (experiment). The data analysis from five experiments for each group is shown in Figure 2f. The SOCE was significantly suppressed in the MetS-VLDL group (0.59 ± 0.03-fold versus control, $P < 0.001$). The SOCE remained unchanged in the normal-VLDL group under the same incubation conditions (0.86 ± 0.10-fold versus control, $P = 0.093$). A positive control experiment was performed through pre-incubation with the STIM1 inhibitor SKF 96365, which suppressed the SOCE. There was also a reduction in TG/caffeine-induced Ca^{2+} release, which presumably was a reduced SR Ca^{2+} store caused by the long-term (48 and 72 h) incubation with SKF 96365 (Figure 2d,e). In Figure 2f, SKF 96365 reduced the SR load without a complete depletion, suggesting a constitutive Ca^{2+} entry through a residual STIM1/Orai1 channel or others. The calcium release-activated channels (CRAC) channel inhibitor, which blocks STIM1–Orai1 coupling and induces more SOCE inhibition, was not applied in this study. The blockers for the voltage-dependent Ca^{2+} channel and Na/Ca exchanger have been shown to not affect the peak of SOCE in HL-1 cells [21]. These blockers were not applied in this study.

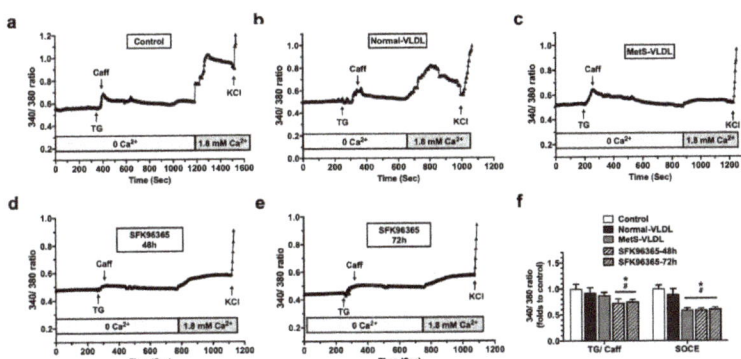

Figure 2. Suppressed store-operated Ca^{2+} entry (SOCE) following sarcoplasmic reticulum (SR) Ca^{2+} depletion in MetS-VLDL-treated HL-1 cardiomyocytes. (**a–c**) Representative ratiometric tracings in fluorescence measurements in control, normal-VLDL, and MetS-VLDL-treated HL-1 cells during SOCE testing. (**d–e**) Representative ratiometric tracings from STIM-1 inhibited HL-1 cells. SKF 96365, a STIM1 inhibitor. (**f**) Analysis of data from the ratiometric fluorescence 340:380 ratio for the peak response to thapsigargin/caffeine (TG/Caff) ($n = 5$ experiments; $^\$ P = 0.024$, $^\# P < 0.001$, $^* P < 0.01$, all vs. control) and the peak of SOCE ($n = 5$ experiments; all $^\# P < 0.001$ vs. control; all $^* P < 0.001$ vs. normal-VLDLs).

3.4. MetS-VLDLs Inhibited the Calcineurin–NFAT Pathway

To confirm if the calcineurin–NFAT pathway downstream of SOCE could be inhibited by MetS-VLDLs, western blots were used to assess the protein expression of cytosolic and nuclear calcineurin and NFAT (Figure 3a). In the MetS-VLDL group, nuclear expression of calcineurin was significantly reduced (0.48 ± 0.09-fold vs. control, Figure 3b), while cytosolic expression was unchanged (0.98 ± 0.53-fold vs. control, Figure 3c). Nuclear NFAT was significantly reduced by MetS-VLDLs (0.51 ± 0.05-fold vs. control, Figure 3d). Phosphorylated NFAT in cytosol was increased in the MetS-VLDL group (1.53 ± 0.5-fold vs. control, Figure 3e). Calcineurin activity was examined using a colorimetric assay (Figure 1f) and was significantly reduced in the MetS-VLDL group (0.71 ± 0.07-fold vs. control, $P = 0.0001$). All of the above changes were absent in the normal-VLDL group. These results revealed that MetS-VLDLs inhibited calcineurin-mediated NFAT dephosphorylation and NFAT nuclear importation and resulted in reduced calcineurin activity.

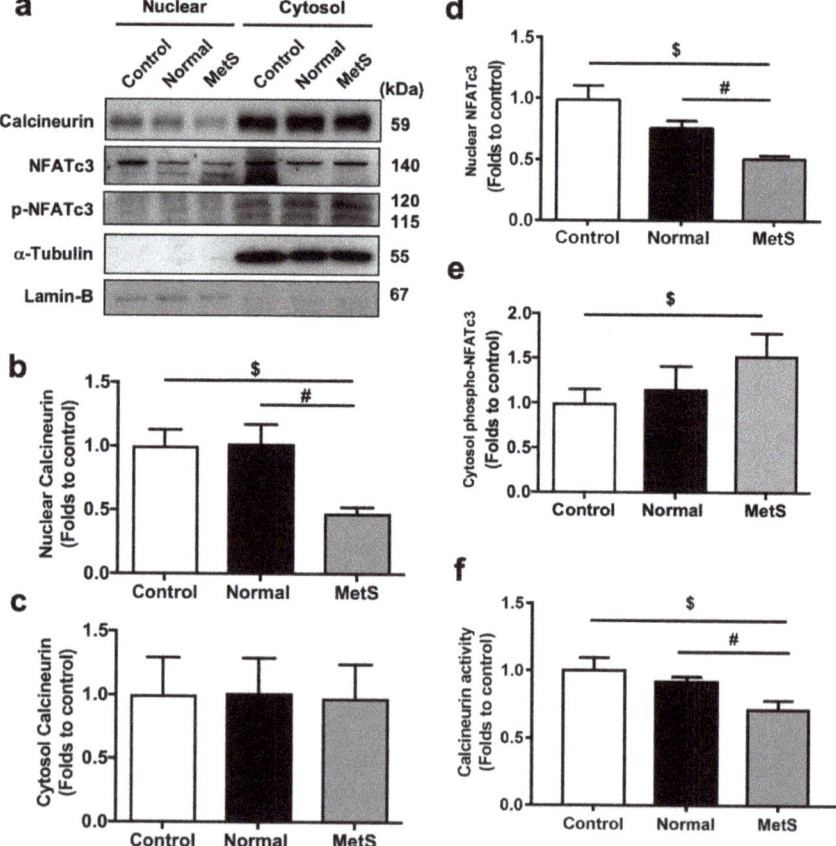

Figure 3. MetS-VLDLs suppressed calcineurin–nuclear factor of activated T-cells (NFAT) signaling pathways. (**a**) Representative bands of western blots ($n = 4$ for each group) for nuclear and cytosolic fractions of calcineurin, NFAT, and phosphorylated NFAT in proteins. (**b**) Reduced nuclear calcineurin in the MetS-VLDL group (MetS) ($n = 4$; $^\$ P = 0.037$ vs. control, $^\# P = 0.04$ vs. normal-VLDL group (Normal)). (**c**) Unchanged cytosolic expression of calcineurin protein ($n = 4$, $P = 0.9377$). (**d**) Reduced nuclear NFAT in the MetS group ($n = 4$; $^\$ P = 0.007$, $^\# P = 0.009$). (**e**) Increased phosphorylated NFAT in the cytoplasm of the MetS group ($n = 4$, $^\$ P = 0.04$). (**f**) Reduced calcineurin activity in the MetS group ($n = 6$; $^\$ P = 0.0001$, $^\# P = 0.0001$).

3.5. MetS-VLDLs Affected Myofilament Protein Expression and Caused Sarcomere Derangement

Given that the calcineurin–NFAT pathway mediates cardiac hypertrophy, we explored whether MetS-VLDLs could affect myofilament protein expression in HL-1 cells and in vivo as well. The VLDL injection did not cause a significant increase in body weight (control 32.3 ± 1.8, normal-VLDL 33.2 ± 1.9, MetS-VLDL 35.1 ± 3.9 g), but mice injected with VLDLs extracted from MetS patients had a significantly increased heart weight at the time of sacrifice (control 0.22 ± 0.04, normal-VLDL 0.19 ± 0.11, MetS-VLDL 0.30 ± 0.04 g, $P < 0.01$ for control vs. MetS-VLDL) (Table S1). The observation of heart chamber enlargement (left atria and left ventricles) and a reduced left ventricular ejection fraction (Table S1) was consistent with our previous study [18]. There was no significant change in circulatory triglyceride and total cholesterol. The data from biochemistry analysis of the animal blood samples collected at their sacrifice are shown in Table S1.

Because the murine atrial tissue was too small to perform multiple protein western blotting, ProQ Diamond Stain in combination with SYPRO stain was used. This method enables simultaneous quantitative analysis of multiple contractile and myofilament phosphoproteins using small amounts of atrial tissue [26]. The expression of phosphorylated troponin I (TnI) and troponin T (TnT) was increased in the MetS-VLDL groups of HL-1 cells and atrial tissues (Figure 4b,d). The expression of phosphorylated myosin regulatory light chain 2 (MLC2) was reduced in MetS-VLDL groups (Figure 4b,d). The expression of desmin was increased in the atrial tissues (Figure 4d), and the result was consistent in immunoblotting using the specific antibody (Figure 4e,f). These changes were consistent with changes upon administration of the STIM1 inhibitor SKF 96365 (72 h incubation) or the calcineurin inhibitor FK506 (24 h incubation) (Figure 4a,b). The opposite change was shown for myosin-binding protein C (cMyBPC), which was significantly reduced in MetS-VLDL-injected mice (msVLDL in Figure 4d) atrial tissues but not in HL-1 cells after MetS-VLDL treatment. Of note, there was no change in myofilament protein expression with short durations of SKF96365 treatment (24 h). It is noteworthy that in addition to targeting STIM1, SKF96365 has been found to exhibit nonspecific inhibition in transient receptor potential-canonical (TRPC) channels, voltage-gated Ca^{2+} channels, and some potassium channels [27]. Therefore, the possibility of nonspecific inhibition from SKF96365 on mediating other channels to affect SOCE in the present study cannot be excluded.

To see if alteration of myofilament protein expression coexisted with sarcomere derangement, TEM was applied. The images showed disorganized Z lines of sarcomeres in atrial tissues of mice receiving a MetS-VLDL injection (Figure 4e). The results indicated that MetS-VLDLs altered atrial myofilament proteins and induced sarcomere derangement.

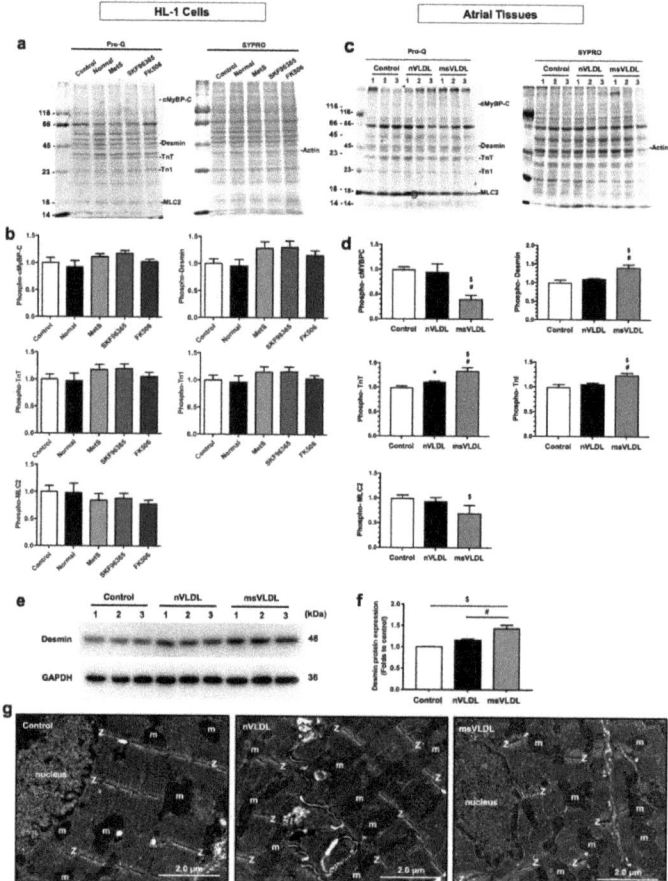

Figure 4. MetS-VLDLs altered myofilament protein expression and induced sarcomere derangement. (**a**) Phosphorylated cardiac myosin-binding protein C (cMyBPC), cardiac troponin I (TnI) and T (TnT), and myosin light chain 2 (MLC2) on 1D-gradient gels stained with ProQ Diamond reagent (left) and total protein expression shown on the gel subsequently stained with SYPRO Ruby (right). SKF 96365, a STIM1-inhibtor; FK-506, a calcineurin-inhibitor; $n = 4$ for each group. (**b**). Densitometry analyses from gels with ProQ and SYPRO staining. (**c**) ProQ Diamond staining gels of mouse atrial proteins ($n = 3$ for each group: Control; Normal-VLDL-injected mice, nVLDL; and MetS-VLDL-injected mice, msVLDL). (**d**) Densitometry analyses for phosphorylated cMyBPC, desmin, TnT, TnI, and MLC2. $ $P < 0.05$ msVLDL versus control; # $P < 0.05$ msVLDL versus nVLDL. (**e,f**) Western blot and densitometry analysis for desmin in atrial tissues. (**g**) Representative transmission electron microscopy (TEM) pictures (at 5000× magnification) showing disorganized Z lines (Z, highlighted with dashed lines) in the atrial tissue of mice receiving a MetS-VLDL injection (msVLDL) compared to normal Z lines in the controls and in mice receiving normal-VLDLs (nVLDL) ($n = 3$ for each group). Atrial sarcomeres are aligned with mitochondria (m).

4. Discussions

The key findings of this study were that MetS-VLDLs reduced STIM1 on the transcriptional and translational levels and enhanced the O-GlcNAcylation modification on STIM1. VLDL-induced STIM1 modulation in turn suppressed SOCE and the downstream calcineurin–NFAT pathway, along with alterations of myofilament proteins and sarcomere derangement in mouse atrial tissues.

It has been suggested that STIM1-Orai1-dependent SOCE assists in maintaining intracellular Ca^{2+} in HL-1 cardiomyocytes [21]. Consistently, STIM1 and Orai1 expression was clearly demonstrated in our experiments through western blots, and SOCE could be assessed when cells were re-perfused with a physiological concentration of Ca^{2+} solution after SR Ca^{2+} depletion by TG and caffeine. Coinciding with this manuscript preparation, there have been more recent reports regarding the regulation of STIM1 expression [28–30]. The importance of SOCE and STIM1 signaling in heart physiology has also been more and more noticed [31]. Although the present study did not determine the specific mechanism by which the MetS-VLDLs induced Orai1-independent STIM1 suppression, the results contribute some understanding to how SOCE could act as a mediator in linking the pathogenesis from VLDLs to atrial myopathy.

A link between the regulation of cellular O-GlcNAcylation and Ca^{2+} signaling has been proven [13]. In Zhu-Mauldin's study, increased O-GlcNAcylation of STIM1 prevented STIM1 puncta formation and blunted STIM1-mediated SOCE. The observation of enhanced O-GlcNAcylation of STIM1 was coincidental with the MetS-VLDL-suppressed SOCE, suggesting that O-GlcNAcylation of STIM1 may affect SOCE. On the other hand, O-GlcNAcylation per se did not affect the protein expression of STIM1 in the present study. O-GlcNAcylation synthesis has been thoroughly proven to impair SOCE-mediated transcription in hyperglycemia and diabetes [15,32–34]. For the first time, this study reports MetS-VLDLs as mediators in enhancing the O-GlcNAcylation of STIM1. Additional studies are needed to better understand how MetS-VLDLs enhance O-GlcNAcylation in atrial cardiomyocytes. This understanding may reveal a novel mechanism linking the metabolic and calcium signaling pathways in cardiac lipotoxicity.

In addition to mediating cardiac hypertrophy, short-term adaptation of energy metabolism enzymes to mechanical loads was shown to critically depend on the calcineurin pathway [35]. The calcineurin–NFAT pathway is suggested to be critical in both pathological hypertrophy and cardiac adaptation to biomechanical stress [35]. In patients and animal models with atrial fibrillation, calcineurin activity and expression are increased [36]. The upregulation of calcineurin is suggested to occur in response to atrial fibrillation-related tachycardia [37], which is different from our study, which identified calcineurin changes in the lipotoxicity of VLDLs at a very early stage of atrial cardiomyopathy. For a reduction of overall calcineurin protein, more studies are needed to elucidate other regulatory pathways. NFAT can also be phosphorylated by a large family of kinases, such as JNK, p38, GSK3β, casein kinase I and II, protein kinase, and possibly also ERK [38]. We suggest that the reduction of nucleus NFAT by MetS-VLDLs resulted from suppressed SOCE-calcineurin-mediated dephosphorylation.

Changes in sarcomere proteins in myofilaments have been shown to be associated with different pathophysiological conditions, such as aging hearts, cardiac hypertrophy, heart failure, and cardiomyopathies [39]. Our assessment confirmed that MetS-VLDLs could influence myofilament protein expression (Figure 4a–d). These changes were consistent with changes upon administration of the STIM1 inhibitor SKF 96365, which also suppressed SOCE in the same incubation conditions (Figure 4a,b and Figure 2d,e). Sarcomere organization and integrity are controlled by complex and dynamic mechanisms [40]. Moreover, the remodeling of myofilament phosphorylation in response to atrial fibrillation and atrial dilatation is complicated [37]. Further studies are needed to elucidate changes in myofilament phosphorylation at a different stage of VLDL-induced atrial cardiomyopathy.

The MetS-VLDLs were isolated from blood samples of patients who had been receiving regular and appropriate medical treatment. The management of treatment was basically in accordance with clinical guidelines, with a goal set of HbA1c in the range of 6.5% to 7% (estimated average glucose level 140 to 154 mg/dL), LDL cholesterol <100 mg/dL, and blood pressure ≤130/80 mmHg. A lipid-lowering agent was not prescribed for elevated triglyceride unless the level was over 500 mg/dL. Although it was not determined how the presence of diabetes mellitus contributed to the distinct effects from the MetS-VLDLs, we believe the results from MetS-VLDLs in the present study were reflective of MetS. This can probably be proven by comparing samples between diabetes alone (noncomplicated type 1 diabetes mellitus) and diabetes with combined MetS.

Some limitations need to be addressed. First, the alterations in the SOCE signaling pathway were not the same in the HL-1 cells and in the atrial tissue with different durations of VLDL application (72 h for the in vitro and 6 weeks for the in vivo). Second, immunoprecipitation was not feasible with the limited protein sample amount (to examine O-GlcNAcylation in murine atrial tissue). Third, we did not examine other calcium regulation proteins, such as Cav 1.2, that can possibly be modulated upon chronic exposure to VLDLs or the STIM1 inhibitor SKF. It remains undetermined how other calcium-related channels or proteins intervene in the effects of MetS-VLDLs on the SOCE signaling pathway. Another limitation is the absence of data on other mediators of SOCE, such as STIM2, Orai2, and Orai3; data on the coupling of STIM1 with Orai1/3; and data on other voltage-dependent Ca^{2+} channels and TRPC channels, which have recently been reported with potential arrhythmogenic roles in mouse ventricular myocytes [41]. Lastly, the concentrations of total cholesterol, low-density-lipoprotein-cholesterol, and VLDL-cholesterol in mice are lower than in humans. Therefore, the biochemistry data (Table S1) cannot be extrapolated to humans.

Clinical Implications

Considering the vulnerability of MetS individuals to develope atrial fibrillation, this study sheds some light on the pathogenesis of VLDL-mediated atrial remodeling in MetS (Figure 5). MetS-VLDLs induced alterations in myofilament protein expression along with the suppression of SOCE. MetS-VLDLs have been shown to induce excessive lipid accumulation, atrial remodeling, and delayed intra-atrial conduction. Moreover, mice injected with MetS-VLDLs developed atrial fibrillation [19,20]. In a human study of patients with valve heart diseases and diabetes, calcineurin–NFATc3 signaling was shown to correlate with the presence of atrial fibrillation [36]. It is possible that STIM1–SOCE regulation changes during the progression of early atrial myopathy, even turning into a transition after the stage of persistent atrial fibrillation. Before the occurrence of atrial fibrillation, we suggest that VLDL triggers and enhances the progression of atrial remodeling (Figure 5). Human studies are mandatory to elucidate whether currently available lipid-lowering agents, such as fibrates, or any other compounds can reduce the cardiac lipotoxicity from VLDL-mediated lipid accumulation to improve atrial cardiomyopathy and to prevent atrial fibrillation in MetS.

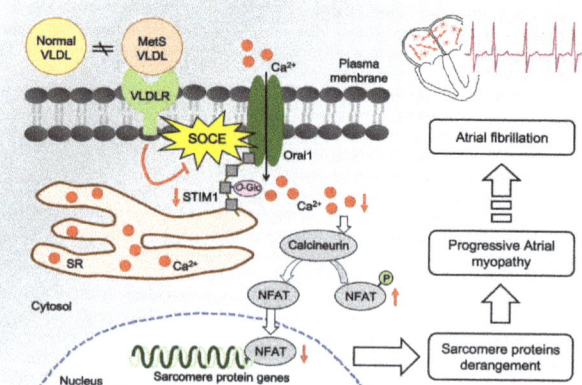

Figure 5. Lipotoxicity of VLDLs on mediating maladaptation of calcium regulation to derangement of sarcomere proteins in atrial myopathy. In metabolic syndrome (MetS), VLDLs undergo biochemical property changes and become different from VLDLs of normal conditions [23]. MetS-VLDLs reduce STIM1 expression and enhance O-GlcNAcylation on STIM1 protein. These changes in concert suppress SOCE and the downstream calcineurin–NFAT pathway, resulting in alteration of myofilament protein expression, disruption of sarcomere organization, and atrial myopathy [35]. The progression of atrial myopathy ultimately leads to atrial fibrillation.

5. Conclusions

MetS-VLDLs reduced STIM1 expression at the transcriptional and translational levels. MetS-VLDLs also modified STIM1 via enhanced O-GlcNAcylation. This STIM1 modulation suppressed SOCE and inhibited the Ca^{2+}–calcineurin–NFAT pathway, resulting in the alteration of sarcomere protein expression in atrial myocytes. These findings may partially explain the pathogenesis of atrial myopathy in MetS. For controlling atrial myopathy in its progression to prevent atrial fibrillation, we suggest a therapeutic target on VLDLs, especially for individuals with MetS.

Supplementary Materials: The following are available online at http://www.mdpi.com/2077-0383/8/6/881/s1, Table S1: The body and heart weights, echocardiographic measurements and biochemistry data in Normal-VLDL and MetS-VLDL injected mice.

Author Contributions: All authors have approved the submitted version and agree to be personally accountable for the author's own contributions. Author contributions: Conceptualization, H.-C.L.; data curation, H.-C.L., Y.-L.S., and H.-T.L.; formal analysis, H.-C.L.; funding acquisition, H.-C.L.; investigation, H.-C.L., L.-Y.K., B.-N.W., S.-J.S., C.-H.C., W.-C.T., and C.-H.C.; methodology, H.-C.L., Y.-L.S., and H.-T.L.; project administration, H.-C.L.; resources, H.-C.L.; software, H.-C.L., Y.-L.S., and H.-T.L.; supervision, H.-C.L.; validation, H.-C.L. and Y.-L.S.; visualization, H.-C.L.; writing—original draft, H.-C.L. and Y.-L.S.; writing—review and editing, H.-C.L.

Funding: This study was supported by Kaohsiung Medical University Hospital research grants (KMUH103-3T03, KMUH104-4T04), Kaohsiung Medical University (KMU-TP104D04), and Taiwan Ministry of Science and Technology grants (MOST 104-2314-B-037 -080 -MY3 to HCL).

Acknowledgments: The authors thank Chung-Ya Wang for VLDL sample isolation and purification.

Conflicts of Interest: The authors declare no conflict of interest.

References

1. Nattel, S.; Dobrev, D. The multidimensional role of calcium in atrial fibrillation pathophysiology: Mechanistic insights and therapeutic opportunities. *Eur. Heart J.* **2012**, *33*, 1870–1877. [CrossRef] [PubMed]
2. Hunton, D.L.; Lucchesi, P.A.; Pang, Y.; Cheng, X.; Dell'Italia, L.J.; Marchase, R.B. Capacitative calcium entry contributes to nuclear factor of activated T-cells nuclear translocation and hypertrophy in cardiomyocytes. *J. Biol. Chem.* **2002**, *277*, 14266–14273. [CrossRef] [PubMed]
3. Palty, R.; Raveh, A.; Kaminsky, I.; Meller, R.; Reuveny, E. SARAF inactivates the store operated calcium entry machinery to prevent excess calcium refilling. *Cell* **2012**, *149*, 425–438. [CrossRef] [PubMed]
4. Luo, X.; Hojayev, B.; Jiang, N.; Wang, Z.V.; Tandan, S.; Rakalin, A.; Rothermel, B.A.; Gillette, T.G.; Hill, J.A. STIM1-dependent store-operated Ca(2)(+) entry is required for pathological cardiac hypertrophy. *J. Mol. Cell Cardiol.* **2012**, *52*, 136–147. [CrossRef] [PubMed]
5. Calloway, N.; Owens, T.; Corwith, K.; Rodgers, W.; Holowka, D.; Baird, B. Stimulated association of STIM1 and Orai1 is regulated by the balance of PtdIns(4,5)P(2) between distinct membrane pools. *J. Cell Sci.* **2011**, *124*, 2602–2610. [CrossRef] [PubMed]
6. Onohara, N.; Nishida, M.; Inoue, R.; Kobayashi, H.; Sumimoto, H.; Sato, Y.; Mori, Y.; Nagao, T.; Kurose, H. TRPC3 and TRPC6 are essential for angiotensin II-induced cardiac hypertrophy. *EMBO J.* **2006**, *25*, 5305–5316. [CrossRef] [PubMed]
7. Collins, H.E.; Zhu-Mauldin, X.; Marchase, R.B.; Chatham, J.C. STIM1/Orai1-mediated SOCE: Current perspectives and potential roles in cardiac function and pathology. *Am. J. Physiol. Heart Circ. Physiol.* **2013**, *305*, H446–H458. [CrossRef] [PubMed]
8. Cahalan, M.D. STIMulating store-operated Ca(2+) entry. *Nat. Cell Biol.* **2009**, *11*, 669–677. [CrossRef]
9. Soboloff, J.; Rothberg, B.S.; Madesh, M.; Gill, D.L. STIM proteins: Dynamic calcium signal transducers. *Nat. Rev. Mol. Cell Biol.* **2012**, *13*, 549–565. [CrossRef]
10. Feske, S.; Prakriya, M. Conformational dynamics of STIM1 activation. *Nat. Struct. Mol. Biol.* **2013**, *20*, 918–919. [CrossRef]
11. Vaidyanathan, K.; Wells, L. Multiple tissue-specific roles for the O-GlcNAc post-translational modification in the induction of and complications arising from type II diabetes. *J. Biol. Chem.* **2014**, *289*, 34466–34471. [CrossRef] [PubMed]
12. Marsh, S.A.; Collins, H.E.; Chatham, J.C. Protein O-GlcNAcylation and Cardiovascular (Patho)physiology. *J. Biol. Chem.* **2014**, *289*, 34449–34456. [CrossRef] [PubMed]

13. Zhu-Mauldin, X.; Marsh, S.A.; Zou, L.; Marchase, R.B.; Chatham, J.C. Modification of STIM1 by O-linked N-acetylglucosamine (O-GlcNAc) attenuates store-operated calcium entry in neonatal cardiomyocytes. *J. Biol. Chem.* **2012**, *287*, 39094–39106. [CrossRef] [PubMed]
14. Nagy, T.; Champattanachai, V.; Marchase, R.B.; Chatham, J.C. Glucosamine inhibits angiotensin II-induced cytoplasmic Ca2+ elevation in neonatal cardiomyocytes via protein-associated O-linked Nacetylglucosamine. *Am. J. Physiol. Cell Physiol.* **2006**, *290*, C57–C65. [CrossRef]
15. Clark, R.J.; McDonough, P.M.; Swanson, E.; Trost, S.U.; Suzuki, M.; Fukuda, M.; Dillmann, W.H. Diabetes and the Accompanying Hyperglycemia Impairs Cardiomyocyte Calcium Cycling through Increased Nuclear O-GlcNAcylation. *J. Biol. Chem.* **2003**, *278*, 44230–44237. [CrossRef] [PubMed]
16. Erickson, J.R.; Pereira, L.; Wang, L.; Han, G.; Ferguson, A.; Dao, K.; Copeland, R.J.; Despa, F.; Hart, G.W.; Ripplinger, C.M.; et al. Diabetic hyperglycaemia activates CaMKII and arrhythmias by O-linked glycosylation. *Nature* **2013**, *502*, 372–376. [CrossRef] [PubMed]
17. Bond, M.R.; Hanover, J.A. A little sugar goes a long way: The cell biology of O-GlcNAc. *J. Cell Biol.* **2015**, *208*, 869–880. [CrossRef]
18. Yokoe, S.; Asahi, M.; Takeda, T.; Otsu, K.; Taniguchi, N.; Miyoshi, E.; Suzuki, K. Inhibition of phospholamban phosphorylation by O-GlcNAcylation: Implications for diabetic cardiomyopathy. *Glycobiology* **2010**, *20*, 1217–1226. [CrossRef]
19. Lee, H.C.; Lin, H.T.; Ke, L.Y.; Wei, C.; Hsiao, Y.L.; Chu, C.S.; Lai, W.T.; Shin, S.J.; Chen, C.H.; Sheu, S.H.; et al. VLDL from Metabolic Syndrome Individuals Enhanced Lipid Accumulation in Atria with Association of Susceptibility to Atrial Fibrillation. *Int. J. Mol. Sci.* **2016**, *17*, 134. [CrossRef]
20. Lee, H.C.; Chen, C.C.; Tsai, W.C.; Lin, H.T.; Shiao, Y.L.; Sheu, S.H.; Wu, B.N.; Chen, C.H.; Lai, W.T. Very-Low-Density Lipoprotein of Metabolic Syndrome Modulates Gap Junctions and Slows Cardiac Conduction. *Sci. Rep.* **2017**, *7*, 12050. [CrossRef]
21. Touchberry, C.D.; Elmore, C.J.; Nguyen, T.M.; Andresen, J.J.; Zhao, X.; Orange, M.; Weisleder, N.; Brotto, M.; Claycomb, W.C.; Wacker, M.J. Store-operated calcium entry is present in HL-1 cardiomyocytes and contributes to resting calcium. *Biochem. Biophys. Res. Commun.* **2011**, *416*, 45–50. [CrossRef] [PubMed]
22. Executive Summary of the Third Report of The National Cholesterol Education Program (NCEP) Expert Panel on Detection, Evaluation, And Treatment of High Blood Cholesterol In Adults (Adult Treatment Panel III). *JAMA* **2001**, *285*, 2486–2497. [CrossRef]
23. Chen, C.H.; Lu, J.; Chen, S.H.; Huang, R.Y.; Yilmaz, H.R.; Dong, J.; Elayda, M.A.; Dixon, R.A.; Yang, C.Y. Effects of electronegative VLDL on endothelium damage in metabolic syndrome. *Diabetes Care* **2012**, *35*, 648–653. [CrossRef] [PubMed]
24. White, S.M.; Constantin, P.E.; Claycomb, W.C. Cardiac physiology at the cellular level: Use of cultured HL-1 cardiomyocytes for studies of cardiac muscle cell structure and function. *Am. J. Physiol. Heart Circ. Physiol.* **2004**, *286*, H823–H829. [CrossRef] [PubMed]
25. Zhou, Y.; Wang, X.; Wang, X.; Loktionova, N.A.; Cai, X.; Nwokonko, R.M.; Vrana, E.; Wang, Y.; Rothberg, B.S.; Gill, D.L. STIM1 dimers undergo unimolecular coupling to activate Orai1 channels. *Nat. Commun.* **2015**, *6*, 8395. [CrossRef] [PubMed]
26. Zaremba, R.; Merkus, D.; Hamdani, N.; Lamers, J.M.; Paulus, W.J.; Dos Remedios, C.; Duncker, D.J.; Stienen, G.J.; van der Velden, J. Quantitative analysis of myofilament protein phosphorylation in small cardiac biopsies. *Proteom. Clin. Appl.* **2007**, *1*, 1285–1290. [CrossRef] [PubMed]
27. Singh, A.; Hildebrand, M.E.; Garcia, E.; Snutch, T.P. The transient receptor potential channel antagonist SKF96365 is a potent blocker of low-voltage-activated T-type calcium channels. *Br. J. Pharm.* **2010**, *160*, 1464–1475. [CrossRef] [PubMed]
28. Kappel, S.; Borgstrom, A.; Stoklosa, P.; Dorr, K.; Peinelt, C. Store-operated calcium entry in disease: Beyond STIM/Orai expression levels. *Semin. Cell Dev. Biol.* **2019**. [CrossRef] [PubMed]
29. Go, C.K.; Gross, S.; Hooper, R.; Soboloff, J. EGR-mediated control of STIM expression and function. *Cell Calcium* **2019**, *77*, 58–67. [CrossRef] [PubMed]
30. Fang, M.; Li, Y.; Wu, Y.; Ning, Z.; Wang, X.; Li, X. miR-185 silencing promotes the progression of atherosclerosis via targeting stromal interaction molecule 1. *Cell Cycle* **2019**, *18*, 682–695. [CrossRef]
31. Rosenberg, P.; Katz, D.; Bryson, V. SOCE and STIM1 signaling in the heart: Timing and location matter. *Cell Calcium* **2019**, *77*, 20–28. [CrossRef] [PubMed]

32. Marsh, S.A.; Dell'Italia, L.J.; Chatham, J.C. Activation of the hexosamine biosynthesis pathway and protein O-GlcNAcylation modulate hypertrophic and cell signaling pathways in cardiomyocytes from diabetic mice. *Amino Acids* **2011**, *40*, 819–828. [CrossRef] [PubMed]
33. Hu, Y.; Belke, D.; Suarez, J.; Swanson, E.; Clark, R.; Hoshijima, M.; Dillmann, W.H. Adenovirus-mediated overexpression of O-GlcNAcase improves contractile function in the diabetic heart. *Circ. Res.* **2005**, *96*, 1006–1013. [CrossRef] [PubMed]
34. Fulop, N.; Marchase, R.B.; Chatham, J.C. Role of protein O-linked N-acetyl-glucosamine in mediating cell function and survival in the cardiovascular system. *Cardiovasc. Res.* **2007**, *73*, 288–297. [CrossRef] [PubMed]
35. Schott, P.; Asif, A.; Gräf, C.; Toischer, K.; Hasenfuss, G.; Kögler, H. Myocardial adaptation of energy metabolism to elevated preload depends on calcineurin activity. *Basic Res. Cardiol.* **2008**, *103*, 232–243. [CrossRef] [PubMed]
36. Zhao, Y.; Cui, G.M.; Zhou, N.N.; Li, C.; Zhang, Q.; Sun, H.; Han, B.; Zou, C.W.; Wang, L.J.; Li, X.D.; et al. Calpain-Calcineurin-Nuclear Factor Signaling and the Development of Atrial Fibrillation in Patients with Valvular Heart Disease and Diabetes. *J. Diabetes Res.* **2016**, *2016*, 4639654. [CrossRef] [PubMed]
37. Heijman, J.; Ghezelbash, S.; Wehrens, X.H.; Dobrev, D. Serine/Threonine Phosphatases in Atrial Fibrillation. *J. Mol. Cell. Cardiol.* **2017**, *103*, 110–120. [CrossRef] [PubMed]
38. Molkentin, J.D. Calcineurin–NFAT signaling regulates the cardiac hypertrophic response in coordination with the MAPKs. *Cardiovasc. Res.* **2004**, *63*, 467–475. [CrossRef] [PubMed]
39. Machackova, J.; Barta, J.; Dhalla, N.S. Myofibrillar remodelling in cardiac hypertrophy, heart failure and cardiomyopathies. *Can. J. Cardiol.* **2006**, *22*, 953–968. [CrossRef]
40. Willis, M.S.; Schisler, J.C.; Portbury, A.L.; Patterson, C. Build it up–Tear it down: Protein quality control in the cardiac sarcomere. *Cardiovasc. Res.* **2009**, *81*, 439–448. [CrossRef] [PubMed]
41. Wen, H.; Zhao, Z.; Fefelova, N.; Xie, L.H. Potential Arrhythmogenic Role of TRPC Channels and Store-Operated Calcium Entry Mechanism in Mouse Ventricular Myocytes. *Front. Physiol.* **2018**, *9*, 1785. [CrossRef] [PubMed]

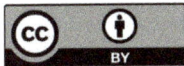

© 2019 by the authors. Licensee MDPI, Basel, Switzerland. This article is an open access article distributed under the terms and conditions of the Creative Commons Attribution (CC BY) license (http://creativecommons.org/licenses/by/4.0/).

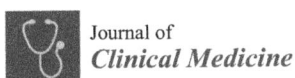 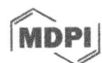

Article

High TSH Level within Normal Range Is Associated with Obesity, Dyslipidemia, Hypertension, Inflammation, Hypercoagulability, and the Metabolic Syndrome: A Novel Cardiometabolic Marker

Yi-Cheng Chang [1,2,3,4], Shih-Che Hua [5], Chia-Hsuin Chang [1,2,6], Wei-Yi Kao [7], Hsiao-Lin Lee [1,2], Lee-Ming Chuang [1,2,6,8], Yen-Tsung Huang [9,*] and Mei-Shu Lai [6,*]

[1] Department of Internal Medicine, National Taiwan University Hospital, Taipei 100, Taiwan; b83401040@gmail.com (Y.-C.C.); chiahsuin123@yahoo.com.tw (C.-H.C.); leehsiaolin1103@gmail.com (H.-L.L.); leeming@ntu.edu.tw (L.-M.C.)
[2] Department of Medicine, College of Medicine, National Taiwan University, Taipei 100, Taiwan
[3] Graduate Institute of Medical Genomics and Proteomics, National Taiwan University, Taipei 100, Taiwan
[4] Institute of Biomedical Science, Academia Sinica, Taipei 115, Taiwan
[5] Division of Endocrinology and Metabolism, Department of Internal Medicine, St. Martin De Porres Hospital, ChiaYi 600, Taiwan; tedshua@gmail.com
[6] Institute of Epidemiology and Preventive Medicine, College of Public Health, National Taiwan University, Taipei 100, Taiwan
[7] MJ Health Screening Center, Taipei 100, Taiwan; cutesttuna@gmail.com
[8] Graduate Institute of Molecular Medicine, National Taiwan University Hospital, Taipei 100, Taiwan
[9] Institute of Statistical Science, Academia Sinica, Taipei 115, Taiwan
* Correspondence: ythuang@stat.sinica.edu.tw (Y.-T.H.); mslai@ntu.edu.tw (M.-S.L.); Tel.: +886-2-2787-5600 (Y.-T.H.); +886-2-3322-8018 (M.-S.L.); Fax: +886-2-2788-6833 (Y.-T.H.); + 886-2-2392-0456 (M.-S.L.)

Received: 6 May 2019; Accepted: 5 June 2019; Published: 7 June 2019

Abstract: (1) Background: Overt and subclinical hypothyroidism has been associated with increased cardiometabolic risks. Here we further explore whether thyroid function within normal range is associated with cardiometabolic risk factors in a large population-based study. (2) Methods: We screened 24,765 adults participating in health examinations in Taiwan. Participants were grouped according to high-sensitive thyroid-stimulating hormone (hsTSH) level as: <50th percentile (0.47–1.48 mIU/L, the reference group), 50–60th percentile (1.49–1.68 mIU/L), 60–70th percentile (1.69–1.94 mIU/L), 70–80th percentile (1.95–2.3 mIU/L), 80–90th percentile (2.31–2.93 mIU/L), and >90th percentile (>2.93 mIU/L). Cardiometabolic traits of each percentile were compared with the reference group. (3) Results: Elevated hsTSH levels within normal range were dose-dependently associated with increased body mass index, body fat percentage, waist circumferences, blood pressure, hemoglobin A1c (HbA1c), fasting insulin, homeostasis model assessment of insulin resistance (HOMA-IR), high homeostasis model of assessment of beta-cell (HOMA-β), triglycerides, total cholesterols, fibrinogen, and uric acids (p-for-trend <0.001), but not with fasting glucose levels. The association remained significant after adjustment of age, sex, and lifestyle. As compared to the reference group, subjects with the highest hsTSH percentile had significantly increased risk of being overweight (adjusted odds ratio (adjOR): 1.35), increased body fat (adjOR: 1.29), central obesity (adjOR: 1.36), elevated blood pressure (adjOR: 1.26), high HbA1c (adjOR: 1.20), hyperinsulinemia (adjOR: 1.75), increased HOMA-IR (adjOR: 1.45), increased HOMA-β (adjOR: 1.40), hypertriglyceridemia (adjOR: 1.60), hypercholesterolemia (adjOR: 1.25), elevated hsCRP (adjOR: 1.34), increased fibrinogen (adjOR: 1.45), hyperuricemia (adjOR: 1.47), and metabolic syndrome (adjOR: 1.42), but significant risk of low fasting glucose (adjOR: 0.89). Mediation analysis indicates that insulin resistance mediates the majority of the association between thyroid hormone status and the metabolic syndrome. (4) Conclusion: Elevated hsTSH within the normal range is a cardiometabolic risk marker associated with central obesity, insulin resistance, elevated blood pressure, dyslipidemia, hyperuricemia, inflammation, and hypercoagulability.

Keywords: thyroid-stimulating hormone; cardiometabolic risks; metabolic syndrome; obesity; hypertension

1. Introduction

Thyroid hormones exert profound effects on systemic metabolism, thermogenesis, and cardiovascular function [1]. Mice lacking thyroid hormone receptors develop hypotension, cold intolerance, and bradycardia [2]. Thyroid hormones enhance lipolysis in fat tissue and fatty acid oxidation in skeletal muscle, leading to improved insulin sensitivity in these tissues [3,4]. Thyroid hormones promote hepatic gluconeogenesis [3,5,6]. Therefore, clinically-overt hyperthyroid status is characterized by impaired glucose tolerance and elevated fasting glucose. Thyroid hormones exert complex effects on cholesterol metabolism in the liver [5–7]. Clinical hypothyroid status is associated with hypercholesterolemia due to impaired hepatic lipid clearance. Collectively, experimental and clinical studies show that thyroid hormones promote metabolic rate, thermogenesis, and weight loss, increase heart rate and blood pressure, reduce serum lipids levels, and improve insulin sensitivity in muscle and fat but elevate hepatic gluconeogenesis and fasting glucose.

Clinically-overt hypothyroidism is characterized by weight gain, cold intolerance, fluid retention, bradycardia, and hypercholesterolemia. Recent evidences demonstrate that subclinical hypothyroidism, defined as elevated thyroid-stimulating hormone (TSH) levels beyond normal range with normal thyroxine levels, is also associated with increased blood pressure, serum cholesterols [8–11], and cardiovascular disease risk [12–14]. In this study, we further explore whether TSH level within the normal limit is associated with cardiometabolic risk factors including central obesity, insulin resistance, high blood pressure, dyslipidemia, and inflammation in a large population-based study.

2. Materials and Methods

2.1. Study Population

Participants of this study were recruited from individuals who participated in a self-paying comprehensive health examination program offered by the MJ Health Management Institute in Taiwan between 2011 and 2016. The data used in this study were held and approved by MJ Health Management Institute, Taiwan. The authorization code is MJHRF2019007C. To comply with regulations related to the privacy of personal electronic data, the identity of every patient was delinked and all data was analyzed anonymously. The protocol was approved by the Research Ethics Committee in St. Martin De Porres Hospital in Taiwan. The ethics committee reference number is 18B-009. All methods were performed in accordance with the relevant guidelines and regulations of the Declaration of Helsinki.

2.2. Inclusion and Exclusion Criteria

Participants who had complete questionnaire information and complete metabolic, inflammation, and thyroid hormone assessment during 2011–2016 ($N = 32,357$) were included. We excluded (1) participants with age <20 years ($N = 290$); (2) those who reported to have received thyroid surgery or thyroid medications ($N = 878$); (3) those who already had hyperthyroidism (high-sensitive thyroid-stimulating hormone (hsTSH) level < 0.47 mIU/L) at the baseline ($N = 1049$); (4) those who already had overt hypothyroidism ($N = 12$); and (5) duplicated cases ($N = 5363$).

Participants were classified into those with high-sensitive thyroid-stimulating hormone (hsTSH) level <50th percentile (0.47–1.48 mIU/L), 50–60th percentile (1.49–1.68 mIU/L), 60–70th percentile (1.69–1.94 mIU/L), 70–80th percentile (1.95–2.3 mIU/L), 80–90th percentile (2.31–2.93 mIU/L), and >90th percentile (>2.93 mIU/L). Participants with TSH <50th percentile were used as the reference group. The normal upper limit of hsTSH is 5.0 mIU/L in the MJ Health Management Institute. The number of participantswith hsTSH higher than normal range (5.0 mIU/L) was only 325 (1.31%) in our study.

2.3. Data Collection

Self-reported questionnaire for lifestyle factors and past medical history were offered by each participant. Each participant undertook a standard panel of history taking, physical examinations, and laboratory tests. Details of the data collection were described elsewhere [15,16]. Overnight fasting blood were collected and analyzed. Alcohol consumption was defined by drinking more than 1 to 2 times a week. Physical inactivity was defined by exercising for less than 1 h a week. Cigarette smoking was defined by currently smoking more than 1 to 2 times a week.

The laboratory method for determination of TSH is a two-step immunoassay using chemiluminescent microparticle immunoassay (Abbott ARCHITECT I2000). In the first step, sample and anti-β TSH antibody-coated paramagnetic microparticles were combined. After washing, anti-α TSH acridinium labeled conjugate was added in the second step. The resulting chemiluminescent reaction was measured. The quality control requirement was a single sample of all control levels tested once every 24 h each day of use. The laboratory of MJ Health Management Institute has passed the ISO 9001:2000 requirements.

2.4. Definition of Cardiometabolic Risk Factors

Overweight was defined as body mass index (BMI) >24 kg/m^2. Increased body fat (%) was defined as: body fat ≥20% in men and ≥25% in women with age ≤30 years and body fat ≥25% in men and ≥30% in women with age >30 years [17]. Increased waist circumference was defined as >90 cm in men and >80 cm in women. Elevated blood pressure was defined as systolic blood pressure >130 mmHg or diastolic blood pressure >85 mmHg. Elevated fasting glucose was defined as ≥100 mg/dL [18]. High HbA1c was defined as HbA1c >5.7%. Hyperinsulinemia was defined as fasting insulin ≥15 mIU/L. High homeostasis model of assessment of insulin resistance (HOMA-IR) was defined as HOMA-IR >3.0 mU/L·mM [19]. High homeostasis model of assessment of beta-cell (HOMA-β) was defined as HOMA-β >75th percentile of the study participants [20]. Hypertriglyceridemia was defined as fasting triglycerides ≥150 mg/dL [18]. Hypercholesterolemia was defined as total cholesterol >200 mg/dL. Low high-density lipoprotein cholesterol (HDL-C) was defined as ≤40 mg/dL in men and ≤50 mg/dL in women [18]. High low-density lipoprotein cholesterol (LDL-C) was defined as LDL-C ≥130 mg/dL. High triglyceride/HDL-C ratio was defined as TG/HDL-C >2.75 in men and >1.65 in women [21]. Elevated high sensitivity C-reactive protein (hsCRP) was defined as ≥3 mg/dL [21]. Elevated serum fibrinogen level was defined as >400 mg/dL [22]. Hyperuricemia was defined as >7.2 mg/dL in men and >6.0 mg/dL in women. Metabolic syndrome was defined according to the International Diabetes Federation (IDF) worldwide definition of the metabolic syndrome [18].Past history of diabetes mellitus was defined by self-reported medical history of diabetes mellitus or history of taking anti-diabetic drugs. Past history of hypertension was defined by self-reported medical history of hypertension or history of taking anti-hypertensive drugs. Past history of dyslipidemia was defined by self-reported medical history of dyslipidemia and history of taking lipid-lowering drugs. Past history of cardiovascular diseases was defined by self-reported medical history of cardiovascular diseases and history of taking cardiovascular drugs.

2.5. Statistical Analyses

Differences in the baseline characteristics of study participants across all hsTSH percentile groups were compared by using the trend test without and with adjustment for age, sex, smoking, alcohol drinking, and physical inactivity. The relation between dichotomous traits including increased adiposity, elevated blood pressure level, hyperglycemia, insulin resistance, dyslipidemia, inflammatory markers, and metabolic syndrome, and across all hsTSH categories, were further evaluated. Multinomial logistic regression was performed to calculate the adjusted odds ratio and 95% confidence intervals without and with controlling for age, sex, smoking, alcohol drinking, and physical inactivity. The optimal cut-off values of hsTSH for each cardiometabolic risk factor were calculated according to the Youden index (sensitivity + specificity − 1) [23]. Statistical analyses were performed using SAS version 9.4 (SAS Institute, Cary, NC, USA). A two-sided *p*-value of <0.05 was considered as statistically significant.

2.6. Mediation Analyses

We further investigated the mediation effects of insulin resistance (measured by HOMA-IR) linking low normal thyroid function (measured by hsTSH or free T4) to metabolic syndrome. More specifically, using mediation modeling, we evaluated the effect of low normal thyroid function on metabolic syndrome risk that is explained by insulin resistance. Mediation analyses were conducted using an existing method [24]. We briefly summarize the analyses in the following. First, we assume a joint model for the mediator and the outcome:

$$\text{logit } \mathbf{P}(Y=1|A,M,X) = \beta_X^T X + \beta_A A + \beta_M M + \beta_{AM} A \times M \quad (1)$$

$$\text{logit } \mathbf{P}(M=1|A,X) = \alpha_X^T X + \alpha_A A \quad (2)$$

where $Y, A, M,$ and X, respectively, are the metabolic syndrome (i.e., the outcome), the hsTSH, HOMA-IR (i.e., the mediator), and the covariates, respectively. Direct and indirect effects of the thyroid function on the risk of metabolic syndrome in relation to insulin resistance can be calculated on the scale of risk difference:

$$\text{Direct effect} = \Gamma(a_1 = 1, a_2 = 0, x) | \Gamma(a_1 = 0, a_2 = 0, x) \quad (3)$$

$$\text{Indirect effect} = \Gamma(a_1 = 1, a_2 = 1, x) | \Gamma(a_1 = 1, a_2 = 0, x) \quad (4)$$

The direct and indirect effects have a causal interpretation provided that the adjustment of covariates satisfies the no-unmeasured confounding assumptions for identifiability: The indirect effect is the effect of the thyroid function on the risk of metabolic syndrome mediated by insulin resistance, and the direct effect is the effect not mediated through affecting insulin resistance. We also measured proportion of mediation as the logarithm of the indirect effect divided by the logarithm of the product of the direct and indirect effects. The proportion of mediation measured the percentage of the effect of the thyroid function on the risk of metabolic syndrome was mediated through insulin resistance, on the scale of log risk ratio. Confidence intervals of 95% of the measurement were calculated using bootstrapping.

3. Results

The study flow is depicted in Figure 1. After exclusion, a total of 24,765 participants were recruited. Their baseline characteristics are listed in Table 1.

Table 1. Baseline characteristics of participants (N = 24,765).

Characteristics	Mean (SD)
Male (number, %)	11,811 (47.69)
Age (years)	44.43 (12.41)
High-sensitive thyroid stimulating hormone (hsTSH) (mIU/L)	1.74 (1.08)
Free T4 (μU/mL)	1.06 (0.13)
Body mass index (kg/m^2)	23.77 (3.97)
Body fat (%)	27.55 (7.31)
Waist circumference (cm)	78.57 (10.95)
Systolic blood pressure (mmHg)	115.64 (17.80)

Table 1. Cont.

Characteristics	Mean (SD)
Diastolic blood pressure (mmHg)	73.86 (11.21)
Fasting glucose (mg/dL)	104.69 (23.30)
Hemoglobin A1c (%)	5.34 (0.78)
Fasting Insulin (mIU/L)	7.94 (6.61)
Homeostasis model assessment of insulin resistance (HOMA-IR) (mU/L·mM)	2.13 (2.29)
Homeostasis model assessment of beta-cell (HOMA-β) (mU/L/mM)	72.44 (51.91)
Triglycerides (mg/dL)	118.23 (105.00)
Total cholesterol (mg/dL)	199.06 (36.46)
High-density lipoprotein cholesterol (mg/dL)	58.57 (15.11)
Low-density lipoprotein cholesterol (mg/dL)	117.95 (33.55)
Triglycerides/High-density lipoprotein cholesterol ratio	2.33 (3.27)
High-sensitive C-reactive protein (mg/L)	1.97 (4.38)
Fibrinogen (mg/dL)	289.64 (56.42)
Uric acid (mg/dL)	5.68 (1.54)
Alcohol consumption (number, %)	4151 (17.39)
Cigarette smoking (number, %)	4004 (16.75)
Physical inactivity (number, %)	15,538 (65.77)
History of diabetes mellitus (number, %)	1017 (4.11)
History of hypertension (number, %)	2736 (11.07)
History of dyslipidemia (number, %)	769 (3.11)
History of cardiovascular diseases (number, %)	1211 (4.9)

SD: Standard deviation; alcohol consumption was defined by drinking more than 1 to 2 times a week; physical inactivity was defined by exercising for less than 1 h a week. Cigarette smoking was defined by currently smoking more than 1 to 2 times a week.

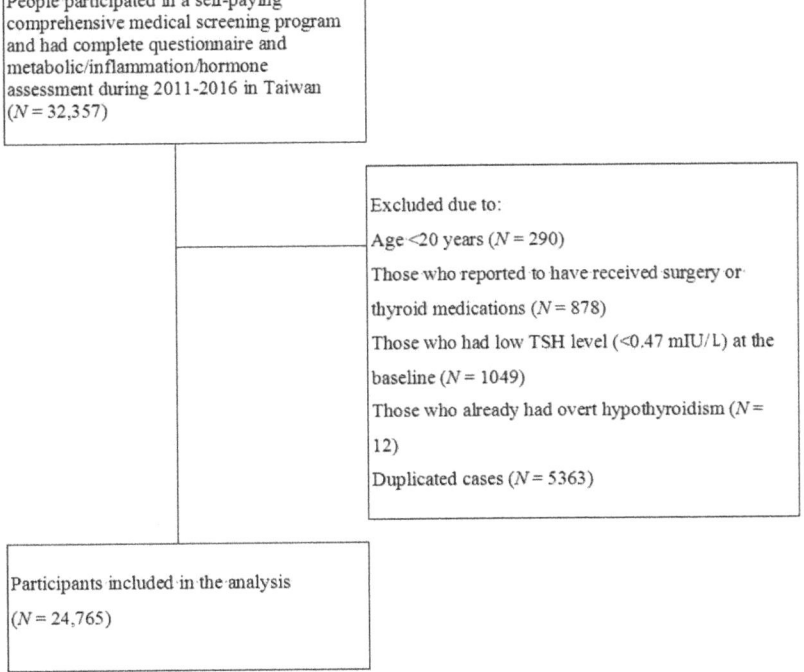

Figure 1. Study flow.

We first examined continuous traits across different hsTSH percentile groups. The crude and adjusted *p*-for-trend is summarized in Table 2. As expected, free T4 levels decreased as hsTSH levels increased (*p*-for-trend < 0.0001). Increased hsTSH was associated with a higher proportion of females (*p*-for-trend < 0.0001) and older ages (*p*-for-trend < 0.0001). Increased hsTSH, even within normal range, was significantly associated with increased BMI, body fat percentage, waist circumference, systolic and diastolic blood pressure, HbA1c, fasting insulin, HOMA-IR, HOMA-β, triglycerides, total cholesterols, HDL-C, LDL-C, triglycerides/HDL-C ratio, fibrinogen, and uric acid, but was not associated with fasting glucose levels after adjustment for age, sex, smoking, alcohol drinking, and physical activity (Table 2). There was also a trend of positive association between hsTSH and hsCRP (*p*-for-trend = 0.083).

We examined the association between hsTSH levels and dichotomous cardiometabolic risk traits. The crude odds ratios (ORs) is listed in Supplementary Table S1 and Figure 2. Briefly, subjects with the highest hsTSH percentile had significantly increased ORs of overweight, high body fat percentage, central obesity, elevated blood pressure, high HbA1c, hyperinsulinemia, high HOMA-β, increased HOMA-IR, hypertriglyceridemia, hypercholesterolemia, high LDL-C, high triglycerides/HDL-C, elevated hsCRP, increased fibrinogen, hyperuricemia, and metabolic syndrome, but low fasting glucose and low HDL-C as compared with the reference group. There was no clear dose-responsive association of past history of hypertension, dyslipidemia, and cardiovascular disease with hsTSH levels. Only a trend of association of past history of diabetes mellitus with hsTSH was found.

We next calculated the optimal cut-off value of hsTSH for each metabolic phenotype according to the Youden index (Supplementary Table S1). The optimal cutoff of hsTSH ranged from 1.147 mIU/L for overweight (BMI > 24 kg/m^2) to 2.225 mIU/L for hypercoagulability (fibrinogen > 400 mg/dL). These results suggest the upper limit of "normal" hsTSH with respect to cardiometabolic risk might need to be reset within this range.

The adjusted ORs are summarized in Table 3 and Figure 2. Similarly, subjects with the highest hsTSH percentile had significantly increased risk of overweight (adjusted OR (adjOR): 1.36, 95% confidence interval (CI) = (1.24, 1.50); $p < 0.0001$), high body fat percentage (adjOR: 1.31, 95% CI = (1.19–1.43), $p < 0.0001$), central obesity (adjOR: 1.37, 95% CI = (1.24–1.53), $p < 0.0001$), elevated blood pressure (adjOR:1.28, 95% CI = (1.14–1.43), $p < 0.0001$), high HbA1c (adjOR: 1.23, 95% CI = (1.08–1.40), $p = 0.0015$), hyperinsulinemia (adjOR: 1.78, 95% CI = (1.51–2.08), $p < 0.0001$), high HOMA-β (adjOR:1.40, 95% CI = (1.27–1.55), $p < 0.0001$), increased HOMA-IR (adjOR: 1.48, 95% CI = (1.32–1.67), $p < 0.0001$), hypertriglyceridemia (adjOR: 1.67, 95% CI = (1.50–1.86), $p < 0.0001$), hypercholesterolemia (adjOR: 1.26, 95% CI = (1.15–1.39), $p < 0.0001$), high LDL-C (adjOR:1.19, 95% CI = (1.08–1.31), $p = 0.0005$), high triglycerides/HDL-C ratio (adjOR: 1.55, 95% CI = (1.41–1.70) $p < 0.0001$), elevated hsCRP (adjOR: 1.36, 95% CI = (1.21–1.52), $p < 0.0001$), increased fibrinogen (adjOR: 1.30, 95% CI = (1.03–1.63), $p = 0.02$), hyperuricemia (adjOR: 1.54, 95% CI = (1.38–1.72), $p < 0.0001$), and metabolic syndrome (adjOR: 1.47, 95% CI = (1.30–1.65), $p < 0.0001$), but had significant risk of low fasting glucose (adjOR: 0.88, 95% CI = (0.80–0.97), $p = 0.0091$) and low HDL-C (adjOR: 1.25, 95% CI = (1.11–1.40), $p = 0.0002$) as compared with the reference group.

Table 2. Characteristics of study participants with different hsTSH levels ($N = 24,765$).

Characteristic	<50th Percentile 0.47–1.48	50–60th Percentile 1.49–1.68	60–70th Percentile 1.69–1.94	70–80th Percentile 1.95–2.3	80–90th Percentile 2.31–2.93	>90th Percentile >2.93	Crude p Value for Trend	Adjusted p Value for Trend *
Number	12,004	2676	2510	2646	2506	2423	-	-
Male (number, %)	6161 (51.32)	1320 (49.33)	1203 (47.93)	1216 (45.96)	1025 (40.90)	886 (36.57)	<0.0001	-
Age (year)	44.05 (12.07)	44.34 (12.42)	44.96 (12.3)	44.61 (12.68)	44.97 (12.72)	45.09 (13.43)	<0.0001	-
Free T4 (ng/dL)	1.068 (0.134)	1.063 (0.118)	1.058 (0.114)	1.056 (0.1165)	1.0522 (0.119)	1.0365 (0.121)	<0.0001	<0.0001
BMI (kg/m2)	23.60 (3.78)	23.88 (4.08)	23.88 (3.96)	24 (4.16)	23.89 (4.18)	24.02 (4.24)	<0.0001	<0.0001
Body fat (%)							<0.0001	<0.0001
Man	24.38 (5.82)	24.74 (6.19)	25.02 (5.98)	25.06 (6.37)	25.13 (6.19)	25.01 (6.47)		
Women	29.59 (7.07)	30.30 (7.63)	30.08 (7.11)	30.56 (7.53)	30.96 (7.76)	31.33 (7.85)	0.46	<0.0001
Waist circumference (cm)								
Men	84.40 (9.07)	85.02 (9.58)	85.54 (9.50)	85.59 (10.03)	86.01 (9.80)	85.95 (10.33)		
Women	72.17 (8.43)	72.63 (8.68)	72.60 (8.52)	73.15 (8.73)	73.32 (8.86)	73.97 (9.74)		
Systolic blood pressure (mmHg)	115.1 (17.34)	116.4 (18.04)	115.7 (17.57)	116.14 (18.27)	115.95 (18.34)	116.35 (18.77)	0.0383	<0.0001
Diastolic blood pressure (mmHg)	73.76 (11.08)	74.10 (11.35)	73.89 (11.14)	74.03 (11.44)	73.7 (11.19)	74.02 (11.5)	0.88	<0.0001
Fasting glucose (mg/dL)	104.78 (23.19)	104.69 (22.24)	104.6 (21.77)	104.48 (23.78)	104.51 (24)	104.74 (25.19)	0.78	0.24
HbA1c (%)	5.33 (0.77)	5.33 (0.75)	5.33 (0.75)	5.35 (0.77)	5.36 (0.81)	5.36 (0.81)	0.034	0.0002
Fasting Insulin (mIU/L)	7.78 (7.02)	7.98 (5.84)	8.01 (5.43)	7.99 (5.26)	8.14 (5.86)	8.39 (8.29)	0.0002	<0.0001
HOMA-IR (mU/L·mM)	2.09 (2.50)	2.13 (1.78)	2.15 (1.82)	2.14 (1.89)	2.18 (2.02)	2.27 (2.73)	0.0015	<0.0001
HOMA-β(mU/L/mM)	70.58 (54.02)	72.99 (54.39)	72.74 (41.95)	73.42 (42.39)	74.93 (47.05)	77.12 (60.83)	<0.0001	<0.0001
TG (mg/dL)	113.67 (95.68)	117.25 (93.75)	122.97 (111.16)	121.91 (147.42)	124.42 (103.92)	126.59 (98.4)	<0.0001	<0.0001
Total cholesterol (mg/dL)	197.44 (35.66)	199.81 (37.65)	199.6 (35.04)	199.32 (37.71)	202.27 (37.84)	202.1 (37.19)	<0.0001	<0.0001
HDL-C (mg/dL)	58.54 (15.24)	58.67 (14.81)	58.09 (15)	57.92 (14.48)	59.16 (15.42)	59.2 (15.23)	0.031	<0.0001
LDL-C (mg/dL)	117.03 (33.25)	118.72 (33.92)	118.33 (32.96)	118.49 (34.51)	119.6 (33.96)	118.96 (33.68)	0.0088	<0.0001
TG/HDL-C	2.24 (3.06)	2.28 (2.34)	2.45 (3.01)	2.45 (5.53)	2.42 (2.66)	2.47 (2.57)	0.0008	<0.0001
hs-CRP (mg/L)	1.94 (4.95)	1.93 (3.82)	2.01 (4.06)	2.05 (3.95)	1.95 (3.14)	2.08 (3.7)	0.1850	0.0883
Fibrinogen (mg/dL)	287.67 (56.23)	289.8 (56.54)	289.84 (56.89)	291.94 (55.99)	292.8 (56.71)	293.24 (56.57)	<0.0001	0.0188
Uric acid (mg/dL)	5.67 (1.52)	5.71 (1.57)	5.71 (1.56)	5.73 (1.58)	5.65 (1.53)	5.68 (1.57)	0.6316	<0.0001

* Adjusted for age, sex, smoking, alcohol drinking, and physical inactivity. hsTSH: High-sensitive thyroid-stimulating hormone. BMI: body mass index; HbA1c: hemoglobin A1c; HOMA-IR: Homeostasis Model Assessment of Insulin Resistance; HOMA-β: Homeostasis Model Assessment of Beta-Cell; TG: triglycerides; HDL-C: high-density lipoprotein cholesterol; LDL-C: low-density lipoprotein cholesterol; hs-CRP: high-sensitive C-reactive protein.

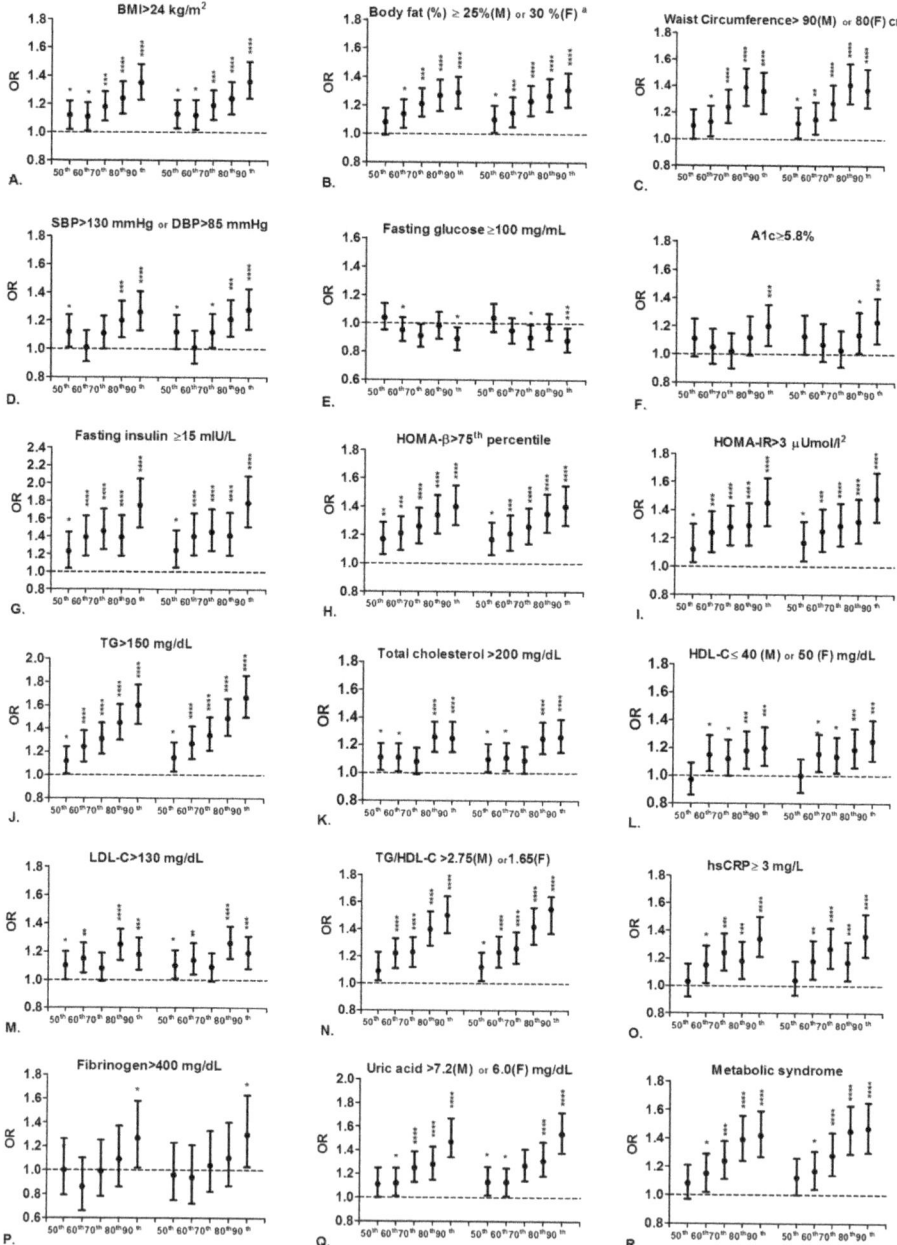

Figure 2. Crude (left panel) and adjusted (right panel) odds ratio for central obesity (**A–C**), elevated blood pressure (**D**), hyperglycemia (**E,F**), insulin resistance (**G–I**), dyslipidemia (**J–N**), inflammation (**O**), hypercoagulability (**P**), hyperuricemia (**Q**) and metabolic syndrome (**R**) among participants with different thyroid-stimulating hormone (TSH) levels ($N = 24,765$). * $p < 0.05$, ** $p < 0.01$, *** $p < 0.001$, **** $p < 0.0001$.

Table 3. The adjusted odds ratio for increased adiposity, elevated blood pressure, dyslipidemia, insulin resistance, hyperglycemia, inflammatory markers, and metabolic syndrome among participants with different high-sensitive thyroid-stimulating hormone (hsTSH) levels (N = 24,765).

Variable	Multinomial Logistic Regression hsTSH Level (mIU/L)							
	1.49–1.68 vs. 0.47–1.48		1.69–1.94 vs. 0.47–1.48		1.95–2.3 vs. 0.47–1.48		>2.93 vs. 0.47–1.48	
	adjOR (95% CI)	p Value	adjOR (95% CI)	p Value	adjOR (95% CI)	p Value	adjOR (95% CI)	p Value
							2.31–2.93 vs. 0.47–1.48 || >2.93 vs. 0.47–1.48	
BMI > 24 kg/m²	1.13 (1.03, 1.23)	0.01	1.12 (1.02, 1.23)	0.02	1.19 (1.09, 1.30)	0.0002	1.24 (1.13, 1.36)	<0.0001	1.36 (1.24, 1.50)	<0.0001
Body fat (%): ≤30 years: male ≥20%; female ≥25% >30 years: male ≥25%; female ≥30%	1.10 (1.01, 1.20)	0.03	1.15 (1.05, 1.26)	0.0022	1.23 (1.13, 1.34)	<0.0001	1.27 (1.16, 1.39)	<0.0001	1.31 (1.19, 1.43)	<0.0001
Waist circumference: Men > 90 cm; women > 80 cm	1.12 (1.01, 1.24)	0.03	1.15 (1.04, 1.28)	0.0082	1.27 (1.15, 1.41)	<0.0001	1.41 (1.27, 1.57)	<0.0001	1.37 (1.24, 1.53)	<0.0001
Systolic blood pressure > 130 mmHg or Diastolic blood pressure > 85 mmHg	1.12 (1.00, 1.24)	0.04	1.01 (0.90, 1.13)	0.86	1.12 (1.01, 1.25)	0.03	1.21 (1.09, 1.35)	0.0006	1.28 (1.14, 1.43)	<0.0001
Fasting glucose ≥ 100 mg/dL	1.04 (0.94, 1.14)	0.45	0.95 (0.86, 1.04)	0.26	0.90 (0.82, 0.99)	0.03	0.97 (0.88, 1.07)	0.54	0.88 (0.80, 0.97)	0.0091
HbA1c ≥ 5.8 %	1.13 (1.00, 1.28)	0.05	1.07 (0.95, 1.22)	0.28	1.03 (0.91, 1.17)	0.68	1.14 (1.01, 1.30)	0.04	1.23 (1.08, 1.40)	0.0015
Fasting insulin ≥ 15 mIU/L	1.24 (1.05, 1.47)	0.01	1.40 (1.19, 1.66)	<0.0001	1.45 (1.24, 1.71)	<0.0001	1.41 (1.19, 1.67)	<0.0001	1.78 (1.51, 2.08)	<0.0001
HOMA-β > 75th percentile	1.17 (1.06, 1.29)	0.0022	1.21 (1.09, 1.34)	0.0003	1.26 (1.14, 1.39)	<0.0001	1.35 (1.22, 1.49)	<0.0001	1.40 (1.27, 1.55)	<0.0001
HOMA-IR > 3.0 (mU/L·mM)	1.17 (1.04, 1.32)	0.0082	1.25 (1.11, 1.41)	0.0002	1.29 (1.15, 1.45)	<0.0001	1.32 (1.17, 1.48)	<0.0001	1.48 (1.32, 1.67)	<0.0001
TG ≥ 150 mg/dL	1.15 (1.03, 1.28)	0.01	1.27 (1.14, 1.42)	<0.0001	1.34 (1.21, 1.50)	<0.0001	1.49 (1.34, 1.66)	<0.0001	1.67 (1.50, 1.86)	<0.0001
Total Cholesterol > 200 mg/dL	1.10 (1.01, 1.21)	0.03	1.11 (1.02, 1.22)	0.02	1.09 (1.00, 1.19)	0.06	1.25 (1.14, 1.37)	<0.0001	1.26 (1.15, 1.39)	<0.0001
HDL-C: men ≤ 40 or women ≤ 50 mg/dL	1.00 (0.88, 1.12)	0.96	1.16 (1.03, 1.30)	0.01	1.14 (1.02, 1.28)	0.02	1.19 (1.06, 1.34)	0.0037	1.25 (1.11, 1.40)	0.0002
LDL-C ≥ 130 mg/dL	1.10 (1.01, 1.21)	0.04	1.14 (1.04, 1.26)	0.0051	1.09 (0.99, 1.19)	0.08	1.26 (1.15, 1.38)	<0.0001	1.19 (1.08, 1.31)	0.0005
TG/HDL-C: men > 2.75 or women > 1.65	1.12 (1.02, 1.23)	0.01	1.23 (1.12, 1.35)	<0.0001	1.26 (1.15, 1.38)	<0.0001	1.42 (1.29, 1.56)	<0.0001	1.55 (1.41, 1.70)	<0.0001
hs-CRP ≥ 3 mg/dL	1.04 (0.93, 1.18)	0.49	1.18 (1.05, 1.33)	0.0057	1.27 (1.13, 1.42)	<0.0001	1.17 (1.04, 1.32)	0.0087	1.36 (1.21, 1.52)	<0.0001
Fibrinogen > 400 mg/dL	0.96 (0.75, 1.23)	0.75	0.94 (0.72, 1.21)	0.61	1.04 (0.82, 1.33)	0.73	1.10 (0.87, 1.40)	0.43	1.30 (1.03, 1.63)	0.02
Uric acid: men > 7.2 or women > 6.0 mg/dL	1.13 (1.02, 1.26)	0.03	1.13 (1.01, 1.27)	0.03	1.27 (1.14, 1.41)	<0.0001	1.31 (1.18, 1.47)	<0.0001	1.54 (1.38, 1.72)	<0.0001
Metabolic syndrome	1.12 (1.00, 1.26)	0.05	1.17 (1.04, 1.31)	0.01	1.28 (1.14, 1.44)	<0.0001	1.45 (1.29, 1.63)	<0.0001	1.47 (1.30, 1.65)	<0.0001
History of diabetes mellitus	1.07 (0.85, 1.34)	0.54	1.01 (0.80, 1.27)	0.93	1.05 (0.83, 1.31)	0.68	1.16 (0.93, 1.45)	0.18	1.32 (1.05, 1.63)	0.013
History of hypertension	1.15 (0.99, 1.32)	0.056	1.11 (0.95, 1.28)	0.16	1.03 (0.89, 1.20)	0.68	1.19 (1.03, 1.38)	0.018	1.08 (0.92, 256)	0.35
History of dyslipidemia	1.14 (0.88, 1.45)	0.32	1.21 (0.94, 1.55)	0.12	1.30 (1.03, 1.65)	0.03	1.03 (0.79, 1.35)	0.81	1.17 (0.91, 1.52)	0.23
History of cardiovascular diseases	1.21 (0.99, 1.47)	0.05	1.02 (0.82, 1.25)	0.88	0.96 (0.78, 1.19)	0.72	1.28 (1.06, 1.56)	0.012	1.18 (0.96, 1.45)	0.11

* Adjusted for age, sex, smoking, alcohol drinking, and physical inactivity. Past history of diabetes mellitus was defined by self-reported medical history of diabetes mellitus or history of taking anti-diabetic drugs. Past history of hypertension was defined by self-reported medical history of hypertension or history of taking anti-hypertensive drugs. Past history of dyslipidemia was defined by self-reported medical history of dyslipidemia and history of taking lipid-lowering drugs. Past history of cardiovascular diseases was defined by self-reported medical history of cardiovascular diseases and history of taking cardiovascular drugs. BMI: body mass index; HbA1c: hemoglobin A1c; HOMA-IR: Homeostasis Model Assessment of Insulin Resistance; HOMA-β: Homeostasis Model Assessment of Beta-Cell; TG: triglycerides; HDL-C: high-density lipoprotein cholesterol; LDL-C: low-density lipoprotein cholesterol; hs-CRP: high-sensitive C-reactive protein; adjOR: Adjusted odds ratio; CI: Confidence interval.

Since insulin resistance had been proposed as the unifying underlying cause of metabolic syndrome [18], we next conducted mediation analyses to model the relationship between thyroid hormone status, insulin resistance, and metabolic syndrome. Specifically, we studied the effect of hsTSH or free T4 on the risk of metabolic syndrome mediated through insulin resistance as measured by HOMA-IR (Supplementary Table S2). In comparison to patients with lower hsTSH levels than the median, those with higher hsTSH levels than the median had a higher risk of metabolic syndrome mediated by HOMA-IR, with a significant effect (indirect effect) measured on the scale of risk difference being 0.63% (95% confidence interval = (0.45%, 0.83%); p-value < 0.0001). The direct effect of high hsTSH (versus low hsTSH) on the risk of metabolic syndrome not mediated through HOMA-IR also revealed a positive effect, with a risk difference of 0.74% (95% CI = (0.42%, 1.05%), p < 0.0001) (Supplementary Table S2). Of the overall hsTSH effect on metabolic syndrome, 46.0% were mediated through HOMA-IR, suggesting that insulin resistance is an important mediator for the effect of thyroid function on metabolic syndrome (Supplementary Table S2).

In addition to hsTSH, we also investigated the effect of lower free T4 levels than the median level, which showed a similar pattern (Supplementary Table S2). In comparison to those with high free T4 (greater than the median level), patients with low free T4 were more likely to develop metabolic syndrome, either mediated by HOMA-IR or not, with indirect and direct effects on the scale of risk difference being 0.54% (95% CI = (0.36%, 0.74%), p < 0.0001) and 0.26% (95% CI = (−0.08%, 0.60%), p = 0.066), respectively. The proportion of the free T4 effect on metabolic syndrome mediated by HOMA-IR was 67.2%, even higher than that of hsTSH (Supplementary Table S2). Taken together, mediation analyses suggest that the effect of thyroid hormone status on metabolic syndrome is significantly mediated by insulin resistance and such a mediation explained the majority of the effect (46.0% for hsTSH; 67.2% for free T4).

4. Discussion

In this large population-based study involving 24,765 subjects, we found that increased hsTSH levels, even within the normal range, is associated with increased risk of central obesity, insulin resistance, elevated blood pressure, hyperglycemia, hyperlipidemia, hyperuricemia, inflammation, hypercoagulability, and metabolic syndrome, suggesting hsTSH as a novel cardiometabolic risk marker. The association was probably mediated through insulin resistance. To our knowledge, this study is the largest study to investigate the association of hsTSH within normal levels in a range of comprehensive cardiometabolic traits using mediation analysis.

Consistently, in a cross-sectional study involving 2703 euthyroid participants from Netherlands, TSH levels were positively associated with insulin resistance and triglycerides levels [25]. In another study involving 1283 euthyroid Chinese, those with TSH levels between 1.91 to 4.80 mIU/L had significantly larger waist circumferences, higher BMI, and a trend of higher serum triglycerides, but a trend of lower prevalence of hyperglycemia than those with TSH between 0.30 to 0.99 mIU/L [26]. In a study involving 2760 Korean euthyroid women, TSH levels were positively associated with waist circumference, blood pressure, and triglycerides, but no fasting glucose or HDL-C [27]. Another study involving 2153 euthyroid Bulgarians showed that the highest TSH quartiles were associated with higher triglycerides, lower HDL-C, and metabolic syndrome, but not with abdominal obesity, hypertension, or diabetes/prediabetes in comparison to the lowest quartiles [28]. In a study involving 201 Italian women, TSH was positively associated with waist circumference [29]. In a study involving 1333 euthyroid Germans, TSH in the upper normal range was associated with higher BMI, higher triglycerides, and metabolic syndrome, but not fasting glucose in comparison to those with TSH in the lower normal range [30]. Another study involving 2771 euthyroid Mexicans showed that TSH was positively associated with waist circumference, systolic blood pressure, total cholesterols, LDL-C, triglycerides, fasting insulin, and HOMA-IR, but not with HDL-C, diastolic pressure, and fasting glucose [31]. In another study involving 3755 euthyroid Iranians, TSH was positively associated with waist circumference, triglycerides, but not with total cholesterol, LDL-C, HDL-C, systolic and diastolic blood pressure, and fasting blood glucose [32]. Collectively, in most studies, higher TSH level is associated with central obesity, elevated blood pressure, increased triglycerides, and insulin resistance, but not with fasting glucose. The mechanism by which elevated TSH is associated with reduced fasting glucose is probably related to the thyroid hormones' action to promote hepatic gluconeogenesis [3,5,6]. It is well-established that the thyroid hormone stimulates gluconeogenesis through up-regulating phosphoenolpyruvate carboxykinase (PEPCK) [33] and increasing sympathetic input to the liver [6]. Rodents with the mutant thyroid receptor display reduced hepatic glucose output [34]. This is consistent with our findings, and other clinical findings, that elevated TSH is associated with lower fasting glucose. Whether this finding will affect the overall cardiovascular risk is currently unknown.

In an analysis targeted to analyze the association of TSH with serum lipids in 30,656 euthyroid Norwegians, there was a linear and significant increase in total cholesterols, LDL-C, and triglycerides with increasing TSH [35]. In another study targeted to analyze the association of TSH with serum lipids in 3664 euthyroid Chinese, TSH was linearly positivity associated with total cholesterols and triglycerides [36]. In another study analyzing the association of TSH with serum lipids, TSH was significantly associated with total cholesterols, triglyceride, and LDL-C, but not with HDL-C, in 7270 euthyroid Koreans [37]. In another analysis targeted to investigate the association between TSH and blood pressure in 30,728 euthyroid Norwegians, increased TSH was significantly associated with increased blood pressure. Higher TSH (3.0–3.5 mIU/L) was associated with increased risk of hypertension in men and women [38].

We observed increased TSH levels within the normal range were significantly associated with increased hsCRP. There is little information mentioning the association between TSH and hsCRP. In a Brazilian study of 12,284 subjects with THS within euthyroid and subclinical hypothyroidism, TSH levels were not associated with CRP [39]. In a Turkey study involving 77 subclinical hypothyroid cases and 50 euthyroid controls, subclinical hypothyroidism was associated with elevated hsCRP [40].

We also observed increased TSH levels were significantly associated with hypercoagulability. Consistently, in a study of 959 French subjects, free T4 levels were inversely correlated with serum fibrinogen level [41]. Conversely, another population-based study in 3804 Germans found that low serum TSH was associated with high fibrinogen levels [42]. Our results strongly support that elevated TSH within the euthyroid range is associated with low-grade inflammation and hypercoagulability, probably related to increased adiposity.

In contrast to our findings, two large cross-sectional studies found a negative association between TSH with measures of obesity [43,44]. A study involving 5998 participants from general Korean population showed that TSH levels were negatively associated with waist circumference and HDL-C, and positively with triglycerides [42]. In another study involving 13,496 euthyroid Koreans, TSH as negatively related to BMI, HDL-C, fasting glucose, and HbA1c [44]. The reason for the discrepancy of TSH association with measures of obesity is not currently known.

Instead of TSH, several studies investigated the association of thyroxine levels with cardiometabolic risk factors. A study involving 303 euthyroid Greeks showed that free T4 levels were negatively associated with subcutaneous fat mass [45]. Another study involving 44,196 euthyroid Koreans showed that normal high free T4 was associated with lower waist circumference [46]. Intriguingly another study involving 941 euthyroid Belgian men showed free T4 levels were positively associated with whole body fat mass and trunk fat mass, but negatively associated with whole body lean mass and radius muscle mass [47]. In conclusion, low normal thyroxine may be associated with increased fat mass.

Using mediation analysis, we found that insulin resistance mediates the association between the metabolic syndrome and free T4 (67.2%) or hsTSH (46.0%). This is consistent with the established action of thyroxine to promote insulin sensitivity of fat and skeletal muscle in experimental models. Because of the difference in measurement techniques, serum hsTSH is a much more sensitive marker than free T4 for assessing thyroid status. Our study showed that hsTSH is a highly sensitive marker of thyroid status associated with metabolic syndrome through the thyroxine's action on insulin resistance.

Our study has some unique strengths. First, this is the largest study investigating the association of high normal TSH with the most comprehensive coverage of cardiometabolic risk factors and the mechanism using mediation analyses. In addition, the lab tests are performed as screening tests rather than for a clinical indication, which prevents the confounding by indication. Our detailed questionnaires coverage of lifestyle enables adjustments for multiple confounding factors and mediation analysis.

Our study has several limitations. First, a longitudinal follow-up study is required in the future since this is a cross-sectional study. Second, although we adjusted various lifestyle factors, residual confounding factors may still exist. Third, the participants are recruited from voluntary health examinations but not from random sampling. Therefore, the risk estimation may not be applicable for the general population.

5. Conclusions

A linear dose-dependent association was found between hsTSH within the normal range with central obesity, dyslipidemia, elevated blood pressure, inflammation, hypercoagulability, and metabolic syndrome, but not with fasting glucose, in a large population. The association is probably mediated through the thyroid hormone's action on insulin sensitivity. Our results suggest high hsTSH within the euthyroid range is a novel cardiometabolic risk marker.

Supplementary Materials: The following are available online at http://www.mdpi.com/2077-0383/8/6/817/s1, Table S1: The crude odds ratio for increased adiposity, elevated blood pressure, dyslipidemia, insulin resistance, hyperglycemia, inflammatory markers, and metabolic syndrome among participants with different TSH levels ($N = 24,765$); Table S2: Mediation analysis modeling the relationship between thyroid function, insulin resistance, and metabolic syndrome.

Author Contributions: Y.-C.C., C.-H.C. and Y.-T.H. conducted the study and drafted the manuscript. L.-M.C. and M.-S.L. conceptualized the research, designed the study, and approved the final version of the manuscript. M.-S.L. and S.-C.H. provided the data and processed the ethical approval process; H.-L.L. wrote the manuscript. W.-Y.K. and Y.-T.H. performed the statistical analyses.

Acknowledgments: We are grateful to all participants in this study. All or part of the data used in this research were authorized by, and received from MJ Health Research Foundation. Any interpretation or conclusion described in this paper does not represent the views of MJ Health Research Foundation.

Conflicts of Interest: The authors declare no conflicts of interest.

References

1. Silva, J.E. Thyroid hormone control of thermogenesis and energy balance. *Thyroid* **1995**, *5*, 481–492. [CrossRef] [PubMed]
2. Wikström, L.; Johansson, C.; Saltó, C.; Barlow, C.; Campos Barros, A.; Baas, F.; Forrest, D.; Thorén, P.; Vennström, B. Abnormal heart rate and body temperature in mice lacking thyroid hormone receptor alpha 1. *EMBO J.* **1998**, *17*, 455–461. [CrossRef] [PubMed]
3. Mullur, R.; Liu, Y.Y.; Brent, G.A. Thyroid hormone regulation of metabolism. *Physiol. Rev.* **2014**, *94*, 355–382. [CrossRef] [PubMed]
4. Klieverik, L.P.; Coomans, C.P.; Endert, E.; Sauerwein, H.P.; Havekes, L.M.; Voshol, P.J.; Rensen, P.C.; Romijn, J.A.; Kalsbeek, A.; Fliers, E. Thyroid hormone effects on whole-body energy homeostasis and tissue-specific fatty acid uptake in vivo. *Endocrinology* **2009**, *150*, 5639–5648. [CrossRef]
5. Sinha, R.A.; Singh, B.K.; Yen, P.M. Thyroid hormone regulation of hepatic lipid and carbohydrate metabolism. *Trends Endocrinol. Metab.* **2014**, *25*, 538–545. [CrossRef] [PubMed]
6. Klieverik, L.P.; Janssen, S.F.; van Riel, A.; Foppen, E.; Bisschop, P.H.; Serlie, M.J.; Boelen, A.; Ackermans, M.T.; Sauerwein, H.P.; Fliers, E.; et al. Thyroid hormone modulates glucose production via a sympathetic pathway from the hypothalamic paraventricular nucleus to the liver. *Proc. Natl. Acad. Sci. USA* **2009**, *106*, 5966–5971. [CrossRef]
7. Gullberg, H.; Rudling, M.; Saltó, C.; Forrest, D.; Angelin, B.; Vennström, B. Requirement for thyroid hormone receptor beta in T3 regulation of cholesterol metabolism in mice. *Mol. Endocrinol.* **2002**, *16*, 1767–1777. [CrossRef] [PubMed]

8. Mehran, L.; Amouzegar, A.; Rahimabad, P.K.; Tohidi, M.; Tahmasebinejad, Z.; Azizi, F. Thyroid Function and Metabolic Syndrome: A Population-Based Thyroid Study. *Horm. Metab. Res.* **2017**, *49*, 192–200. [CrossRef]
9. Waring, A.C.; Rodondi, N.; Harrison, S.; Kanaya, A.M.; Simonsick, E.M.; Miljkovic, I.; Satterfield, S.; Newman, A.B.; Bauer, D.C.; Health, Ageing, and Body Composition (Health ABC) Study. Thyroid function and prevalent and incident metabolic syndrome in older adults: The Health, Ageing and Body Composition Study. *Clin. Endocrinol.* **2012**, *76*, 911–918. [CrossRef]
10. Yang, L.; Lv, X.; Yue, F.; Wei, D.; Liu, W.; Zhang, T. Subclinical hypothyroidism and the risk of metabolic syndrome: A meta-analysis of observational studies. *Endocr. Res.* **2016**, *41*, 158–165. [CrossRef]
11. Lu, Y.H.; Xia, Z.L.; Ma, Y.Y.; Chen, H.J.; Yan, L.P.; Xu, H.F. Subclinical hypothyroidism is associated with metabolic syndrome and clomiphene citrate resistance in women with polycystic ovary syndrome. *Gynecol. Endocrinol.* **2016**, *32*, 852–855. [CrossRef] [PubMed]
12. Delitala, A.P.; Fanciulli, G.; Maioli, M.; Delitala, G. Subclinical hypothyroidism, lipid metabolism and cardiovascular disease. *Endocr. Res.* **2016**, *41*, 158–165. [CrossRef] [PubMed]
13. Floriani, C.; Gencer, B.; Collet, T.H.; Rodondi, N. Subclinical thyroid dysfunction and cardiovascular diseases: 2016 update. *Eur. Heart J.* **2018**, *39*, 503–507. [CrossRef] [PubMed]
14. Tseng, F.Y.; Lin, W.Y.; Lin, C.C.; Lee, L.T.; Li, T.C.; Sung, P.K.; Huang, K.C. Subclinical hypothyroidism is associated with increased risk for all-cause and cardiovascular mortality in adults. *J. Am. Coll. Cardiol.* **2012**, *60*, 730–737. [CrossRef] [PubMed]
15. Wu, D.M.; Pai, L.; Chu, N.F.; Sung, P.K.; Lee, M.S.; Tsai, J.T.; Hsu, L.L.; Lee, M.C.; Sun, C.A. Prevalence and clustering of cardiovascular risk factors among healthy adults in a Chinese population: The MJ Health Screening Center Study in Taiwan. *Int. J. Obes. Relat. Metab. Disord.* **2001**, *25*, 1189–1195. [CrossRef] [PubMed]
16. Wen, C.P.; Cheng, T.Y.; Tsai, M.K.; Chang, Y.C.; Chan, H.T.; Tsai, S.P.; Chiang, P.H.; Hsu, C.C.; Sung, P.K.; Hsu, Y.H.; et al. All-cause mortality attributable to chronic kidney disease: A prospective cohort study based on 462 293 adults in Taiwan. *Lancet* **2008**, *371*, 2173–2182. [CrossRef]
17. Ho-Pham, L.T.; Lai, T.Q.; Nguyen, M.T.; Nguyen, T.V. Relationship between Body Mass Index and Percent Body Fat in Vietnamese: Implications for the Diagnosis of Obesity. *PLoS ONE* **2015**, *10*, e0127198. [CrossRef]
18. Alberti, K.G.; Zimmet, P.; Shaw, J. Metabolic syndrome—A new world-wide definition. A Consensus Statement from the International Diabetes Federation. *Diabet. Med.* **2006**, *23*, 469–480. [CrossRef]
19. Yin, J.; Li, M.; Xu, L.; Wang, Y.; Cheng, H.; Zhao, X.; Mi, J. Insulin resistance determined by Homeostasis Model Assessment (HOMA) and associations with metabolic syndrome among Chinese children and teenagers. *Diabetol. Metab. Syndr.* **2013**, *5*, 71. [CrossRef]
20. Song, D.K.; Hong, Y.S.; Sung, Y.A.; Lee, H. Insulin resistance according to β-cell function in women with polycystic ovary syndrome and normal glucose tolerance. *PLoS ONE* **2017**, *12*, e0178120. [CrossRef]
21. Gaziano, J.M.; Hennekens, C.H.; O'Donnell, C.J.; Breslow, J.L.; Buring, J.E. Fasting triglycerides, high-density lipoprotein, and risk of myocardial infarction. *Circulation* **1997**, *96*, 2520–2525. [CrossRef] [PubMed]
22. Yu, W.; Wang, Y.; Shen, B. An elevated preoperative plasma fibrinogen level is associated with poor overall survival in Chinese gastric cancer patients. *Cancer Epidemiol.* **2016**, *42*, 39–45. [CrossRef] [PubMed]
23. Youden, W.J. Index for rating diagnostic tests. *Cancer* **1950**, *3*, 32–35. [CrossRef]
24. Shih, S.; Huang, Y.T.; Yang, H.I. A multiple mediator approach to quantify the effects of ADH1B and ALDH2 genes on hepatocellular carcinoma risk. *Genet. Epidemiol.* **2018**, *42*, 394–404. [CrossRef] [PubMed]
25. Roos, A.; Bakker, S.J.; Links, T.P.; Gans, R.O.; Wolffenbuttel, B.H. Thyroid function is associated with components of the metabolic syndrome in euthyroid subjects. *J. Clin. Endocrinol. Metab.* **2007**, *92*, 491–496. [CrossRef] [PubMed]
26. Lai, Y.; Wang, J.; Jiang, F.; Wang, B.; Chen, Y.; Li, M.; Liu, H.; Li, C.; Xue, H.; Li, N.; et al. The relationship between serum thyrotropin and components of metabolic syndrome. *Endocr. J.* **2011**, *58*, 23–30. [CrossRef] [PubMed]
27. Oh, J.Y.; Sung, Y.A.; Lee, H.J. Elevated thyroid stimulating hormone levels are associated with metabolic syndrome in euthyroid young women. *Korean J. Intern. Med.* **2013**, *28*, 180–186. [CrossRef] [PubMed]
28. Shinkov, A.; Borissova, A.M.; Kovatcheva, R.; Atanassova, I.; Vlahov, J.; Dakovska, L. The prevalence of the metabolic syndrome increases through the quartiles of thyroid stimulating hormone in a population-based sample of euthyroid subjects. *Arq. Bras. Endocrinol. Metabol.* **2014**, *58*, 926–932. [CrossRef]

29. De Pergola, G.; Ciampolillo, A.; Paolotti, S.; Trerotoli, P.; Giorgino, R. Free triiodothyronine and thyroid stimulating hormone are directly associated with waist circumference, independently of insulin resistance, metabolic parameters and blood pressure in overweight and obese women. *Clin. Endocrinol. (Oxf)* **2007**, *67*, 265–269. [CrossRef]
30. Ruhla, S.; Weickert, M.O.; Arafat, A.M.; Osterhoff, M.; Isken, F.; Spranger, J.; Schöfl, C.; Pfeiffer, A.F.; Möhlig, M. A high normal TSH is associated with the metabolic syndrome. *Clin. Endocrinol. (Oxf)* **2010**, *72*, 696–701. [CrossRef]
31. De Jesus Garduño-Garcia, J.; Alvirde-Garcia, U.; López-Carrasco, G.; Padilla Mendoza, M.E.; Mehta, R.; Arellano-Campos, O.; Choza, R.; Sauque, L.; Garay-Sevilla, M.E.; Malacara, J.M. TSH and free thyroxine concentrations are associated with differing metabolic markers in euthyroid subjects. *Eur. J. Endocrinol.* **2010**, *163*, 273–278. [CrossRef] [PubMed]
32. Mehran, L.; Amouzegar, A.; Tohidi, M.; Moayedi, M.; Azizi, F. Serum free thyroxine concentration is associated with metabolic syndrome in euthyroid subjects. *Thyroid* **2014**, *24*, 1566–1574. [CrossRef] [PubMed]
33. Li, Y.; Wang, L.; Zhou, L.; Song, Y.; Ma, S.; Yu, C.; Zhao, J.; Xu, C.; Gao, L. Thyroid stimulating hormone increases hepatic gluconeogenesis via CRTC2. *Mol. Cell Endocrinol.* **2017**, *446*, 70–80. [CrossRef] [PubMed]
34. Jornayvaz, F.R.; Lee, H.Y.; Jurczak, M.J.; Alves, T.C.; Guebre-Egziabher, F.; Guigni, B.A.; Zhang, D.; Samuel, V.T.; Silva, J.E.; Shulman, G.I. Thyroid hormone receptor-α gene knockout mice are protected from diet-induced hepatic insulin resistance. *Endocrinology* **2012**, *153*, 583–591. [CrossRef] [PubMed]
35. Asvold, B.O.; Bjøro, T.; Vatten, L.J. Associations of TSH levels within the reference range with future blood pressure and lipid concentrations: 11-year follow-up of the HUNT study. *Eur. J. Endocrinol.* **2013**, *169*, 73–82. [CrossRef] [PubMed]
36. Wang, F.; Tan, Y.; Wang, C.; Zhang, X.; Zhao, Y.; Song, X.; Zhang, B.; Guan, Q.; Xu, J.; Zhang, J.; et al. Thyroid-stimulating hormone levels within the reference range are associated with serum lipid profiles independent of thyroid hormones. *J. Clin. Endocrinol. Metab.* **2012**, *97*, 2724–2731. [CrossRef] [PubMed]
37. Lee, Y.K.; Kim, J.E.; Oh, H.J.; Park, K.S.; Kim, S.K.; Park, S.W.; Kim, M.J.; Cho, Y.W. Serum TSH level in healthy Koreans and the association of TSH with serum lipid concentration and metabolic syndrome. *Korean J. Intern. Med.* **2011**, *26*, 432–439. [CrossRef] [PubMed]
38. Asvold, B.O.; Bjøro, T.; Nilsen, T.I.; Vatten, L.J. Association between blood pressure and serum thyroid-stimulating hormone concentration within the reference range: A population-based study. *J. Clin. Endocrinol. Metab.* **2007**, *92*, 841–845. [CrossRef] [PubMed]
39. Peixoto de Miranda, É.J.F.; Bittencourt, M.S.; Santos, I.S.; Lotufo, P.A.; Benseñor, I.M. Thyroid Function and High-Sensitivity C-Reactive Protein in Cross-Sectional Results from the Brazilian Longitudinal Study of Adult Health (ELSA-Brasil): Effect of Adiposity and Insulin Resistance. *Eur. Thyroid J.* **2016**, *5*, 240–246. [CrossRef]
40. Tuzcu, A.; Bahceci, M.; Gokalp, D.; Tuzun, Y.; Gunes, K. Subclinical hypothyroidism may be associated with elevated high-sensitive c-reactive protein (low grade inflammation) and fasting hyperinsulinemia. *Endocr. J.* **2005**, *52*, 89–94. [CrossRef] [PubMed]
41. Chadarevian, R.; Bruckert, E.; Giral, P.; Turpin, G. Relationship between thyroid hormones and fibrinogen levels. *Blood Coagul. Fibrinolysis* **1999**, *10*, 481–486. [CrossRef] [PubMed]
42. Dörr, M.; Robinson, D.M.; Wallaschofski, H.; Schwahn, C.; John, U.; Felix, S.B.; Völzke, H. Low serum thyrotropin is associated with high plasma fibrinogen. *J. Clin. Endocrinol. Metab.* **2006**, *91*, 530–534. [CrossRef] [PubMed]
43. Park, S.B.; Choi, H.C.; Joo, N.S. The relation of thyroid function to components of the metabolic syndrome in Korean men and women. *J. Korean Med. Sci.* **2011**, *26*, 540–545. [CrossRef] [PubMed]
44. Kim, H.J.; Bae, J.C.; Park, H.K.; Byun, D.W.; Suh, K.; Yoo, M.H.; Kim, J.H.; Min, Y.K.; Kim, S.W.; Chung, J.H. Triiodothyronine Levels Are Independently Associated with Metabolic Syndrome in Euthyroid Middle-Aged Subjects. *Endocrinol. Metab. (Seoul)* **2016**, *31*, 311–319. [CrossRef] [PubMed]
45. Alevizaki, M.; Saltiki, K.; Voidonikola, P.; Mantzou, E.; Papamichael, C.; Stamatelopoulos, K. Free thyroxine is an independent predictor of subcutaneous fat in euthyroid individuals. *Eur. J. Endocrinol.* **2009**, *161*, 459–465. [CrossRef] [PubMed]

46. Kim, B.J.; Kim, T.Y.; Koh, J.M.; Kim, H.K.; Park, J.Y.; Lee, K.U.; Shong, Y.K.; Kim, W.B. Relationship between serum free T4 (FT4) levels and metabolic syndrome (MS) and its components in healthy euthyroid subjects. *Clin. Endocrinol. (Oxf)* **2009**, *70*, 152–160. [CrossRef]
47. Roef, G.; Lapauw, B.; Goemaere, S.; Zmierczak, H.G.; Toye, K.; Kaufman, J.M.; Taes, Y. Body composition and metabolic parameters are associated with variation in thyroid hormone levels among euthyroid young men. *Eur. J. Endocrinol.* **2012**, *167*, 719–726. [CrossRef]

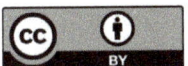

© 2019 by the authors. Licensee MDPI, Basel, Switzerland. This article is an open access article distributed under the terms and conditions of the Creative Commons Attribution (CC BY) license (http://creativecommons.org/licenses/by/4.0/).

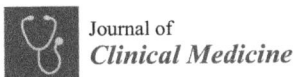 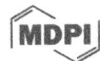

Article

Plasma microRNA Profiling Reveals Novel Biomarkers of Epicardial Adipose Tissue: A Multidetector Computed Tomography Study

David de Gonzalo-Calvo [1,2,3,*], David Vilades [4], Pablo Martínez-Camblor [5], Àngela Vea [2], Andreu Ferrero-Gregori [3,6], Laura Nasarre [2], Olga Bornachea [1,2], Jesus Sanchez Vega [4], Rubén Leta [4], Núria Puig [7,8], Sonia Benítez [7], Jose Luis Sanchez-Quesada [7,9], Francesc Carreras [3,4] and Vicenta Llorente-Cortés [1,2,3,*]

1. Institute of Biomedical Research of Barcelona (IIBB) - Spanish National Research Council (CSIC), 08036 Barcelona, Spain; olgabornachea79@gmail.com
2. Biomedical Research Institute Sant Pau (IIB Sant Pau), 08041 Barcelona, Spain; angelavea@gmail.com (À.V.); lnasarre@santpau.cat (L.N.)
3. CIBERCV, Institute of Health Carlos III, 28029 Madrid, Spain; AFerrero@santpau.cat (A.F.-G.); FCarreras@santpau.cat (F.C.)
4. Cardiac Imaging Unit, Cardiology Department, Hospital de la Santa Creu i Sant Pau, 08041 Barcelona, Spain; DVilades@santpau.cat (D.V.); JSanchezV@santpau.cat (J.S.V.); RLeta@santpau.cat (R.L.)
5. Geisel School of Medicine, Dartmouth College, Hanover, NH 03755, USA; pablo.martinez.camblor@dartmouth.edu
6. Cardiology Service, Hospital de la Santa Creu i Sant Pau, Universitat Autònoma de Barcelona (UAB), 08041 Barcelona, Spain
7. Cardiovascular Biochemistry, Biomedical Research Institute Sant Pau (IIB Sant Pau), 08041 Barcelona, Spain; NPuigG@santpau.cat (N.P.); SBenitez@santpau.cat (S.B.); JSanchezQ@santpau.cat (J.L.S.-Q.)
8. Molecular Biology and Biochemistry Department, Universitat Autònoma de Barcelona (UAB), 08193 Cerdanyola del Valles, Spain
9. CIBERDEM, Institute of Health Carlos III, 28029 Madrid, Spain
* Correspondence: david.degonzalo@gmail.com (D.d.G.-C.); cllorente@santpau.cat (V.L.-C.); Tel.: +34-935-565-891 (D.d.G.-C.); +34-935-565-888 (V.L.-C.)

Received: 6 May 2019; Accepted: 28 May 2019; Published: 1 June 2019

Abstract: Epicardial adipose tissue (EAT) constitutes a novel parameter for cardiometabolic risk assessment and a target for therapy. Here, we evaluated for the first time the plasma microRNA (miRNA) profile as a source of biomarkers for epicardial fat volume (EFV). miRNAs were profiled in plasma samples from 180 patients whose EFV was quantified using multidetector computed tomography. In the screening study, 54 deregulated miRNAs were identified in patients with high EFV levels (highest tertile) compared with matched patients with low EFV levels (lowest tertile). After filtering, 12 miRNAs were selected for subsequent validation. In the validation study, miR-15b-3p, miR-22-3p, miR-148a-3p miR-148b-3p and miR-590-5p were directly associated with EFV, even after adjustment for confounding factors (p value < 0.05 for all models). The addition of miRNA combinations to a model based on clinical variables improved the discrimination (area under the receiver-operating-characteristic curve (AUC) from 0.721 to 0.787). miRNAs correctly reclassified a significant proportion of patients with an integrated discrimination improvement (IDI) index of 0.101 and a net reclassification improvement (NRI) index of 0.650. Decision tree models used miRNA combinations to improve their classification accuracy. These results were reproduced using two proposed clinical cutoffs for epicardial fat burden. Internal validation corroborated the robustness of the models. In conclusion, plasma miRNAs constitute novel biomarkers of epicardial fat burden.

Keywords: biomarker; cardiometabolic disease; epicardial adipose tissue; epicardial fat; epicardial fat volume; microRNA

1. Introduction

MicroRNAs (miRNAs) are evolutionarily conserved small noncoding RNAs (ncRNAs) that posttranscriptionally regulate gene expression playing a critical role in cellular pathways involved in development, homeostasis and the response to stress [1]. In addition to their intracellular localization, miRNAs have also been detected in the extracellular space and circulation [2]. Extracellular miRNAs can be easily assayed by analyzing bodily fluids, they are stable against degradation, have a long half-life in biological samples, and can be detected with techniques readily available in clinical laboratories [3]. Thus, miRNA-based tests provide an interesting opportunity to develop novel tools to assist in clinical decision-making [3]. A number of publications have proposed the use of circulating miRNAs as biomarkers for a wide range of medical conditions [4,5]. Indeed, monitoring alterations in the patterns of circulating miRNAs could be useful in the diagnosis and prognostic stratification within diverse cardiovascular and metabolic disorders [6,7].

Epicardial adipose tissue (EAT), the visceral fat depot located between the myocardium and visceral pericardium, is a metabolically active tissue that regulates cardiovascular homeostasis under physiological conditions [8]. However, under pathological conditions, excessive accumulation of EAT surrounding the myocardium and the coronary arteries actively contributes to the development and progression of cardiovascular disease [9]. Although the mechanisms are not fully understood, EAT has been directly implicated in different pathological processes via secretion of pro-inflammatory, pro-fibrotic and metabolic mediators [10,11]. The relationship between epicardial fat burden and cardiovascular disease has recently gained attention among the medical community. Multiple clinical studies have demonstrated that epicardial fat is a risk factor for coronary artery disease (CAD) [12], heart failure (HF) [13] and atrial fibrillation (AF) [14]. A prognostic value for major adverse cardiovascular events and mortality has also been reported [15]. Furthermore, epicardial fat accumulation has been correlated with metabolic diseases including diabetes and metabolic syndrome [16]. Consequently, EAT constitutes a novel parameter for cardiometabolic risk assessment and a target for therapy [17,18].

Epicardial adipose tissue can be clinically measured using different imaging techniques such as transthoracic echocardiography, cardiovascular magnetic resonance (CMR) and computed tomography (CT). However, the need for specialized centers and trained personnel, in addition to the operating expenses, limit the applicability of this methodology. Surprisingly, there are limited studies investigating non-invasive and easily accessible biomarkers to quantify EAT [19,20]. Despite the potential of miRNAs as clinical indicators, they have not yet been used to assess the epicardial fat burden. Here, we address this important gap by evaluating the plasma miRNA profile to identify biomarkers for epicardial fat volume (EFV).

2. Experimental Section

2.1. Study Population

This is a prospective study including clinically stable patients referred for coronary computed tomography angiography (CCTA) in the Cardiac Imaging Unit of the Hospital de la Santa Creu i Sant Pau (Barcelona, Spain). According to miRNA profiling data, accepting a significance level of 0.05 and a power of 80% in a two-sided test, and assuming a common standard deviation (SD) of 0.9, 51 subjects were necessary in both study groups to recognize as statistically significant a difference greater than or equal to 0.5 arbitrary units (au). EAT assessment was performed after blood collection. Therefore, the sample size used was higher to ensure the necessary number of patients. Finally, 180 consecutive patients were enrolled in the study. Exclusion criteria included suspected acute coronary syndrome, contraindications to CCTA imaging, any survival-limiting disease or any severe infectious disease. Detailed demographic, anthropometric, clinical and pharmacological information was obtained from electronic medical records. All subjects gave written informed consent before participating in the study.

The study protocol was approved by the local ethical committee of the Hospital de la Santa Creu i Sant Pau. The study was performed in accordance with the Helsinki Declaration.

2.2. Coronary Computed Tomography Angiography (CCTA)

A CCTA exam using a 256-slice CT scanner (Brilliance iCT 256; Philips Healthcare, Amsterdam, the Netherlands) was performed on all participants. A contrast-enhanced scan was performed to assess CAD and EFV. The scan was prospectively triggered at 75% of the RR interval using 100 kV (120 kV in patients with a body mass index >30 kg m^{-2}) if the heart rate was below 65 beats per min (bpm), and retrospectively gated (helical acquisition) if the heart rate was higher than 65 bpm. Iodinated contrast (Xenetix 350; Guerbet, Aulnay-sous-Bois, France) was administered at a dose of 0.7–1 mL kg^{-1} (range 50–120) and followed by a 40 mL saline flush, and both injected at a rate of 5–6 mL/s. CCTA studies were subsequently analyzed off-line. Coronary artery plaques were defined as any tissue structure >1 mm^2 that existed either within the coronary artery lumen or adjacent to the coronary artery lumen that could be distinguished from the surrounding pericardial tissue, epicardial fat, or the lumen itself. Coronary artery disease was quantified for stenosis by quantitative coronary angiography (CT-QCA) in any luminal diameter narrowing ≥50% of the reference luminal diameter. The methodology to calculate EFV was performed with a dedicated software as follows (OsiriX MD, v 6.5, FDA cleared, Pixmeo): first, the upper and lower slice limits of pericardium were manually defined in an axial view. Then, the EFV was marked in each slice by drawing regions of interest with voxel densities between −150 to −30 Hounsfield units (corresponding to adipose tissue). A contiguous 3-dimensional volume render was then performed and quantified in cubic centimeters (cm^3), and indexed to body surface area (cm^3 m^{-2}) to produce an EFV-index (EFVi). Body surface area data was available for 160 patients. Patients were stratified according EFV tertiles: first and second tertiles (11.93–118.00 cm^3) and third tertile (118.74–257.35 cm^3). Additionally, we used two binary cutoffs previously proposed as clinically relevant: EFV > 125 cm^3 [15] and EFVi > 68.1 cm^3 m^{-2} [21].

2.3. Blood Collection

Blood collection and processing were performed using standardized protocols [22]. Blood samples were obtained in K$_2$-ethylenediaminetetra-acetic acid (EDTA) blood collection tubes (BD) by venipuncture after a night of fasting and before beginning any interventional procedure or administration of contrast agents. The blood was processed within 2 h after isolation. To obtain plasma, blood samples were fractionated by centrifugation at 1300 × g for 15 min at room temperature. After centrifugation, plasma supernatant was aliquoted into 1.5 mL DNA LoBind tubes and stored at −80 °C until analysis.

2.4. Epicardial Adipose Tissue (EAT)

Epicardial adipose tissue explants were obtained from patients undergoing cardiac surgery ($N = 8$). Patients were diagnosed with either CAD ($N = 4$) or valve disease ($N = 4$). 100 mg pieces of EAT were incubated for 24 h in 1 mL serum-free DMEM supplemented with antibiotics in 5% CO$_2$. miRNAs were isolated from tissue and from the conditioned media.

2.5. High-Sensitive C-Reactive Protein (CRP) Concentration

High-sensitive C-reactive protein (hs-CRP) concentrations were determined using an immunoturbidimetry method on the Roche Cobas c501 analyzer (Roche Diagnostics, Mannheim, Germany). The hs-CRP assay has an analytic range from 0.3 to 350 mg L^{-1}. The assay had interrun coefficients of variation that ranged from 1.2 to 3.6%.

2.6. MicroRNA Isolation

Profiling of miRNA was conducted in the same laboratory and under the same conditions. Experienced staff blinded to clinical data performed all laboratory measurements. Total RNA was isolated from 150 µL of frozen plasma samples or conditioned medium samples using miRNeasy Serum/Plasma Kit (Qiagen, Hilden, Germany), according to the manufacturer's instructions. For EAT, total RNA was isolated from 100 mg of tissue using the miRNeasy Mini Kit (Qiagen). For normalization of extracellular miRNAs, synthetic *Caenorhabditis elegans* miR-39-3p (cel-miR-39-3p), lacking sequence homology to human miRNAs, was added as an external reference miRNA (1.6×10^8 copies µL^{-1}). The mixture was also supplemented with 1 µg of MS2 carrier RNA (Roche, Merck, Darmstadt, Germany) to improve extracellular miRNA yield. Purification of RNA was performed with RNeasy MinElute or RNeasy Mini Spin columns according to the manufacturer's instructions. RNA was eluted in nuclease-free H$_2$O and stored in a -80 °C freezer.

2.7. Quantification of MicroRNA

Quantitative polymerase chain reaction (qPCR) was performed according to the protocol for the miRCURY LNA Universal RT microRNA PCR System (Exiqon, Qiagen, Hilden, Germany), which offers an optimal performance [23]. According to the manufacturer's instructions, different protocols for cDNA synthesis were used for extracellular or tissue miRNAs. The RNA in the plasma and conditioned media cannot be accurately quantified. Therefore, we used the same starting sample volume rather than RNA quantity (2 µL of RNA). For tissue, total RNA concentration was determined with a NanoDrop ND-1000 spectrophotometer (NanoDrop Technologies). Then, RNA samples were adjusted to a concentration of 5 ng µL^{-1} using nuclease-free H$_2$O. RNA was reverse transcribed in 10 µL reactions using the Universal cDNA Synthesis Kit II (Exiqon). The RT reaction was performed with the following conditions: incubation for 60 min at 42 °C followed by heat-inactivation for 5 min at 95 °C; the reaction was then immediately cooled to 4 °C. cDNA was stored at -20 °C.

For the screen, we used the 384 well Serum/Plasma Focus microRNA PCR Panel V4 (Exiqon). The panel included primer sets for 179 miRNAs commonly found in serum and plasma samples. Each selected miRNA was validated in plasma, conditioned media and tissue using 384-well Pick-&-Mix microRNA PCR Plates (V4) (Exiqon). qPCR was performed in 10 µL reactions using the 7900HT Fast Real-Time PCR System (Applied Biosystems, Thermo Fisher Scientific, Waltham, Massachusetts, USA) with the following cycling conditions: 10 min at 95 °C, 40 cycles of 10 s at 95 °C and 1 min at 60 °C, followed by a melting curve analysis. The synthetic UniSp3 assay was analyzed as interplate calibrator. The SDS v2.3 software was used to determine the quantification cycle number (Cq) and perform the melting curve analysis. The Cq was defined as the fractional cycle number at which the fluorescence exceeded a given threshold. The specificity of the qPCR was corroborated by melting curve analysis. miRNAs were considered to be expressed at Cq values < 35. Relative quantification was performed using the 2^{-dCq} method, where $dCq = Cq_{miRNA} - Cq_{cel\text{-}miR\text{-}39\text{-}3p}$ for extracellular miRNAs and $Cq_{miRNA} - Cq_{SNORD48}$ for tissue miRNAs. Expression levels were log$_2$-transformed for statistical analyses.

2.8. Statistical Analysis

Statistical analysis was performed using the statistical software package R version 3.5.2. Descriptive statistics were used to summarize the characteristics of the study population. The Kolmogorov–Smirnov test was used to test normality. Data were described as the mean ± SD and median (P25–P75) for continuous variables. Frequency (percentage) was used for categorical variables. Continuous variables were compared between groups using the Student's *t*-test and Mann–Whitney U test for normally distributed and nonnormally distributed variables, respectively. Categorical variables were compared between groups using Fisher's exact test. Spearman's rho coefficient was used to assess the correlation between continuous variables. In the screen, heat map visualization was used to determine whether plasma miRNAs can differentiate between patients according to EFV tertile [24]. In the validation study, logistic regression analyses were used to investigate whether plasma miRNAs were independently associated with EFV.

Backward stepwise regression models were used to explore the performance of plasma miRNAs, in combination with clinical covariates, as biomarkers of EFV. Clinical covariates were chosen based on statistical differences observed between study groups (p value < 0.1): age, sex, body mass index (BMI) and diabetes mellitus. The results were presented as an odds ratio (OR) and 95% confidence intervals (CI). Receiver-operating-characteristic (ROC) curves were constructed to assess the global discriminative ability. The results were presented as the area under the ROC curve (AUC) and 95% CI. The added discrimination capacity of plasma miRNA over the multiparameter clinical model was tested by the DeLong test [25]. The Integrated Discrimination Improvement (IDI) index and Net Reclassification Improvement (NRI) index were computed to assess the reclassification capacity of plasma miRNAs [26]. The internal validity of the final models was tested for 500 bootstrap resamples, using the 'rms' package by Frank Harrell [27] in the R Project for Statistical Computing. The calibration of the models was assessed by the corresponding plots using the same package.

Decision tree models were developed using a chi-squared automatic interaction detector (CHAID) algorithm [28]. The CHAID algorithm utilizes statistical significance from Chi-square tests to establish a hierarchy of predictors, here the parameters that composed our clinical model and plasma miRNAs. CHAID analysis identifies potential interactions among the predictors and selects the optimal combination of variables and cutoff values for classification. The two-tailed significance level was set at p value < 0.05.

3. Results

3.1. Study Population

Table 1 shows the characteristics of the study population. The mean age was 65.0 ± 12.8 years, and 104 patients (58%) were male. The prevalence for hypertension, dyslipidemia, diabetes mellitus and active or former smoker was 62%, 57%, 21% and 33%, respectively. Patients underwent multiple pharmacological therapies including antiplatelet drugs (41%), statins (48%), beta-blockers (32%), angiotensin-converting-enzyme (ACE) inhibitors (54%) and diuretics (27%).

Standardized quantitative categories for EFV are currently lacking. Therefore, the study population was stratified according to EFV tertiles: patients in the first and second tertiles (low-medium epicardial fat burden) and patients in the third tertile (high epicardial fat burden). Compared to patients in the first and second tertiles of EFV, patients in the third tertile were typically older, more frequently male with a higher BMI and prevalence of diabetes mellitus (Table 1). The use of statin, an antiplatelet drug, and beta-blockers was also higher in patients in the third tertile.

Table 1. Characteristics of the study population.

Variable	All N = 180	Tertile 1&2 N = 120	Tertile 3 N = 60	p Value
Clinical characteristics				
Age (years), mean ± SD	65.0 ± 12.8	63.5 ± 13.8	68.1 ± 9.9	0.011
Male, N (%)	104 (58)	63 (53)	41 (68)	0.055
Body mass index (kg m^{-2}), median (P25–P75)	27.0 (24.8–30.3)	25.9 (24.2–29.2)	29.4 (26.3–32.1)	<0.001
Body surface area (m^2), median (P25–P75) N = 160	1.8 (1.7–2.0)	1.8 (1.7–1.9)	1.9 (1.9–2.1)	0.001
Hypertension, N (%)	111 (62)	70 (58)	41 (68)	0.255
Dyslipidemia, N (%)	102 (57)	66 (55)	36 (60)	0.632
Diabetes mellitus, N (%)	37 (21)	18 (15)	19 (32)	0.011
Active or former smoker, N (%)	59 (33)	36 (30)	23 (38)	0.310
hs-CRP (mg L^{-1}), median (P25–P75)	2.00 (0.97–4.07)	1.90 (0.85–4.00)	2.10 (1.11–4.62)	0.590
Coronary artery disease, N (%)	55 (30.6)	35 (29.2)	20 (33.3)	0.608
Glomerular filtration rate < 60 mL/mi/1.73 m^2, N (%)	16 (9)	11 (9)	5 (8)	1.000
Medication use				
Antiplatelet drugs, N (%)	73 (41)	43 (36)	40 (50)	0.071
Statins, N (%)	87 (48)	52 (43)	35 (58)	0.052
Beta-blockers, N (%)	58 (32)	34 (28)	24 (40)	0.086
Angiotensin-converting-enzyme inhibitors, N (%)	97 (54)	64 (53)	33 (55)	0.746
Diuretics, N (%)	48 (27)	31 (26)	17 (28)	0.718
Epicardial fat burden				
Epicardial fat volume (cm^3), median (P25–P75)	96.0 (66.5–130.6)	79.3 (55.8–96.4)	146.4 (130.5–178.4)	<0.001
Epicardial fat volume-indexed (cm^3 m^{-2}), median (P25–P75) N = 160	50.0 (38.2–67.2)	42.0 (32.1–52.4)	76.3 (67.4–92.9)	<0.001

Data are presented as frequencies (percentages) for categorical variables. Continuous variables are presented as mean ± standard deviation (SD) or median (P25–P75). Differences between groups were analyzed using Student's t-test, Mann–Whitney U test or Fisher's exact test. hs-CRP: High-sensitive C-reactive protein.

3.2. Profiling of Plasma MicroRNAs

To determine whether the plasma miRNAs were differentially expressed between study groups, we first profiled the expression of 179 miRNAs in patients with low (first EFV tertile, N = 8) and high epicardial fat burden (third EFV tertile, N = 8) (Table S1). Due to the sample size and in order to gain statistical power, patients in the second EFV tertile were not included in this phase. To minimize potential confounding variables, we also restricted our analysis to patients in the first and third tertiles who matched according to age, sex, BMI, cardiovascular risk factors and hs-CRP levels. The expression level of miR-208a-3p was below the limit of detection in 94% of the samples and was excluded from additional analyses. Unsupervised hierarchical clustering based on miRNA expression profile clearly separated patients in the third tertile from patients in the first tertile (Figure 1A). Analysis of the data identified 54 significantly differentially expressed miRNAs (Figure 1B, Table S2). To identify potential biomarkers, we selected 8 miRNAs (miR-15b-3p, miR-15b-5p, miR-22-3p, miR-27b-3p, miR-146a-5p, miR-148b-3p, miR-339-3p and miR-590-5p) for further validation based on their statistical significance ($p \leq 0.01$) and abundance in the circulation (median Cq < 30, maximum Cq = 32 and detected in all samples) (Figure 1C, Table S2). Several differentially expressed miRNAs belonged to the same family as our candidates: miR-21-5p, miR-27a-3p, miR-148a-3p (p value = 0.065) and miR-152-3p (Figure 1C, Table S2). Members within the same miRNA family share seed sequences and could be functionally related (Table S3). Thus, these miRNAs were also selected for further validation in order to test whether the combination of all family members could have higher potential as biomarker than individual members. These miRNAs were all abundantly expressed in the circulation, meeting the established criteria. Except for miR-15b-3p and miR-15b-5p, all of the candidates were derived from different miRNA genomic clusters (>10 kb) (Table S3).

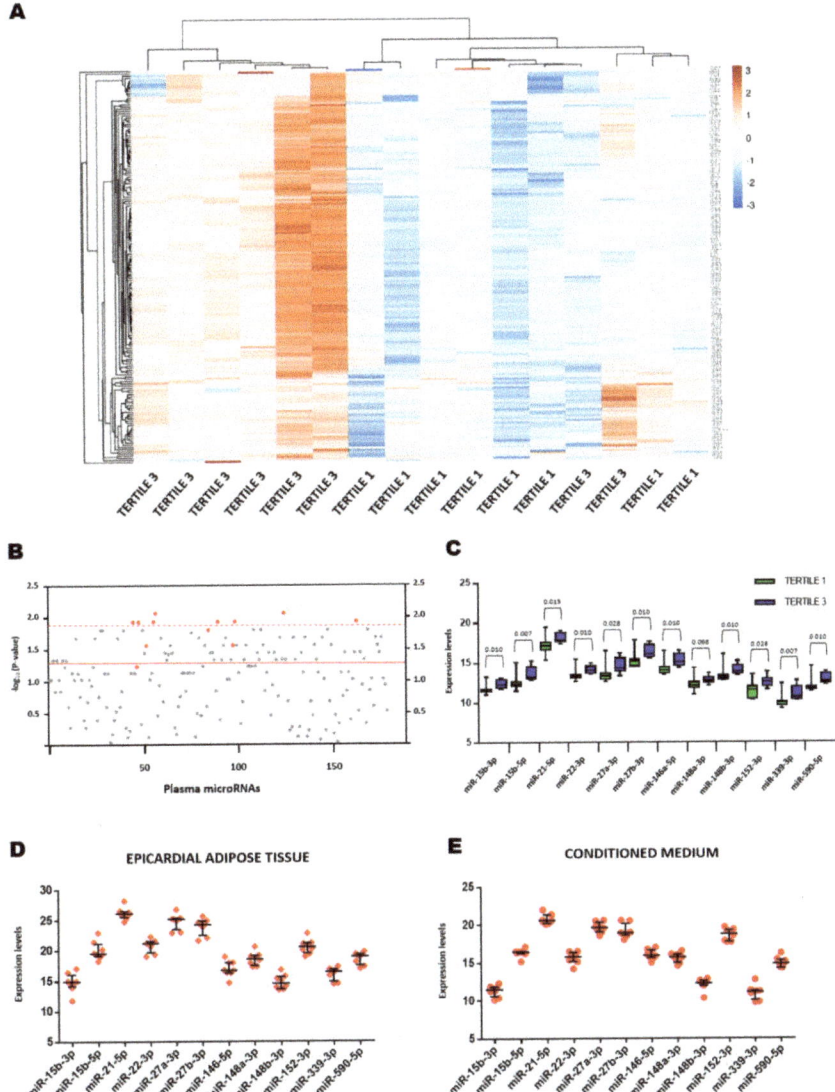

Figure 1. Plasma microRNA (miRNA) profiling. (**A**) Unsupervised hierarchical clustering. The heat map diagram shows the result of a two-way hierarchical clustering of patients and miRNAs. Each column represents a patient (Tertile 1 of epicardial fat volume vs. Tertile 3 of epicardial fat volume). Each row represents a miRNA. The patient clustering tree is shown on top. The miRNA clustering tree is shown on the left. The color scale illustrates the relative expression level of miRNAs. The expression intensity of each miRNA in each sample varies from red to blue, which indicates relatively high or low expression, respectively. (**B**) p value for the comparison between study groups. Each point represents a miRNA. Red dots represent the selected candidates. (**C**) Plasma expression levels of miRNAs in study groups. (**D**) Expression levels of miRNAs in epicardial adipose tissue explants. Each point represents a sample. (**E**) Expression levels of miRNAs in conditioned media exposed to epicardial adipose tissue explants. Each point represents a sample. Relative quantification was performed using cel-miR-39-3p as the external standard for extracellular miRNAs and SNORD48 as the internal standard for tissue miRNAs. MicroRNA levels were log2-transformed. MicroRNA expression levels are expressed as arbitrary units. Differences between groups were analyzed using the Mann–Whitney U test. p values describe the significance level of differences for each comparison.

To further characterize the potential of these miRNAs as biomarkers of EFV, we evaluated their expression levels in human EAT explants and in conditioned media that was exposed to human EAT explants. The miRNA profiles were similar in both sample sets, and all of the miRNAs were detected in all tissue and conditioned media samples (Cq < 35) (Figure 1D,E).

3.3. Plasma MicroRNAs and Epicardial Fat Volume

Selected miRNAs from the screen were validated in the whole study population ($N = 180$). To do that, patients were stratified into two categories: low-medium epicardial fat burden (patients in the first and second EFV tertiles, $N = 120$) and high epicardial fat burden (patients in the third EFV tertile, $N = 60$). Representative patients in the first-second and third EFV tertiles are shown in Figure 2A,B. As shown in Figure 2C, the plasma expression levels of miR-15b-3p, miR-22-3p, miR-148a-3p, miR-148b-3p and miR-590-5p were significantly higher in patients in the third tertile compared with those in the first and second tertiles. Plasma miR-15b-3p, miR-22-3p, miR-148a-3p and miR-148b-3p were directly correlated with EFV (Table S4).

Logistic regression models were used to evaluate the associations between EFV (first and second tertiles vs. third tertile) and miRNAs (Table 2). Using unadjusted logistic regression models (model 1), the plasma levels of miR-15b-3p, miR-22-3p, miR-148a-3p, miR-148b-3p and miR-590-5p were directly associated with EFV. After correcting for confounding factors including age, sex, BMI, diabetes mellitus, medication use (antiplatelet drugs, statin use and beta-blockers use) and CAD (models 2, 3 and 4), the association between the EFV and these miRNAs remained statistically significant.

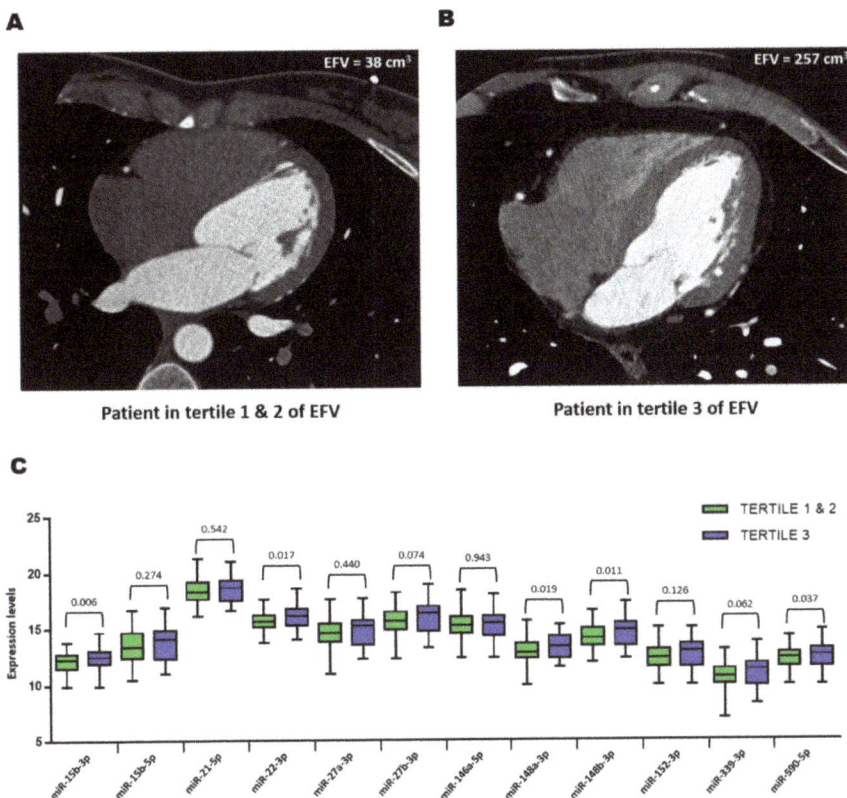

Figure 2. Plasma microRNA (miRNA) validation. (**A–B**) Examples of multidetector computed tomography scans and the corresponding epicardial fat volume of patients in the first-second and third tertiles of epicardial fat volume. (**C**) Plasma expression levels of miRNAs in study groups. MicroRNA levels were $\log_2$-transformed. MicroRNA expression levels are expressed as arbitrary units. Differences between groups were analyzed using Student's *t*-test for independent samples. *p* values describe the significance level of differences for each comparison. EFV: epicardial fat volume.

Table 2. Association between circulating microRNAs and epicardial fat volume.

	Model 1		Model 2		Model 3		Model 4	
	OR (95% CI)	p Value	OR (95% CI)	p Value	OR (95% CI)	p Value	OR (95% CI)	p Value
miR-15b-3p	1.701 (1.158–2.500)	0.007	1.800 (1.177–2.753)	0.007	1.832 (1.181–2.844)	0.007	1.793 (1.174–2.738)	0.007
miR-15b-5p	1.132 (0.907–1.412)	0.273	1.183 (0.923–1.516)	0.185	1.168 (0.905–1.507)	0.234	1.182 (0.922–1.515)	0.188
miR-21-5p	1.092 (0.824–1.446)	0.540	1.169 (0.856–1.596)	0.327	1.127 (0.816–1.555)	0.468	1.168 (0.855–1.596)	0.329
miR-22-3p	1.551 (1.075–2.239)	0.019	1.677 (1.113–2.527)	0.013	1.655 (1.089–2.516)	0.018	1.669 (1.109–2.514)	0.014
miR-27a-3p	1.100 (0.865–1.398)	0.438	1.146 (0.880–1.492)	0.311	1.120 (0.852–1.471)	0.417	1.142 (0.877–1.488)	0.324
miR-27b-3p	1.269 (0.976–1.651)	0.076	1.331 (0.994–1.781)	0.055	1.320 (0.977–1.782)	0.070	1.325 (0.989–1.774)	0.059
miR-146a-5p	1.010 (0.781–1.305)	0.942	1.066 (0.805–1.410)	0.657	1.027 (0.768–1.372)	0.858	1.062 (0.801–1.406)	0.677
miR-148a-3p	1.387 (1.052–1.829)	0.020	1.417 (1.045–1.921)	0.025	1.429 (1.045–1.955)	0.025	1.417 (1.045–1.923)	0.025
miR-148b-3p	1.444 (1.081–1.929)	0.013	1.563 (1.130–2.161)	0.007	1.527 (1.096–2.128)	0.012	1.558 (1.127–2.154)	0.007
miR-152-3p	1.222 (0.945–1.581)	0.127	1.310 (0.982–1.748)	0.066	1.283 (0.953–1.728)	0.101	1.306 (0.979–1.744)	0.070
miR-339-3p	1.304 (0.985–1.726)	0.064	1.350 (0.992–1.838)	0.056	1.317 (0.960–1.806)	0.088	1.344 (0.988–1.830)	0.060
miR-590-5p	1.449 (1.018–2.062)	0.039	1.571 (1.062–2.324)	0.024	1.541 (1.030–2.306)	0.036	1.564 (1.059–2.312)	0.025

Model 1: Unadjusted; Model 2: Adjusted for age, sex, body mass index and diabetes mellitus; Model 3: Model 2 adjusted for antiplatelet drugs, statins use and beta-blockers use; Model 4: Model 2 adjusted for coronary artery disease. OR: odds ratio; 95% CI: 95% confidence interval.

3.4. Performance of Plasma MicroRNAs as Biomarkers of Epicardial Fat Volume

The AUC was used to assess the discriminative capacity of plasma miRNAs as biomarkers for EFV. As shown in Figure 3A, all of the individual miRNAs showed poor discrimination ability (AUC = 0.518–0.625). The discrimination capacity was also modest for the combination of miRNAs in pairs or families (AUC = 0.590–0.642).

To further explore the role of plasma miRNAs as potential biomarkers for EFV, we evaluated the effect of adding our miRNAs on the discrimination capacity of a model originally based on clinical variables: age, sex, BMI and diabetes mellitus (clinical model). When the miRNAs were added as independent variables (clinical model + plasma miRNAs), miR-27a-3p and miR-148b-3p were significant predictors of EFV (Figure 3B). Comparison of ROC curves showed that the AUC for the clinical model + plasma miRNAs was significantly higher (9.2%) than that of the clinical model alone: AUC = 0.721 vs. 0.787. Adding both miRNAs to the clinical model also led to a significant reclassification of the patients: IDI = 0.101 and NRI = 0.650. Bootstrap internal validation supported the robustness of the model including plasma miRNAs (Figure S1A).

Decision tree models were constructed using the CHAID algorithm. First, we included the variables from the clinical model. As shown in Figure 3C, the decision tree identified the cutoff values for BMI and age. The first variable selected was BMI. For patients with a BMI >25.8 kg m^{-2}, age was the next most relevant predictor with a cutoff value of 54 years. Second, in addition to the variables from the clinical model, we included the miRNA candidates (Figure 3D). Again, BMI was the first variable selected. In this case, miR-148b-3p was the next most significant predictor for patients with BMI >25.8 kg m^{-2}. A cutoff expression value of 14.29 arbitrary units (au) allowed the enrichment in two subgroups of patients in the first and second tertiles (70.9%) and the third tertile (61.1%). In patients with a BMI >25.8 kg m^{-2} and miR-148b-3p expression levels ≤14.29 au, a miR-146a-5p expression level >14.65 au increased the percentage of patients in the first and second tertiles to 91.3%. In patients with BMI >25.8 kg m^{-2} and miR-148b-3p expression levels >14.29 au, age was the most significant predictor, increasing the percentage of patients older than 59 years that belonged to the third tertile to 74.4%.

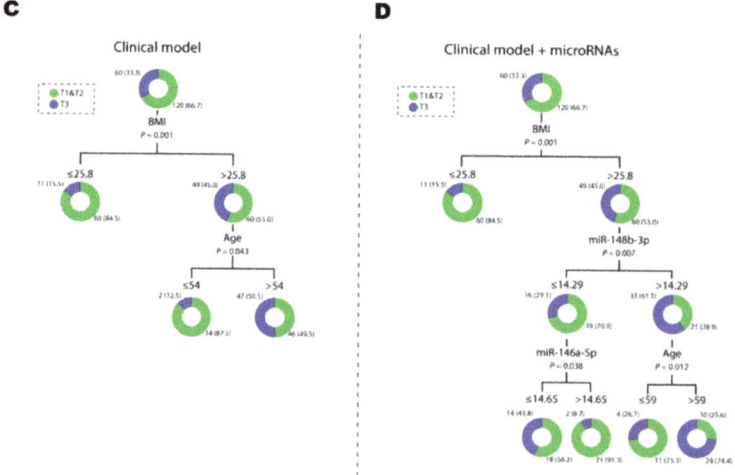

Figure 3. Plasma microRNAs (miRNAs) as biomarkers of epicardial fat volume, according to EFV tertiles. (**A**) Area under the ROC curve (AUC) for each individual miRNAs and for combinations of miRNAs in pairs or families. (**B**) Performance of plasma miRNAs as biomarkers. (**C,D**) Decision trees calculated by chi-squared automatic interaction detector (CHAID) algorithm. The following variables were included in the clinical model: age, sex, body mass index and diabetes mellitus. MicroRNA levels were $\log_2$-transformed. For logistic regression models, data are presented as an odds ratio (OR) and 95% confidence intervals (CI). For discrimination analysis, data are presented as the AUC and 95% CI. For reclassification analysis, data are presented as the Integrated Discrimination Improvement (IDI) index and Net Reclassification Improvement (NRI) index and their respective and 95% CI. For decision trees, data are shown as frequency (percentage) of patients in each study group.

3.5. Validation Using Alternative Cutoffs of Epicardial Fat Volume

To validate these findings, we evaluated the ability of our miRNAs to serve as biomarkers using previously published binary cutoffs of epicardial fat burden: Spearman et al. (EFV ≤125 cm^3 vs. EFV >125 cm^3) [15] (Figure 4) and Shmilovich et al. (EFVi ≤68.1 cm^3 m^{-2} vs. (EFVi >68.1 cm^3 m^{-2}) [21] (Figure S2). The discrimination capacity was modest for all individual miRNAs and when combined in pairs or families for both clinical ranges (Figure 4A, Figure S2A). In support of the above findings, adding the candidates to the clinical models demonstrated that plasma miRNAs, in particular miR-27a-3p, miR-146a-5p, miR-148b-3p and miR-152-3p, were significant predictors of EFV and EFVi (Figure 4B, Figure S2B). The addition of miRNAs significantly augmented the discriminative power of the clinical models and reclassify a significant proportion of the patients (Figure 4B, Figure S2B). The robustness of the models including miRNAs was confirmed by bootstrap (Figure S1B,C).

The decision tree model identified several plasma miRNAs, miR-27b-3p, miR-146a-5p and miR-148b-3p for classification using the clinical range proposed by Spearman et al. (Figure 4C,D). miR-27a-3p and miR-339-3p were also selected using the clinical range proposed by Shmilovich et al. (Figure S2C,D).

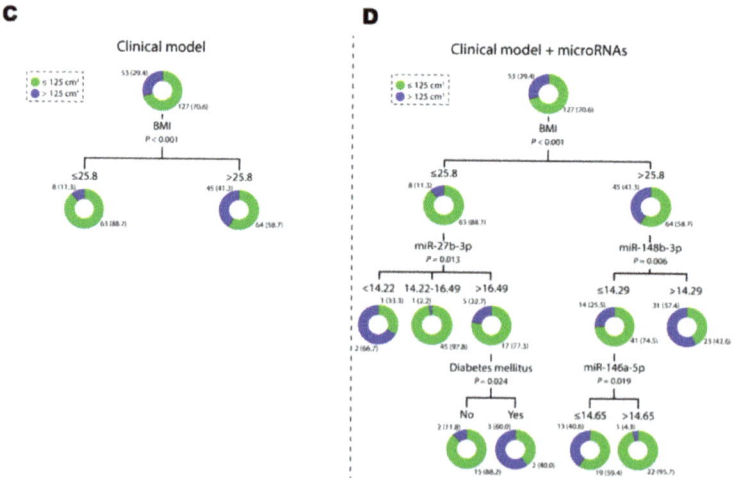

Figure 4. Plasma microRNAs (miRNAs) as biomarkers of epicardial fat volume, according to the cutoff values proposed by Spearman et al. [15]. (**A**) Area under the ROC curve (AUC) for each individual miRNAs and for combinations of miRNAs in pairs or families. (**B**) Performance of plasma miRNAs as biomarkers. (**C,D**) Decision trees calculated by Chi-squared Automatic Interaction Detector (CHAID) algorithm. The following variables were included in the clinical model: age, sex, body mass index and diabetes mellitus. MicroRNA levels were $\log_2$-transformed. For logistic regression models, data are presented as an odds ratio (OR) and 95% confidence intervals (CI). For discrimination analysis, data are presented as the AUC and 95% CI. For reclassification analysis, data are presented as the Integrated Discrimination Improvement (IDI) index and Net Reclassification Improvement (NRI) index and their respective 95% CI. For decision trees, data are shown as frequency (percentage) of patients in each study group.

4. Discussion

Our study provides the first insight into the value of the circulating miRNA signature as a source of clinical indicators for epicardial fat assessment.

First, we showed that patients with high EFV had higher plasma levels of miR-15b-3p, miR-22-3p, miR-148a-3p, miR-148b-3p and miR-590-5p. Plasma miR-15b-3p, miR-22-3p, miR-148a-3p and miR-148b-3p were also directly correlated with EFV. Importantly, these miRNAs were associated with EFV even after extensive adjustment for demographic, anthropometric and clinical variables, including medication use. The results support the previously suggested link between circulating miRNAs and different fat depots [29–34]. Indeed, we have recently demonstrated that serum levels of the cardiomyocyte-enriched miR-1 and miR-133a-3p are positively correlated with myocardial steatosis in type 2 diabetes patients [35]. We then evaluated the performance of plasma miRNAs as biomarkers of EFV and EFVi. The expression of miRNAs, individually, pairwise, or in families, showed modest discrimination values for all EFV and EFVi cutoffs. The substantial overlap in plasma miRNA levels between patients with high or low levels of epicardial fat suggests that miRNAs should not be used alone to predict EFV. Conversely, the comparison of ROC curves showed that different combinations of miR-27a-3p, miR-146a-5p, miR-148b-3p and miR-152-3p improved the discrimination ability over a clinical model that included significant predictors of EFV: age, sex, BMI and diabetes mellitus. The same miRNAs correctly reclassify patients misclassified by the clinical model alone. Decision tree models supported these findings. As expected, BMI was the most powerful predictor for both EFV and EFVi in those decision trees when considering clinical variables. The inclusion of plasma miRNAs in the decision tree models yielded more specific patient subgroups. These results were observed using three independent EFV cutoffs: EFV tertiles in our study population, the EFV clinical range proposed by Spearman et al. [15] and the EFVi clinical range proposed by Shmilovich et al. [21].

According to our findings, the addition of certain miRNA signatures to clinical variables may help classify patients by their EFV. It seems that the ideal scenario for miRNA testing is based on the concept of several miRNAs-one disease contrary to the one miRNA-one disease concept, at least for EAT assessment. Therefore, the use of miRNA signatures may provide more comprehensive information for a clinical decision than the analysis of individual miRNAs. Additionally, our results suggest a potential of circulating miRNAs as biomarkers of EFV in specific patient subpopulations. These results are consistent with a new strategy that recommends the clinical application of biomarkers in individuals or subgroups of individuals as an alternative to the classical one size fits all. Overall, this study provides useful hypothesis-generating data. Using signatures of miRNAs is a promising strategy to identify biomarkers for EFV or EFVi, and subsequently, cardiometabolic disease. Because different pharmacological interventions and lifestyle changes have been proposed to treat epicardial fat accumulation [36,37], our results may have a clinical impact. The quantification of EFV is important in stratifying patients according to their cardiometabolic risk profile and evaluating the effect of treatments. However, imaging techniques are limited by methodology and operating expenses. In this context, miRNA-based tests have emerged as a cost-effective alternative for risk assessment and disease monitoring [38]. Therefore, the incorporation of a diagnostic assessment tool that combines information from clinical variables and plasma miRNA signatures into clinical workflows could provide substantial health and economic benefits in the management of cardiometabolic disease (e.g., as gatekeeper for the inclusion or exclusion of patients in subsequent imaging studies).

Epicardial fat is a source of signaling molecules that can modulate the structure and function of adjacent tissues, i.e., myocardium and vasculature. The secretion of pro-inflammatory adipocytokines from EAT into the circulatory system may also affect the systemic inflammatory state [39]. Extracellular miRNAs have been proposed to function as paracrine and endocrine signals [40,41]. Here, we have demonstrated that our miRNAs are secreted from human EAT explants and are presented in the circulation. Although the understanding of circulating ncRNA biology is still at an early stage [42], it is possible to speculate about the role of miRNAs in the cross-talk between EAT and target tissues. Indeed, miRNAs secreted from fat tissue may be novel adipokines that can regulate metabolism in distant tissues [34,43]. Previous findings are consistent with this hypothesis. miR-27a derived from adipocytes of high-fat diet mice induced insulin resistance in skeletal muscle cells, which suggests that this miRNA mediates cross-talk between adipose tissue and skeletal muscle [44]. Exosomes derived from miR-146a-modified adipose-derived stem cells attenuated myocardial damage in an acute myocardial infarction model in rats [45]. Thus, the miRNAs identified in this study may participate in regulating molecular pathways implicated in cardiometabolic physiology and pathology. Further investigation to determine the mechanisms are warranted, with a special focus on the precise role of plasma miRNAs in intercellular communication.

The strengths of this study include the use of CCTA to quantify epicardial fat, an accurate imaging method widely used in clinical studies [46], and the complete volumetric analysis of epicardial fat instead of using markers such as linear thickness. The use of plasma miRNAs as potential biomarkers was explored using three distinct classifications for epicardial fat burden, including quantitative methods proposed for standardization. In addition, decision tree models were incorporated in the evaluation of plasma miRNAs as indicators. However, the results of our study should be interpreted with respect to the study design and its limitations. First, the study population was a heterogeneous group of patients referred for CCTA. Although these patients represented a group at high cardiometabolic risk, the application of the results to other populations is limited. The results require further corroboration in a real-world setting. Nonetheless, our intention was to test the potential of using circulating miRNAs as biomarkers of epicardial fat content. Second, the classification used for the evaluation of miRNAs as biomarkers was arbitrary: EFV tertiles. As stated above, the cutoffs proposed by the bibliography have been reported as clinically relevant. However, they have not been widely accepted by clinical practice. Therefore, patients were divided into two categories: first and second EFV tertiles (low-medium epicardial fat burden) vs. third EFV tertile (high epicardial fat burden). Third, only 12 of all the candidates initially identified in the screen were further validated in the patient population. Other miRNAs may be potential biomarkers. Fourth, although EAT has unique metabolic properties and is associated with cardiovascular risk independent of other indicators of adiposity [14], it remains possible that other visceral fat depots may be confounding factors. Fifth, we cannot exclude the impact caused by physiological and pathological conditions that were not recorded in the plasma miRNA profile [47].

In any case, our results established the strength of plasma miRNAs as biomarkers for the evaluation of EFV. This investigation provides a rationale for larger and multicentric studies focused on the use of miRNAs in the routine quantification of epicardial fat burden.

Supplementary Materials: The following are available online at http://www.mdpi.com/2077-0383/8/6/780/s1: Table S1: Characteristics of the study population (Screening), Table S2: Plasma microRNA screening, Table S3: microRNA candidates, Table S4: Correlations between epicardial fat volume and plasma microRNAs, Figure S1: Calibration plots (with internal validation), Figure S2: Plasma microRNAs as biomarkers of epicardial fat volume-indexed (EFVi), according to the cutoff proposed by Shmilovich et al.

Author Contributions: Conceptualization, D.d.G.-C., D.V., F.C. and V.L.-C.; methodology, D.d.G.-C., P.M.-C., À.V., A.F.-G., L.N., O.B., J.S.V., R.L. and N.P.; software, P.M.-C. and A.F-G.; investigation, D.d.G.-C., D.V., P.M.-C., À.V., A.F.-G., L.N., J.S.V., R.L., N.P., S.B. and J.L.S.-Q.; resources, D.V., R.L., S.B., J.L.S.-Q. and F.C.; writing—original draft preparation, D.d.G.-C. and D.V.; writing—review and editing, P.M.-C., A.F.-G., S.B., J.L.S.-Q., V.L.-C. and F.C.; supervision, D.d.G.-C. and V.L.-C.; project administration, D.d.G.-C. and V.L.-C.; funding acquisition, D.d.G.-C., S.B., J.L.S.-Q., V.L.-C. and F.C.

Funding: D.d.G.-C. was a recipient of a Juan de la Cierva-Incorporación grant from the Ministerio de Economía y Competitividad (IJCI-2016-29393). O.B. (Project 201521-10) and N.P. (Project 201716) were recipients of Fundació Marató TV3. S.B. and J.L.S.-Q. (2017-SGR-1149) and D.d.G.-C., L.N., À.V., D.V., R.L. and V.L.-C. (2017-SGR-946) are members of Quality Research Groups from Generalitat de Catalunya. S.B., J.L.S.-Q., N.P., V.L.-C. and D.d.G.-C. are members of the Group of Vascular Biology of the Spanish Society of Atherosclerosis (SEA). This work was funded by FIS PI14/01729 (to V.L.-C.), FIS PI16/00471 (to J.L.S.-Q.) & FIS PI18/01584 (to V.L.-C.) grants from Instituto Salud Carlos III, co-financed by the European Fund for Regional Development (EFRD) and by Project 201521-10 from Fundació MARATÓ TV3 (to V.L.-C.). CIBERCV (CB16/11/00403 to V.L.-C. and D.d.G.-C. and CB16/11/00276 to A.F.-G.) and CIBERDEM (CB07/08/0016 to J.L.S.-Q.) are projects from Instituto de Salud Carlos III.

Acknowledgments: The authors thank the Cardiac Imaging Unit and Cardiac Surgery Service personnel from the Hospital de la Santa Creu i Sant Pau (Barcelona, Spain) for their excellent work.

Conflicts of Interest: The authors declare no conflict of interest.

References

1. Mendell, J.T.; Olson, E.N. MicroRNAs in stress signaling and human disease. *Cell* **2012**, *148*, 1172–1187. [CrossRef]
2. Mitchell, P.S.; Parkin, R.K.; Kroh, E.M.; Fritz, B.R.; Wyman, S.K.; Pogosova-Agadjanyan, E.L.; Peterson, A.; Noteboom, J.; O'Briant, K.C.; Allen, A.; et al. Circulating microRNAs as stable blood-based markers for cancer detection. *Proc. Natl. Acad. Sci. USA* **2008**, *105*, 10513–10518. [CrossRef]
3. De Gonzalo-Calvo, D.; Vea, A.; Bar, C.; Fiedler, J.; Couch, L.S.; Brotons, C.; Llorente-Cortes, V.; Thum, T. Circulating non-coding RNAs in biomarker-guided cardiovascular therapy: A novel tool for personalized medicine? *Eur. Heart J.* **2019**, *40*, 1643–1650. [CrossRef] [PubMed]
4. Bianchi, F.; Nicassio, F.; Marzi, M.; Belloni, E.; Dall'olio, V.; Bernard, L.; Pelosi, G.; Maisonneuve, P.; Veronesi, G.; Di Fiore, P.P. A serum circulating miRNA diagnostic test to identify asymptomatic high-risk individuals with early stage lung cancer. *EMBO Mol. Med.* **2011**, *3*, 495–503. [CrossRef]
5. Ralfkiaer, U.; Hagedorn, P.H.; Bangsgaard, N.; Lovendorf, M.B.; Ahler, C.B.; Svensson, L.; Kopp, K.L.; Vennegaard, M.T.; Lauenborg, B.; Zibert, J.R.; et al. Diagnostic microRNA profiling in cutaneous T-cell lymphoma (CTCL). *Blood* **2011**, *118*, 5891–5900. [CrossRef]
6. De Gonzalo-Calvo, D.; Iglesias-Gutierrez, E.; Llorente-Cortes, V. Epigenetic Biomarkers and Cardiovascular Disease: Circulating MicroRNAs. *Rev. Esp. Cardiol.* **2017**, *70*, 763–769. [CrossRef] [PubMed]
7. Guay, C.; Regazzi, R. Circulating microRNAs as novel biomarkers for diabetes mellitus. *Nat. Rev. Endocrinol.* **2013**, *9*, 513–521. [CrossRef] [PubMed]
8. Iacobellis, G. Local and systemic effects of the multifaceted epicardial adipose tissue depot. *Nat. Rev. Endocrinol.* **2015**, *11*, 363–371. [CrossRef] [PubMed]
9. Packer, M. The epicardial adipose inflammatory triad: Coronary atherosclerosis, atrial fibrillation, and heart failure with a preserved ejection fraction. *Eur. J. Heart Fail.* **2018**, *20*, 1567–1569. [CrossRef]
10. Ansaldo, A.M.; Montecucco, F.; Sahebkar, A.; Dallegri, F.; Carbone, F. Epicardial adipose tissue and cardiovascular diseases. *Int. J. Cardiol.* **2019**, *278*, 254–260. [CrossRef]
11. Blumensatt, M.; Fahlbusch, P.; Hilgers, R.; Bekaert, M.; Herzfeld de Wiza, D.; Akhyari, P.; Ruige, J.B.; Ouwens, D.M. Secretory products from epicardial adipose tissue from patients with type 2 diabetes impair mitochondrial beta-oxidation in cardiomyocytes via activation of the cardiac renin-angiotensin system and induction of miR-208a. *Basic Res. Cardiol.* **2017**, *112*, 2. [CrossRef]
12. Mancio, J.; Azevedo, D.; Saraiva, F.; Azevedo, A.I.; Pires-Morais, G.; Leite-Moreira, A.; Falcao-Pires, I.; Lunet, N.; Bettencourt, N. Epicardial adipose tissue volume assessed by computed tomography and coronary artery disease: A systematic review and meta-analysis. *Eur. Heart J. Cardiovasc. Imaging* **2018**, *19*, 490–497. [CrossRef] [PubMed]
13. Nyman, K.; Graner, M.; Pentikainen, M.O.; Lundbom, J.; Hakkarainen, A.; Siren, R.; Nieminen, M.S.; Taskinen, M.R.; Lundbom, N.; Lauerma, K. Cardiac steatosis and left ventricular function in men with metabolic syndrome. *J. Cardiovasc. Magn. Reson.* **2013**, *15*, 103. [CrossRef]
14. Bos, D.; Vernooij, M.W.; Shahzad, R.; Kavousi, M.; Hofman, A.; van Walsum, T.; Deckers, J.W.; Ikram, M.A.; Heeringa, J.; Franco, O.H.; et al. Epicardial Fat Volume and the Risk of Atrial Fibrillation in the General Population Free of Cardiovascular Disease. *JACC Cardiovasc. Imaging* **2017**, *10*, 1405–1407. [CrossRef]
15. Spearman, J.V.; Renker, M.; Schoepf, U.J.; Krazinski, A.W.; Herbert, T.L.; De Cecco, C.N.; Nietert, P.J.; Meinel, F.G. Prognostic value of epicardial fat volume measurements by computed tomography: A systematic review of the literature. *Eur. Radiol.* **2015**, *25*, 3372–3381. [CrossRef] [PubMed]
16. Pierdomenico, S.D.; Pierdomenico, A.M.; Cuccurullo, F.; Iacobellis, G. Meta-analysis of the relation of echocardiographic epicardial adipose tissue thickness and the metabolic syndrome. *Am. J. Cardiol.* **2013**, *111*, 73–78. [CrossRef]
17. Beltowski, J. Epicardial adipose tissue: The new target for statin therapy. *Int. J. Cardiol.* **2019**, *274*, 353–354. [CrossRef]

18. Iacobellis, G.; Mohseni, M.; Bianco, S.D.; Banga, P.K. Liraglutide causes large and rapid epicardial fat reduction. *Obesity* **2017**, *25*, 311–316. [CrossRef] [PubMed]
19. De Gonzalo-Calvo, D.; Vilades, D.; Nasarre, L.; Carreras, F.; Leta, R.; Garcia-Moll, X.; Llorente-Cortes, V. Circulating levels of soluble low-density lipoprotein receptor-related protein 1 (sLRP1) as novel biomarker of epicardial adipose tissue. *Int. J. Cardiol.* **2016**, *223*, 371–373. [CrossRef]
20. Gonzalo-Calvo, D.; Colom, C.; Vilades, D.; Rivas-Urbina, A.; Moustafa, A.H.; Perez-Cuellar, M.; Sanchez-Quesada, J.L.; Perez, A.; Llorente-Cortes, V. Soluble LRP1 is an independent biomarker of epicardial fat volume in patients with type 1 diabetes mellitus. *Sci. Rep.* **2018**, *8*, 1054. [CrossRef]
21. Shmilovich, H.; Dey, D.; Cheng, V.Y.; Rajani, R.; Nakazato, R.; Otaki, Y.; Nakanishi, R.; Slomka, P.J.; Thomson, L.E.; Hayes, S.W.; et al. Threshold for the upper normal limit of indexed epicardial fat volume: Derivation in a healthy population and validation in an outcome-based study. *Am. J. Cardiol.* **2011**, *108*, 1680–1685. [CrossRef] [PubMed]
22. Tuck, M.K.; Chan, D.W.; Chia, D.; Godwin, A.K.; Grizzle, W.E.; Krueger, K.E.; Rom, W.; Sanda, M.; Sorbara, L.; Stass, S.; et al. Standard operating procedures for serum and plasma collection: early detection research network consensus statement standard operating procedure integration working group. *J. Proteome Res.* **2009**, *8*, 113–117. [CrossRef] [PubMed]
23. Mestdagh, P.; Hartmann, N.; Baeriswyl, L.; Andreasen, D.; Bernard, N.; Chen, C.; Cheo, D.; D'Andrade, P.; DeMayo, M.; Dennis, L.; et al. Evaluation of quantitative miRNA expression platforms in the microRNA quality control (miRQC) study. *Nat. Methods* **2014**, *11*, 809–815. [CrossRef] [PubMed]
24. Metsalu, T.; Vilo, J. ClustVis: A web tool for visualizing clustering of multivariate data using Principal Component Analysis and heatmap. *Nucleic Acids Res.* **2015**, *43*, W566–W570. [CrossRef]
25. DeLong, E.R.; DeLong, D.M.; Clarke-Pearson, D.L. Comparing the areas under two or more correlated receiver operating characteristic curves: A nonparametric approach. *Biometrics* **1988**, *44*, 837–845. [CrossRef]
26. Pencina, M.J.; D'Agostino, R.B., Sr.; Steyerberg, E.W. Extensions of net reclassification improvement calculations to measure usefulness of new biomarkers. *Stat. Med.* **2011**, *30*, 11–21. [CrossRef] [PubMed]
27. Harrell, F.E. *Regression Modeling Strategies. Springer Series in Statistics*; Springer: Cham, Germany; New York, NY, USA, 2015.
28. Kass, G. An exploratory technique for investigating large quantities of categorical data. *Appl. Stat.* **1980**, *29*, 119–127. [CrossRef]
29. Chen, Y.; Buyel, J.J.; Hanssen, M.J.; Siegel, F.; Pan, R.; Naumann, J.; Schell, M.; van der Lans, A.; Schlein, C.; Froehlich, H.; et al. Exosomal microRNA miR-92a concentration in serum reflects human brown fat activity. *Nat. Commun.* **2016**, *7*, 11420. [CrossRef]
30. Cui, X.; You, L.; Zhu, L.; Wang, X.; Zhou, Y.; Li, Y.; Wen, J.; Xia, Y.; Wang, X.; Ji, C.; et al. Change in circulating microRNA profile of obese children indicates future risk of adult diabetes. *Metabolism* **2018**, *78*, 95–105. [CrossRef]
31. Heneghan, H.M.; Miller, N.; McAnena, O.J.; O'Brien, T.; Kerin, M.J. Differential miRNA expression in omental adipose tissue and in the circulation of obese patients identifies novel metabolic biomarkers. *J. Clin. Endocrinol. Metab.* **2011**, *96*, E846–E850. [CrossRef]
32. Pek, S.L.; Sum, C.F.; Lin, M.X.; Cheng, A.K.; Wong, M.T.; Lim, S.C.; Tavintharan, S. Circulating and visceral adipose miR-100 is down-regulated in patients with obesity and Type 2 diabetes. *Mol. Cell Endocrinol.* **2016**, *427*, 112–123. [CrossRef] [PubMed]
33. Prats-Puig, A.; Ortega, F.J.; Mercader, J.M.; Moreno-Navarrete, J.M.; Moreno, M.; Bonet, N.; Ricart, W.; Lopez-Bermejo, A.; Fernandez-Real, J.M. Changes in circulating microRNAs are associated with childhood obesity. *J. Clin. Endocrinol. Metab.* **2013**, *98*, E1655–E1660. [CrossRef] [PubMed]
34. Thomou, T.; Mori, M.A.; Dreyfuss, J.M.; Konishi, M.; Sakaguchi, M.; Wolfrum, C.; Rao, T.N.; Winnay, J.N.; Garcia-Martin, R.; Grinspoon, S.K.; et al. Adipose-derived circulating miRNAs regulate gene expression in other tissues. *Nature* **2017**, *542*, 450–455. [CrossRef] [PubMed]
35. De Gonzalo-Calvo, D.; van der Meer, R.W.; Rijzewijk, L.J.; Smit, J.W.; Revuelta-Lopez, E.; Nasarre, L.; Escola-Gil, J.C.; Lamb, H.J.; Llorente-Cortes, V. Serum microRNA-1 and microRNA-133a levels reflect myocardial steatosis in uncomplicated type 2 diabetes. *Sci. Rep.* **2017**, *7*, 47. [CrossRef]
36. Nakazato, R.; Rajani, R.; Cheng, V.Y.; Shmilovich, H.; Nakanishi, R.; Otaki, Y.; Gransar, H.; Slomka, P.J.; Hayes, S.W.; Thomson, L.E.; et al. Weight change modulates epicardial fat burden: A 4-year serial study with non-contrast computed tomography. *Atherosclerosis* **2012**, *220*, 139–144. [CrossRef]

37. Parisi, V.; Petraglia, L.; D'Esposito, V.; Cabaro, S.; Rengo, G.; Caruso, A.; Grimaldi, M.G.; Baldascino, F.; De Bellis, A.; Vitale, D.; et al. Statin therapy modulates thickness and inflammatory profile of human epicardial adipose tissue. *Int. J. Cardiol.* **2019**, *274*, 326–330. [CrossRef]
38. Walter, E.; Dellago, H.; Grillari, J.; Dimai, H.P.; Hackl, M. Cost-utility analysis of fracture risk assessment using microRNAs compared with standard tools and no monitoring in the Austrian female population. *Bone* **2018**, *108*, 44–54. [CrossRef]
39. Packer, M. Epicardial Adipose Tissue May Mediate Deleterious Effects of Obesity and Inflammation on the Myocardium. *J. Am. Coll. Cardiol.* **2018**, *71*, 2360–2372. [CrossRef] [PubMed]
40. Bang, C.; Batkai, S.; Dangwal, S.; Gupta, S.K.; Foinquinos, A.; Holzmann, A.; Just, A.; Remke, J.; Zimmer, K.; Zeug, A.; et al. Cardiac fibroblast-derived microRNA passenger strand-enriched exosomes mediate cardiomyocyte hypertrophy. *J. Clin. Invest.* **2014**, *124*, 2136–2146. [CrossRef] [PubMed]
41. Shan, Z.; Qin, S.; Li, W.; Wu, W.; Yang, J.; Chu, M.; Li, X.; Huo, Y.; Schaer, G.L.; Wang, S.; et al. An Endocrine Genetic Signal Between Blood Cells and Vascular Smooth Muscle Cells: Role of MicroRNA-223 in Smooth Muscle Function and Atherogenesis. *J. Am. Coll. Cardiol.* **2015**, *65*, 2526–2537. [CrossRef]
42. Bär, C.; Thum, T.; de Gonzalo-Calvo, D. Circulating miRNAs as mediators in cell-to-cell communication. *Epigenomics* **2019**, *11*, 111–113. [CrossRef] [PubMed]
43. Ying, W.; Riopel, M.; Bandyopadhyay, G.; Dong, Y.; Birmingham, A.; Seo, J.B.; Ofrecio, J.M.; Wollam, J.; Hernandez-Carretero, A.; Fu, W.; et al. Adipose Tissue Macrophage-Derived Exosomal miRNAs Can Modulate In Vivo and In Vitro Insulin Sensitivity. *Cell* **2017**, *171*, 372–384. [CrossRef] [PubMed]
44. Yu, Y.; Du, H.; Wei, S.; Feng, L.; Li, J.; Yao, F.; Zhang, M.; Hatch, G.M.; Chen, L. Adipocyte-Derived Exosomal MiR-27a Induces Insulin Resistance in Skeletal Muscle Through Repression of PPARgamma. *Theranostics* **2018**, *8*, 2171–2188. [CrossRef] [PubMed]
45. Pan, J.; Alimujiang, M.; Chen, Q.; Shi, H.; Luo, X. Exosomes derived from miR-146a-modified adipose-derived stem cells attenuate acute myocardial infarction-induced myocardial damage via downregulation of early growth response factor 1. *J. Cell. Biochem.* **2018**, *120*, 4434–4443. [CrossRef] [PubMed]
46. Raggi, P. Epicardial adipose tissue as a marker of coronary artery disease risk. *J. Am. Coll. Cardiol.* **2013**, *61*, 1396–1397. [CrossRef]
47. De Gonzalo-Calvo, D.; Davalos, A.; Fernandez-Sanjurjo, M.; Amado-Rodriguez, L.; Diaz-Coto, S.; Tomas-Zapico, C.; Montero, A.; Garcia-Gonzalez, A.; Llorente-Cortes, V.; Heras, M.E.; et al. Circulating microRNAs as emerging cardiac biomarkers responsive to acute exercise. *Int. J. Cardiol.* **2018**, *264*, 130–136. [CrossRef]

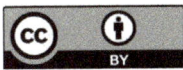

© 2019 by the authors. Licensee MDPI, Basel, Switzerland. This article is an open access article distributed under the terms and conditions of the Creative Commons Attribution (CC BY) license (http://creativecommons.org/licenses/by/4.0/).

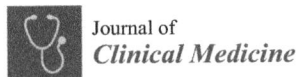

Article

CA125 as a Marker of Heart Failure in the Older Women: A Population-Based Analysis

Weronika Bulska-Będkowska [1,*], Elżbieta Chełmecka [2], Aleksander J. Owczarek [2], Katarzyna Mizia-Stec [3], Andrzej Witek [4], Aleksandra Szybalska [5], Tomasz Grodzicki [6], Magdalena Olszanecka-Glinianowicz [7] and Jerzy Chudek [1,8]

1. Department of Internal Diseases and Oncological Chemotherapy, School of Medicine in Katowice, Medical University of Silesia, 40-027 Katowice, Poland; chj@poczta.fm
2. Department of Statistics, Department of Instrumental Analysis, School of Pharmacy and Laboratory Medicine in Sosnowiec, Medical University of Silesia, 41-200 Sosnowiec, Poland; echelmecka@sum.edu.pl (E.C.); aowczarek@paintbox.com.pl (A.J.O.)
3. First Department of Cardiology, School of Medicine in Katowice, Medical University of Silesia, 40-635 Katowice, Poland; kmizia@op.pl
4. Department of Gynecology and Obstetrics, School of Medicine in Katowice, Medical University of Silesia, 40-752 Katowice, Poland; awitek@sum.edu.pl
5. International Institute of Molecular and Cell Biology, Warsaw 02-109, Poland; a.szybalska@iimcb.gov.pl
6. Department of Internal Medicine and Gerontology, Jagiellonian University Medical College, 31-531 Cracow, Poland; tomekg@su.krakow.pl
7. Health Promotion and Obesity Management Unit, Department of Pathophysiology, School of Medicine in Katowice, Medical University of Silesia, 40-752 Katowice, Poland; magols@esculap.pl
8. Pathophysiology Unit, Department of Pathophysiology, School of Medicine in Katowice, Medical University of Silesia, 40-752 Katowice, Poland
* Correspondence: lek.weronikabulska@gmail.com; Tel.: +48-322-526-091

Received: 17 February 2019; Accepted: 30 April 2019; Published: 3 May 2019

Abstract: (1) Background: Cancer antigen 125 (CA125) is a glycoprotein that is expressed by tissue derived from coelomic epithelium in the pleura, peritoneum, pericardium. It has been shown that CA125 concentrations are correlated with NT-proBNP in older people with congestive heart failure (HF). We conducted a study on the association between concentrations of CA125 and NT-proBNP in a population-based cohort of older Polish women. (2) Methods: The current research is sub-study of a large, cross-sectional research project (PolSenior). The study group consisted of 1565 Caucasian women aged 65–102 years. To assess the relationship between CA125 and other variables a stepwise backward multivariate normal and skew-t regression analyses were performed. (3) Results: The median of CA125 concentration was 13.0 U/mL and values over the upper normal range limit (35 U/mL) were observed in 5.1% ($n = 79$) of the study cohort. The concentration of CA125 was positively related to age, hospitalization for HF and history of atrial fibrillation and chronic obstructive pulmonary disease, levels of NT-proBNP, IL-6, hs-CRP and triglycerides. We found in the multivariate analyses, that increased CA125 levels were independently associated with $\log_{10}$ (IL-6) ($\beta = 11.022$), history of hospitalization for HF ($\beta = 4.619$), $\log_{10}$ (NT-proBNP) ($\beta = 4.416$) and age ($\beta = 3.93$ for 10 years). (4) Conclusions: Despite the association between CA125 and NT-proBNP, the usefulness of CA125 for the detection of HF in older women is limited by factors such as inflammatory status and age.

Keywords: carbohydrate antigen-125; heart failure; inflammatory marker; older women

1. Introduction

Cancer antigen 125 (CA125) is a glycoprotein that is expressed by tissue derived from coelomic epithelium and has a molecular weight estimated to range from 110 to more than 2000 kD [1].

The CA125 serum level has been shown to be increased in women with ovarian cancer and less often in breast [2], lung [3] and gastrointestinal cancers [4]. However, it is not a screening test for malignancies as it may also be elevated in a variety of benign conditions (such as pregnancy, endometriosis, uterine leiomyomata, pelvic inflammatory disease, cirrhosis, peritonitis, pleuritis, pancreatitis, and tuberculosis) [5]. Several recent studies have shown that serum CA125 levels are also elevated in heart failure (HF), atrial fibrillation (AF), and ischemic heart disease [6–8]. Only a few studies that have assessed the CA125 levels in selected groups of patients after cardiac surgery (cardiac transplantation, transcatheter aortic valve implantation) have been published so far [9,10]. It seems that neurohormonal and inflammatory activation, as well as increased central venous volume and congestion, are the factors that increase the level of CA125 [11,12].

It is worth noting that the serum concentration of CA125 was associated with the severity of clinical conditions and poor short-term prognosis in patients with cardiovascular disease [13]. Ma et al. [14] showed a significant correlation between serum concentration of CA125 and the clinical status of patients aged 85 and older with congestive HF as well as the usefulness of CA125 as a prognostic factor of death and rehospitalization. Moreover, Yucel et al. [15] reported that the serum concentration of CA125 may be used to predict AF in patients with systolic HF. In addition, a significant correlation between CA125 and NT-proBNP levels was found in Chinese older patients only with congestive HF. Moreover, it should be noted that this group included only less than 16% of women [14]. It is well known that the clinical course of cardiovascular diseases differs between men and women [16], thus the separate analysis of biomarkers and risk factors in men and women seems reasonable. Furthermore, the impact of chronic diseases and inflammatory markers on CA125 levels in a population-based cohort has not been studied, yet.

The main aim of this study was to assess the relationships between the serum concentration of CA125 and NT-proBNP in a population-based cohort of older Polish women.

2. Materials and Methods

The current study was part of the PolSenior project, which was a large, cross-sectional, multicenter, interdisciplinary research project performed among the older Polish adult population (4979 respondents aged 65 and older, including 2412 women). Only women aged 65 and older with an assessed serum level of CA125 (n = 1951) were included in this sub-study. The exclusion criteria were as follow: (1) history of neoplastic disease (n = 125), (2) hepatitis B virus or hepatitis C virus infection (n = 52), (3) lack of information about the cardiovascular disease (n = 158), (4) lack of NT-pro BNP assessment (n = 51). Finally, the study group consisted of 1565 older Polish women (Figure A1).

The PolSenior project consisted of three stages: (1) conducting a health and socioeconomic survey by nurses trained for this purpose nurses that included comprehensive geriatric assessment, (2) measurements of body mass, height, waist circumference and blood pressure, (3) the collection of blood and urine samples.

The study was approved by the Bioethics Committee of the Medical University of Silesia in Katowice (KNW/0022/KB1/38/II/08/10; KNW-6501-38/I/08). Before enrollment, written and informed consent was obtained from all subjects or their caregivers.

2.1. Biochemical Measurements

Serum concentrations of CA125 and NT-proBNP were measured by the electrochemiluminescence method (ECLIA) using an Elecsys 2010 (CA125) and Cobas E411 (NT-proBNP) analyzers (Roche Diagnostics GmbH, Mannheim, Germany), with an intermediate precision of <4.2%, and 4.6%, respectively. The sensitivity of the method for CA125 was 0.6 U/mL. According to the current guidelines, a value of NT-proBNP below 125 pg/mL was considered as the exclusion criteria for the diagnosis of heart failure [17].

Serum levels of C-reactive protein were assessed by the latex-enhanced immunoturbidimetric assay using an automated system (Modular PPE, Roche Diagnostics GmbH, Mannheim, Germany) with a limit of quantification (LoQ) of 0.11 mg/L and intermediate precision of <5.7%. The biochemical tests such as total cholesterol, high-density lipoprotein (HDL), low-density lipoprotein (LDL), triglycerides, creatinine (Jaffa method) were also measured using an automated system (Modular PPE) with intermediate precisions of <1.7%, <1.3%, 1.2%, <1.8% and <2.3%, respectively.

Urinalysis by the Combur-Test (Roche Diagnostics, Mannheim, Germany) was performed in all urine samples using the Miditron M system (Roche Diagnostics, Mannheim, Germany). Albuminuria was diagnosed if the albumin concentration in the urine was >30 mg/L. If albuminuria was not detected in the urine strip test, the albumin concentration was measured by the immunoturbidimetric method (Roche Diagnostics, Mannheim Germany) with high sensitivity (LoQ of 3 mg/L).

Plasma interleukin 6 (IL-6) was assessed by ELISA using a kit produced by R and D Systems (Minneapolis, MN, USA) with a LoQ of 0.11 pg/mL and intermediate precision of <6.5%. Serum insulin levels were assessed by the electrochemiluminescence method (ECLIA) using commercially available kits on a Cobas E411 analyzer (Roche Diagnostics GmbH, Mannheim, Germany) with an intermediate precision of <3.8%.

2.2. Data Analysis

Hospitalization for HF and/or myocardial infarction, diagnosis of AF and/or coronary artery disease and/or chronic obstructive pulmonary disease (COPD), currently applied treatment and smoking status were collected from the questionnaire survey.

Diagnosis of diabetes was based on medical history, medication use, and fasting serum glucose above 125 mg/dL. Participants were considered to have hypertension if they had a mean systolic blood pressure (SBP) ≥140 mmHg and/or diastolic blood pressure (DBP) ≥90 mmHg or used antihypertensive medications [18].

The body mass index (BMI) was calculated as the weight (kg) divided by the square of the height (meters).

Estimated glomerular filtration rate (eGFR; mL/min/1.73 m^2) was calculated according to the short MDRD (modification of diet in renal disease) formula.

The albumin-to-creatinine ratio (ACR; mg/g) was calculated as the urine albumin concentration divided by the urine creatinine concentration.

The homeostatic model assessment (HOMA-IR) was used to evaluate insulin resistance (fasting serum insulin (µU/mL) × fasting plasma glucose (mmol/L)/22.5). Insulin resistance was diagnosed if HOMA-IR was 2.5 or higher.

2.3. Statistical Analysis

Statistical analyses were performed using STATISTICA 10.0 PL (TIBCO Software Inc, Palo Alto, CA, USA) and StataSE 12.0 (StataCorp LP, TX, USA). Statistical significance was set at a *p*-value below 0.05. All tests were two-tailed. Nominal and ordinal data were expressed as percentages, while interval data were expressed as a mean value ± standard deviation in the case of a normal distribution, or as median (lower quartile–upper quartile) in the event of data with a skewed or non-normal distribution. To assess the relationship between CA125 and other variables, a stepwise backward multivariate normal and skew-t regression analyses were used, due to the heavily skewed distribution of some variables. The range of serum CA125 concentration was shown with the histogram and was modelled with the kernel density plot with the Epanechnikov kernel function (Figure A2).

3. Results

3.1. Characteristics of the Study Population

Our sub-study consisted of 1565 Polish women aged between 65–102 years. The average age was 78 ± 9 years. Characteristics of the study population according to age, medical conditions, biochemical parameters and medication used are shown in Table 1.

The study cohort included: 1218 (78.2%) women diagnosed with hypertension, 291 (18.6%) with coronary artery disease, 160 (10.2%) previously hospitalized for heart failure, 105 (6.7%) with past myocardial infarction and 297 (19%) with a history of atrial fibrillation.

As a consequence of diagnosed cardiovascular diseases, a large percentage of study participants were taking medications, including angiotensin-converting-enzyme inhibitors (ACE-I) and angiotensin II receptor blockers (ARB) ($n = 764$; 48.8%), β-blockers ($n = 603$; 38.5%), diuretics ($n = 513$; 32.8%), and the mineralocorticoid receptor blocker–spironolactone ($n = 193$; 12.3%). Every fourth woman received lipid-lowering drugs, mostly statins ($n = 382$; 24.4%) and very rarely fibrates ($n = 19$; 1.2%).

Table 1. Characteristics of the study population according to age, medical conditions, biochemical parameters and medication used. Data are provided as mean ± standard deviation (SD), median (1–3 Q) or numbers (percentage).

	All ($n = 1565$)
Age (years)	78 ± 9
65–69 years, n (%)	293 (18.7)
70–74 years, n (%)	321 (20.5)
75–79 years, n (%)	259 (16.5)
80–84 years, n (%)	229 (14.6)
85–90 years, n (%)	233 (14.9)
>90 years, n (%)	230 (14.7)
BMI (kg/m^2)	29.1 ± 5.5
<18.5 kg/m^2, n (%)	16 (1.1)
18.5–24.9 kg/m^2, n (%)	324 (2.2)
25–29.9 kg/m^2, n (%)	527 (36.2)
≥30 kg/m^2, n (%)	590 (40.5)
Current smoker, n (%)	67 (4.3)
Hypertension, n (%)	1218 (78.2)
Coronary artery disease, n (%)	291 (18.6)
Hospitalization for MI, n (%)	105 (6.7)
Hospitalization for HF, n (%)	160 (10.2)
AF, n (%)	297 (19.0)
Diabetes, n (%)	384 (24.5)
COPD, n (%)	249 (15.9)
Glucose, mg/dL	94.5 (85.7–107.1)
Impaired fasting glucose, n (%)	558 (35.6)
HOMA-IR	1.44 (0.74–2.76)
Total cholesterol, mg/dL	211.1 ± 47.2
LDL-cholesterol, mg/dL	124.9 ± 41.3
HDL-cholesterol, mg/dL	52.9 ± 13.8
Triglycerydes, mg/dL	121.5 (93.1–158.9)
eGFR-MDRD short, mL/min/1.73 m^2	73.5 ± 21.1
eGFR < 60 mL/min/1.73 m^2, n (%)	387 (24.7)
ACR	5.56 (2.36–15.75)
ACR ≥ 300, n (%)	39 (2.7)

Table 1. *Cont.*

	All (*n* = 1565)
hs-CRP, mg/dL	2.47 (1.21–4.88)
Il-6, pg/mL	2.2 (1.5–3.7)
NT-proBNP, pg/mL	225 (114–504)
Ca125, U/mL	13.0 (9.7–17.6)
Ca125 > 35 U/mL, *n* (%)	79 (5.1)
β-blockers, *n* (%)	603; 38.5%
ACE-I or ARB, *n* (%)	764 (48.8)
Diuretics, *n* (%)	513 (32.8)
Spironolactone, *n* (%)	193 (12.3)
Statins, *n* (%)	382 (24.4)
Fibrates, *n* (%)	19 (1.2)

Abbreviations: BMI—body mass index, MI—myocardial infarction, HT—heart failure, AF—atrial fibrillation, COPD—chronic obstructive pulmonary disease, HOMAR-IR—homeostatic model assessment, ACR—albumin-to-creatinine ratio, hsCRP—high-sensitivity C-reactive protein, Il-6—interleukin 6, ACE-I—angiotensin-converting-enzyme inhibitor, ARB—angiotensin receptor blockers. Data provided as mean ± standard deviation (SD), median (1–3 Q) or numbers (percentage).

3.2. Serum CA125 Concentration

The median of CA125 serum concentration was 13.0 U/mL (lower and upper quartile: 9.72–17.60, range: 1.1–225.9 U/mL). CA125 levels over the upper normal range limit (35 U/mL) were found in 79 women (5.1%, see Figure A2).

In a univariate analysis serum concentration of CA125 was positively related to age, hospitalization for HF and history of AF and COPD as well as the serum levels of NT-proBNP, IL-6, hsCRP, and triglycerides (Figure 1). The CA125 concentration was inversely related to BMI, the concentration of HDL-cholesterol and eGFR values (Table 2). There was no association between CA125 concentration and the occurrence of diabetes, hypertension, coronary heart disease and history of myocardial infarction as well as used cardiac medication (Table 2).

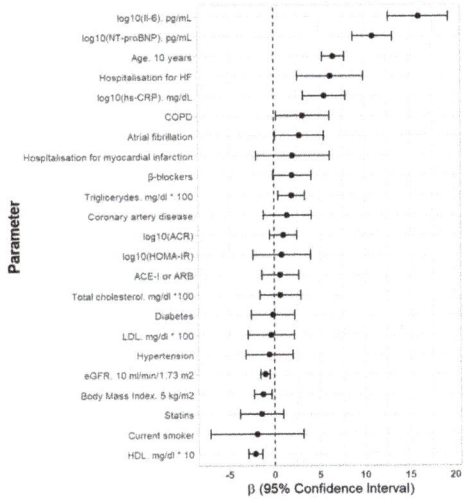

Figure 1. Univariate parameters associated with serum CA125 concentrations in older Polish

women. Abbreviations: Il-6—interleukin 6, HF—heart failure, hs-CRP—high sensitivity C-reactive protein, COPD—chronic obstructive pulmonary disease, ACR—albumin-to-creatinine ratio, HOMAR-IR—homeostatic model assessment, ACE-I—angiotensin-converting-enzyme inhibitor, ARB—angiotensin receptor blockers.

To assess the factors affecting CA125 serum concentration, a multivariate stepwise backward skew-t regression model was used with independent factors selected based on univariate analyses, and the results are shown in Table 2. We found that increased concentration of CA125 was independently associated with $\log_{10}$ (Il-6) ($\beta = 11.022$), history of hospitalization for HF ($\beta = 4.619$), $\log_{10}$ (NT-proBNP) ($\beta = 4.416$) and age ($\beta = 3{,}93$ for 10 years), as shown in Figure 2.

Table 2. Univariate and multivariate, stepwise, backward skew-t regression analyses of factors associated with increased CA125 serum concentrations in older Polish women.

$\log_{10}$ (CA125 U/mL) * 100	Univariate			Multivariate		
	β	95% CI: β	p	β	95% CI: β	p
Age (years)	0.656	0.534–0.777	<0.001	0.393	0.255–0.532	<0.001
BMI (kg/m^2)	−0.260	−0.454–−0.066	<0.01	-	-	-
Current smoker (Yes)	−1.950	−7.107–3.206	0.46	-	-	-
AF (Yes)	2.805	0.081–5.528	<0.05	-	-	-
Coronary artery disease (Yes)	1.438	−1.222–4.098	0.29	-	-	-
Hospitalization for MI (Yes)	2.040	−2.043–6.124	0.33	-	-	-
Hospitalization for HF (Yes)	6.249	2.615–9.882	<0.01	4.619	1.042–8.196	<0.05
Hypertension (Yes)	−0.577	−3.218–2.065	0.67	-	-	-
Diabetes (Yes)	−0.183	−2.603–2.237	0.88	-	-	-
COPD (Yes)	3.173	0.234–6.111	<0.05	2.607	−0.281–5.495	0.08
Total cholesterol (mg/dL) *100	0.636	−1.635–0.291	0.58	-	-	-
LDL-cholesterol (mg/dL) * 100	−0.366	−2.931–2.198	0.78	-	-	-
HDL-cholesterol (mg/dL)	−0.218	−0.945–−0.142	<0.001	-	-	-
Triglycerides (mg/dL) * 100	1.937	0.461–3.413	<0.05	-	-	-
$\log_{10}$ (NT-proBNP (pg/mL))	10.928	8.701–13.156	<0.001	4.416	1.904–6.927	<0.001
eGFR (mL/min/1.73 m^2)	−0.107	−0.158–−0.055	<0.001	-	-	-
$\log_{10}$ (IL-6 (pg/mL))	16.028	12.691–19.365	<0.001	11.022	7.608–14.436	<0.001
$\log_{10}$ (hs-CRP (mg/dL))	5.570	3.255–7.884	<0.001	-	-	-
$\log_{10}$ (HOMA-IR)	0.809	−2.404–4.021	0.62	-	-	-
$\log_{10}$ (ACR)	1.002	−0.533–2.537	0.20	-	-	-
Medication						
β-blockers, n (%)	1.980	−0.138–4.099	0.07	-	-	-
ACE-I or ARB, n (%)	0.654	−1.419–2.727	0.54	-	-	-
Statins, n (%)	−1.436	−3.837–0.966	0.24	-	-	-

Abbreviations: BMI—body mass index, AF—atrial fibrillation, MI—myocardial infarction, HT—heart failure, COPD—chronic obstructive pulmonary disease, IL-6—interleukin 6, hsCRP—high-sensitivity C-reactive protein, HOMAR-IR—homeostatic model assessment, ACR—albumin-to-creatinine ratio, ACE-I—angiotensin-converting-enzyme inhibitor, ARB—angiotensin receptor blockers. * Statistical significance was set at a p-value below 0.05.

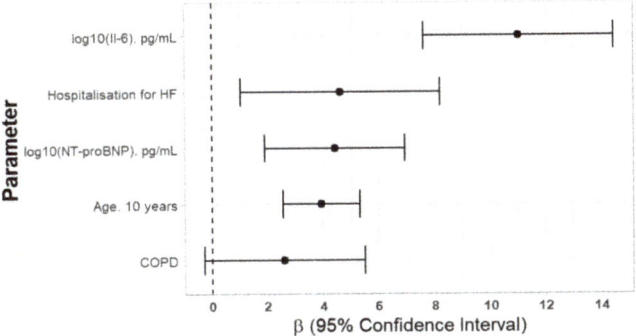

Figure 2. Independent factors affecting serum CA125 concentrations. Abbreviations: Il-6—interleukin 6, HF—heart failure, COPD—chronic obstructive pulmonary disease.

4. Discussion

To the best of our knowledge, the current study was the first to investigate the association between CA125 and NT-proBNP levels in a population-based cohort of older Caucasian women. Ma et al. [14] conducted a similar study, but among Chinese patients hospitalized for chronic HF aged 85 years and older, with the majority of the study group being men (84%). It should be noted that race is an independent factor influencing CA125 levels. Pauler et al. [19] showed that CA125 levels were the highest in Caucasians, lower in Asians and the lowest in African healthy postmenopausal women.

We found that the serum concentration of CA125 was independently associated with NT-proBNP. This association may suggest a similar release mechanism related to an elevation in intracavitary pressures, venous pressure and stress of cardiac walls [20].

Nunez et al. [21] showed that the simultaneous increase in the values of CA125 and NT-proBNP was associated with the highest risk of mortality due to acute HF and that the increase of the value of one marker was also related to the indirect risk. Mendez et al. [22] suggested that the value of CA125 over 60 U/L (higher than the upper range of normal values) may identify patients in chronic HF with poor outcome. However, there are insufficient studies to determine the limit of CA125 value for the assessment of mortality risk in patients with HF. On the basis of our results, the assessment of CA125 usefulness as a marker of HF severity and mortality for HF is not possible. The association between CA125 and NT-proBNP levels is not enough to prove its' usefulness in the work-up of HF. Nevertheless, the findings of other researchers that have shown an association between CA125 and New York Heart Association (NYHA) functional classification scale [13,23–25], ejection fraction of the left ventricle [15,26,27], systolic pulmonary artery pressure [13,15,25,28,29], pulmonary artery wedge pressure [13], right atrial pressure [13], left atrial volume index [30], are interesting and stimulate for further studies.

The obtained results also showed that serum CA125 levels were independently associated with the history of hospitalization for HF and increased levels of IL-6. This is in accordance with studies that have shown that the increased CA125 concentration in HF is associated with mechanical stress and systemic inflammation [31]. In addition, it has been shown that inflammatory cytokines activate CA125 synthesis by the mesothelial cells [32]. In HF, high venous pressure can lead to the congestion and increased hydrostatic pressure on the mesothelium [33], stimulating the release of inflammatory markers such as IL-6 or IL-10, TNF-α [11,12]. We have found a statistical association between CA125 and IL-6, supporting the hypothesis that elevated levels of IL-6 in cardiovascular diseases may play a leading role in the stimulation of CA125-producing cells in a damaged mesothelium. Other studies have also confirmed the association between cytokines and CA125 levels in subjects with HF [12,34].

In the present study, the serum levels of CA125 were positively related to the history of atrial fibrillation (AF), but we did not demonstrate its independent association in a multivariate analysis.

AF was found in up to 30% of subjects with HF [28], therefore we supposed that AF may have a secondary role in the increase of CA125 values. In addition, Sekiguchi et al. [35] revealed that a high CA125 concentration was an independent predictor of new-onset AF in healthy postmenopausal women without HF. It has also been shown that increased levels of cytokines such as IL-2, IL-6, IL-8, TNF-α in subjects with new-onset AF, can stimulate mesothelial cells to produce CA125 [36]. Recently published studies have demonstrated the independent effect of permanent AF on CA125 levels [28]. Despite the observed results in our study of an association between CA125 and IL-6, we could not verify whether CA125 is a predictor of AF in the course of HF.

In addition, we did not find an independent association between the occurrence of coronary heart disease and a history of myocardial infarction and CA125 serum concentration. This is in contrast to the results obtained by Yalta et al. [37], which revealed increased CA125 concentration in patients with acute myocardial infarction within 72 h of the incident. It is possible that the damage to the myocardium caused a decline in myocardial performance with an increase in central venous pressure in some patients and inflammatory response that stimulated mesothelial cells.

We also found an association between the occurrence of chronic obstructive pulmonary disease and CA125 concentration. Other studies have also confirmed a relationship between COPD and CA125 levels [38–40]. Chronic obstructive pulmonary disease is characterized by abnormal enlargement of the right ventricular (RV), leading to heart failure. Yilmez et al. [41] suggested that high CA125 levels were associated with RV failure. The high concentrations of CA125 in COPD are probably caused by increased systolic pulmonary artery pressure, which is considered equal to the RV systolic pressure. However, our data cannot support this observation.

Finally, this study demonstrated the independent association of CA125 concentration with age. Our study showed a positive association between age and the serum levels of CA125. This study was the first one to analyze a large group of Caucasian women with a wide age span (65–102 years). In a previous study, Johnson et al. [42] observed similar results among multi-ethnic women without cardiac disease aged between 55–74 years. Pauler et al. [19] demonstrated the opposite results, where a decrease in CA125 concentrations with aging in postmenopausal women during the 12-year follow-up period. However, the study was carried out among a group of younger and healthy women aged between 40–60 years. In addition, Sikaris et al. [43] described that the CA125 concentration gradually increased after the age of 70 years, both in men and in women.

In summary, our study showed the relationship between CA 125 and NT-proBNP levels. In addition, we observed that increased CA125 levels may be related to numerous factors such as age, hospitalization for HF, history of AF and COPD, as well as increased levels of inflammatory markers (IL-6, hs-CRP). Thus, the clinical usefulness of CA125 as a marker of HF diagnosis and severity is limited. The usefulness of CA125 as a prognostic marker for HF severity and mortality in Caucasian women population requires further study.

This study has some limitations, mostly related to the lack of objective measures of the severity of HF. We did not evaluate echocardiographic metrics as it is difficult to apply in population-based studies performed in the participants' place of living. Hospital discharge cards shown by participants do not exclude the occurrence of compensated HF and past asymptomatic myocardial infarction in some participants. Moreover, CA125 was not assessed in men. This is why the final results cannot be generalized for the whole population aged over 65 years.

The strength of this study was the inclusion of the oldest women representative of the Polish population. The study group included women aged between 65 and 102, which allowed the conclusion that age affects the value of the marker. Moreover, we were the first to examine the association between CA125 and NT-proBNP levels in a large population-based cohort of Caucasian women and assess the factors affecting the circulating CA125 levels.

5. Conclusions

Despite the association between CA125 and NT-proBNP, the usefulness of CA125 for the detection of HF in the older women is limited by factors such as inflammatory status and age.

Author Contributions: Conceptualization, W.B.-B. and J.C.; formal analysis, A.J.O. and E.C.; investigation, A.S., J.C., M.O.-G., T.G.; writing—original draft preparation, W.B.-B. and J.C.; writing—review and editing, W.B.-B. J.C., M.O.-G, K.M.-S., A.S., A.W.; visualization, W.B.-B., J.C., A.J.O.; supervision, J.C.; project administration, A.S.

Funding: This research was funded by Ministry of Science and Higher Education (Poland), No. PBZ-MEIN-9/2/2006.

Conflicts of Interest: The authors declare no conflicts of interest.

Appendix A

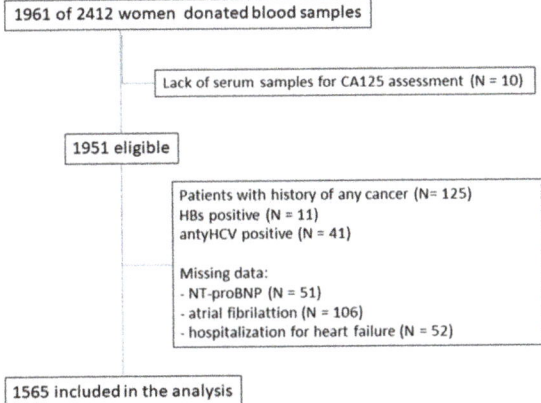

Figure A1. Study flow.

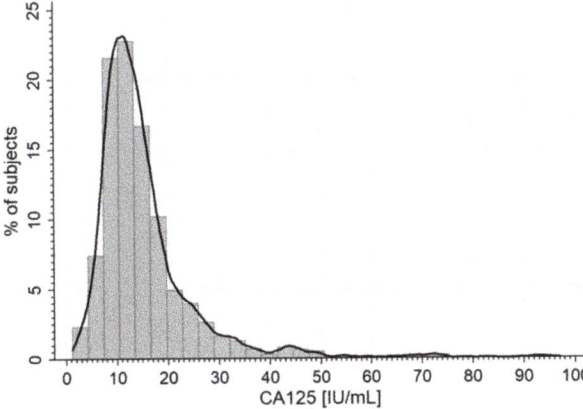

Figure A2. The range of CA125 serum concentration.

References

1. Weiland, F.; Fritz, K.; Oehler, M.K.; Hoffmann, P. Methods for identification of CA125 from ovarian cancer ascites by high resolution mass spectrometry. *Int. J. Mol. Sci.* **2012**, *13*, 9942–9958. [CrossRef] [PubMed]
2. Fang, C.; Cao, Y.; Liu, X.; Zeng, X.-T.; Li, Y. Serum CA125 is a predictive marker for breast cancer outcomes and correlates with molecular subtypes. *Oncotarget* **2017**, *8*, 63963–63970. [CrossRef]

3. Zhu, Y.; Yang, Y.; Wang, Y.; Zhang, L. Role of serum CA125 and CA199 concentration in diagnosis and prognosis evaluation of lung cancer patients. *Int. J. Clin. Exp. Pathol.* **2016**, *9*, 5388–5396.
4. Polat, E.; Duman, U.; Duman, M.; Derya Peker, K.; Akyuz, C.; Fatih Yasar, N.; Uzun, O.; Akbulut, S.; Birol Bostanci, E.; Yol, S. Preoperative serum tumor marker levels in gastric cancer. *Pak. J. Med. Sci.* **2014**, *30*, 145–149.
5. Meden, H.; Fattahi-Meibodi, A. CA 125 in benign gynecological conditions. *Int. J. Biol. Markers.* **1998**, *13*, 231–237. [CrossRef] [PubMed]
6. Li, K.H.C.; Gong, M.; Li, G.; Baranchuk, A.; Liu, T.; Wong, M.C.S.; Jesuthasan, A.; Lai, R.W.C.; Lai, J.C.L.; Lee, A.P.W.; et al. Cancer antigen-125 and outcomes in acute heart failure: A systematic review and meta-analysis. *Heart Asia* **2018**, *10*, e011044. [CrossRef] [PubMed]
7. Cheung, A.; Gong, M.; Bellanti, R.; Ali-Hasan-Al-Saegh, S.; Li, G.; Roig, E.; Núñez, J.; Stamos, T.D.; Yilmaz, M.B.; Hakki, K.; et al. Cancer antigen-125 and risk of atrial fibrillation: A systematic review and meta-analysis. *Heart Asia* **2018**, *10*, e010970. [CrossRef] [PubMed]
8. Li, X.; He, M.; Zhu, J.; Yao, P.; Li, X.; Yuan, J.; Min, X.; Lang, M.; Yang, H.; Hu, F.B.; et al. Higher carbohydrate antigen 125 levels are associated with increased risk of coronary heart disease in elderly chinese: a population-based case-control study. *PLoS ONE* **2013**, *8*, e81328. [CrossRef]
9. Becerra-Muñoz, V.M.; Sobrino-Márquez, J.M.; Rangel-Sousa, D.; Fernández-Cisnal, A.; Lage-Gallé, E.; García-Pinilla, J.M.; Martínez-Martínez, Á.; de Teresa-Galván, E. Long-term prognostic role of CA-125 in noncongestive patients undergoing a cardiac transplantation. *Biomark Med.* **2017**, *11*, 239–243.
10. Rheude, T.; Pellegrini, C.; Reinhard, W. Determinants of elevated carbohydrate antigen 125 in patients with severe symptomatic aortic valve stenosis referred for transcatheter aortic valve implantation. *Biomarkers* **2018**, *23*, 299–304. [CrossRef] [PubMed]
11. Hamdy, N.M. Relationship between pro-anti-inflammatory cytokines, T-cell activation and CA 125 in obese patients with heart failure. *Med. Sci. Monit.* **2011**, *17*, CR174–CR179. [CrossRef]
12. Kosar, F.; Aksoy, Y.; Ozguntekin, G.; Ozerol, I.; Varol, E. Relationship between cytokines and tumour markers in patients with chronic heart failure. *Eur. J. Heart Fail* **2006**, *8*, 270–274. [CrossRef]
13. D'Aloia, A.; Faggiano, P.; Aurigemma, G.; Bontempi, L.; Ruggeri, G.; Metra, M.; Nodari, S.; Dei Cas, L. Serum levels of carbohydrate antigen 125 in patients with chronic heart failure: Relation to clinical severity, hemodynamic and Doppler echocardiographic abnormalities, and short-term prognosis. *J. Am. Coll. Cardiol.* **2003**, *41*, 1805–1811. [CrossRef]
14. Ma, J.; Zhao, Y.; Wang, Y.; Guo, Y.; Li, J. Tumor marker levels in patients aged 85 years and older chronic heart failure. *Eur. J. Intern. Med.* **2013**, *24*, 440–443. [CrossRef]
15. Yucel, H.; Kaya, H.; Zorlu, A.; Yıldırımlı, K.; Sancakdar, E.; Gunes, H.; Kurt, R.; Ozgul, U.; Turgut, O.O.; Yilmaz, M.B. Cancer antigen 125 levels and increased risk of new-onset atrial fibrillation. *Herz* **2015**, *40* (Suppl. 2), 119–124. [CrossRef]
16. Möller-Leimkühler, A.M. Gender differences in cardiovascular disease and comorbid depression. *Dialogues. Clin. Neurosci.* **2007**, *9*, 71–83. [PubMed]
17. Ponikowski, P.; Voors, A.A.; Anker, S.D.; Bueno, H.; Cleland, J.G.F.; Coats, A.J.S.; Falk, V.; Gonzalez-Juanatey, J.R.; Harjola, V.P.; Jankowska, E.A.; et al. 2016 ESC guidelines for the diagnosis and treatment of acute and chronic heart failure. *Rev. Esp. Cardiol.* **2016**, *69*, 1167.
18. Zdrojewski, T.; Wizner, B.; Więcek, A.; Ślusarczyk, P.; Chudek, J.; Mossakowska, M.; Bandosz, P.; Bobak, M.; Kozakiewicz, K.; Broda, G.; et al. Prevalence, awareness, and control of hypertension in elderly and very elderly in Poland: Results of a cross-sectional representative survey. *J. Hypertens.* **2016**, *34*, 532–538. [CrossRef] [PubMed]
19. Pauler, D.K.; Menon, U.; McIntosh, M.; Symecko, H.L.; Skates, S.J.; Jacobs, I.J. Factors influencing serum CA125II levels in healthy postmenopausal women. *Cancer Epidemiol. Biomarkers Prev.* **2001**, *10*, 489–493. [PubMed]
20. Palazzuoli, A.; Gallotta, M.; Quatrini, I.; Nuti, R. Natriuretic peptides (BNP and NT-proBNP): Measurement and relevance in heart failure. *Vasc. Health Risk Manag.* **2010**, *6*, 411–418. [CrossRef]
21. Núñez, J.; Núñez, E.; Bayés-Genís, A.; Fonarow, G.C.; Miñana, G.; Bodí, V.; Pascual-Figal, D.; Santas, E.; Garcia-Blas, S.; Chorro, F.J.; et al. Long-term serial kinetics of N-terminal pro B-type natriuretic peptide and carbohydrate antigen125 for mortality risk prediction following acute heart failure. *Eur. Heart J. Acute Cardiovasc. Care.* **2017**, *6*, 685–696. [CrossRef] [PubMed]

22. Méndez, A.B.; Ordoñez-Llanos, J.; Ferrero, A. Prognostic value of increased carbohydrate antigen in patients with heart failure. *World J. Cardiol.* **2014**, *6*, 205–212. [CrossRef] [PubMed]
23. Kouris, N.T.; Kontogianni, D.D.; Papoulia, E.P.; Goranitou, G.S.; Zaharos, I.D.; Grassos, H.A.; Kalkandi, E.M.; Sifaki, M.D.; Babalis, D.K. Clinical and prognostic value of elevated CA125 levels in patients with congestive heart failure. *Hellenic J. Cardiol.* **2006**, *47*, 269–274. [PubMed]
24. Amorim, S.; Campelo, M.; Moura, B.; Martins, E.; Rodrigues, J.; Barroso, I.; Faria, M.; Guimarães, T.; Macedo, F.; Silva-Cardoso, J.; et al. The role of biomarkers in dilated cardiomyopathy: Assessment of clinical severity and reverse remodeling. *Rev. Port. Cardiol.* **2017**, *36*, 709–716. [CrossRef]
25. Kouris, N.T.; Zacharos, I.D.; Kontogianni, D.D.; Goranitou, G.S.; Sifaki, M.D.; Grassos, H.E.; Kalkandi, E.M.; Babalis, D.K. Significance of CA125 levels in patients with chronic congestive heart failure. Correlation with clinical and echocardiographic parameters. *Eur. J. Heart Fail.* **2005**, *7*, 199–203. [CrossRef] [PubMed]
26. Ding, Y.; Wang, Q.; Yang, Y.; Wang, L. Diagnostic value of copeptin and cancer antigen 125 in acute heart failure patients with atrial fibrillation and their correlations with short-term cardiovascular events. *Zhonghua Wei Zhong Bing Ji Jiu Yi Xue* **2018**, *30*, 1024–1028.
27. Yilmaz, M.B.; Zorlu, A.; Tandogan, I. Plasma CA-125 level is related to both sides of the heart: A retrospective analysis. *Int. J. Cardiol.* **2011**, *149*, 80–82. [CrossRef]
28. Kaya, H.; Zorlu, A.; Yucel, H.; Tatlisu, M.A.; Kivrak, T.; Coskun, A.; Yilmaz, M.B. Higher cancer antigen 125 level is associated with the presence of permanent atrial fibrillation in systolic heart failure patients. *Acta Cardiol.* **2016**, *71*, 61–66. [CrossRef]
29. Vizzardi, E.; Nodari, S.; D'Aloia, A.; Chiari, E.; Faggiano, P.; Metra, M.; Dei Cas, L. CA 125 tumoral marker plasma levels relate to systolic and diastolic ventricular function and to the clinical status of patients with chronic heart failure. *Echocardiography* **2008**, *25*, 955–960. [CrossRef]
30. Duman, D.; Palit, F.; Simsek, E.; Bilgehan, K. Serum carbohydrate antigen 125 levels in advanced heart failure: Relation to B-type natriuretic peptide and left atrial volume. *Eur. J. Heart Fail.* **2008**, *10*, 556–559. [CrossRef]
31. Huang, F.; Chen, J.; Liu, Y.; Zhang, K.; Wang, J.; Huang, H. New mechanism of elevated CA125 in heart failure: The mechanical stress and inflammatory stimuli initiate CA125 synthesis. *Med. Hypotheses* **2012**, *79*, 381–383. [CrossRef]
32. Zeillemaker, A.M.; Verbrugh, H.A.; Hoynck van Papendrecht, A.A.; Leguit, P. CA-125 secretion by peritoneal mesothelial cells. *J. Clin. Pathol.* **1994**, *47*, 263–265. [CrossRef] [PubMed]
33. Duman, C.; Ercan, E.; Tengiz, I.; Bozdemir, H.; Ercan, H.E.; Nalbantgil, I. Elevated serum CA 125 levels in mitral stenotic patients with heart failure. *Cardiology* **2003**, *100*, 7–10. [CrossRef] [PubMed]
34. Stanciu, A.E.; Stanciu, M.M.; Vatasescu, R.G. NT-proBNP and CA 125 levels are associated with increased pro-inflammatory cytokines in coronary sinus serum of patients with chronic heart failure. *Cytokine* **2018**, *111*, 13–19. [CrossRef] [PubMed]
35. Sekiguchi, H.; Shimamoto, K.; Takano, M.; Kimura, M.; Takahashi, Y.; Tatsumi, F.; Watanabe, E.; Jujo, K.; Ishizuka, N.; Kawana, M.; et al. Cancer antigen-125 plasma level as a biomarker of new-onset atrial fibrillation in postmenopausalwomen. *Heart* **2017**, *103*, 1368–1373. [CrossRef]
36. De Gennaro, L.; Brunetti, D.; Montrone, D.; De Rosa, F.; Cuculo, A.; Di Biase, M. Inflammatory activation and carbohydrate antigen-125 levels in subjects with atrial fibrillation. *Eur. J. Clin. Invest.* **2012**, *42*, 371–375. [CrossRef]
37. Yalta, K.; Yilmaz, A.; Turgut, O.O.; Erselcan, T.; Yilmaz, M.B.; Karadas, F.; Yontar, C.; Tandogan, I. Evaluation of tumor markers CA-125 and CEA in acute myocardial infarction. *Adv. Ther.* **2006**, *23*, 1052–1059. [CrossRef]
38. Zhang, M.; Li, Y.L.; Yang, X.; Shan, H.; Zhang, Q.H.; Feng, X.L.; Xie, Y.Y.; Tang, J.J.; Zhang, J. Clinical significance of serum carbohydrate antigen 125 in acute exacerbation of chronic obstructive pulmonary disease. *Nan Fang Yi Ke Da Xue Xue Bao* **2016**, *36*, 1386–1389. [PubMed]
39. Li, S.; Ma, H.; Gan, L.; Ma, X.; Wu, S.; Li, M.; Tang, C.H.; Tsai, H.C. Cancer antigen-125 levels correlate with pleural effusions and COPD-related complications in people living at high altitude. *Medicine* **2018**, *97*, e12993. [CrossRef]
40. Barouchos, N.; Papazafiropoulou, A.; Iacovidou, N.; Vrachnis, N.; Barouchos, N.; Armeniakou, E.; Dionyssopoulou, V.; Mathioudakis, A.G.; Christopoulou, E.; Koltsida, S.; et al. Comparison of tumor markers and inflammatory biomarkers in chronic obstructive pulmonary disease (COPD) exacerbations. *Scand. J. Clin. Lab Invest.* **2015**, *75*, 126–132. [CrossRef]

41. Yilmaz, M.B.; Zorlu, A.; Dogan, O.T.; Karahan, O.; Tandogan, I.; Akkurt, I. Role of CA-125 in identification of right ventricular failure in chronic obstructive pulmonary disease. *Clin. Cardiol.* **2011**, *34*, 244–248. [CrossRef] [PubMed]
42. Johnson, C.C.; Kessel, B.; Riley, T.L.; Ragard, L.R.; Williams, C.R.; Xu, J.L.; Buys, S.S.; ProsTate, Lung, Colorectal and Ovarian Cancer Project Team. The epidemiology of CA-125 in women without evidence of ovarian cancer in the prostate, lung, colorectal and ovarian cancer (PLCO). *Screening Trial. Gynecol. Oncol.* **2008**, *110*, 383–389. [CrossRef] [PubMed]
43. Sikaris, K.A. CA125-A test with a change of heart. *Heart Lung Circ.* **2011**, *20*, 634–640. [CrossRef] [PubMed]

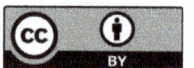

© 2019 by the authors. Licensee MDPI, Basel, Switzerland. This article is an open access article distributed under the terms and conditions of the Creative Commons Attribution (CC BY) license (http://creativecommons.org/licenses/by/4.0/).

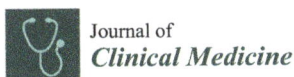 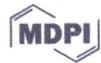

Article

Associations of Adiposity and Diet Quality with Serum Ceramides in Middle-Aged Adults with Cardiovascular Risk Factors

Margaret A. Drazba [1], Ida Holásková [2], Nadine R. Sahyoun [3] and Melissa Ventura Marra [1,*]

1. Division of Animal and Nutritional Sciences, West Virginia University, Morgantown, WV 26506, USA; madrazba@mix.wvu.edu
2. Office of Statistics, West Virginia University, Davis College of Agriculture, Natural Resources and Design, West Virginia Agriculture and Forestry Experiment Station, Morgantown, WV 26506-6108, USA; iholaskova@mail.wvu.edu
3. Department of Nutrition and Food Science, University of Maryland, College Park, MD 20742, USA; nsahyoun@umd.edu
* Correspondence: melissa.marra@mail.wvu.edu; Tel.: +1-304-293-2690

Received: 22 March 2019; Accepted: 16 April 2019; Published: 17 April 2019

Abstract: Rates of adverse cardiovascular events have increased among middle-aged adults. Elevated ceramides have been proposed as a risk factor for cardiovascular events. Diet quality and weight status are inversely associated with several traditional risk factors; however, the relationship to ceramides is less clear. This study aimed to determine associations of adiposity and diet quality with circulating ceramides in middle-aged adults ($n = 96$). Diet quality was estimated using the Healthy Eating Index 2015 (HEI-2015). Serum ceramide concentrations were determined by liquid chromatography–mass spectrometry. A ceramide risk score was determined based on ceramides C16:0, C18:0, and C24:1 and their ratios to C24:0. Participants who were classified as at 'moderate risk' compared to 'lower-risk' based on a ceramide risk score had significantly higher body mass index (BMI) values, as well as higher rates of elevated fibrinogen levels, metabolic syndrome, and former smoking status. BMI was positively associated with the ceramide C18:0 ($R^2 = 0.31$, $p < 0.0001$), the ratio between C18:0/C24:0 ceramides ($R^2 = 0.30$, $p < 0.0001$), and the ceramide risk score ($R^2 = 0.11$, $p < 0.009$). Total HEI-2015 scores ($R^2 = 0.42$, $p = 0.02$), higher intakes of vegetables ($R^2 = 0.44$, $p = 0.02$) and whole grains ($R^2 = 0.43$, $p = 0.03$), and lower intakes of saturated fats ($R^2 = 0.43$, $p = 0.04$) and added sugar ($R^2 = 0.44$, $p = 0.01$) were associated with lower C22:0 values. These findings suggest that circulating ceramides are more strongly related to adiposity than overall diet quality. Studies are needed to determine if improvements in weight status result in lower ceramides and ceramide risk scores.

Keywords: diet quality; ceramides; obesity; cardiovascular risk; healthy eating index

1. Introduction

Cardiovascular disease (CVD) and major CVD events such as myocardial infarction (MI) and stroke are largely preventable, yet they remain leading causes of death, disability, and health care spending in the United States (U.S.) [1]. In 2016, a third of all MIs and strokes in the U.S. occurred in 35 to 64-year-old adults [1]. As a result, CVD mortality rates are increasing in middle-aged adults despite declines in the general population over the past few decades [2]. Prevention efforts focus on identifying and treating modifiable risk factors such as dyslipidemia, diabetes, hypertension, and obesity [2]. However, traditional risk factors are not always strong predictors of events. Many patients hospitalized for an MI or stroke have low-density lipoprotein (LDL) levels within a normal range [3], suggesting that those at CVD risk are not being identified before the disease progresses to an event. There is emerging evidence that a class of lipids—ceramides—may play an important role in the pathogenesis of CVD, and may better predict CVD events than some traditional risk factors [4–6].

Ceramides are a bioactive class of lipids that are synthesized via several molecular pathways, of which the most characterized is de novo synthesis. De novo synthesis begins with palmitoyl CoA and the amino acid L-serine. Then, the resulting sphingoid base is attached to fatty acid side chains of different lengths and degrees of unsaturation, leading to a group of molecules [7] that are diverse in structure and function [8,9]. Ceramides play a role in cell membrane integrity, inflammation, and apoptosis [10], and when they accumulate, they are thought to contribute to the progression of chronic disease, including atherosclerosis [11]. Their low levels in biological samples, large biodiversity, and polar nature made it difficult to quantify ceramides [7]. However, recent advances in mass spectroscopy now allow for the quantification of these small-molecule metabolites, some of which may be prognostic markers for CVD [12].

Elevated circulating concentrations of three specific ceramides: N-palmitoyl-sphingosine (C16:0), N-stearoyl-sphingosine (C18:0), and N-nervonoyl-sphingosine (C24:1) were found to be predictive of CVD events in patients with coronary artery disease independent of traditional risk factors [4]. The predictive value was found to be greater when the ceramides were normalized to N-lignoceroyl-sphingosine (C24:0), which is a ceramide that is abundant in the circulation but thought not to be related to CVD [4]. In 2016, the Mayo Clinic began offering a diagnostic test to measure ceramides and assign the risk of a future CVD event based on a ceramide risk score. The risk score is based on six values: C16:0, C18:0, and C24:1, and the ratio of each to C24:0 [5]. Participants classified at higher risk based on their ceramide risk score were four times more likely to suffer a CVD event than those at lower risk [4] independent of age, sex, smoking status, and LDL cholesterol [4,5].

Evidence-based clinical care guidelines for reducing elevated ceramide levels and the risk score are not available [13]. It has been suggested that changes in diet may help lower ceramides, and thus CVD risk; however, controlled studies have not been conducted in humans. Higher diet quality and adherence to healthy dietary patterns have been associated with lower CVD risk and mortality [14]. However, no studies have assessed the relationship of diet quality or adherence to United States (U.S.) Dietary Guidelines for Americans (DGAs) as measured by the Healthy Eating Index 2015 (HEI-2015) on circulating ceramides or the ceramide risk score. It is plausible that interventions effective in reducing traditional risk factors also modify circulating ceramides. Studies have shown that circulating ceramides can be modified through exercise [15], statin use [16,17], and weight loss post-bariatric surgery [18,19]. Short-term intervention studies in small samples of healthy humans have shown that caloric excess and increased saturated fat intake increase ceramide levels [20–22]. However, there were no significant changes in ceramides after one year in participants at high CVD risk in the PREDIMED (Prevention with Mediterranean Diet) study [23].

The relationship between adiposity, diet quality, and ceramides that make up the ceramide risk score is largely unknown. In the U.S., people living in the state of West Virginia experience higher rates of obesity, type 2 diabetes, and hypertension [24], and lower rates of adequate fruit and vegetable intake [25] than any other state in the nation. CVD risk reduction is a public health priority in the state. Middle-aged adults represent a priority population in national health campaigns. The purpose of this study was to determine if diet quality (e.g., adherence to the U.S DGAs), and adiposity were associated with serum ceramides and the ceramide risk score in middle-aged West Virginians with at least one risk factor for CVD.

2. Materials and Methods

2.1. Study Design and Sample

In this cross-sectional study, data were analyzed from 96 middle-aged adults (45 to 64 years old) who took part in a larger diet and cardiovascular risk assessment study. Participants were recruited from two counties in north-central West Virginia by word-of-mouth and community advertising. Exclusion criteria included current smokers; diagnosis of cancer or kidney, heart, or liver disease; surgery six months prior; and anti-inflammatory or anticoagulant medications.

The study consisted of three modes of data collection: multiple telephone interviews to assess dietary intake; an online survey administered using REDCap (Research Electronic Data Capture), which is a secure web-based application designed to support data capture for research studies [26]; and an in-person health assessment. At the in-person health assessment, anthropometric and blood pressure measurements were taken by research staff, and a trained phlebotomist performed a fasting venous blood draw. The study protocol was approved by the West Virginia University (WVU) Institutional Review Board. All the participants provided informed consent before participation and received a $100 gift card upon completion of the study.

2.2. Demographic and Health-Related Data

Demographic data and smoking history were self-reported via the online survey. Participants also provided health and medication history at the in-person visit. Blood collected was analyzed by WVU Hospital lab for LDL cholesterol, high-density lipoprotein (HDL) cholesterol, non-HDL cholesterol, triglycerides, glucose, insulin, C-reactive protein (CRP), and fibrinogen. Insulin sensitivity was calculated using the homeostatic model assessment of insulin resistance (HOMA-IR) as fasting insulin (mU L^{-1}) × fasting glucose (mmol L^{-1})/22.5 [27] using measured fasting glucose and insulin values. Participants were classified as having a health condition if at least one of the following criteria was met: (1) they reported being diagnosed by a health care provider, (2) they reported taking a medication that is used to treat the condition, or (3) the measured laboratory values or blood pressure (BP) met standard diagnostic cut-off values. The cut-off values for the diagnoses were as follows: pre-diabetes or diabetes, fasting plasma glucose >100 mg/dL [28]; dyslipidemia, LDL ≥100 mg/dL or triglycerides ≥150 mg/dL; hypertension, systolic BP >120 or diastolic BP >80 mm Hg [29]; and a diagnoses of metabolic syndrome required meeting three of the 5 factors defined by the National Cholesterol Education Program Adult Treatment Panel III [30].

Blood pressure was measured using the Omron HEM-907XL Intellisense® Automatic Oscillatory Digital Blood Pressure monitor (Omron Health Care, Lake Forest, IL, USA) [31]. A single assessor performed all the blood pressure measurements. Arm circumference was measured to the nearest 0.1 cm to determine appropriate cuff size based on manufacturer recommendations. With the participant in a seated upright position and after an initial rest of 5 min, the machine took three blood pressure measurements at 30-second intervals; the average reading was used for analysis [32]. Anthropometric and body composition measurements were taken using standardized protocols, with participants fasted, lightly clothed, and without shoes. Measurements were recorded in duplicate, and averages were used for analysis. Height (cm) was measured using the Seca 274 digital mobile stadiometer (Seca, Hamburg, Germany). Weight (kg) and fat mass index (FMI) (kg/m^2) were measured using the Seca medical Bioelectrical Composition Analyzer (mBCA) 514 (Seca, Hamburg, Germany). Body mass index (BMI) was calculated as weight (kg)/height (m^2) and was classified using World Health Organization classifications [33]. Waist and hip circumferences (cm) were measured using a Gulick II Tape Measure. Waist circumference (WC) was measured at the iliac crest; values >102 cm for men and >88 cm for women were classified 'at risk' [33]. Hip circumference was measured at the maximum point of protuberance of the buttocks. Waist–hip ratio (WHR) was calculated as waist circumference (cm)/hip circumference (cm); values were classified as 'at risk' if WHR was ≥0.90 cm for men and ≥0.85 cm for women [33].

2.3. Diet Quality Assessment

Dietary intake data were collected and analyzed using three 24-hour dietary recalls and Nutrition Data Systems for Research (NDSR) software version 15 (2015) developed by the Nutrition Coordinating Center, University of Minnesota, Minneapolis, MN. Self-reported dietary intake was obtained via telephone interview by trained research personnel using the NDSR four-pass method on non-consecutive days (one weekend and two weekdays). Food and nutrient data was transformed into the HEI-2015 metric, which measures adherence to the 2015–2020 Dietary Guidelines for Americans (DGAs) [34] based on 13 components (nine adequacies and four moderation). To calculate the HEI-2015 scores, NDSR output data was transformed into HEI component variables using NDSR's unpublished guide [35]. Food group servings (total fruits, whole fruits, total vegetables, greens and beans, whole grains, dairy, total protein foods, seafood and plant proteins, and refined grains) were converted to total servings per 1000 kilocalories and sodium intake was converted to mg per 1000 kilocalories. A ratio of polyunsaturated fatty acids (PUFAs) and monounsaturated fatty acids (MUFAs) to saturated fatty acids (SFAs) was generated by dividing the sum of PUFAs and MUFAs by SFAs. Added sugars and saturated fats were assessed as percent of kilocalories. For the four moderation components—refined grains, sodium, added sugars, and saturated fats—higher scores represent lower intakes. Once the NDSR components were in units consistent with the HEI metric, the simple HEI scoring algorithm method for multiple days of intake data was applied [36]. Component scores were summed for a total score ranging from 0–100, with higher scores indicating better adherence to the 2015–2020 U.S. DGAs.

2.4. Ceramides Analysis

Lipidomics analysis was conducted by the WVU Metabolomics Core using liquid chromatography–mass spectrometry (LC-MS). Serum samples were extracted using a modified Bligh and Dyer procedure using C12:0-ceramide as an internal standard (Avanti Polar Lipids, Alabaster, AL, USA) using previously described methods [37,38]. Following liquid–liquid extraction, the organic layer was dried under nitrogen gas (Organomation Associates Inc., Berlin, MA, USA) and resuspended in pure methanol before analysis. Ceramides were separated by gradient elution using ultra high-pressure liquid chromatography (ExionLC AD, SCIEX, Framingham, MA, USA) on a C18 reverse-phase column (Phenomenex, Torrence, CA, USA). Ceramides were detected using electrospray ionization tandem mass spectrometry (ESI-MS/MS) as previously described (QTRAP 5500, SCIEX) [39]. Ionspray source voltage was 5000 V at a temperature of 500 °C. Nebulizer, heater, curtain, and collision gas pressures were maintained at 70, 60, 28, and 9 psi, respectively. Ceramide ionization parameters were optimized individually, ranging from a declustering potential of 30 to 50 V, an entrance potential of 10 to 15 V, collision energy of 32 to 37 V, and a collision cell exit potential of 13 to 17 V. Ceramides were measured by multiple reaction monitoring of the protonated molecular ion with a transition ion of 264.2 m/z. Eleven-point calibration curves (0.1 ng/mL to 10 µg/mL) were constructed by plotting the area under the curve for C16:0-ceramide, C18:0-ceramide, C22:0-ceramide, and C24:0-ceramide (Avanti Polar Lipids). Fluctuations in extraction and ionization efficiencies were controlled by normalizing to the C12:0-ceramide response, and samples were re-run if the internal standard response deviated more than 20% from its median value. Concentrations were determined by curve fitting the identified ceramide species based on acyl-chain length. Standards were injected in duplicate to ensure similar response (the overall mean CV was 12.08%; $R^2 \geq 0.985$). Instrument control and quantitation were performed using Analyst 1.6.3 and MultiQuant 3.0.2 software, respectively (SCIEX).

2.5. Ceramides Risk Score

The ceramides used in this analysis included the six variables that make up the ceramide risk score (C16:0, C18:0, C24:1, C16:0/C24:0, C18:0/C24:0, and C24:1/C24:0) [40] and two additional ceramides (C20:0 and C22:0) that were identified in the literature as being related to diet [20,41], adiposity [42], or CVD risk [15,23,43]. Ceramides (ng/mL) were converted to units that were consistent with the ceramide risk score (µmol/L). Ceramide risk scores were calculated by assigning a value between 0–2 to each of the six risk score components based on published cut-off values [4,5]. The six component scores were summed for a total ceramide risk score ranging from 0 to 12, with higher scores indicating a higher risk of adverse cardiovascular events. The scores were categorized into risk groups: lower risk (0–2), moderate risk (3–6), and increased risk (7–9) [4]. No participant scores met a fourth category:

higher risk (10–12). For analysis purposes in this study, the 'increased risk' category was combined into the 'moderate risk', as only three participants had scores in the increased risk category.

2.6. Statistical Analysis

Demographic and health-related data were reported as means and standard errors of the mean (SEM) or frequency with percentage, when appropriate. Ceramides and risk factors for CVD (i.e., cholesterol, triglycerides, glucose) were log-transformed to achieve a normal distribution for analysis. Medians and interquartile ranges were reported for non-normally distributed variables. To assess differences between ceramide risk score categories for all the demographic and clinical characteristics, Student's *t*-test or Chi-square tests were performed when appropriate. Bivariate analysis was performed to assess the relationship between potential confounding variables (demographics, health conditions, CVD biomarkers, inflammatory markers, and lifestyle factors) and each ceramide and the ceramide risk score. The Benjamini–Hochberg procedure was performed to control for excessive Type I error due to multiple analyses, with a false discovery rate set to 10%. The variables that remained significant after the Benjamini–Hochberg procedure were entered into a stepwise regression model, with alpha-to-enter set at 0.15 and alpha-to-remove set at 0.15. This enabled us to estimate the effect of multiple variables on ceramides and the ceramide risk score. The variables that remained significant were included in the adjusted model. Multiple linear regression models were done to assess the hypothesized relationship between the HEI-2015 diet quality score and BMI on a continuous scale with individual ceramides along with the ceramide risk score. These models enabled us to assess if the HEI-2015 or BMI were associated with ceramide levels when adjusted for other significant clinical, demographic, or lifestyle characteristics. The 13 HEI-2015 components were analyzed further using multiple linear regression models with individual ceramides and the ceramide risk score. BMI was further analyzed categorically against each individual ceramide and the ceramide risk score using one-way ANOVA and Tukey's HSD (honestly significant difference) test for comparison of BMI categories (normal, overweight, and obese).

All data analyses were performed using JMP and SAS software (JMP®, Version Pro 12.2, SAS Institute Inc., Cary, NC, USA, Copyright ©2015; SAS®, Version 9.4, SAS Institute Inc., Cary, NC, USA, Copyright ©2002–2012). Power of the test was determined as 80% for the relationship of BMI and the ceramide risk score. Significance criterion alpha for all tests was 0.05.

3. Results

3.1. Participant Characteristics by Ceramide Risk Category

Overall, most participants were non-Hispanic white (95.8%), college educated (57.3%), and had annual household incomes >$50,000 (67.4%). Demographic and health-related characteristics by ceramide risk category are presented in Table 1. The mean age of the sample was 54 ± 4.7 years old Over half were women (57.3%). The mean BMI was 30.85 ± 7.23; 51.1% were classified as obese. All the participants had at least one cardiovascular risk factor; 92% had dyslipidemia (controlled and uncontrolled). Participants classified at 'moderate risk' compared to 'low-risk' based on ceramide risk category had significantly higher BMI ($p = 0.003$), WC ($p = 0.005$), and FMI ($p = 0.004$), elevated fibrinogen levels (35.0% versus 14.3%, $p = 0.02$), higher rates of metabolic syndrome (52.5% versus 28.6%, $p = 0.02$), and had formerly smoked (62.5% versus 1.1%, $p = 0.04$).

The most abundant circulating ceramides were C24:0 followed by C22:0 and C24:1. Ceramide risk scores ranged from 0 to 8 out of a possible 12 points; 58.3% were in the low-risk group, and 41.7% were in the moderate risk or increased risk groups. Supplemental Table S1 shows quantities of ceramides by risk category.

Table 1. Participant characteristics by ceramide risk category.

	All N = 96	Lower Risk [1] n = 56	Moderate Risk [2] n = 40	p-Value [3]
Demographic Factors				
Age, year	54.30 ± 0.47	53.95 ± 0.55	54.8 ± 0.84	0.40
Sex, women	55 (57.3%)	33 (58.9%)	22 (55.0%)	0.70
Health-Related Factors				
Adiposity				
Body Mass Index, kg/m^2	30.85 ± 0.74	29.22 ± 0.92	33.13 ± 1.13	0.003
Waist Circumference, cm	103.35 ± 1.67	99.41 ± 2.07	108.87 ± 2.55	0.005
Elevated Waist Circumference [4]	70 (72.9%)	37 (66.1%)	33 (82.5%)	0.07
Waist-to-Hip Ratio, cm	0.90 ± 0.008	0.89 ± 0.01	0.91 ± 0.01	0.16
Elevated Waist-to-Hip Ratio [5]	63 (65.6%)	36 (64.3%)	27 (67.5%)	0.74
Fat Mass Index, kg/m^2	12.26 ± 0.55	11.00 ± 0.65	14.02 ± 0.89	0.004
Laboratory Values				
Total Cholesterol ≥200 mg/dL	52 (54.2%)	30 (53.6%)	22 (55.0%)	0.89
LDL ≥100 mg/dL	77 (81.1%)	43 (76.8%)	34 (87.2%)	0.20
Low HDL [6]	22 (22.9%)	12 (21.4%)	10 (25.0%)	0.68
Triglycerides ≥150 mg/dL	18 (18.8%)	9 (16.1%)	9 (22.5%)	0.43
Glucose >100 mg/dL	35 (36.5%)	19 (33.9%)	16 (40.0%)	0.54
Insulin >24 mg/dL	4 (4.17%)	1 (1.8%)	3 (7.5%)	0.17
HOMA-IR	2.18 (0.17)	1.97 (0.19)	2.48 (0.31)	0.19
CRP ≥8 mg/dL	16 (16.7%)	9 (16.1%)	7 (17.5%)	0.85
Fibrinogen >400 mg/dL	22 (22.9%)	8 (14.3%)	14 (35.0%)	0.02
Medical Conditions				
Metabolic Syndrome	37 (38.5%)	16 (28.6%)	21 (52.5%)	0.02
Diabetes	39 (40.6%)	22 (39.3%)	17 (42.5%)	0.75
Dyslipidemia	88 (91.7%)	50 (89.3%)	38 (95.0%)	0.32
Hypertension	37 (38.5%)	18 (32.1%)	19 (47.5%)	0.13
Statin use	23 (24.0%)	13 (23.2%)	10 (25.0%)	0.84
Lifestyle Factors				
Former Smoker	48 (50.0%)	23 (41.1%)	25 (62.5%)	0.04
HEI-2015 Diet Scores	54.05 ± 1.45	55.27 ± 1.73	52.36 ± 2.49	0.34

Values are means ± SEM for continuous variables or n (%) for categorical variables. Abbreviations: LDL, low-density lipoprotein; HDL, high-density lipoprotein; HOMA-IR, homeostatic model assessment of insulin resistance; CRP, C-reactive protein; HEI-2015, Healthy Eating Index 2015. [1] Lower risk: ceramide risk score 0–2. [2] Moderate risk: ceramide risk score 3–6, and three participants with scores of 7 (n = 2) and 8 (n = 1). [3] Student's t-test or chi-square tests were used to test significance; significant p-value <0.05. [4] Elevated waist circumference is >102 cm for men and >88 cm for women. [5] Elevated waist-to-hip ratio is ≥0.90 cm for men and ≥0.85 cm for women. [6] Low HDL is <40 mg/dL for men and <50 mg/dL for women.

3.2. Relationship between Potential Covariates and Ceramide

Age, gender, income, statin use, and hypertension were not significantly associated with any of the ceramides or the risk score. All of the adiposity measures (i.e., WC, WHR, and FMI); several laboratory values (LDL, HDL, non-HDL, triglycerides, glucose, insulin, HOMA-IR, fibrinogen, and CRP); having a diagnosis of diabetes or metabolic syndrome, and being a former smoker were each significantly associated with at least one ceramide or the risk score. However, after stepwise regression, only LDL, HDL, non-HDL, glucose, FMI, fibrinogen, and smoking status remained significantly associated with individual ceramides or the risk score, and therefore were the only covariates included in the adjusted models. Supplemental Table S2 depicts the results of bivariate analyses of associations between traditional CVD risk factors and ceramides.

3.3. Relationship of BMI (Adiposity) and HEI (Diet Quality) with Ceramides

Table 2 shows the associations between BMI and HEI scores with ceramides. BMI was associated with C18:0, C16:0/24:0, C18:0/C24:0, and the ceramide risk score in unadjusted models, and remained positively associated with C18:0, C18:0/C24:0, and the ceramide risk score after adjusting for covariates.

The diet quality scores measured by HEI-2015 ranged from 25.6 to 87.7 out of 100 points. The mean score was 54.05 ± 1.45, indicating 'needing improvement' (HEI scores 51–80). Diet quality was inversely associated with only one ceramide, C22:0, in both unadjusted and adjusted models. It was not associated with any of the ceramides that make up the risk score. Ceramides C16:0, C24:0, and C24:1/24:0 were not associated with any of the outcome variables.

Table 2. Associations between BMI (adiposity) and HEI-2015 (diet quality) with ceramides.

Outcome Variables	Ceramides Included in the Ceramide Risk Score				Ceramide Risk Score	Other Ceramides	
	C18:0	C24:1	C16:0/24:0	C18:0/24:0		C20:0	C22:0
Unadjusted Model							
BMI (kg/m^2)	0.80; 0.19 (<0.001)	NS	0.36; 0.07 (0.006)	1.02; 0.26 (<0.001)	5.97; 0.07 (0.006)	NS	NS
HEI-2015	NS	NS	NS	NS	NS	NS	−0.002; 0.06 (0.009)
Adjusted Models							
BMI (kg/m^2)	0.81; 0.31 (<0.0001)	NS	NS	0.91; 0.30 (<0.0001)	5.58; 0.11 (0.009)	NS	NS
HEI-2015	NS	NS	NS	NS	NS	NS	−0.002; 0.42 (0.02)

Values reported are slope per unit change; coefficient of determination R^2 and (significant p-value). Abbreviations: HEI-2015, Healthy Eating Index 2015; BMI, body mass index; NS, not significant. Covariates used in adjusted models varied by ceramide: C18:0 (HDL-C, glucose); C24:1 (LDL, non-HDL); C16:0/24:0 (glucose, fibrinogen); C18:0/24:0 (glucose); C24:1/24:0 (smoking); ceramide risk score (smoking); C20:0 (LDL, non-HDL); C22:0 (LDL, non-HDL).

Table 3 depicts the associations between individual HEI-2015 component scores and ceramides. After adjusting for confounding risk factors, HEI scores that represent the recommended intakes for total vegetables, whole grains, saturated fats, and added sugars were each inversely associated with C22:0. That is, higher intakes of vegetables and whole grains and lower intakes of saturated fats and added sugar were associated with lower C22:0 values. Absolute saturated fat intake (grams per day) was significantly and positively associated with C22:0 (R^2 = 0.41, p = 0.04). Individual HEI components (i.e., whole fruit, total fruit, greens and beans, dairy, total protein foods, seafood and plant protein, unsaturated to saturated fatty acid ratio, and sodium) were not associated with any ceramides or the ceramide risk score.

Table 3. Associations between the Healthy Eating Index (HEI-2015) components and ceramides.

HEI Component	Ceramides in Risk Score			Other Ceramides	
	C16:0	C24:1	C16:0/24:0	C20:0	C22:0
Unadjusted Models					
Total Vegetables	−0.02; 0.04 (0.02)	NS	NS	NS	−0.03; 0.05 (0.01)
Whole Grains	NS	NS	NS	−0.01; 0.04 (0.03)	−0.01; 0.04 (0.03)
Refined Grains	NS	NS	−0.007; 0.04 (0.03)	NS	NS
Saturated Fats	NS	−0.01; 0.05 (0.01)	NS	−0.02; 0.06 (0.01)	−0.02; 0.08 (0.003)
Added Sugar	NS	NS	NS	NS	−0.01; 0.07 (0.007)
Adjusted Models					
Total Vegetables	NS	NS	NS	NS	−0.02; 0.44 (0.02)
Whole Grains	NS	NS	NS	NS	−0.007; 0.43 (0.03)
Saturated Fats	NS	NS	NS	NS	−0.008; 0.43 (0.03)
Added Sugar	NS	NS	NS	NS	−0.009; 0.44 (0.01)

Values reported are slope per unit change; coefficient of determination R^2 and (p-value). Abbreviations: HEI-2015, Healthy Eating Index 2015; NS, not significant. Ceramides not significant with any HEI-2015 components were C18:0, C24:0, C18:0/24:0, C24:1/24:0 or the ceramide risk score (not shown). Covariates used in adjusted models varied by ceramide: C16:0 (HDL, non-HDL, glucose); C24:1 (LDL, non-HDL); C16:0/24:0 (glucose, fibrinogen); C20:0 (LDL, non-HDL); C22:0 (LDL, non-HDL). Significant p-value <0.05.

Figure 1 depicts ceramide concentrations by BMI category. Of the 96 participants, 22.9% were classified as normal weight, 26.0% were classified as overweight, and 51.0% were classified as obese. Five of the six values that make up the ceramide risk score (C16:0, C18:0, C16:0/24:0, C18:0/24:0, C24:1/24:0, and C20:0) were all significantly higher in participants classified as obese compared to normal weight. Four of the six values in the risk score (C16:0, C18:0, C16:0/24:0, and C18:0/24:0) were significantly higher in participants classified as overweight compared to normal weight. Figure 2 shows the ceramide risk score by BMI category. The risk score increased by BMI category and was significantly higher between participants classified as normal weight versus obese (1.36 ± 0.24 versus 3.14 ± 0.31, $p = 0.001$).

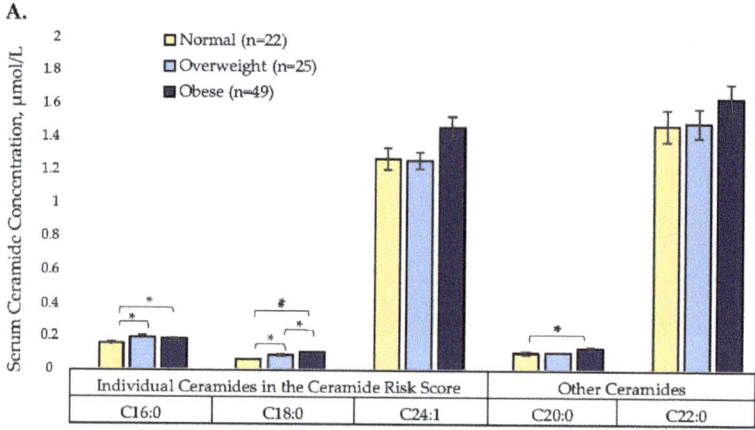

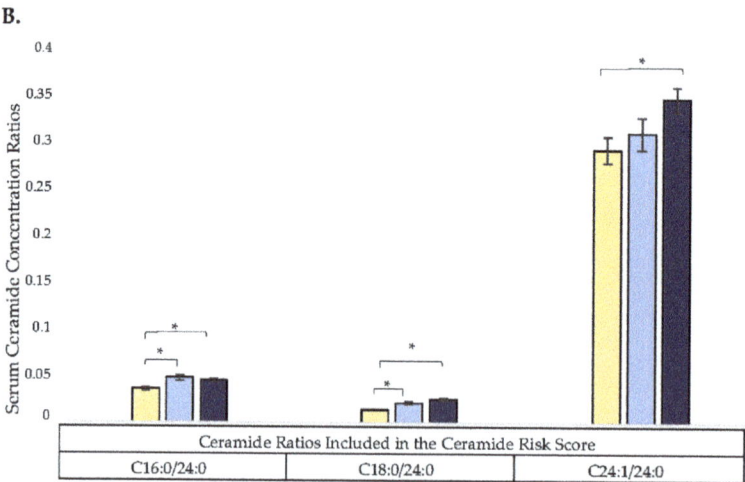

Figure 1. (**A**) Serum ceramide concentrations (μmol/L) by BMI category: normal weight (18.5–24.9 kg/m^2), overweight (25–29.9 kg/m^2), and obese (≥30 kg/m^2). Values reported are mean concentrations. (**B**) Ceramide ratios included in the risk score by BMI category. Values are means of ratios. Tukey's honestly significant difference (HSD) was used to test significance between the three BMI categories. * Significant p-values < 0.05.

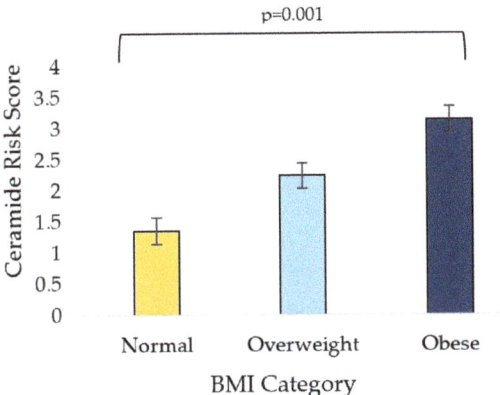

Figure 2. Ceramide risk score by BMI category: normal (18.5–24.9 kg/m^2), overweight (25–29.9 kg/m^2), and obese ($\geq$30 kg/m^2). Values represent means and SEM. Tukey's HSD was used to test significance between categories.

4. Discussion

This is the first study to examine the cross-sectional associations of adiposity and diet quality with the ceramide risk score, which is an emerging risk factor for CVD. We detected that even between the two lowest ceramide risk score categories, there were significant differences between groups for adiposity (BMI and FMI), and rates of elevated fibrinogen (a proinflammatory mediator), metabolic syndrome, and former smoker status. BMI was positively associated with the ceramide risk score and two of the six ceramide values in the risk score (C18:0 and C18:0/24:0). Total HEI-2015 scores and four diet component scores (total vegetables, whole grains, saturated fats, and added sugars) were inversely associated with only one ceramide, C22:0, which is a ceramide associated in the literature with diet [20,41] but not included in the ceramide risk score. Higher diet component scores indicate improvements in diet quality. That is, higher scores represent higher intakes of vegetables and whole grains, but lower intakes of saturated fats and added sugar.

Similar to other studies, the most abundant serum ceramides were C24:0 and C24:1 [44,45]. Ceramide C24:0 was positively associated with LDL, non-HDL, and triglycerides, as has been reported in other studies [4], but inversely associated with fibrinogen in our population. We did not see associations between statin use and ceramides. Study results have been inconsistent, with some studies showing lower circulating ceramides in participants taking statins [42,46] and others such as ours, did not [42]. In our population, 91.7% of participants had dyslipidemia. However, 24% reported statin use, but of those, 60.9% still had high lipid levels, suggesting that the statins were ineffective or that participants were not regularly taking their medications. Additionally, significantly more participants with metabolic syndrome were in the moderate ceramide risk category compared to the low-risk category. This finding is consistent with other studies that ceramides may be inducers of metabolic disorders [47].

4.1. Associations between Adiposity and Ceramides

BMI was positively associated with the ceramide risk score, C18:0, and C18:0/24:0 after adjusting for confounding variables. To our knowledge, no other studies have compared BMI with this specific total ceramide risk score, but studies have reported an association between BMI and various circulating ceramide species. Circulating C18:0 was associated with BMI in several studies [4,42,44]. Consistent with our study, Meeusen et al. reported an association between BMI and two of the six risk components of the risk score (C18:0 and C18:0/24:0); however, the association was minimal (R^2 value <3%) compared to the 30% in this study [4]. Differences in populations and overall sample size (n = 495 versus n = 96) may account for variation in the strength of the associations. In contrast, Mielke et al. reported additional associations of BMI with C16:0, C24:1, C20:0, and C22:0 among middle-aged subjects with an average BMI of 26 kg/m^2 (overweight) [42] that we did not detect. In a small sample, Haus et al. detected higher concentrations of C18:0, C20:0, and C24:1 ceramides in subjects with type 2 diabetes and obesity (n = 13) compared to lean healthy control subjects (n = 14) [44]. A possible mechanism for increased serum ceramides is that in obese humans, circulating free fatty acids, which serve as substrates for ceramide synthesis via the de novo pathway, are elevated, leading to an overproduction of ceramides [48,49]. Ceramides can be synthesized in several different tissues, but those synthesized in the liver can be readily incorporated in very low-density lipoprotein (VLDL) particles and released into the circulation [50]. Ceramides circulate in the blood mainly associated with lipoprotein particles, VLDL and LDL [50]. Thus, overproduction in the liver is a potential source for elevated circulating ceramides. Excess ceramides are postulated to be the mechanistic link between obesity and obesity-related chronic conditions. Thus, our research adds to literature suggesting a link between obesity and a potential overproduction and accumulation of C18:0 species and the overall ceramide risk score. Studies are needed that determine if dietary interventions for weight loss result in a reduction of the ceramides in the risk score.

4.2. Associations between Diet Quality and Ceramides

We did not detect associations between diet quality and ceramide species in individual ceramides in the risk score or total risk score; however, greater HEI scores were associated with lower C22:0 concentrations after adjusting for LDL and non-HDL cholesterol. We found that 42% of the variation in C22:0—a very-long-chain ceramide with a saturated acyl chain—was explained by the HEI scores indicating a strong association. There is limited research on the associations between diet and ceramides. This was the first study to assess the relationship between the a priori HEI metric of diet quality and ceramides as a marker for CVD risk. However, other studies have shown that the HEI score was related to reductions in other CVD risk factors such as LDL [51] and reductions in CVD mortality [14,52].

While C22:0 is not part of the ceramide risk score, previous studies showed that it is positively associated with CVD risk in humans [23,43]. Two intervention studies that measured C22:0 found that it was modifiable by diet [20,41]. One intervention of 200 subjects who were between 30–65 years old with metabolic syndrome aimed to determine how a Nordic diet affected the lipidomic profile compared to control subjects. Subjects in the intervention consumed a dietary pattern of higher amounts of fiber, vegetables, fruits, berries, and fish, lower intakes of salt and sugar, and a higher quality of dietary fat than the control for 18 to 24 weeks. The control group received low-fiber cereal products and dairy fat such as butter [41]. Results indicated a significant decrease in C22:0, C23:0, and C24:0 concentrations compared to the control group after 12 weeks, but not after 24 weeks [41]. In another study, Heilbronn et al. also observed an elevation in C22:0 by 25% in subjects overfed by 1250 kilocalories per day for 28 days [20].

When assessing individual HEI components, we found that participants had higher scores, indicating that better adherence to recommendations for saturated fat intake (≤8% of energy intake) had lower C22:0 concentrations. Additionally, participants who consumed higher amounts of absolute saturated fat (grams per day) had higher C22:0. De novo ceramide synthesis depends on the availability of free fatty acids, specifically the saturated fat palmitate [10]. The overconsumption of this saturated fat may result in excess ceramide accumulation [10]. Additionally, in our population, better adherence to the DGAs for total vegetable intake, whole grain intake, and added sugar intake was also associated with lower C22:0. This suggests that multiple components of the diet work synergistically, and that dietary patterns should be studied in relationship to ceramides in larger samples. Future studies on the relationship between ceramides and diet quality are needed, specifically long-term intervention studies to assess changes in ceramides after improvements in diet quality.

4.3. Limitations

There are several limitations to this study. First, our sample size was small and used a convenience sample whose ceramide risk scores fell largely within the two lowest groups of risk. A larger sample may have included a broader range of risk scores, and associations may have been detected when the lowest versus highest scores are compared. Second, the majority of participants were non-Hispanic white, which is representative of the population in West Virginia, but makes it difficult to generalize findings to other populations. Third, the cross-sectional study design does not allow for cause–effect relationships. Studies are needed to investigate long-term changes in ceramides over time. Lastly, the study used self-reported data, such as dietary intake, medications, and medical conditions. There are inherent limitations with self-reported intake data, specifically the under-reporting of dietary intake or failing to report all the medications used.

4.4. Clinical implications

Laboratory tests are currently available that quantify ceramides and categorize risk of CVD events.. However, studies have not yet been conducted to inform evidence-based guidelines on treatments to effectively modify ceramides should they be elevated. It is plausible that diet, lifestyle, and lipid-lowering medications known to reduce traditional risk factors may also be effective in lowering ceramides. Large epidemiological studies to confirm the relationship between specific ceramides and CVD events, and interventional studies to determine the effectiveness of treatment strategies in reducing ceramides and CVD events are urgently needed. Until this data is available, it seems premature to use ceramides as a therapeutic target in clinical practice.

5. Conclusions

This study showed that middle-aged adults with obesity had higher circulating C18:0 and C18:0/24:0, and higher ceramide risk scores than those who were normal weight or overweight. Higher BMI remained independently associated with higher ceramide levels after adjusting for confounding variables. Future studies are needed to determine if a reduction in weight status results in lower ceramide risk scores in humans, and if interventions to improve diet quality would be effective in lowering ceramides and the ceramide risk score.

Supplementary Materials: The following are available online at http://www.mdpi.com/2077-0383/8/4/527/s1, Table S1: Ceramides concentrations and ceramide risk scores (CRS) by risk category; Table S2: Bivariate analysis of ceramides by risk factors for cardiovascular disease to assess for possible covariates.

Author Contributions: Conceptualization, Methodology, Data Curation, Project Administration and Funding Acquisition, M.V.M.; Data Analysis, M.A.D. and I.H.; Writing—Original Draft Preparation, M.A.D. and M.V.M.; Writing—Review & Editing, all authors.

Funding: This work was supported by the WVU Provost's Office through the Health Disparities Mountains of Excellence flash fund award; the USDA National Institute of Food and Agriculture (NIFA) Hatch/Multi-State project 1009924 (WVU), and the West Virginia Agricultural and Forestry Experiment Station. The software was provided by the West Virginia Clinical and Translational Science Institute (National Institute of General Medical Sciences of the National Institutes of Health under Award Number 2U54GM104942-02). The content is solely the responsibility of the authors, and does not necessarily represent the official views of any of the funding sources.

Acknowledgments: The authors would like to thank WVU research assistants' Wijdan Dabeek, Corey Coe, Paige Starrett, Brittany Abruzzino, Stephanie Thompson, and Michelle Campion for their contributions to the study. They would also like to express their gratitude to the men and women who participated in the study.

Conflicts of Interest: The authors declare no conflict of interest.

References

1. CDC. Prevent 1 Million Heart Attacks & Strokes. Available online: https://www.cdc.gov/vitalsigns/million-hearts/index.html (accessed on 17 December 2018).
2. Wall, H.K. Vital Signs: Prevalence of Key Cardiovascular Disease Risk Factors for Million Hearts 2022—United States, 2011–2016. *MMWR Morb. Mortal. Wkly. Rep.* **2018**, *67*, 983–991. [PubMed]

3. Sachdeva, A.; Cannon, C.P.; Deedwania, P.C.; Labresh, K.A.; Smith, S.C.; Dai, D.; Hernandez, A.; Fonarow, G.C. Lipid levels in patients hospitalized with coronary artery disease: An analysis of 136,905 hospitalizations in Get with the Guidelines. *Am. Heart J.* **2009**, *157*, 111–117.e2.
4. Meeusen, J.W.; Donato, L.J.; Bryant, S.C.; Baudhuin, L.M.; Berger, P.B.; Jaffe, A.S. Plasma Ceramides: A Novel Predictor of Major Adverse Cardiovascular Events After Coronary Angiography. *Arterioscler. Thromb. Vasc. Biol.* **2018**, *38*. [CrossRef]
5. Laaksonen, R.; Ekroos, K.; Sysi-Aho, M.; Hilvo, M.; Vihervaara, T.; Kauhanen, D.; Suoniemi, M.; Hurme, R.; März, W.; Scharnagl, H.; et al. Plasma ceramides predict cardiovascular death in patients with stable coronary artery disease and acute coronary syndromes beyond LDL-cholesterol. *Eur. Heart J.* **2016**, *37*, 1967–1976.
6. Havulinna, A.S.; Sysi-Aho, M.; Hilvo, M.; Kauhanen, D.; Hurme, R.; Ekroos, K.; Salomaa, V.; Laaksonen, R. Circulating Ceramides Predict Cardiovascular Outcomes in the Population-Based FINRISK 2002 Cohort. *Arterioscler. Thromb. Vasc. Biol.* **2016**, *36*, 2424–2430.
7. Cremesti, A.E.; Fischl, A.S. Current methods for the identification and quantitation of ceramides: An overview. *Lipids* **2000**, *35*, 937–945. [PubMed]
8. Park, J.-W.; Park, W.-J.; Futerman, A.H. Ceramide synthases as potential targets for therapeutic intervention in human diseases. *Biochim. Biophys. Acta* **2014**, *1841*, 671–681.
9. Wattenberg, B.W. The long and the short of ceramides. *J. Biol. Chem.* **2018**, *293*, 9922–9923. [PubMed]
10. Bikman, B.T.; Summers, S.A. Ceramides as modulators of cellular and whole-body metabolism. *J. Clin. Investig.* **2011**, *121*, 4222–4230.
11. Bismuth, J.; Lin, P.; Yao, Q.; Chen, C. Ceramide: A common pathway for atherosclerosis? *Atherosclerosis* **2008**, *196*, 497–504.
12. Mundra, P.A.; Shaw, J.E.; Meikle, P.J. Lipidomic analyses in epidemiology. *Int. J. Epidemiol.* **2016**, *45*, 1329–1338.
13. Summers, S.A. Could Ceramides Become the New Cholesterol? *Cell Metab.* **2018**, *27*, 276–280. [PubMed]
14. Reedy, J.; Krebs-Smith, S.M.; Miller, P.E.; Liese, A.D.; Kahle, L.L.; Park, Y.; Subar, A.F. Higher diet quality is associated with decreased risk of all-cause, cardiovascular disease, and cancer mortality among older adults. *J. Nutr.* **2014**, *144*, 881–889.
15. Bergman, B.C.; Brozinick, J.T.; Strauss, A.; Bacon, S.; Kerege, A.; Bui, H.H.; Sanders, P.; Siddall, P.; Kuo, M.S.; Perreault, L. Serum sphingolipids: Relationships to insulin sensitivity and changes with exercise in humans. *Am. J. Physiol. Endocrinol. Metab.* **2015**, *309*, E398–E408.
16. Tarasov, K.; Ekroos, K.; Suoniemi, M.; Kauhanen, D.; Sylvänne, T.; Hurme, R.; Gouni-Berthold, I.; Berthold, H.K.; Kleber, M.E.; Laaksonen, R.; et al. Molecular lipids identify cardiovascular risk and are efficiently lowered by simvastatin and PCSK9 deficiency. *J. Clin. Endocrinol. Metab.* **2014**, *99*, E45–E52.
17. Ng, T.W.K.; Ooi, E.M.M.; Watts, G.F.; Chan, D.C.; Weir, J.M.; Meikle, P.J.; Barrett, P.H.R. Dose-dependent effects of rosuvastatin on the plasma sphingolipidome and phospholipidome in the metabolic syndrome. *J. Clin. Endocrinol. Metab.* **2014**, *99*, E2335–E2340.
18. Huang, H.; Kasumov, T.; Gatmaitan, P.; Heneghan, H.M.; Kashyap, S.R.; Schauer, P.R.; Brethauer, S.A.; Kirwan, J.P. Gastric bypass surgery reduces plasma ceramide subspecies and improves insulin sensitivity in severely obese patients. *Obesity* **2011**, *19*, 2235–2240.
19. Özer, H.; Aslan, İ.; Oruç, M.T.; Çöpelci, Y.; Afşar, E.; Kaya, S.; Aslan, M. Early postoperative changes of sphingomyelins and ceramides after laparoscopic sleeve gastrectomy. *Lipids Health Dis.* **2018**, *17*, 269.
20. Heilbronn, L.K.; Coster, A.C.F.; Campbell, L.V.; Greenfield, J.R.; Lange, K.; Christopher, M.J.; Meikle, P.J.; Samocha-Bonet, D. The effect of short-term overfeeding on serum lipids in healthy humans. *Obesity* **2013**, *21*, E649–E659.
21. Luukkonen, P.K.; Sädevirta, S.; Zhou, Y.; Kayser, B.; Ali, A.; Ahonen, L.; Lallukka, S.; Pelloux, V.; Gaggini, M.; Jian, C.; et al. Saturated Fat Is More Metabolically Harmful for the Human Liver Than Unsaturated Fat or Simple Sugars. *Diabetes Care* **2018**, *41*, 1732–1739.
22. Kien, C.L.; Bunn, J.Y.; Poynter, M.E.; Stevens, R.; Bain, J.; Ikayeva, O.; Fukagawa, N.K.; Champagne, C.M.; Crain, K.I.; Koves, T.R.; et al. A lipidomics analysis of the relationship between dietary fatty acid composition and insulin sensitivity in young adults. *Diabetes* **2013**, *62*, 1054–1063.
23. Wang, D.D.; Toledo, E.; Hruby, A.; Rosner, B.A.; Willett, W.C.; Sun, Q.; Razquin, C.; Zheng, Y.; Ruiz-Canela, M.; Guasch-Ferré, M.; et al. Plasma Ceramides, Mediterranean Diet, and Incident Cardiovascular Disease in the PREDIMED Trial. *Circulation* **2017**, *135*, 2028–2040.

24. Segal, L.M.; Rayburn, J.; Beck, S.E. *The State of Obesity: Better Policies for a Healthier America 2017*; Trust for America's Health, The Robert Wood Johnson Foundation: Washington, DC, USA, 2017; pp. 1–108. Available online: https://www.tfah.org/report-details/the-state-of-obesity-2017 (accessed on 16 April 2019).
25. Lee-Kwan, S.H.; Moore, L.V.; Blanck, H.M.; Harris, D.M.; Galuska, D. Disparities in State-Specific Adult Fruit and Vegetable Consumption—United States, 2015. *MMWR Morb. Mortal. Wkly. Rep.* **2017**, *66*, 1241–1247. [PubMed]
26. Harris, P.A.; Taylor, R.; Thielke, R.; Payne, J.; Gonzalez, N.; Conde, J.G. Research electronic data capture (REDCap)—A metadata-driven methodology and workflow process for providing translational research informatics support. *J. Biomed. Inform.* **2009**, *42*, 377–381.
27. Gutch, M.; Kumar, S.; Razi, S.M.; Gupta, K.K.; Gupta, A. Assessment of insulin sensitivity/resistance. *Indian J. Endocrinol. Metab.* **2015**, *19*, 160–164.
28. National Institute of Health Diabetes & Prediabetes Tests|NIDDK. Available online: https://www.niddk.nih.gov/health-information/diagnostic-tests/diabetes-prediabetes (accessed on 30 July 2018).
29. National Institute of Health. High Blood Pressure. Available online: http://www.nia.nih.gov/health/high-blood-pressure (accessed on 30 July 2018).
30. Grundy, S.M.; Bryan Brewer, J.H.; Cleeman, J.I.; Sidney, C.; Smith, J.; Lenfant, C. Definition of Metabolic Syndrome. *Circulation* **2004**, *109*, 433–438.
31. Ostchega, Y.; Nwankwo, T.; Sorlie, P.D.; Wolz, M.; Zipf, G. Assessing the validity of the Omron HEM-907XL oscillometric blood pressure measurement device in a National Survey environment. *J. Clin. Hypertens.* **2010**, *12*, 22–28.
32. Viera, A.J.; Zhu, S.; Hinderliter, A.L.; Shimbo, D.; Person, S.D.; Jacobs, D.R. Diurnal blood pressure pattern and development of prehypertension or hypertension in young adults: The CARDIA study. *J. Am. Soc. Hypertens.* **2011**, *5*, 48–55.
33. World Health Organization. *Waist Circumference and Waist-Hip Ratio: Report of a WHO Expert Consultation, Geneva, 8–11 December 2008*; vi; World Health Organization: Geneva, Switzerland, 2008; ISBN 978-92-4-150149-1.
34. U.S. Department of Health and Human Services and U.S. Department of Agriculture 2015–2020 Dietary Guidelines for Americans—health.gov. Available online: https://health.gov/dietaryguidelines/2015/ (accessed on 27 June 2018).
35. Nutrition Coordination Center (NCC), University of Minnesota. Guide to Creating Variables, Needed to Calculate Scores for Each Component of the Healthy Eating Index-2015 (HEI-2015). Available online: http://www.ncc.umn.edu/ndsrsupport/hei2015.pdf (accessed on 16 August 2017).
36. National Cancer Institute Division of Cancer Control and Population Sciences. The Healthy Eating Index Research Uses: Overview of the Methods & Calculations. Available online: https://epi.grants.cancer.gov/hei/hei-methods-and-calculations.html (accessed on 2 July 2018).
37. Rico, J.E.; Bandaru, V.V.R.; Dorskind, J.M.; Haughey, N.J.; McFadden, J.W. Plasma ceramides are elevated in overweight Holstein dairy cows experiencing greater lipolysis and insulin resistance during the transition from late pregnancy to early lactation. *J. Dairy Sci.* **2015**, *98*, 7757–7770. [PubMed]
38. Haughey, N.J.; Cutler, R.G.; Tamara, A.; McArthur, J.C.; Vargas, D.L.; Pardo, C.A.; Turchan, J.; Nath, A.; Mattson, M.P. Perturbation of sphingolipid metabolism and ceramide production in HIV-dementia. *Ann. Neurol.* **2004**, *55*, 257–267. [PubMed]
39. Meikle, P.J.; Wong, G.; Barlow, C.K.; Weir, J.M.; Greeve, M.A.; MacIntosh, G.L.; Almasy, L.; Comuzzie, A.G.; Mahaney, M.C.; Kowalczyk, A.; et al. Plasma lipid profiling shows similar associations with prediabetes and type 2 diabetes. *PLoS ONE* **2013**, *8*, e74341.
40. Mayo Clinic. *Plasma Ceramides: A Novel Biomarker of Unstable Atherosclerotic Cardiovascular Disease*; Mayo Foundation for Medical Education and Research: Rochester, MN, USA, 2016; pp. 1–4. Available online: https://cdn.prod-carehubs.net/n1/96e99366cea7b0de/uploads/2016/07/ceramides-brochure-final-0616.pdf (accessed on 16 April 2019).
41. Lankinen, M.; Schwab, U.; Kolehmainen, M.; Paananen, J.; Nygren, H.; Seppänen-Laakso, T.; Poutanen, K.; Hyötyläinen, T.; Risérus, U.; Savolainen, M.J.; et al. A Healthy Nordic Diet Alters the Plasma Lipidomic Profile in Adults with Features of Metabolic Syndrome in a Multicenter Randomized Dietary Intervention. *J. Nutr.* **2016**, *146*, 662–672.

42. Mielke, M.M.; Bandaru, V.V.R.; Han, D.; An, Y.; Resnick, S.M.; Ferrucci, L.; Haughey, N.J. Demographic and clinical variables affecting mid- to late-life trajectories of plasma ceramide and dihydroceramide species. *Aging Cell* **2015**, *14*, 1014–1023. [PubMed]
43. Mantovani, A.; Bonapace, S.; Lunardi, G.; Salgarello, M.; Dugo, C.; Canali, G.; Byrne, C.D.; Gori, S.; Barbieri, E.; Targher, G. Association between plasma ceramides and inducible myocardial ischemia in patients with established or suspected coronary artery disease undergoing myocardial perfusion scintigraphy. *Metabolism* **2018**, *85*, 305–312. [PubMed]
44. Haus, J.M.; Kashyap, S.R.; Kasumov, T.; Zhang, R.; Kelly, K.R.; Defronzo, R.A.; Kirwan, J.P. Plasma ceramides are elevated in obese subjects with type 2 diabetes and correlate with the severity of insulin resistance. *Diabetes* **2009**, *58*, 337–343.
45. Ichi, I.; Nakahara, K.; Miyashita, Y.; Hidaka, A.; Kutsukake, S.; Inoue, K.; Maruyama, T.; Miwa, Y.; Harada-Shiba, M.; Tsushima, M.; et al. Association of ceramides in human plasma with risk factors of atherosclerosis. *Lipids* **2006**, *41*, 859–863. [PubMed]
46. Peterson, L.R.; Xanthakis, V.; Duncan, M.S.; Gross, S.; Friedrich, N.; Völzke, H.; Felix, S.B.; Jiang, H.; Sidhu, R.; Nauck, M.; et al. Ceramide Remodeling and Risk of Cardiovascular Events and Mortality. *J. Am. Heart Assoc.* **2018**, *7*, e007931. [PubMed]
47. Chaurasia, B.; Summers, S.A. Ceramides—Lipotoxic Inducers of Metabolic Disorders. *Trends Endocrinol. Metab. TEM* **2015**, *26*, 538–550.
48. Boden, G. Obesity and Free Fatty Acids (FFA). *Endocrinol. Metab. Clin. N. Am.* **2008**, *37*, 635–646.
49. Fucho, R.; Casals, N.; Serra, D.; Herrero, L. Ceramides and mitochondrial fatty acid oxidation in obesity. *FASEB J.* **2017**, *31*, 1263–1272. [PubMed]
50. Iqbal, J.; Walsh, M.T.; Hammad, S.M.; Hussain, M.M. Sphingolipids and Lipoproteins in Health and Metabolic Disorders. *Trends Endocrinol. Metab. TEM* **2017**, *28*, 506–518.
51. Loprinzi, P.D.; Branscum, A.; Hanks, J.; Smit, E. Healthy Lifestyle Characteristics and Their Joint Association with Cardiovascular Disease Biomarkers in US Adults. *Mayo Clin. Proc.* **2016**, *91*, 432–442. [PubMed]
52. Schwingshackl, L.; Bogensberger, B.; Hoffmann, G. Diet Quality as Assessed by the Healthy Eating Index, Alternate Healthy Eating Index, Dietary Approaches to Stop Hypertension Score, and Health Outcomes: An Updated Systematic Review and Meta-Analysis of Cohort Studies. *J. Acad. Nutr. Diet.* **2018**, *118*, 74–100.e11. [PubMed]

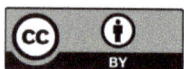

© 2019 by the authors. Licensee MDPI, Basel, Switzerland. This article is an open access article distributed under the terms and conditions of the Creative Commons Attribution (CC BY) license (http://creativecommons.org/licenses/by/4.0/).

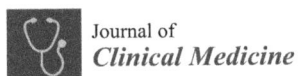

Review

Classic and Novel Biomarkers as Potential Predictors of Ventricular Arrhythmias and Sudden Cardiac Death

Zornitsa Shomanova [1], Bernhard Ohnewein [2], Christiane Schernthaner [2], Killian Höfer [2], Christian A. Pogoda [1], Gerrit Frommeyer [3], Bernhard Wernly [2], Mathias C. Brandt [2], Anna-Maria Dieplinger [4], Holger Reinecke [1], Uta C. Hoppe [2], Bernhard Strohmer [2], Rudin Pistulli [1,†] and Lukas J. Motloch [2,†,*]

1. Department of Cardiology I, Coronary and Peripheral Vascular Disease, Heart Failure, University Hospital Muenster, Albert Schweitzer Campus 1, A1, 48149 Muenster, Germany; zornitsa.shomanova@ukmuenster.de (Z.S.); christian.pogoda@ukmuenster.de (C.A.P.); holger.reinecke@ukmuenster.de (H.R.); rudin.pistulli@ukmuenster.de (R.P.)
2. Clinic II for Internal Medicine, Paracelsus Medical University, Muellner Hauptstrasse 48, 5020 Salzburg, Austria; b.ohnewein@salk.at (B.O.); c.schernthaner@salk.at (C.S.); k.hoefer@salk.at (K.H.); b.wernly@salk.at (B.W.); m.brandt@salk.at (M.C.B.); u.hoppe@salk.at (U.C.H.); b.strohmer@salk.at (B.S.)
3. Department of Cardiology II, Electrophysiology, University Hospital Muenster, Albert-Schweitzer-Campus 1, A1, D-48149 Muenster, Germany; gerrit.frommeyer@ukmuenster.de
4. Institute for Nursing and Practice, Paracelsus Medical University, Muellner Strubergasse 21, 5020 Salzburg, Austria; anna.dieplinger@pmu.ac.at
* Correspondence: lukas.motloch@stud.pmu.ac.at
† These authors contributed equally to this work.

Received: 31 January 2020; Accepted: 14 February 2020; Published: 20 February 2020

Abstract: Sudden cardiac death (SCD), most often induced by ventricular arrhythmias, is one of the main reasons for cardiovascular-related mortality. While coronary artery disease remains the leading cause of SCD, other pathologies like cardiomyopathies and, especially in the younger population, genetic disorders, are linked to arrhythmia-related mortality. Despite many efforts to enhance the efficiency of risk-stratification strategies, effective tools for risk assessment are still missing. Biomarkers have a major impact on clinical practice in various cardiac pathologies. While classic biomarkers like brain natriuretic peptide (BNP) and troponins are integrated into daily clinical practice, inflammatory biomarkers may also be helpful for risk assessment. Indeed, several trials investigated their application for the prediction of arrhythmic events indicating promising results. Furthermore, in recent years, active research efforts have brought forward an increasingly large number of "novel and alternative" candidate markers of various pathophysiological origins. Investigations of these promising biological compounds have revealed encouraging results when evaluating the prediction of arrhythmic events. To elucidate this issue, we review current literature dealing with this topic. We highlight the potential of "classic" but also "novel" biomarkers as promising tools for arrhythmia prediction, which in the future might be integrated into clinical practice.

Keywords: sudden cardiac death; ventricular arrhythmia; ventricular tachycardia; biomarkers; cardiac biomarkers; heart failure

1. Introduction

According to the World Health Organization, cardiovascular disease (CVD) is the number one cause of death. Around 18 million people died of cardiac causes in 2016, accounting for over 30% of all mortality worldwide [1]. Sudden cardiac death (SCD), most often induced by ventricular arrhythmias, is one of the main reasons for CVD-related deaths. Coronary artery disease (CAD) remains the leading cause of SCD with up to 80% of all patients suffering from SCD. Cardiomyopathies like dilated cardiomyopathy account for around 15% of the SCD population, while especially in younger populations genetic disorders are overrepresented [2,3]. Consequently, high-risk populations have been identified, one of the most prominent being heart failure with reduced left ventricular ejection fraction (HFrEF) [4].

Even in this high-risk population, which is prone to develop malignant episodes of ventricular arrhythmias with consecutive SCD [5], antiarrhythmic drug therapy often increases or at best has a neutral effect on cardiac-related mortality [6]. With the beginning of the implantable cardiac defibrillator (ICD) era, a new effective tool for prevention of SCD was available. Indeed, the MADIT- and SCDHEFT trials showed high therapeutic primary prevention efficiency in a high-risk population [7,8]. Patients with severe reduced left ventricular function with ischemic but also with non-ischemic etiology presented a reduced overall mortality after ICD implantation. Based on such promising data, ICD therapy for the prevention of SCD is considered a class I indication in patients with severe impaired left ventricular ejection fraction (LVEF < 35%) [9].

Of note, device therapy is designed to convert tachyarrhythmias following their onset. Therefore, it does not cure the arrhythmogenic disorder. On the other hand, inappropriate ICD-mediated shocks can substantially reduce patients' quality of life by causing a variety of psychopathological disorders [10]. To add insult to injury, device therapy is associated with frequent surgical complications as well as device and lead failures [11]. Consequently, a significant number of patients receive ICD therapy without any benefit, while suffering adverse events. Therefore, improvements in risk stratification for SCD remain one of the main goals in daily clinical practice. Nevertheless, despite many efforts to enhance the efficiency of risk-stratification strategies by application of electrocardiogram (ECG) parameters, genetic testing, measurements of the autonomic nervous system and novel imaging tools like magnetic resonance imaging (MRI), up to date confirmation of severe LVEF reduction seems to be the only efficient tool [12]. However, while the majority of SCD patients present with preserved left ventricular ejection fraction, this strategy shows a low sensitivity in the general population.

Ventricular tachyarrhythmias are caused by different pathophysiological mechanisms including enhanced automaticity, triggered activity and/or reentry [13,14]. The first two are provoked by cellular phenomena. Enhanced automaticity is characterized by an acceleration of the spontaneous firing rate of the action potential. Consequently, increased automaticity of ventricular myocytes can lead to irregular activation patterns of the myocardium. Triggered activity is characterized by calcium-mediated premature action potentials that arise from early or delayed afterdepolarizations. On the other hand, the most common mechanism of cardiac reentry is a multicellular process involving excitation wave fronts that propagate around zones with impaired conduction and refractory tissue.

These pro-arrhythmic effects are caused by electrophysiological remodeling processes with consequent impaired heterogeneity of cardiac ion channel expression and function within the different regions and layers of the heart. Furthermore, fibrotic processes influence the electrophysiological characteristics of the cardiomyocyte and have a major impact on cardiac conduction [13,14]. All these processes are presented in major cardiac pathologies with increased risk of ventricular arrhythmias, including heart failure (HF) and cardiac ischemia, as well as inherited arrhythmogenic disorders like hypertrophic cardiomyopathy (HCM), arrhythmogenic right ventricular dysplasia (ARVD) or Brugada syndrome. Of note, these mechanisms are often modulated or/and induced by different processes like myocardial necrosis, inflammation, myocardial stress or neurohormonal activation with the involvement of various biological signal proteins. While these proteins are often released during signaling processes, their levels can be measured in patient serum as indicator of signaling activation. Consequently, they can be useful for characterization of normal or pathogenic processes of the heart including electrophysiological remodeling. Indeed, biomarkers have become a useful tool, which refers to a broad subcategory of quantifiable and reproducible characteristics of biological signs. Therefore, they can and should be used for cardiac risk stratification.

Indeed, since the incorporation of aspartate transaminase in the diagnosis of acute myocardial infarction (MI) in the late 1950s, the predictive value of cardiac biomarkers has been an important field of ongoing research. Consequently, "classic" cardiac biomarkers like BNP or troponin, but also inflammatory biomarkers like C-reactive protein (CRP) or high-sensitive (hsCRP), have improved general diagnostic efficiency in various cardiovascular diseases like CAD or HF [15]. This leads to their broad clinical implication in the cardiovascular field. In addition, emerging biomarkers and further on the horizon of categories like myocardial necrosis, inflammation, plaque instability, platelet activation, myocardial stress and neurohormonal activation were investigated in recent years. Indeed, "novel" cardiac biomarkers, like the soluble suppression of tumorigenicity 2 (sST2) protein, have been uncovered as additional tools to improve the management of cardiac disease [16].

While focusing on cardiac arrhythmias, various studies have already explored the implication of the "classic" biomarkers in risk stratification of ventricular arrhythmias and SCD indicating promising results. Furthermore, recent trials have also focused on the potential of the application of "novel" cardiac biomarkers in this clinically important field. However, to the best of our knowledge, research results were not reviewed, yet.

Therefore, in this review we will summarize how biomarkers of cardiac and non-cardiac origin might help predict the risk of ventricular cardiac arrhythmias in different risk populations. Furthermore, besides the potential clinical implication of the "classic" cardiac biomarkers, we review recent results, which investigated the implication of "novel" cardiac biomarkers as potential predictors of fatal ventricular arrhythmias. Of note, further investigations in this exciting field might be translated into novel risk assessment approaches in the future.

2. 'Classic' Inflammatory Biomarkers as Potential Predictors of Ventricular Arrhythmias

Inflammation is known to play a pivotal role in the pathophysiology of atherosclerosis with consequent CVD. Consequently, "classic" inflammatory biomarkers like CRP and interleukins have been already evaluated in the setting of coronary heart disease [17]. Indeed, chronic inflammation and thrombosis can transform a stable atherosclerotic plaque to an unstable lesion [17]. While CAD is one of the main risk factors for SCD, an association between classic markers of inflammation and malignant ventricular arrhythmias was already investigated in various clinical trials [18]. This topic will be discussed in the following chapter.

2.1. C-Reactive Protein (CRP) and High-Sensitive (hs) CRP

Initially discovered as a pathogenic factor, CRP has been known in medicine since 1930. Nowadays CRP is understood to be an inflammatory acute-phase protein, of which levels increase in case of injury or infection. In humans, it is mainly produced in the liver following increased levels of interleukin 6 (IL-6). Furthermore, it is also released by smooth muscle cells of the aorta as well as by fat tissue [19]. The role of CRP in the development of atherosclerotic plaques is well established [20]. CRP stimulates the absorption of low-density lipoprotein (LDL) in the macrophages of endothelial cells, thus contributing to the progression of atherosclerotic plaques and their conversion from stable to unstable condition. This can cause coronary plaque rupture with following ventricular arrhythmias (ventricular tachycardia/ventricular fibrillation (VT/VF)) with consequent SCD [21]. Inflammation, on the other hand, induces structural remodeling of the heart, which promotes an arrhythmogenic substrate [22,23].

Furthermore, inflammation plays an important role in the pathology of ischemic heart disease and HF. Therefore, it is easy to speculate a link between inflammatory markers and CAD or/and HF related arrhythmias. Consequently, previous investigations focused on the association between CRP and/or high-sensitive CRP (CRP assessed by a more sensitive assay to estimate the risk of CAD) and ventricular arrhythmias related to ischemic heart disease or/and ischemic HF. Although the link between inflammation and (ventricular) arrhythmias via ischemic heart disease seems well documented, the question remains whether these inflammatory markers are directly related to the intrinsic pathomechanisms of these malignant events.

The association of inflammatory markers including CRP with MI and SCD has been described in several epidemiological studies. During a follow-up of 13 years of 5888 elderly subjects (aged over 65 years) baseline levels of CRP but also interleukin 6 (IL-6) were linked to the long-term risk of SCD [24]. Similar results were observed in 9758 middle-aged men, when CRP, IL-6 and fibrinogen plasma levels were linked to MI-related death. Nevertheless, in this trial only increased IL-6 levels were found to be an independent risk factor [25]. Further investigations focused on the incidence of ventricular arrhythmias during the acute phase of MI. Hodzic and colleagues observed a positive correlation with increased troponin, but also with CRP [26].

The levels of CRP were also investigated in patients carrying ICDs. Of note, this population at risk has a reliable rhythm monitoring due to the implanted devices. As it turns out, an association between the occurrence of VT/VF with increased serum CRP levels was also described in these patients [27,28].

Furthermore, CRP levels were also investigated in patients with purely non-CAD related arrhythmogenic disorders. A study investigated inflammatory markers in patients with arrhythmogenic right-ventricular dysplasia (ARVD). This inherited rare cardiomyopathy is characterized by scar formation in the right ventricle favoring the incidence of malignant ventricular arrhythmias. When compared to another group of patients with idiopathic right outflow VT, ARVD patients had significantly higher levels of serum CRP. Also, within the ARVD group, Bonny and colleagues observed increased serum levels of CRP 24 h after VT incidence. Interestingly, infiltrates of T lymphocytes were found in myocardial biopsies of ARVD patients, thus suggesting a mechanistic link between inflammatory markers, inflammation and arrhythmias [29]. Other interesting results were described in patients experiencing torsade de pointes (TdP) tachycardia. Of note, this malignant arrhythmia is often promoted by QT-interval prolongation on ECG. Interestingly, CRP elevation corresponded to QT-Interval prolongation. Consequently, the authors speculated that inflammatory cytokines might influence ion channel function with consequent alteration of the QT interval [30].

High-sensitivity C-reactive protein (hsCRP) assays can detect CRP concentrations much lower than conventional CRP assays (down to < 0.04 mg/L). Therefore, they facilitate the detection of low-grade inflammation [31,32]. For this reason, several studies investigating CRP as a potential predictive risk factor for SCD used hsCRP assays for estimation of low-grade inflammatory activity.

The prognostic value of hsCRP for the occurrence of SCD has been evaluated in an epidemiological trial. In healthy men, increased baseline hsCRP levels were associated with a 2.8-fold increased risk of SCD, thus indicating the possibility using this inflammatory marker for identifying high-risk patients [21]. Further trials focused on patients with implanted ICD. Of note, when investigated in patient cohorts following ICD implantation (for primary or secondary prevention), baseline hsCRP levels in patients with appropriate ICD therapy were significantly higher compared to those without ICD therapy. This relationship consisted during the follow-up of 24 months. A baseline hsCRP >3 mg/L was independently associated with appropriate ICD therapy. In contrast, baseline levels of brain natriuretic peptide (BNP) did not show such association, although an increase of BNP during follow-up was significantly associated with appropriate ICD therapy [33]. Blangy and colleagues reported increased levels of BNP and hsCRP in patients experiencing VT amongst 121 ICD patients with history of otherwise stable CAD and a prior history of MI [34]. Furthermore, when investigated in 100 patients with structural heart disease (ischemic or idiopathic dilated cardiomyopathy) who experienced electrical storms compared to those with single episodes of VT/VF or without ICD intervention, higher baseline, hsCRP but also IL-6 and NT-proBNP levels were reported [35].

On the other hand, despite the above evidence regarding hsCRP as a risk predictor of malignant arrhythmias and SCD, some studies did not find such an association. Indeed, in a multicenter prospective observational study performed in 268 patients after MI (>30 days) and LVEF ≤30%, who were indicated for ICD- or cardiac resynchronization therapy-defibrillator (CRT-D)-implantation, no correlation between the occurrence of SCD and/or VT/VF and increased hsCRP was observed (follow-up of two years). Nevertheless, increased hsCRP levels were associated with all-cause mortality, death due to HF and first hospitalization for HF. Therefore, the authors suggested that increased hsCRP levels might predict SCD only in low cardiovascular risk populations [36]. In accordance with this suggestion, Konstantinos et al. found no significant difference in levels of hsCRP, IL-6, tumor necrosis factor alpha (TNF-α) and BNP in stable HF with implanted ICD when comparing patients with ventricular tachyarrhythmia to the arrhythmia free population [37].

A further study investigated hsCRP levels in dialysis patients. These patients commonly have several risk factors for SCD, such as atherosclerosis, left-ventricular hypertrophy with associated fibrosis and endothelial dysfunction. Therefore, they represent a special group with increased risk of SCD. Indeed. Parekhand and colleagues reported higher levels of hsCRP and IL-6 as potential predictors of SCD in this population. Of note, higher levels of these biomarkers were associated with twice the risk of SCD (follow-up of 9.5 years) when compared to patients with lower levels [38].

2.2. Interleukin 6 (IL-6)

The cytokine IL-6 is a small signaling protein with inflammatory properties. It is an important mediator of the acute phase response. In atherosclerosis, IL-6 is produced by macrophages in atherosclerotic plaques. Furthermore, it is released by visceral adipose tissue and in the sub-endothelial space. Of note, IL-6 causes an increase of CRP-levels and starts the inflammation cascade [39,40].

As already mentioned above, there is data indicating the predictive role of IL-6 for the occurrence of SCD in epidemiological trials [24,25]. Furthermore, its association with ventricular arrhythmias has been also observed in patients with established CAD. Safranow et al. investigated the interaction between inflammation, metabolic syndrome and arrhythmias in 167 CAD patients. CRP and IL-6 were found to be independent predictors of symptoms of advanced CAD including the incidence of ventricular arrhythmias. The occurrence of metabolic syndrome was strongly related to IL-6. This observation was linked to the contribution of the inflammatory biomarkers in the evolution of insulin resistance, leading to manifestation of metabolic syndrome. Regarding episodes of VT or/and VF, the investigators found a strong association with increased IL-6 and CRP levels. The authors speculated that inflammatory biomarkers could be involved in the transformation of the atherosclerotic plaques into instable lesions, leading to ischemia and respective malignant arrhythmias [40].

As already pointed out above, data on the predictive value of IL-6 in the ICD population is controversial [35,37]. Nevertheless, Streitner and colleagues reported promising results. In 47 patients with implanted ICD (ischemic or dilated cardiomyopathy), significantly higher IL-6 levels were reported at baseline and during follow-up (nine months) in patients experiencing arrhythmic episodes. Indeed, elevated IL-6 serum concentrations were associated with a higher risk of spontaneous VT/VF events [41]. These observations were reassured by the results presented by Cheng and colleagues who investigated a multimarker approach [42]. Nevertheless, this trial will be discussed in the following chapter.

3. 'Classic' Cardiac Biomarkers as Potential Predictors of Ventricular Arrhythmias

The use of biological markers has been able to improve the accuracy of diagnosis and therapy in cardiovascular patients. In various cardiovascular pathologies, this approach promotes stratification of cardiovascular risk, both during the hospitalization period and the long-term observation period. Indeed, levels of several biomarkers indicate the incidence of malignant cardiovascular events, reflect the dynamics of disease and enhance the efficacy of therapy regimes. "Classic" biomarkers like Troponins are well integrated clinical tools in identifying cardiac damage, but also correlate with the long-term outcome of cardiac patients [43]. The serum level of BNP, a protein secreted by cardiomyocytes during cardiac stress, constitutes a tool already routinely applied in the diagnosis and monitoring of HF patients [44].

Therefore, the role of the described "classic" biomarkers was already extensively investigated in various cardiac pathologies. Interestingly, in the past, several studies dealing with diverse cardiac pathologies associated with ventricular arrhythmias have also focused on their potential role for the prediction of these malignant disorders. These investigations revealed promising results [45].

Consequently, this chapter will focus on the clinical potential of "classic" cardiac biomarkers BNP and NT-proBNP as well as Troponins in dealing with malignant ventricular arrhythmias.

3.1. Brain Natriuretic Peptides (BNP and Non-Terminal (NT)-proBNP)

The pre-pro brain natriuretic peptide (pre-proBNP) is a hormone consisting of 134 amino acids, released by ventricular cardiomyocytes during mechanical stress situations like increased volume, stretch and hypertrophy. A part of this protein (consisting of 108 amino acids) splits from the pre-proBNP molecule, resulting in the prohormone BNP (proBNP). ProBNP is further split into two molecules: the biologically active BNP (32 amino acids) and the inactive non-terminal (NT)-proBNP (76 amino acids). NT-proBNP circulates longer in the blood (and thus has a higher concentration) compared to BNP, making it easier to measure in laboratory tests. BNP induces vessel dilation and diuresis, thus reducing preload and afterload, and consequently reducing myocardial stress. It is eliminated by binding to cells expressing BNP-receptors, while NT-proBNP is eliminated through the kidneys. Therefore, patients with renal disease have increased NT-proBNP levels, making its clinical interpretation significantly more difficult. Both BNP and NT-proBNP are established biomarkers of structural heart conditions. Interestingly, their association with ventricular arrhythmias and SCD was also investigated in various trials, while in their elegant meta-analysis Scott and colleagues already highlighted its application in HF patients [46]. Furthermore, novel trials investigated the potential application for risk stratification of ventricular arrhythmogenic disorders when combined with "novel" cardiac biomarkers. However, these studies will be discussed in the next chapter of this review dealing with "novel" biomarker candidates.

Several studies have found an association between increased BNP levels and the occurrence of malignant ventricular arrhythmias or/and SCD [47–49]. Furthermore, in their elegant study performed in 521 patients following acute MI, Tapanainen and colleagues elucidated that besides low LVEF, also increased levels of BNP are significant predictors of SCD. Interestingly, the SCD survival curves of patients with and without BNP elevation started to diverge at 20 months after MI, with the split further increasing during the 43 months of follow-up. Consequently, the authors speculated that BNP would indicate ventricular stretch, hypertrophy and fibrosis, which in the long run induce tissue fibrosis and other arrhythmia-related changes of the myocardium. Therefore, BNP could play a role as an indirect predictor of malignant ventricular arrhythmias, as it reflects malignant electrophysiological remodeling processes [50].

Another research group investigated the role of BNP levels in predicting SCD in a high-risk population of 452 patients with HFrEF. During a follow-up of three years, the authors were able to identify BNP as an independent predictor of SCD. In line with Tapanainen and colleagues, they also speculated BNP levels reflect the stage of cardiac remodeling, since the release of this hormone is provoked by similar etiologies, which promote this pathophysiological process (stretch, increased intraventricular pressure etc.) [51]. These results were confirmed by further investigations. Indeed, Watanabe and colleagues found an increased risk of SCD in HFrEF patients when increased BNP levels were combined with left ventricular impairment and dilation parameters as well as non-sustained VTs and diabetes [52]. Furthermore, in this same context, various smaller single-center studies observed potential value of increased BNP levels when used for the prediction of ventricular tachyarrhythmias in the ICD HFrEF population [28,34,53–56].

There is also evidence that if effective HF therapies can lower BNP, it translates to a better prognosis in terms of malignant ventricular arrhythmias and SCD. Such was the case in the MADIT-CRT study. Effective CRT-D therapy was able to reduce BNP levels after one year. Patients, whose BNP levels were reduced by more than one-third of the baseline value, had a significantly lower risk of subsequent VT/VF or death. The authors suggested that cardiac resynchronization probably led to reverse ventricular remodeling, which in turn reduced the risk of malignant arrhythmias [53].

Based on the promising results described above, it would be tempting to link BNP to specific mechanisms of ventricular arrhythmias, such as the prolongation of the membrane action potential. Of note, in HF this pathology leads to prolonged QTc on ECG with consequent increased risk of VTs and SCD. Vrtovec and his group investigated this exciting topic. In SCD patients, they observed an association between increased levels of BNP and prolonged QTc. Because QT interval is mainly affected by ventricular repolarization, the authors hypothesized that patients with elevated BNP may develop prolonged action potential duration and therefore QT-interval prolongation. They speculated additional BNP induced alterations on a cellular level. Consequently, the authors suggested BNP regulates cardiac calcium metabolism leading to increased calcium entry with resulting electrophysiological abnormalities and ventricular tachyarrhythmias [57].

Further investigations focused on the application of BNP levels in inherited arrhythmogenic disorders such as HCM. This inherited condition is characterized by severe ventricular hypertrophy with or without left outflow obstruction leading to cardiac stress with particularly increased risk of SCD. Consequently, risk stratification in this population is one of the main clinical objectives. Two research groups from Japan investigated the prognostic potential of elevated BNP in HCM patients revealing promising results. Indeed, elevated cTnI but also BNP levels were associated with an increased risk of the incidence of cardiovascular events including VT. Interestingly, combination of both was able to boost the predictive value when compared to a single-marker approach [58]. Minami and colleagues could confirm this observation. The authors observed also a relationship between increased BNP levels and SCD in this population ($n = 346$) indicating BNP as a promising tool for the prediction of malignant arrhythmic events in this inherited arrhythmogenic pathology [59].

Based on its longer half-life and higher concentrations in the peripheral blood (compared to BNP), NT-proBNP is the cardiac marker commonly used to diagnose and control the progression of HF in the daily clinical practice. In accordance with the results described above for BNP and already summarized in the meta-analysis by Scott and colleagues [46], various investigations presented also promising results for NT-proBNP, when applied as predictor of SCD in the HF population.

Elevated intraventricular volume and pressure eventually leads to dilation of the left atrium (LA). Whether such a dilation of LA also has a predictive role for SCD was the research topic of a study group from Spain. In 494 HF patients Bayes-Genis et al. found that, the combination of both increased LA size (>26 mm/m^2) and NT-proBNP (>908 ng/L) was associated with an eight-fold increased risk of SCD, resulting in a 25% risk of this event in the follow-up period of 36 months. Consequently, the authors suggested a high specificity of this approach, although the underlying mechanisms for their observations remain unknown [60].

Indeed, higher NT-proBNP levels seem to be associated with increased occurrence of ventricular arrhythmias and/or SCD in patients with HF due to ischemic and non-ischemic etiology [61,62]. However, there is yet insufficient evidence, whether any cardiac biomarker qualifies as a powerful risk predictor for malignant arrhythmias and/or SCD in this population. Nevertheless, prediction of these malignant events in HF patients is one of the main objectives of present translational research. In an ideal clinical scenario, the decision whether a prophylactic ICD implantation is indicated in HF patients, should depend on their assessed risk of malignant arrhythmias and/or SCD. As of today, HF patients undergo prophylactic ICD implantation based on present cardiac societies' guidelines (HF symptoms combined with a significantly reduced LVEF). Therefore, in order to investigate an additive application of biomarkers in this population, several biomarker studies (including NT-proBNP) tested their potential as predictors of mortality and/or arrhythmias following ICD-implantation, with encouraging results [35,63–67]. Notably, arrhythmic events are easy to monitor in this population, due to the implanted device systems. In one of the larger studies, Cheng and colleagues investigated 1189 patients with HFrEF following ICD implantation for primary prevention of SCD. During a follow-up period of four years, 137 patients had appropriate ICD shocks while 343 patients suffered from death for various reasons. Nevertheless, in this study only higher IL-6 levels were able to predict the occurrence of appropriate ICD shocks while all investigated biomarkers (CRP, IL-6, TNF-α, NT-proBNP and troponin T) presented a higher risk of all-cause mortality. Therefore, based on their results, the investigators suggested a combined biomarker score reflecting all-cause mortality, in order to identify patients who are unlikely to benefit from primary prevention through ICD [42].

Following out-of-hospital resuscitation, measured NT-proBNP show distinguishing properties between underlying ischemic und non-ischemic heart disease, as well as in terms of survival of patients. Aarsetøy and colleagues investigated the application of serum copeptin and hscTnT but also NT-proBNP in the event of SCD. They collected blood samples from 77 patients following out-of-hospital resuscitation due to VF, and observed promising results for NT-proBNP. Of note, the biomarker was significantly higher in patients with heart disease without MI and in non-survivors compared to survivors, which also in this population supports the hypothesis of its predictive value [68].

Because NT-proBNP, in contrast to BNP, undergoes renal elimination, its serum levels are also increased due to renal dysfunction [69]. Therefore, several studies focused on NT-proBNP in patients with kidney disease. An association was found between SCD and elevated NT-proBNP, but also cTnI levels, in hemodialysis patients [70–72]. However, different cut-off serum levels were suggested. Winkler et al. concluded serum levels over 9252 pg/mL being predictive of SCD (two-fold increased risk) [72], while Kruzan et al. proposed a cut-off > 7350 pg/mL (three-fold higher risk of SCD) [71]. Of note, this group also observed a higher predictive value for NT-proBNP than for cTnI. The authors speculated that volume overload with consequent ventricular stretching, may drive NT-proBNP elevation. Nevertheless, they did not exclude decreased renal clearance as a potential reason for the NT-proBNP elevation in this patient group [71]. On the other hand, when measuring levels of NT-proBNP during a four-year follow-up in dialysis patients with type 2 diabetes mellitus, Winkler et al. were able to identify subgroups of patients with increased risk of SCD. Of note, patients with higher baseline NT-proBNP, which decreased over 10 percent in the follow-up measurements, had lower adjusted relative risk of SCD than patients with stable levels [72].

Some further research was performed in patients with HCM. Nevertheless, when investigated in 847 HCM patients, NT-proBNP levels were a significant predictor of HF and transplant-related deaths but not for SCD or appropriate ICD shocks [73]. Similar findings were revealed by Rajter-Salwa and his group who investigated the relationship between biomarkers (hs-TnI and NT-proBNP) and the calculated five-year risk score for SCD in 46 HCM patients [9]. Notably, no difference between patients with higher and lower NT-proBNP levels was noted, indicating NT-proBNP to be a poor predictor of ventricular arrhythmogenic events in the HCM population [74].

As previously mentioned, as an established biomarker in management of HF, NT-proBNP seems also to be an additive useful tool, when applied for risk stratification for ventricular arrhythmias or/and SCD in this population. Nevertheless, promising results were also revealed when applied in the "healthy" population. Of note, NT-proBNP levels seem to be associated with increased frequency of ventricular ectopy [75,76]. Furthermore, when investigated in a prospective case-control study in 32,828 healthy nurses (Nurse Health Study), an association between NT-proBNP at baseline and the risk of SCD during 16 years of follow-up was observed. NT-proBNP levels over the cut-off of 389 pg/mL had a five-fold increased risk of SCD, indicating even in the "healthy" population a potential value of this biomarker [77].

3.2. Troponins

The troponin complex includes three subunits and is positioned on the thin filaments of the striated muscles. These subunits are troponin T (TnT), troponin I (TnI) and troponin C (TnC). TnT is a protein, which connects the troponin complex with tropomyosin. TnI controls the binding of actin with myosin. The role of TnC is to connect tropomyosin with calcium. While TnC has the same structure in both the skeletal and heart muscle, in the heart TnT and I have different amino acid compositions. Thus, both cardiac troponins (cTnI and cTnT) can be identified in the blood as specific biomarkers of the heart. Of note, assays for high-sensitivity (hs) Troponins provide a more sensitive measurement allowing the detection of lower concentrations [78]. Therefore, they are implicated in daily clinical practice.

Cardiac troponins (cTnT and cTnI) are biomarkers of myocardial injury mostly released during necrotic processes often caused by myocardial ischemia. Necrosis promotes the replacement of cardiac myocytes with fibrotic tissue as well as further electrophysiological remodeling which predispose ventricular arrhythmias with eventual SCD. However, necrosis is not the only cause for Troponin release. A small free pool of TnT is situated in the cytosol. Therefore, prolonged leakage might be observed during the degeneration of myofilaments in irreversibly injured cells [79]. Besides being markers of cardiac damage, several studies investigated the application of levels of Troponins as potential tools in the risk assessment of malignant arrhythmias.

Indeed, as we describe in the previous chapters of this review, several trials showed promising results when evaluating troponins in terms of the occurrence of ventricular arrhythmias or/and SCD [28,42]. Liu et al. investigated the possible association between levels of Troponin and ventricular arrhythmias in 218 patients with chronic HF. In the setting of severe decompensated HF, patients with positive cTnI (>0.5 ng/mL) were more likely to develop ventricular arrhythmias than patients with negative troponin. The authors speculated that patients with decompensated HF might suffer from minimal myocardial injury or "microinfarction" causing sub endocardial ischemia or increasing wall stress with consequent myocardial necrosis [80].

As already mentioned above, high-sensitivity troponin assays enable the detection of lower troponin levels. Therefore, they facilitate earlier diagnosis of MI or/and other cardiac stress situation. Their application for prediction of malignant arrhythmogenic events was also investigated in several trials.

A larger longitudinal study from the USA evaluated the association between the levels of hsTnT and SCD in 3089 older subjects (ambulatory participants in the Cardiovascular Health Study) during a follow-up of 13 years. Indeed, even after adjustment for typical risk factors, elevated baseline hsTnT levels were associated with the incidence of SCD. The authors speculated hsTnT to reflect cardiomyocyte injury caused by possible ageing processes or unrecognized coronary disease with consequent scar formations as potential substrate for the incidence of ventricular arrhythmias [81].

Of note, this hypothesis is in line with studies performed in CAD patients. When investigated with other biomarkers (hsCRP, sST2, BNP) in 1946 CAD patients with preserved left-ventricular function (mean follow-up of 76 ± 20 months), elevated sST2 but also hsTnT (≥15 ng/mL) were the strongest predictors of SCD (followed by hsCRP and BNP) [49].

Interestingly, besides ischemic heart disease, hs-troponins may also be of predictive value when dealing with other cardiomyopathies. Indeed, patients with non-ischemic cardiomyopathy and increased hsTnT levels may have increased risk of SCD, as well. Two investigator groups investigated this exciting issue in patients with dilated cardiomyopathy. They compared hsTnT to conventional TnT, in terms of predicting cardiovascular events including SCD. Both groups found hsTnT to be a better independent predictor than TnT in multivariate analyses [82,83]

Furthermore, Kubo and colleagues investigated hsTnT as a potential marker for prediction of adverse events in 183 HCM patients. They found that elevated hsTnT, but also the degree of elevation, were associated with a higher risk of adverse cardiovascular events including the incidence of sustained VT. The authors supposed that increased hsTnT in HCM patients may reflect relative myocardial ischemia promoted by an imbalance between the hypertrophy of the myocardium and insufficient coronary arterial supply [84].

4. 'Novel and Alternative' Biomarkers as Potential Predictors of Ventricular Arrhythmias

As already mentioned above, cardiac biomarkers are protein components of cell structures that are released into the blood stream when myocardial injury occurs. Consequently, they have a major impact on the diagnosis, risk stratification, and treatment of patients with various cardiac pathologies and symptoms including chest pain with suspected acute coronary syndrome or during evaluation of acute exacerbations of HF. In recent years, active research efforts have brought forward an increasingly large number of "novel and alternative" candidate markers candidates of various pathophysiological origins. Investigations of these promising biological compounds have revealed exiting and encouraging results when dealing with cardiovascular pathologies. Interestingly, their diagnostic, prognostic and/or therapeutic utility was already investigated in the first clinical trials evaluating ventricular arrhythmogenic disorders. While trials with "classic" biomarkers are summarized in Tables 1–3, new promising biomarkers candidates are presented in Tables 4–6 and will be discussed in the following chapter.

Table 1. Predictive value of "classic" biomarkers in heart failure.

Heart Failure	Biomarker	Underlying Condition	Pacemaker/ICD	Arrhythmias	Outcome	Number of Patients	Study Design	FU-Duration	Specific Endpoint	Effect on SCD
Biasucci et al., 2006 [27]	CRP	ICM	ICD	VT/VF	CRP is associated with VT/VF	65	Prospective, single center	-	Appropriate ICD shocks for sVT/VF	SCD not directly investigated
Theuns et al., 2012 [33]	hsCRP, BNP	CHF	ICD	VA	Independently associated with ICD appropriate therapy	100	Prospective, single center	24 months	Appropriate ICD therapy, VA	Independent predictor of SCD*
Blangy et al., 2007 [34]	hsCRP, BNP	ICM	ICD	VT	hsCRP and BNP associated with VTs	121	Prospective, single center	1 year	VTs	SCD not directly investigated
Streitner et al., 2009 [35]	hsCRP, IL-6, NT-proBNP	DCM, CAD	ICD	VT/VF	Correlation with occurrence of electrical storm	86	Prospective, single center	9 months	VT/VF or electrical storm	SCD not directly investigated
Biasucci et al., 2012 [36]	hsCRP	ICM	ICD/CRT-D	VT/VF	Not associated with SCD or VT/VF	268	Prospective, multicenter (CAMI-GUIDE study)	2 years	VT/VF or SCD	No effect
Kontantino et al., 2007 [37]	IL-6, TNFα, hsCRP, BNP	CHF	ICD	VT/VF	No correlation with VT/VF	50	Prospective, single center	152±44 days	VT/VF	SCD not directly investigated
Streitner et al., 2007 [41]	IL-6	ICM	ICD	VT/VF	Associated with VT/VF	47	Prospective, single center	9 months	VT/VF	SCD not directly investigated
Cheng et al., 2014 [42]	IL-6, CRP, TNFα-receptor II, pro-BNP	CHF	ICD	VA	IL-6 predictive for appropriate ICD shocks	1189	Prospective, multicenter (PROSe-ICD study)	4 years	Appropriate ICD shock	IL-6 independent predictor of SCD*
Berger et al., 2002 [51]	BNP	CHF	None	SCD	Independent predictor of SCD	452	Prospective, single center	3 years	SCD	Independent predictor of SCD

Table 1. Cont.

Heart Failure	Biomarker	Underlying Condition	Pacemaker/ICD	Arrhythmias	Outcome	Number of Patients	Study Design	FU-Duration	Specific Endpoint	Effect on SCD
Watanabe et al., 2006 [52]	BNP	CHF	None	SCD	Associated with SCD when combined with echo parameters, nsVTs and diabetes	680	Prospective, multicenter (CHART study)	-	SCD	Factor associated with SCD
Medina et al., 2016 [53]	BNP	CHF	ICD/CRT-D	VT/VF	Independent predictor of VT/VF	1197	Sub-study, prospective, multicenter (MADIT-CRT study)	1 year	VT/VF	SCD not directly investigated
Christ et al., 2007 [54]	BNP	CHF	ICD	VT/VF	Predictive of VT/VF	123	Prospective, single center	25 months	VT/VF	SCD not directly investigated
Verma et al., 2006 [56]	BNP, CRP	CHF	ICD	Appropriate ICD therapy	BNP predictive of appropriate ICD shocks	345	Prospective cohort single center	13 months	Appropriate ICD shocks	Independent predictor of SCD *
Vrotovec et al., 2013 [57]	BNP	CHF	None	SCD	Not predictive of SCD	512	Prospective single center	1 year	SCD	No effect
Bayes-Genis et al., 2007 [60]	NT-proBNP	CHF	None	SCD	Predictive of SCD	494	Prospective, multicenter (MUSIC study)	36 months	SCD	Independent predictor of SCD
Simon et al., 2008 [62]	NT-proBNP	DCM	None	nsVTs	Correlation with occurrence of nsVTs	30	Prospective, single center	21.6 ± 1.2 months	nsVTs	SCD not directly investigated
Scott et al., 2011 [63]	NT-proBNP, sST2, CRP, IL-6	CHF	ICD	Appropriate ICD therapy	NT-proBNP predictive of appropriate ICD therapy	156	Prospective, single center	15 ± 3 months	Appropriate ICD therapy	Factor associated with SCD *
Klingenberg et al., 2006 [64]	NT-proBNP	ICM	ICD	VA	Independent predictor of ICD therapy	50	Prospective, single center	1 year	Appropriate ICD therapy	Independent predictor for SCD *

Table 1. Cont.

Heart Failure	Biomarker	Underlying Condition	Pacemaker/ ICD	Arrhythmias	Outcome	Number of Patients	Study Design	FU-Duration	Specific Endpoint	Effect on SCD
Manios et al., 2005 [65]	NT-proBNP	ICM	ICD	VA	Predictive of VA	35	Prospective, single center	1 year	VA	SCD not directly investigated
Yu et al., 2007 [66]	NT-proBNP	ICM	ICD	VT/VF	Predictive of VT/VF	99	Prospective, single center	18 months	VT/VF	SCD not directly investigated
Levine et al., 2014 [67]	NT-proBNP, BNP	CHF	ICD	VA	Independently predictive of appropriate ICD therapy	695	Retrospective, multicenter	-	Appropriate ICD therapy	Independent predictor of SCD *

BNP, B-type natriuretic peptide; CAD, coronary artery disease; CHF, chronic heart failure; CMP, cardiomyopathy; CRP, C-reactive protein; CRT-D, cardiac resynchronization therapy – defibrillator; DCM, dilated cardiomyopathy; hsCRP, high sensitive C-reactive protein; ICD, implantable cardiac defibrillator; ICM, ischemic heart disease; IL-6, interleukin 6; nsVT, non sustained ventricular tachycardia; NT-proBNP, N-terminal pro-B-type natriuretic peptide; SCD, sudden cardiac death; sST2, soluble tool-like receptor-2; sVT, sustained ventricular tachycardia; TNFα, tumor necrosis factor alpha; VA, ventricular arrhythmias; VF, ventricular fibrillation; VT, ventricular tachycardia; sVT, sustained ventricular tachycardia; *If patient had ICD, appropriate therapy was defined as sudden cardiac death.

Table 2. Predictive value of "classic" biomarkers in hereditary cardiomyopathies.

Genetic	Biomarker	Underlying Condition	Pacemaker/ICD	Arrhythmias	Outcome	Number of Patients	Study Design	FU-Duration	Specific Endpoint	Effect on SCD
Bonny et al., 2010 [29]	CRP	ARVD/C	None	VT	Associated with VT	91	Prospective, single center	-	VT	SCD not directly investigated
Minami et al., 2018 [59]	BNP	HCM	None	SCD	Independent predictor of SCD	346	Prospective, single center	8.4 years	SCD	Independent predictor of SCD
Coats et al., 2013 [73]	NT-proBNP	HCM	None	SCD	Independent predictor of all-cause mortality but not of SCD	847	Prospective, single center	3.5 years	All-cause mortality (SCD)	No effect

ARVD, arrhythmogenic right-ventricular dysplasia/cardiomyopathy; BNP, N-type natriuretic peptide; CRP, C-reactive protein; HCM, hypertrophic cardiomyopathy; NT-proBNP, N-terminal pro-B-type natriuretic peptide; SCD, sudden cardiac death; VT, ventricular tachycardia.

Table 3. Predictive value of "classic" biomarkers in the general population.

General Population	Biomarker	Underlying Condition	Arrhythmias	Outcome	Number of Patients	Study Design	FU-Duration	Specific Endpoint	Effect on SCD
Hussein et al., 2013 [24]	CRP, IL-6	Adults aged 65 years or older	SCD	CRP and IL-6 are associated with SCD	5888	Subgroup analysis of prospective multicenter (Cardiovascular Health Study)	17 years (median 13.1 years)	SCD	Factor associated with SCD
Albert et al., 2002 [21]	hsCRP	Healthy men	SCD	Associated with SCD	97	Sub-study, prospective (Physician's Healthy Study)	17 years	SCD	Factor associated with SCD
Korngold et al., 2009 [77]	NT-proBNP, hsCRP	Healthy women	SCD	Associated with SCD	32 828	Prospective, nested, case-control study	16 years	SCD	Factor associated with SCD
Hussein et al., 2013 [81]	hs-TnT	Ambulatory participants	SCD	Associated with SCD	4 431	Subgroup analysis of prospective multicenter (Cardiovascular Health Study)	13.1 years	SCD	Factor associated with SCD

AMI, acute myocardial infarction; CRP, C-reactive protein; hsCRP, high-sensitive C-reactive protein; IL-6, Interleukin 6; NT-proBNP, N-terminal pro-B-type natriuretic peptide; SCD, sudden cardiac death; VF, ventricular fibrillation; VT, ventricular tachycardia.

Table 4. Predictive value of novel or alternative biomarkers in heart failure.

Heart Failure	Biomarker	Underlying Condition	Pacemaker/ICD	Arrhythmias	Outcome	Number of Patients	Study Design	FU-Duration	Specific Endpoint	Effect on SCD
Daidoji et al., 2012 [85]	H-FABP	CMP	ICD	Appropriate ICD shocks or cardiac death	Correlation with levels of H-FABP	107	Prospective, single center	33.6 month	appropriate ICD shock or cardiac death	Independent predictor of SCD *
Nodera et al., 2018 [86]	Uric Acid	CHF	ICD	VT	Uric Acid predicts VT	56	Prospective, single center	30 ± 8 months	appropriate ICD shock	Independent predictor of SCD *
Flevari et al., 2012 [87]	MMP-9	CHF	ICD	VT	MMP-9 and PICP are predictive of VT	74	Prospective, single center	1 year	appropriate intervention for sVT	Independent predictor of SCD *
Sardu et al., 2018 [28]	sST2, NT-proBNP, CRP	HF patients with metabolic syndrome	ICD	Appropriate ICD therapy	Prediction of ICD shocks	MS: 99 vs. Non-MS: 107	Prospective, multicenter	1 year	appropriate and inappropriate ICD therapy	Independent predictor of SCD *
Francia et al., 2014 [88]	OPN, galectin-3	CHF	ICD	VF, VT	OPN and galectin-3 predict sVT/VF	75	Prospective, single center	29 ± 17 months	first sVT/VF	Independent predictor of SCD *
Ahmad et al., 2014 [89]	NT-proBNP, sST2, galectin-3	CHF	None	SCD	Positive with NT-proBNP, mildly incremental when combined with novel biomarkers	813	Sub-study, Prospective, multicenter (HF-ACTION)	2.5 years	SCD	Independent predictor of SCD
Skali H et al., 2016 [90]	sST2	HF	CRT Registry	VT	Predictive of VT	684	Sub-study, prospectively, multicenter (MADIT)	1 year	VT/VF or death	SCD not directly investigated
Pascual-Figal et al., 2009 [91]	sST2 NT-proBNP	CHF	None	SCD	Positive when Combined with NT-proBNP levels	36 SCD matched 63 Controls	Sub-group analysis, case-control design of prospective, multicenter MUSIC study	3-years	SCD	Independent predictor of SCD

CMP, cardiomyopathy; CHF, chronic heart failure; CRP, C-reactive protein; CRT, cardiac resynchronization therapy; CVD, cardiovascular death; H-FABP, Heart-type fatty acid binding protein; ICD, implantable cardiac defibrillator; MMP-9, matrix metallo-proteinase; MS, metabolic syndrome; NTproBNP, N-terminal pro-B-type natriuretic peptide; OPN, Osteopontin; PICP, procollagen type I carboxyterminal peptide; SCD, sudden cardiac death; sST2, soluble toll-like receptor-2; sVT, sustained ventricular tachycardia; VT, ventricular tachyarrhythmia; VF, ventricular fibrillation. * If patient had ICD, appropriate ICD therapy was defined as sudden cardiac death.

Table 5. Predictive value of novel or alternative biomarkers in hereditary cardiomyopathies.

Genetic	Biomarker	Underlying Condition	Pacemaker/ICD	Arrhythmias	Outcome	Number of Patients	Study Design	FU-Duration	Specific Endpoint	Effect on SCD
Oz et al., 2017 [92]	Galectin-3	ARVD	ICD	VF, VT	Correlation with Galectin-3	29 vs. 24 controls	Retrospective, multicenter	-	nsVT/sVT	SCD not directly investigated
Daidoji et al., 2016 [93]	H-FABP	Brugada syndrome	ICD	Appropriate ICD shock, VF	Correlation with VA	31	Prospective, single-center	5 years	appropriate ICD shock	Independent predictor of SCD *
Zachariah et al., 2012 [94]	MMP3	HCM	ICD	VT/VF	MMP3 predicts VA	45	Retrospective, single Center	6 months	CA, sVT/VF with ICD shock	SCD not directly investigated
Emet et al., 2018 [95]	Galectin-3	HCM	ICD	SCD	Predictive 5 year risk of SCD	52	Cross-sectional data	-	Correlation between the estimated 5-year risk of SCD	SCD not directly investigated

ARVD, arrhythmogenic right ventricular dysplasia; CA, cardiac arrest; HCM, hypertrophic cardiomyopathy; H-FABP, Heart-type fatty acid binding protein; ICD, implantable cardiac defibrillator; MMP-9, matrix metallo-proteinase; nsVT, non-sustained ventricular tachycardia; SCD, sudden cardiac death; VA, ventricular arrhythmias; VF, ventricular fibrillation; VT ventricular tachycardia. * If patient had ICD, appropriate ICD therapy was defined as sudden cardiac death.

Table 6. Predictive value of novel or alternative biomarkers in the general population.

General Population	Biomarker	Underlying Condition	Arrhythmias	Outcome	Number of Patients	Study Design	FU-Duration	Specific Endpoint	Effect on SCD
Kunutsor et al., 2016 [96]	Fibrinogen	Non	SCD	Fibrinogen is associated with SCD	1773	Prospective cohort study, multicenter	22 years	SCD	Independent predictor of SCD
Yamade at al., 2011 [97]	Uric acid	Non-specific LVH	VT	Uric acid predicts VT	167	Prospective, single center	24 h	Correlation with VT in 24h- Holter ECG	SCD not directly investigated
Deo et al., 2010 [98]	Cystatin C	Age/no cardio-vascular disease	SCD	Correlation with cystatin C	4465	Subgroup analysis of Prospective, multicenter CHS (Cardiovascular health study)	11.2 years	SCD	Independent predictor of SCD
Jouven et al., 2001 [99]	circulating nonesterified fatty acids	Non	SCD	independent risk factor for SCD	5250	Cohort-Study(Paris Prospective Study I)	22 years	SCD	Independent predictor of SCD

ECG, electrocardiogram; LVH, left ventricular hypertrophy; SCD, sudden cardiac death; VT, ventricular tachycardia.

4.1. Soluble ST2 (sST2)

ST2 is a member of the interleukin 1 receptor family. Originally, this protein was linked to myocardial dysfunction, fibrosis, and remodeling [100]. Interestingly, upregulation of soluble ST2 (sST2) was also shown to be related to mechanical stress of the heart with consequent cardiac damage. Of note, there are two known isoforms, which both are associated with cardiac pathologies. While sSt2 is soluble, the second isoform St2 is a receptor, bound to the cell membrane [101]. Their role in cardiac pathophysiological processes involving progression of coronary atherosclerosis, but also cardiac remodeling with consequent fibrosis, has been uncovered in recent years [100]. Of note, their function was shown to depend on interleukin 33 (Il-33). Il-33 binds to the ST2 receptor in order to reduce cardiac damage during cardiac stress. Nevertheless, tethered with sST2, Il-33 is unable to become involved into further cellular pathways, resulting in the potential loss of cardioprotective characteristics [102,103]. Consequently, higher levels of sST2 are linked to more severe stress responses in the heart [103]. On the other hand, sST2 seems to be involved in the pathophysiology of ischemic events. Of note, serum levels are associated with ischemic damage and remain high, even in the post-MI period. Since recovery of left ventricular function is impaired in patients with higher sST2 levels, sST2 is speculated to play an important role in remodeling following an acute ischemic event [104]. Logically, further efforts were made to integrate sST2 into daily clinical practice of dealing with cardiovascular patients.

Indeed, higher sST2 levels (above 36.3 ng/mL) are associated with adverse outcomes in patients with HF [105]. Since NT-proBNP and sST2 are both elevated in this pathology and are part of two different pathological pathways, combining them as part of a risk assessment strategy was the next logical step. In fact, among symptomatic HF patients, sST2 concentrations are strongly predictive of mortality and might be useful in risk stratification when used alone or together with NT-proBNP [106]. Consequently, a moderate benefit in the risk assessment of HF patients was made when measurements of sST2 were combined with NT-proBNP. These results, led to the proposal of a "solid" threshold of sST2 levels in HF patients [106,107].

Since the HF population is known to be at high risk of ventricular arrhythmias with consequent SCD, the application of this strategy was also investigated for the prediction of these malignant events. In their elegant case-control study, by analyzing data from the MUSIC registry (three-year multicenter registry of ambulatory HF patients with New York Heart Association functional class (NYHA) II-III, and LVEF ≤ 45%, Pascual-Dual and colleagues were able to demonstrate that higher sST2 levels are associated with SCD. Indeed, 34% of patients with sST2 levels above 0.15 ng/mL developed SCD while 74% of patients with both increased sST2 and NT-proBNP levels experienced this fatal event. Therefore, the authors postulated that this combination might be a valuable clinical tool for predicting SCD in HF patients [91]. Nevertheless, these enthusiastic results could not be fully reproduced by further trials. In a subgroup analysis of the HF-ACTION trial, adding novel biomarkers such as sST2 and galectin 3 to NT-proBNP levels in the risk calculation model, showed a strong association with death by pump failure. Yet, there was only a weak improvement while assessing for SCD [89].

However, in patients with mildly symptomatic HF evaluated during the MADIT-CRT trial, a 10% elevation of sST2 levels alone over one year, was shown to be predictive of increased risk of onset of ventricular arrhythmias and death. Nevertheless, in the same study it was shown, that an elevated sST2 baseline is not directly predictive of ventricular arrhythmias [90].

Further, investigations were performed in patients treated with ICD for primary prevention. Since the ST2 protein is a marker of myocardial stress, sympathetic hyperactivation and neuro-hormonal axis dysfunction [28], one might speculate that in the ICD population with HF, sST2 levels could reflect alterations of the electrophysiological substrate and thus identify patients at a higher risk of shock therapy. Of note, these pathophysiological alterations are more common in patients suffering from metabolic syndrome. Therefore, in their elegant study Sardu and colleagues focused on this specific population at risk. Interestingly, in these patients, sST2 values could differentiate patients with a higher risk of ICD therapy, and worse prognosis [28].

Other studies focused on further specific risk populations. Mitral annulus disjunction is a displacement of the mitral valve. Since it is accompanied by mitral annular myocardial fibrosis, it is a mechanism proposed for the development of ventricular arrhythmias with potential consequent SCD [108]. In this population, patients suffering from ventricular arrhythmias had higher circulating levels of sST2. Indeed, while combined with LVEF and fibrosis assessed by late gadolinium enhancement on MRI, sST2 measurements were able to improve risk stratification in this specific risk population [109].

4.2. Galectin-3

Galectins are a family of proteins defined by two characteristics: functionally a beta-galactoside affinity and structurally a conserved carbohydrate recognition domain (CRD). Initially, these proteins were only thought to play a significant role in embryogenic processes. However, further research uncovered, galectins are important players in various physiological and pathophysiological processes including immune activation [110].

The galectin family members are expressed in three different structural forms: dimeric, tandem or chimera. Of all discovered chimeric structural forms, galectin-3 is the only protein with a N-terminal protein-binding domain and a C-terminal carbohydrate-recognition domain. The protein is expressed in various tissues including lung, kidney, as well as the heart. Consistent with other members of the lectin family, this soluble beta-galactoside-binding protein is activated as a response to tissue damage [111]. Galectin-3 is active on both the intracellular and/or the extracellular levels. On the cellular level, it regulates messenger ribonucleic acid (mRNA) splicing and contributes to the regulation of anti-apoptotic signaling [112], while extracellularly it is secreted by macrophages and is involved in the recognition of pathogens as well as in acute chronic inflammation processes [113,114]. Furthermore, this protein seems to be a potent mitogen for fibroblasts [115]. Therefore, galectin-3 represents an intriguing link between inflammatory and fibrotic processes, which are frequent findings in various cardiac pathophysiologies, including HF [116].

Indeed, when measured in the general population, elevated levels of galectin-3 are associated with higher incidence of CVD, but also with an elevated risk of all-cause mortality [117]. Especially in recent years, this protein was shown to be a useful complementary biomarker in prognosis and risk stratification of HF patients [118]. However, as already mentioned above, concerning prediction of SCD in this population at risk, first results adding novel biomarkers including galectin-3 to NT-proBNP for risk assessment, showed only weak improvement while assessing for this malignant event [89]. On the other hand, together with osteopontin, Francia and colleagues evaluated a possible association of galectin-3 levels with the incidence of sustained VT/VF in 75 newly implanted ICD-HF-patients. Of note, even after correction for other risk factors, during a follow-up of over two years, plasma levels of galectin-3 predicted sustained VT/VF in HF patients at high risk of SCD [88].

In various arrhythmogenic pathologies including genetic disorders, tissue inflammation and fibrosis are key processes of electrophysiological remodeling. Therefore, one might speculate that there will be further clinical applications of galectin-3 as a potential tool for prediction of ventricular arrhythmias. Consequently, further studies focused on genetic disorders like ARVD and HCM. Of note, both pathologies are mainly characterized by defective genes responsible for connective tissue structure, resulting in remodeling including tissue inflammation and fibrosis with consequent ventricular arrhythmias [92]. Indeed, in a small study (conducted in 24 patients with ARVD vs. 29 control patients) galectin-3 levels were shown to be increased in patients with ARVD. Furthermore, they were predictive for the onset of VT as well as VF. Therefore, the authors postulated, galectin-3 as a potential biomarker involved in the onset of ARVD. A further study investigated a possible association with risk prediction of SCD in HCM. Of note, in this population, five-year risk of SCD is routinely assessed using a standard questionnaire outlined in the 2014 European Society of Cardiology guidelines [9]. The authors observed a positive correlation between the estimated five-year risk of SCD and serum levels of galectin-3, thus indicating an additive tool for SCD-prediction in this population [95].

4.3. Heart-Type Fatty Acid Binding Protein (H-FABP)

Heart fatty acid-binding protein (H-FABP) is ubiquitous in myocardial cells. Therefore, upon myocardial membrane injury H-FABP is released in the bloodstream [119]. Of note, peak levels are observed three hours following an MI [120]. Consequently, H-FABP was established as a marker of ongoing myocardial membrane damage and has been reported to be a useful indicator for future cardiovascular events [121]. Therefore, further trials explored its potential application in predicting arrhythmogenic events in high-risk populations. In 107 consecutive patients with cardiomyopathy, who had received an ICD, circulating serum H-FABP levels >4.3 ng/mL, but not Troponin T levels, were a significant independent prognostic factor for the incidence of appropriate shock therapy or/and cardiac death. Furthermore, assessment of subgroups showed that H-FABP levels could be used to anticipate event-free periods in patients with ICD and additive amiodarone therapy. Indeed, the outcome of patients receiving ICD for primary as well as secondary prevention was predictable via H-FABP levels [85].

A further study investigated the application of myocardial membrane injury assessed by H-FABP levels in Brugada syndrome. Of note, this genetic disorder is defined by inherited sodium channel dysfunction with consequent risk of SCD [122]. Also in this high risk population serum H-FABP levels (>2.4 ng/mL), but not Troponin T levels, were an independent prognostic factor for appropriate ICD shocks due to VF (during a five-year follow up) indicating H-FABP as a promising biomarker for the prediction of malignant ventricular arrhythmias [93].

4.4. Metalloproteinases (MMP) and Procollagens

Metalloproteinases (MMPs) are enzymes mainly concerned with the turnover of extracellular matrix. Their role in the development of post-infarction scar tissue is a growing field of investigation. Indeed, these proteins are key enzymes involved in post-MI remodeling, including processing of cytokines and extracellular matrix (ECM) substrates to regulate the inflammatory and fibrotic components of myocardial wound healing. Furthermore, these enzymes are upstream initiators with regulatory functions in cell signaling cascades [123]. Consequently, in HF patients, levels of diverse MMPs seem to reflect the progression of cardiac remodeling [124]. Therefore, as reflectors of cardiac turnover processes with consequent remodeling, they might be suspected as useful predictors of ventricular arrhythmias. Indeed, in 74 HF patients with implanted ICD, the ratio of MMP-9 and the tissue inhibitor of matrix metalloproteinase 1 was able to predict tachyarrhythmic events necessitating appropriate interventions, indicating further potential future applications in this clinical field [87].

While cardiac remodeling is one the main pathophysiological characteristics of hypertrophic cardiomyopathy, a further study focused on this genetic disorder. Indeed, in a population of adolescent HCM patients, MMP-3 levels were significantly higher in patients prone to ventricular arrhythmias. However, when adjusted for age, the effect was attenuated, indicating the need for further research in this exciting field [94].

Previous investigations already focused on other biomarkers, which were known indicators of excessive turnover of the extracellular mass of the heart. They included circulating procollagens. While these compounds were linked to worsening of HF and the function of the left ventricle, further studies explored possible associations with the incidence of ventricular arrhythmias [125]. Indeed, in ICD patients implanted for spontaneous sustained VT due to ischemic heart disease, incidence of VT could be linked to high type I aminoterminal peptide (PINP) and low procollagen type III aminoterminal peptide (PIIINP) levels. Nevertheless, these markers presented a low specificity.

4.5. Endothelin

As one of the most potent vasoconstrictive peptides, the endothelium-derived factor endothelin became a novel objective of research in the late 1980s [126]. Endothelin 1 (ET 1) not only leads to the stimulation of interleukin expression in monocytes and increases platelet aggregation, but also stimulates expression of growth factors. EtA and EtB are the predominant receptors activated via endothelin. EtA is exclusively expressed on vascular smooth muscle cells and has a greater selectivity for ET1 [127]. Furthermore, endothelin seems to be a contributing factor in the development of chronic hypertension [128]. Nevertheless, in contrast to other myocardial biomarkers, endothelin 1 has very early been the matter of investigation in the pathophysiology of cardiac arrhythmias. Indeed, in animal models, endothelin is associated with the incidence of ventricular arrhythmias [129,130] but also with ECG modulation including QTc prolongation [130]. In addition, endothelin was linked to ischemia induced ventricular arrhythmias [131] and arrhythmogenic responses during myocardial reperfusion [132]. Several mechanisms are proposed to be activated via ET1 to promote arrhytmic events. Nevertheless, early afterdepolarizations triggered by ion channel remodeling, but also sympathetic activation, were suggested to be the main causes of ET1 induced arrhythmias [133–135]. Inspired by these promising results, further research focused on patients with decompensated HF. Of note, this population is characterized by increased neurohumoral activation with a higher rate of ventricular arrhythmias and SCD [4,128,129]. Et1 levels, as well as renin-angiotensin-aldosterone-system (RAAS) activity, but also interleukin 6 and TNF-α were assessed in 83 of those patients. Indeed, 24 h Holter-monitoring revealed an association of Et1 levels and ventricular ectopy [136].

A further study explored the application of ET1 measurement in ICD-patients (implanted for multiple underlying conditions). ET1 levels were significantly increased one hour and even one minute after shock therapy, giving further evidence, that the potential biomarker plays an important role in the development of malignant arrhythmogenic events [137]. Nevertheless, despite promising findings in basic research studies as well as in the first clinical trials, the role of ET1 as potential predictor of ventricular arrhythmias still needs to be evaluated.

4.6. Uric Acid

Uric acid is the final product of the purine metabolism. In recent years, serum uric acid has gained interest as a determinant of cardiovascular risk. Indeed, patients with hyperuricemia are at higher risk of cardiovascular events [138]. Furthermore, high serum levels are a strong, independent marker of poor prognosis in HF [139]. Consequently, they also seem to be associated with the incidence of ventricular arrhythmias in this high-risk population. Indeed, in a smaller trial in 56 HF patients with implanted ICD for primary prevention, higher uric acid levels were linked to the development of ventricular tachyarrhythmias [86]. Similar results were revealed in patients with diagnosed left-ventricular hypertrophy. In this population uric acid levels were shown to be an independent predictor of the occurrence of VT during Holter-monitoring [140].

4.7. Other Promising Biomarkers

Besides the already discussed promising biomarkers, several trials investigated further biomarkers of various origin. Therefore, we would also like to provide a brief overview of this growing topic of ongoing investigation.

Fibrinogen is a glycoprotein involved in clotting processes. Furthermore, it is a known promotor of revascularization and wound healing, but also acts as an acute-phase protein, which is secreted in response to systemic inflammation and tissue injury [141]. Consequently, fibrinogen plasma levels were shown to be higher in patients suffering from CVD, as indicated by a subgroup analysis of the Framingham population [142]. Nevertheless, data available from the PRIME study (multicenter prospective cohort designed to identify risk factors for coronary heart disease) could not reveal an association with SCD when assessed with other biomarkers such as IL-6 or CRP [25]. Differing results were presented by Kunutsor and colleagues [96]. Interestingly, when investigated in a bigger cohort including 1773 middle-aged men who were followed up for 22 years, fibrinogen levels were positively associated with the risk of SCD. However, addition of plasma fibrinogen to a SCD risk prediction model containing established risk factors was not able to improve risk discrimination in this population [96]

Impaired kidney function is a known cardiovascular risk factor. As already mentioned, this population is also at higher risk of SCD [143]. In their elegant trial, Deo and colleagues investigated a possible association between SCD and established biomarkers of renal function in an elderly population without prevalent CVD at baseline. During a follow-up of more than 10 years, the authors were able to uncover that impaired kidney function assessed by cystatin C, but not by creatinine levels or glomerular filtration rate, are linked to SCD events in the future [144].

Osteopontin is an extracellular structural protein. As an organic component of the bone, it is involved in bone-remodeling processes [145]. Furthermore, while it is expressed in a range of immune cells, it is also involved in immunity [146]. One study focused on the possible connection between osteoponin levels and the incidence of ventricular arrhythmias. As already mentioned above, Francia and colleagues investigated levels of osteoponin and galectin-3 in HF patients with implanted ICD. Indeed, higher plasma levels were predictive of the incidence of sustained VT/VF, indicating this potential biomarker as a clinical promising tool requiring further investigation [88].

Growth differentiation factor-15 (GDF-15) is a stress-responsive transforming growth factor-ß-related cytokine. It increases and is independently related to an adverse prognosis in systolic, but also diastolic HF [147]. Furthermore, it was also suggested to be a prognostic biomarker in the evaluation of short- and long-term outcomes in ST-elevation myocardial infarction (STEMI) patients [148]. Interestingly, in STEMI patients with VF complications, levels of GDF 15 seem to be increased and are also predictive when assessing short-term mortality [149].

5. Summary

Recent studies have identified the significance of serum biomarkers as risk factors for ventricular tachyarrhythmias. Beyond the established clinical risk factors, elevations of the "classic" biomarkers like BNP and NT-proBNP, as well as troponins were already elucidated as potential predictors of SCD in various populations at risk. Inflammatory biomarkers seem also to be associated with ventricular arrhythmias and may have a significant role in their pathogenesis. Furthermore, recent studies have investigated "novel" biomarkers originating from various pathophysiological contexts, like sST2, galectin-3 or H-FABP. In the HF population at risk in particular, these substances indicate a promising potential for prediction of malignant arrhythmic events. Furthermore, their application might also be useful in inherited arrhythmogenic pathologies. Combining these biomarkers in a multimarker approach might further improve risk assessment strategies. Nevertheless, further translational research is necessary to elucidate the potential of these promising biological compounds in dealing with ventricular arrhythmias and SCD.

Author Contributions: Conceptualization: Z.S., B.O., C.S., B.W, M.C.B., A.-M.D., B.S., R.P. and L.J.M.; Investigation: Z.S., B.O., K.H., G.F., B.W., R.P. and L.J.M.; Project administration: R.P. and L.J.M.; Resources: H.R., U.C.H., R.P and L.J.M.; Supervision: R.P. and L.J.M.; Original draft writing preparation and writing: Z.S., B.O., C.S., A.-M.D., B.S., R.P and L.J.M.; Writing review and editing: Z.S., B.O., C.S., K.H., C.A.P., G.F., B.W., M.C.B., A.-M.D., H.R., U.C.H., B.S., R.P. and L.J.M. All authors have read and agreed to the published version of the manuscript.

Funding: This research received no external funding.

Conflicts of Interest: We declare no direct or indirect interest (financial or nature) with a private, industrial or commercial organization relationship with the subject presented.

References

1. WHO International. Available online: https://www.who.int/health-topics/cardiovascular-diseases/#tab=tab_1 (accessed on 28 January 2020).
2. Greene, H.L. Sudden arrhythmic cardiac death—Mechanisms, resuscitation and classification: The Seattle perspective. *Am. J. Cardiol.* **1990**, *65*, 4B–12B. [CrossRef]
3. Zipes, D.P.; Wellens, H.J. Sudden cardiac death. *Circulation* **1998**, *98*, 2334–2351. [CrossRef] [PubMed]
4. Schocken, D.D.; Arrieta, M.I.; Leaverton, P.E.; Ross, E.A. Prevalence and mortality rate of congestive heart failure in the United States. *J. Am. Coll. Cardiol.* **1992**, *20*, 301–306. [CrossRef]

5. Tomaselli, G.F.; Beuckelmann, D.J.; Calkins, H.G.; Berger, R.D.; Kessler, P.D.; Lawrence, J.H.; Kass, D.; Feldman, A.M.; Marban, E. Sudden cardiac death in heart failure. The role of abnormal repolarization. *Circulation* **1994**, *90*, 2534–2539. [CrossRef] [PubMed]
6. Echt, D.S.; Liebson, P.R.; Mitchell, L.B.; Peters, R.W.; Obias-Manno, D.; Barker, A.H.; Arensberg, D.; Baker, A.; Friedman, L.; Greene, H.L.; et al. Mortality and morbidity in patients receiving encainide, flecainide, or placebo. The Cardiac Arrhythmia Suppression Trial. *N. Engl. J. Med.* **1991**, *324*, 781–788. [CrossRef] [PubMed]
7. Moss, A.J.; Zareba, W.; Hall, W.J.; Klein, H.; Wilber, D.J.; Cannom, D.S.; Daubert, J.P.; Higgins, S.L.; Brown, M.W.; Andrews, M.L.; et al. Prophylactic implantation of a defibrillator in patients with myocardial infarction and reduced ejection fraction. *N. Engl. J. Med.* **2002**, *346*, 877–883. [CrossRef] [PubMed]
8. Bardy, G.H.; Lee, K.L.; Mark, D.B.; Poole, J.E.; Packer, D.L.; Boineau, R.; Domanski, M.; Troutman, C.; Anderson, J.; Johnson, G.; et al. Amiodarone or an implantable cardioverter-defibrillator for congestive heart failure. *N. Engl. J. Med.* **2005**, *352*, 225–237. [CrossRef]
9. Priori, S.G.; Blomstrom-Lundqvist, C.; Mazzanti, A.; Blom, N.; Borggrefe, M.; Camm, J.; Elliott, P.M.; Fitzsimons, D.; Hatala, R.; Hindricks, G.; et al. 2015 ESC Guidelines for the management of patients with ventricular arrhythmias and the prevention of sudden cardiac Death. The Task Force for the Management of Patients with Ventricular Arrhythmias and the Prevention of Sudden Cardiac Death of the European Society of Cardiology. *G. Ital. Cardiol.* **2016**, *17*, 108–170. [CrossRef]
10. Bostwick, J.M.; Sola, C.L. An updated review of implantable cardioverter/defibrillators, induced anxiety, and quality of life. *Psychiatr. Clin. North. Am.* **2007**, *30*, 677–688. [CrossRef]
11. Gould, P.A.; Krahn, A.D.; Canadian Heart Rhythm Society Working Group on Device Advisories. Complications associated with implantable cardioverter-defibrillator replacement in response to device advisories. *JAMA* **2006**, *295*, 1907–1911. [CrossRef]
12. Lane, R.E.; Cowie, M.R.; Chow, A.W. Prediction and prevention of sudden cardiac death in heart failure. *Heart* **2005**, *91*, 674–680. [CrossRef] [PubMed]
13. Motloch, L.J.; Akar, F.G. Gene therapy to restore electrophysiological function in heart failure. *Expert Opin. Biol. Ther.* **2015**, *15*, 803–817. [CrossRef] [PubMed]
14. Paar, V.; Jirak, P.; Larbig, R.; Zagidullin, N.S.; Brandt, M.C.; Lichtenauer, M.; Hoppe, U.C.; Motloch, L.J. Pathophysiology of Calcium Mediated Ventricular Arrhythmias and Novel Therapeutic Options with Focus on Gene Therapy. *Int. J. Mol. Sci.* **2019**, *20*. [CrossRef] [PubMed]
15. Shaw, R.M.; Rudy, Y. The vulnerable window for unidirectional block in cardiac tissue: Characterization and dependence on membrane excitability and intercellular coupling. *J. Cardiovasc. Electrophysiol.* **1995**, *6*, 115–131. [CrossRef]
16. Yancy, C.W.; Jessup, M.; Bozkurt, B.; Butler, J.; Casey, D.E., Jr.; Drazner, M.H.; Fonarow, G.C.; Geraci, S.A.; Horwich, T.; Januzzi, J.L.; et al. 2013 ACCF/AHA guideline for the management of heart failure: A report of the American College of Cardiology Foundation/American Heart Association Task Force on Practice Guidelines. *J. Am. Coll. Cardiol.* **2013**, *62*, e147–e239. [CrossRef]
17. Tiong, A.Y.; Brieger, D. Inflammation and coronary artery disease. *Am. Heart J.* **2005**, *150*, 11–18. [CrossRef]
18. Mountantonakis, S.; Deo, R. Biomarkers in atrial fibrillation, ventricular arrhythmias, and sudden cardiac death. *Cardiovasc. Ther.* **2012**, *30*, e74–e80. [CrossRef]
19. Calabro, P.; Willerson, J.T.; Yeh, E.T. Inflammatory cytokines stimulated C-reactive protein production by human coronary artery smooth muscle cells. *Circulation* **2003**, *108*, 1930–1932. [CrossRef]
20. Yasojima, K.; Schwab, C.; McGeer, E.G.; McGeer, P.L. Generation of C-reactive protein and complement components in atherosclerotic plaques. *Am. J. Pathol.* **2001**, *158*, 1039–1051. [CrossRef]
21. Albert, C.M.; Ma, J.; Rifai, N.; Stampfer, M.J.; Ridker, P.M. Prospective study of C-reactive protein, homocysteine, and plasma lipid levels as predictors of sudden cardiac death. *Circulation* **2002**, *105*, 2595–2599. [CrossRef]
22. Carnes, C.A.; Chung, M.K.; Nakayama, T.; Nakayama, H.; Baliga, R.S.; Piao, S.; Kanderian, A.; Pavia, S.; Hamlin, R.L.; McCarthy, P.M.; et al. Ascorbate attenuates atrial pacing-induced peroxynitrite formation and electrical remodeling and decreases the incidence of postoperative atrial fibrillation. *Circ. Res.* **2001**, *89*, e32–e38. [CrossRef] [PubMed]
23. Frustaci, A.; Chimenti, C.; Bellocci, F.; Morgante, E.; Russo, M.A.; Maseri, A. Histological substrate of atrial biopsies in patients with lone atrial fibrillation. *Circulation* **1997**, *96*, 1180–1184. [CrossRef] [PubMed]

24. Hussein, A.A.; Gottdiener, J.S.; Bartz, T.M.; Sotoodehnia, N.; DeFilippi, C.; See, V.; Deo, R.; Siscovick, D.; Stein, P.K.; Lloyd-Jones, D. Inflammation and sudden cardiac death in a community-based population of older adults: The Cardiovascular Health Study. *Heart Rhythm* **2013**, *10*, 1425–1432. [CrossRef] [PubMed]
25. Luc, G.; Bard, J.M.; Juhan-Vague, I.; Ferrieres, J.; Evans, A.; Amouyel, P.; Arveiler, D.; Fruchart, J.C.; Ducimetiere, P.; Group, P.S. C-reactive protein, interleukin-6, and fibrinogen as predictors of coronary heart disease: The PRIME Study. *Arter. Thromb. Vasc. Biol.* **2003**, *23*, 1255–1261. [CrossRef] [PubMed]
26. Hodzic, E.; Drakovac, A.; Begic, E. Troponin and CRP as Indicators of Possible Ventricular Arrhythmias in Myocardial Infarction of the Anterior and Inferior Walls of the Heart. *Mater. Sociomed.* **2018**, *30*, 185–188. [CrossRef] [PubMed]
27. Biasucci, L.M.; Giubilato, G.; Biondi-Zoccai, G.; Sanna, T.; Liuzzo, G.; Piro, M.; De Martino, G.; Ierardi, C.; dello Russo, A.; Pelargonio, G.; et al. C reactive protein is associated with malignant ventricular arrhythmias in patients with ischaemia with implantable cardioverter-defibrillator. *Heart* **2006**, *92*, 1147–1148. [CrossRef]
28. Sardu, C.; Marfella, R.; Santamaria, M.; Papini, S.; Parisi, Q.; Sacra, C.; Colaprete, D.; Paolisso, G.; Rizzo, M.R.; Barbieri, M. Stretch, Injury and Inflammation Markers Evaluation to Predict Clinical Outcomes After Implantable Cardioverter Defibrillator Therapy in Heart Failure Patients With Metabolic Syndrome. *Front. Physiol.* **2018**, *9*, 758. [CrossRef]
29. Bonny, A.; Lellouche, N.; Ditah, I.; Hidden-Lucet, F.; Yitemben, M.T.; Granger, B.; Larrazet, F.; Frank, R.; Fontaine, G. C-reactive protein in arrhythmogenic right ventricular dysplasia/cardiomyopathy and relationship with ventricular tachycardia. *Cardiol. Res. Pr.* **2010**, *2010*. [CrossRef]
30. Lazzerini, P.E.; Laghi-Pasini, F.; Bertolozzi, I.; Morozzi, G.; Lorenzini, S.; Simpatico, A.; Selvi, E.; Bacarelli, M.R.; Finizola, F.; Vanni, F.; et al. Systemic inflammation as a novel QT-prolonging risk factor in patients with torsades de pointes. *Heart* **2017**, *103*, 1821–1829. [CrossRef]
31. Jialal, I.; Devaraj, S.; Venugopal, S.K. C-reactive protein: Risk marker or mediator in atherothrombosis? *Hypertension* **2004**, *44*, 6–11. [CrossRef]
32. Helal, I.; Zerelli, L.; Krid, M.; ElYounsi, F.; Ben Maiz, H.; Zouari, B.; Adelmoula, J.; Kheder, A. Comparison of C-reactive protein and high-sensitivity C-reactive protein levels in patients on hemodialysis. *Saudi J. Kidney Dis. Transpl.* **2012**, *23*, 477–483. [PubMed]
33. Theuns, D.A.; Smith, T.; Szili-Torok, T.; Muskens-Heemskerk, A.; Janse, P.; Jordaens, L. Prognostic role of high-sensitivity C-reactive protein and B-type natriuretic peptide in implantable cardioverter-defibrillator patients. *Pacing Clin. Electrophysiol.* **2012**, *35*, 275–282. [CrossRef] [PubMed]
34. Blangy, H.; Sadoul, N.; Dousset, B.; Radauceanu, A.; Fay, R.; Aliot, E.; Zannad, F. Serum BNP, hs-C-reactive protein, procollagen to assess the risk of ventricular tachycardia in ICD recipients after myocardial infarction. *Europace* **2007**, *9*, 724–729. [CrossRef] [PubMed]
35. Streitner, F.; Kuschyk, J.; Veltmann, C.; Ratay, D.; Schoene, N.; Streitner, I.; Brueckmann, M.; Schumacher, B.; Borggrefe, M.; Wolpert, C. Role of proinflammatory markers and NT-proBNP in patients with an implantable cardioverter-defibrillator and an electrical storm. *Cytokine* **2009**, *47*, 166–172. [CrossRef] [PubMed]
36. Biasucci, L.M.; Bellocci, F.; Landolina, M.; Rordorf, R.; Vado, A.; Menardi, E.; Giubilato, G.; Orazi, S.; Sassara, M.; Castro, A.; et al. Risk stratification of ischemic patients with implantable cardioverter defibrillators by C-reactive protein and a multi-markers strategy: Results of the CAMI-GUIDE study. *Eur. Heart J.* **2012**, *33*, 1344–1350. [CrossRef]
37. Konstantino, Y.; Kusniec, J.; Reshef, T.; David-Zadeh, O.; Mazur, A.; Strasberg, B.; Battler, A.; Haim, M. Inflammatory biomarkers are not predictive of intermediate-term risk of ventricular tachyarrhythmias in stable CHF patients. *Clin. Cardiol.* **2007**, *30*, 408–413. [CrossRef]
38. Parekh, R.S.; Plantinga, L.C.; Kao, W.H.; Meoni, L.A.; Jaar, B.G.; Fink, N.E.; Powe, N.R.; Coresh, J.; Klag, M.J. The association of sudden cardiac death with inflammation and other traditional risk factors. *Kidney Int.* **2008**, *74*, 1335–1342. [CrossRef]
39. Schieffer, B.; Schieffer, E.; Hilfiker-Kleiner, D.; Hilfiker, A.; Kovanen, P.T.; Kaartinen, M.; Nussberger, J.; Harringer, W.; Drexler, H. Expression of angiotensin II and interleukin 6 in human coronary atherosclerotic plaques: Potential implications for inflammation and plaque instability. *Circulation* **2000**, *101*, 1372–1378. [CrossRef]

40. Safranow, K.; Dziedziejko, V.; Rzeuski, R.; Czyzycka, E.; Bukowska, H.; Wojtarowicz, A.; Binczak-Kuleta, A.; Jakubowska, K.; Olszewska, M.; Ciechanowicz, A.; et al. Inflammation markers are associated with metabolic syndrome and ventricular arrhythmia in patients with coronary artery disease. *Postep. Hig. Med. Dosw.* **2016**, *70*, 56–66. [CrossRef]
41. Streitner, F.; Kuschyk, J.; Veltmann, C.; Brueckmann, M.; Streitner, I.; Brade, J.; Neumaier, M.; Bertsch, T.; Schumacher, B.; Borggrefe, M.; et al. Prospective study of interleukin-6 and the risk of malignant ventricular tachyarrhythmia in ICD-recipients—A pilot study. *Cytokine* **2007**, *40*, 30–34. [CrossRef]
42. Cheng, A.; Zhang, Y.; Blasco-Colmenares, E.; Dalal, D.; Butcher, B.; Norgard, S.; Eldadah, Z.; Ellenbogen, K.A.; Dickfeld, T.; Spragg, D.D.; et al. Protein biomarkers identify patients unlikely to benefit from primary prevention implantable cardioverter defibrillators: Findings from the Prospective Observational Study of Implantable Cardioverter Defibrillators (PROSE-ICD). *Circ. Arrhythm. Electrophysiol.* **2014**, *7*, 1084–1091. [CrossRef]
43. Ottani, F.; Galvani, M.; Nicolini, F.A.; Ferrini, D.; Pozzati, A.; Di Pasquale, G.; Jaffe, A.S. Elevated cardiac troponin levels predict the risk of adverse outcome in patients with acute coronary syndromes. *Am. Heart J.* **2000**, *140*, 917–927. [CrossRef] [PubMed]
44. Oremus, M.; McKelvie, R.; Don-Wauchope, A.; Santaguida, P.L.; Ali, U.; Balion, C.; Hill, S.; Booth, R.; Brown, J.A.; Bustamam, A.; et al. A systematic review of BNP and NT-proBNP in the management of heart failure: Overview and methods. *Heart Fail. Rev.* **2014**, *19*, 413–419. [CrossRef] [PubMed]
45. Mountantonakis, S.; Gerstenfeld, E.P. Atrial Tachycardias Occurring After Atrial Fibrillation Ablation: Strategies for Mapping and Ablation. *J. Atr. Fibrillation* **2010**, *3*, 290. [CrossRef] [PubMed]
46. Scott, P.A.; Barry, J.; Roberts, P.R.; Morgan, J.M. Brain natriuretic peptide for the prediction of sudden cardiac death and ventricular arrhythmias: a meta-analysis. *Eur J Heart Fail* **2009**, *11*, 958–966. [CrossRef] [PubMed]
47. Golukhova, E.Z.; Gromova, O.; Grigoryan, M.; Merzlyakov, V.; Shumkov, K.; Bockeria, L.; Serebruany, V.L. Noninvasive Predictors of Malignant Arrhythmias. *Cardiology* **2016**, *135*, 36–42. [CrossRef]
48. Suzuki, S.; Yoshimura, M.; Nakayama, M.; Mizuno, Y.; Harada, E.; Ito, T.; Nakamura, S.; Abe, K.; Yamamuro, M.; Sakamoto, T.; et al. Plasma level of B-type natriuretic peptide as a prognostic marker after acute myocardial infarction: A long-term follow-up analysis. *Circulation* **2004**, *110*, 1387–1391. [CrossRef] [PubMed]
49. Lepojarvi, E.S.; Huikuri, H.V.; Piira, O.P.; Kiviniemi, A.M.; Miettinen, J.A.; Kentta, T.; Ukkola, O.; Perkiomaki, J.S.; Tulppo, M.P.; Junttila, M.J. Biomarkers as predictors of sudden cardiac death in coronary artery disease patients with preserved left ventricular function (ARTEMIS study). *PLoS ONE* **2018**, *13*, e0203363. [CrossRef]
50. Tapanainen, J.M.; Lindgren, K.S.; Makikallio, T.H.; Vuolteenaho, O.; Leppaluoto, J.; Huikuri, H.V. Natriuretic peptides as predictors of non-sudden and sudden cardiac death after acute myocardial infarction in the beta-blocking era. *J. Am. Coll. Cardiol.* **2004**, *43*, 757–763. [CrossRef]
51. Berger, R.; Huelsman, M.; Strecker, K.; Bojic, A.; Moser, P.; Stanek, B.; Pacher, R. B-type natriuretic peptide predicts sudden death in patients with chronic heart failure. *Circulation* **2002**, *105*, 2392–2397. [CrossRef]
52. Watanabe, J.; Shinozaki, T.; Shiba, N.; Fukahori, K.; Koseki, Y.; Karibe, A.; Sakuma, M.; Miura, M.; Kagaya, Y.; Shirato, K. Accumulation of risk markers predicts the incidence of sudden death in patients with chronic heart failure. *Eur. J. Heart Fail.* **2006**, *8*, 237–242. [CrossRef] [PubMed]
53. Medina, A.; Moss, A.J.; McNitt, S.; Zareba, W.; Wang, P.J.; Goldenberg, I. Brain natriuretic peptide and the risk of ventricular tachyarrhythmias in mildly symptomatic heart failure patients enrolled in MADIT-CRT. *Heart Rhythm* **2016**, *13*, 852–859. [CrossRef] [PubMed]
54. Christ, M.; Sharkova, J.; Bayrakcioglu, S.; Herzum, I.; Mueller, C.; Grimm, W. B-type natriuretic peptide levels predict event-free survival in patients with implantable cardioverter defibrillators. *Eur. J. Heart Fail.* **2007**, *9*, 272–279. [CrossRef] [PubMed]
55. Nagahara, D.; Nakata, T.; Hashimoto, A.; Wakabayashi, T.; Kyuma, M.; Noda, R.; Shimoshige, S.; Uno, K.; Tsuchihashi, K.; Shimamoto, K. Predicting the need for an implantable cardioverter defibrillator using cardiac metaiodobenzylguanidine activity together with plasma natriuretic peptide concentration or left ventricular function. *J. Nucl. Med.* **2008**, *49*, 225–233. [CrossRef]
56. Verma, A.; Kilicaslan, F.; Martin, D.O.; Minor, S.; Starling, R.; Marrouche, N.F.; Almahammed, S.; Wazni, O.M.; Duggal, S.; Zuzek, R.; et al. Preimplantation B-type natriuretic peptide concentration is an independent predictor of future appropriate implantable defibrillator therapies. *Heart* **2006**, *92*, 190–195. [CrossRef]

57. Vrtovec, B.; Knezevic, I.; Poglajen, G.; Sebestjen, M.; Okrajsek, R.; Haddad, F. Relation of B-type natriuretic peptide level in heart failure to sudden cardiac death in patients with and without QT interval prolongation. *Am. J. Cardiol.* **2013**, *111*, 886–890. [CrossRef]
58. Kubo, T.; Kitaoka, H.; Okawa, M.; Yamanaka, S.; Hirota, T.; Baba, Y.; Hayato, K.; Yamasaki, N.; Matsumura, Y.; Yasuda, N.; et al. Combined measurements of cardiac troponin I and brain natriuretic peptide are useful for predicting adverse outcomes in hypertrophic cardiomyopathy. *Circ. J.* **2011**, *75*, 919–926. [CrossRef]
59. Minami, Y.; Haruki, S.; Kanbayashi, K.; Maeda, R.; Itani, R.; Hagiwara, N. B-type natriuretic peptide and risk of sudden death in patients with hypertrophic cardiomyopathy. *Heart Rhythm* **2018**, *15*, 1484–1490. [CrossRef]
60. Bayes-Genis, A.; Vazquez, R.; Puig, T.; Fernandez-Palomeque, C.; Fabregat, J.; Bardaji, A.; Pascual-Figal, D.; Ordonez-Llanos, J.; Valdes, M.; Gabarrus, A.; et al. Left atrial enlargement and NT-proBNP as predictors of sudden cardiac death in patients with heart failure. *Eur. J. Heart Fail.* **2007**, *9*, 802–807. [CrossRef]
61. Tigen, K.; Karaahmet, T.; Kahveci, G.; Tanalp, A.C.; Bitigen, A.; Fotbolcu, H.; Bayrak, F.; Mutlu, B.; Basaran, Y. N-terminal pro brain natriuretic peptide to predict prognosis in dilated cardiomyopathy with sinus rhythm. *Heart Lung Circ.* **2007**, *16*, 290–294. [CrossRef]
62. Simon, T.; Becker, R.; Voss, F.; Bikou, O.; Hauck, M.; Licka, M.; Katus, H.A.; Bauer, A. Elevated B-type natriuretic peptide levels in patients with nonischemic cardiomyopathy predict occurrence of arrhythmic events. *Clin. Res. Cardiol.* **2008**, *97*, 306–309. [CrossRef]
63. Scott, P.A.; Townsend, P.A.; Ng, L.L.; Zeb, M.; Harris, S.; Roderick, P.J.; Curzen, N.P.; Morgan, J.M. Defining potential to benefit from implantable cardioverter defibrillator therapy: The role of biomarkers. *Europace* **2011**, *13*, 1419–1427. [CrossRef] [PubMed]
64. Klingenberg, R.; Zugck, C.; Becker, R.; Schellberg, D.; Heinze, G.; Kell, R.; Remppis, A.; Schoels, W.; Katus, H.A.; Dengler, T.J. Raised B-type natriuretic peptide predicts implantable cardioverter-defibrillator therapy in patients with ischemic cardiomyopathy. *Heart* **2006**, *92*, 1323–1324. [CrossRef] [PubMed]
65. Manios, E.G.; Kallergis, E.M.; Kanoupakis, E.M.; Mavrakis, H.E.; Kambouraki, D.C.; Arfanakis, D.A.; Vardas, P.E. Amino-terminal pro-brain natriuretic peptide predicts ventricular arrhythmogenesis in patients with ischemic cardiomyopathy and implantable cardioverter-defibrillators. *Chest* **2005**, *128*, 2604–2610. [CrossRef] [PubMed]
66. Yu, H.; Oswald, H.; Gardiwal, A.; Lissel, C.; Klein, G. Comparison of N-terminal pro-brain natriuretic peptide versus electrophysiologic study for predicting future outcomes in patients with an implantable cardioverter defibrillator after myocardial infarction. *Am. J. Cardiol.* **2007**, *100*, 635–639. [CrossRef]
67. Levine, Y.C.; Rosenberg, M.A.; Mittleman, M.; Samuel, M.; Methachittiphan, N.; Link, M.; Josephson, M.E.; Buxton, A.E. B-type natriuretic peptide is a major predictor of ventricular tachyarrhythmias. *Heart Rhythm* **2014**, *11*, 1109–1116. [CrossRef] [PubMed]
68. Aarsetoy, R.; Aarsetoy, H.; Hagve, T.A.; Strand, H.; Staines, H.; Nilsen, D.W.T. Initial Phase NT-proBNP, but Not Copeptin and High-Sensitivity Cardiac Troponin-T Yielded Diagnostic and Prognostic Information in Addition to Clinical Assessment of Out-of-Hospital Cardiac Arrest Patients With Documented Ventricular Fibrillation. *Front. Cardiovasc. Med.* **2018**, *5*, 44. [CrossRef]
69. Luchner, A.; Hengstenberg, C.; Lowel, H.; Riegger, G.A.; Schunkert, H.; Holmer, S. Effect of compensated renal dysfunction on approved heart failure markers: Direct comparison of brain natriuretic peptide (BNP) and N-terminal pro-BNP. *Hypertension* **2005**, *46*, 118–123. [CrossRef]
70. Wang, A.Y.; Lam, C.W.; Chan, I.H.; Wang, M.; Lui, S.F.; Sanderson, J.E. Sudden cardiac death in end-stage renal disease patients: A 5-year prospective analysis. *Hypertension* **2010**, *56*, 210–216. [CrossRef]
71. Kruzan, R.M.; Herzog, C.A.; Wu, A.; Sang, Y.; Parekh, R.S.; Matsushita, K.; Hwang, S.; Cheng, A.; Coresh, J.; Powe, N.R.; et al. Association of NTproBNP and cTnI with outpatient sudden cardiac death in hemodialysis patients: The Choices for Healthy Outcomes in Caring for ESRD (CHOICE) study. *BMC Nephrol.* **2016**, *17*, 18. [CrossRef]
72. Winkler, K.; Wanner, C.; Drechsler, C.; Lilienthal, J.; Marz, W.; Krane, V. Change in N-terminal-pro-B-type-natriuretic-peptide and the risk of sudden death, stroke, myocardial infarction, and all-cause mortality in diabetic dialysis patients. *Eur. Heart J.* **2008**, *29*, 2092–2099. [CrossRef] [PubMed]
73. Coats, C.J.; Gallagher, M.J.; Foley, M.; O'Mahony, C.; Critoph, C.; Gimeno, J.; Dawnay, A.; McKenna, W.J.; Elliott, P.M. Relation between serum N-terminal pro-brain natriuretic peptide and prognosis in patients with hypertrophic cardiomyopathy. *Eur. Heart J.* **2013**, *34*, 2529–2537. [CrossRef] [PubMed]

74. Rajtar-Salwa, R.; Hladij, R.; Dimitrow, P.P. Elevated Level of Troponin but Not N-Terminal Probrain Natriuretic Peptide Is Associated with Increased Risk of Sudden Cardiac Death in Hypertrophic Cardiomyopathy Calculated According to the ESC Guidelines 2014. *Dis. Markers* **2017**, *2017*, 9417908. [CrossRef] [PubMed]
75. Sajadieh, A.; Nielsen, O.W.; Rasmussen, V.; Ole Hein, H.; Hansen, J.F. Increased ventricular ectopic activity in relation to C-reactive protein, and NT-pro-brain natriuretic peptide in subjects with no apparent heart disease. *Pacing Clin. Electrophysiol.* **2006**, *29*, 1188–1194. [CrossRef]
76. Skranes, J.B.; Einvik, G.; Namtvedt, S.K.; Randby, A.; Hrubos-Strom, H.; Brynildsen, J.; Hagve, T.A.; Somers, V.K.; Rosjo, H.; Omland, T. Biomarkers of cardiovascular injury and stress are associated with increased frequency of ventricular ectopy: A population-based study. *BMC Cardiovasc. Disord.* **2016**, *16*, 233. [CrossRef]
77. Korngold, E.C.; Januzzi, J.L., Jr.; Gantzer, M.L.; Moorthy, M.V.; Cook, N.R.; Albert, C.M. Amino-terminal pro-B-type natriuretic peptide and high-sensitivity C-reactive protein as predictors of sudden cardiac death among women. *Circulation* **2009**, *119*, 2868–2876. [CrossRef]
78. Jaffe, A.S.; Ordonez-Llanos, J. High-sensitivity cardiac troponin: From theory to clinical practice. *Rev. Esp. Cardiol.* **2013**, *66*, 687–691. [CrossRef]
79. Sato, Y.; Yamada, T.; Taniguchi, R.; Nagai, K.; Makiyama, T.; Okada, H.; Kataoka, K.; Ito, H.; Matsumori, A.; Sasayama, S.; et al. Persistently increased serum concentrations of cardiac troponin t in patients with idiopathic dilated cardiomyopathy are predictive of adverse outcomes. *Circulation* **2001**, *103*, 369–374. [CrossRef]
80. Liu, Z.Q.; Cui, L.Q. Association between serum cardiac troponin I and myocardial remodeling in patients with chronic heart failure. *Zhonghua Xin Xue Guan Bing Za Zhi* **2006**, *34*, 437–439.
81. Hussein, A.A.; Gottdiener, J.S.; Bartz, T.M.; Sotoodehnia, N.; deFilippi, C.; Dickfeld, T.; Deo, R.; Siscovick, D.; Stein, P.K.; Lloyd-Jones, D. Cardiomyocyte injury assessed by a highly sensitive troponin assay and sudden cardiac death in the community: The Cardiovascular Health Study. *J. Am. Coll. Cardiol.* **2013**, *62*, 2112–2120. [CrossRef]
82. Baba, Y.; Kubo, T.; Yamanaka, S.; Hirota, T.; Tanioka, K.; Yamasaki, N.; Sugiura, T.; Kitaoka, H. Clinical significance of high-sensitivity cardiac troponin T in patients with dilated cardiomyopathy. *Int. Heart J.* **2015**, *56*, 309–313. [CrossRef] [PubMed]
83. Kawahara, C.; Tsutamoto, T.; Nishiyama, K.; Yamaji, M.; Sakai, H.; Fujii, M.; Yamamoto, T.; Horie, M. Prognostic role of high-sensitivity cardiac troponin T in patients with nonischemic dilated cardiomyopathy. *Circ. J.* **2011**, *75*, 656–661. [CrossRef] [PubMed]
84. Kubo, T.; Kitaoka, H.; Yamanaka, S.; Hirota, T.; Baba, Y.; Hayashi, K.; Iiyama, T.; Kumagai, N.; Tanioka, K.; Yamasaki, N.; et al. Significance of high-sensitivity cardiac troponin T in hypertrophic cardiomyopathy. *J. Am. Coll. Cardiol.* **2013**, *62*, 1252–1259. [CrossRef] [PubMed]
85. Daidoji, H.; Arimoto, T.; Nitobe, J.; Tamura, H.; Kutsuzawa, D.; Ishigaki, D.; Ishino, M.; Takahashi, H.; Shishido, T.; Miyashita, T.; et al. Circulating heart-type fatty acid binding protein levels predict the occurrence of appropriate shocks and cardiac death in patients with implantable cardioverter-defibrillators. *J. Card. Fail.* **2012**, *18*, 556–563. [CrossRef]
86. Nodera, M.; Suzuki, H.; Matsumoto, Y.; Kamioka, M.; Kaneshiro, T.; Yoshihisa, A.; Ohira, T.; Takeishi, Y. Association between Serum Uric Acid Level and Ventricular Tachyarrhythmia in Heart Failure Patients with Implantable Cardioverter-Defibrillator. *Cardiology* **2018**, *140*, 47–51. [CrossRef]
87. Flevari, P.; Theodorakis, G.; Leftheriotis, D.; Kroupis, C.; Kolokathis, F.; Dima, K.; Anastasiou-Nana, M.; Kremastinos, D. Serum markers of deranged myocardial collagen turnover: Their relation to malignant ventricular arrhythmias in cardioverter-defibrillator recipients with heart failure. *Am. Heart J.* **2012**, *164*, 530–537. [CrossRef]
88. Francia, P.; Adduci, C.; Semprini, L.; Borro, M.; Ricotta, A.; Sensini, I.; Santini, D.; Caprinozzi, M.; Balla, C.; Simmaco, M.; et al. Osteopontin and galectin-3 predict the risk of ventricular tachycardia and fibrillation in heart failure patients with implantable defibrillators. *J. Cardiovasc. Electrophysiol.* **2014**, *25*, 609–616. [CrossRef]
89. Ahmad, T.; Fiuzat, M.; Neely, B.; Neely, M.L.; Pencina, M.J.; Kraus, W.E.; Zannad, F.; Whellan, D.J.; Donahue, M.P.; Pina, I.L.; et al. Biomarkers of myocardial stress and fibrosis as predictors of mode of death in patients with chronic heart failure. *JACC Heart Fail.* **2014**, *2*, 260–268. [CrossRef]

90. Skali, H.; Gerwien, R.; Meyer, T.E.; Snider, J.V.; Solomon, S.D.; Stolen, C.M. Soluble ST2 and Risk of Arrhythmias, Heart Failure, or Death in Patients with Mildly Symptomatic Heart Failure: Results from MADIT-CRT. *J. Cardiovasc. Transl. Res.* **2016**, *9*, 421–428. [CrossRef]
91. Pascual-Figal, D.A.; Ordonez-Llanos, J.; Tornel, P.L.; Vazquez, R.; Puig, T.; Valdes, M.; Cinca, J.; de Luna, A.B.; Bayes-Genis, A.; Investigators, M. Soluble ST2 for predicting sudden cardiac death in patients with chronic heart failure and left ventricular systolic dysfunction. *J. Am. Coll. Cardiol.* **2009**, *54*, 2174–2179. [CrossRef]
92. Oz, F.; Onur, I.; Elitok, A.; Ademoglu, E.; Altun, I.; Bilge, A.K.; Adalet, K. Galectin-3 correlates with arrhythmogenic right ventricular cardiomyopathy and predicts the risk of ventricular-arrhythmias in patients with implantable defibrillators. *Acta Cardiol.* **2017**, *72*, 453–459. [CrossRef] [PubMed]
93. Daidoji, H.; Arimoto, T.; Iwayama, T.; Ishigaki, D.; Hashimoto, N.; Kumagai, Y.; Nishiyama, S.; Takahashi, H.; Shishido, T.; Miyamoto, T.; et al. Circulating heart-type fatty acid-binding protein levels predict ventricular fibrillation in Brugada syndrome. *J. Cardiol.* **2016**, *67*, 221–228. [CrossRef] [PubMed]
94. Zachariah, J.P.; Colan, S.D.; Lang, P.; Triedman, J.K.; Alexander, M.E.; Walsh, E.P.; Berul, C.I.; Cecchin, F. Circulating matrix metalloproteinases in adolescents with hypertrophic cardiomyopathy and ventricular arrhythmia. *Circ. Heart Fail.* **2012**, *5*, 462–466. [CrossRef] [PubMed]
95. Emet, S.; Dadashov, M.; Sonsoz, M.R.; Cakir, M.O.; Yilmaz, M.; Elitok, A.; Bilge, A.K.; Mercanoglu, F.; Oncul, A.; Adalet, K.; et al. Galectin-3: A Novel Biomarker Predicts Sudden Cardiac Death in Hypertrophic Cardiomyopathy. *Am. J. Med. Sci.* **2018**, *356*, 537–543. [CrossRef]
96. Kunutsor, S.K.; Kurl, S.; Zaccardi, F.; Laukkanen, J.A. Baseline and long-term fibrinogen levels and risk of sudden cardiac death: A new prospective study and meta-analysis. *Atherosclerosis* **2016**, *245*, 171–180. [CrossRef]
97. Yamade, M.; Sugimoto, M.; Uotani, T.; Nishino, M.; Kodaira, C.; Furuta, T. Resistance of Helicobacter pylori to quinolones and clarithromycin assessed by genetic testing in Japan. *J. Gastroenterol. Hepatol.* **2011**, *26*, 1457–1461. [CrossRef]
98. Deo, R.; Sotoodehnia, N.; Katz, R.; Sarnak, M.J.; Fried, L.F.; Chonchol, M.; Kestenbaum, B.; Psaty, B.M.; Siscovick, D.S.; Shlipak, M.G. Cystatin C and sudden cardiac death risk in the elderly. *Circ. Cardiovasc. Qual. Outcomes* **2010**, *3*, 159–164. [CrossRef]
99. Jouven, X.; Charles, M.A.; Desnos, M.; Ducimetiere, P. Circulating nonesterified fatty acid level as a predictive risk factor for sudden death in the population. *Circulation* **2001**, *104*, 756–761. [CrossRef]
100. Pascual-Figal, D.A.; Januzzi, J.L. The biology of ST2: The International ST2 Consensus Panel. *Am. J. Cardiol.* **2015**, *115*, 3B–7B. [CrossRef]
101. Shah, R.V.; Januzzi, J.L., Jr. ST2: A novel remodeling biomarker in acute and chronic heart failure. *Curr. Heart Fail. Rep.* **2010**, *7*, 9–14. [CrossRef]
102. Brint, E.K.; Fitzgerald, K.A.; Smith, P.; Coyle, A.J.; Gutierrez-Ramos, J.C.; Fallon, P.G.; O'Neill, L.A. Characterization of signaling pathways activated by the interleukin 1 (IL-1) receptor homologue T1/ST2. A role for Jun N-terminal kinase in IL-4 induction. *J. Biol. Chem.* **2002**, *277*, 49205–49211. [CrossRef] [PubMed]
103. Kakkar, R.; Lee, R.T. The IL-33/ST2 pathway: Therapeutic target and novel biomarker. *Nat. Rev. Drug Discov.* **2008**, *7*, 827–840. [CrossRef] [PubMed]
104. Weir, R.A.; Miller, A.M.; Murphy, G.E.; Clements, S.; Steedman, T.; Connell, J.M.; McInnes, I.B.; Dargie, H.J.; McMurray, J.J. Serum soluble ST2: A potential novel mediator in left ventricular and infarct remodeling after acute myocardial infarction. *J. Am. Coll. Cardiol.* **2010**, *55*, 243–250. [CrossRef] [PubMed]
105. Mueller, T.; Dieplinger, B.; Gegenhuber, A.; Poelz, W.; Pacher, R.; Haltmayer, M. Increased plasma concentrations of soluble ST2 are predictive for 1-year mortality in patients with acute destabilized heart failure. *Clin. Chem.* **2008**, *54*, 752–756. [CrossRef]
106. Januzzi, J.L., Jr.; Peacock, W.F.; Maisel, A.S.; Chae, C.U.; Jesse, R.L.; Baggish, A.L.; O'Donoghue, M.; Sakhuja, R.; Chen, A.A.; van Kimmenade, R.R.; et al. Measurement of the interleukin family member ST2 in patients with acute dyspnea: Results from the PRIDE (Pro-Brain Natriuretic Peptide Investigation of Dyspnea in the Emergency Department) study. *J. Am. Coll. Cardiol.* **2007**, *50*, 607–613. [CrossRef] [PubMed]
107. Ky, B.; French, B.; McCloskey, K.; Rame, J.E.; McIntosh, E.; Shahi, P.; Dries, D.L.; Tang, W.H.; Wu, A.H.; Fang, J.C.; et al. High-sensitivity ST2 for prediction of adverse outcomes in chronic heart failure. *Circ. Heart Fail.* **2011**, *4*, 180–187. [CrossRef]

108. Dejgaard, L.A.; Skjolsvik, E.T.; Lie, O.H.; Ribe, M.; Stokke, M.K.; Hegbom, F.; Scheirlynck, E.S.; Gjertsen, E.; Andresen, K.; Helle-Valle, T.M.; et al. The Mitral Annulus Disjunction Arrhythmic Syndrome. *J. Am. Coll. Cardiol.* **2018**, *72*, 1600–1609. [CrossRef]
109. Scheirlynck, E.; Dejgaard, L.A.; Skjolsvik, E.; Lie, O.H.; Motoc, A.; Hopp, E.; Tanaka, K.; Ueland, T.; Ribe, M.; Collet, C.; et al. Increased levels of sST2 in patients with mitral annulus disjunction and ventricular arrhythmias. *Open Heart* **2019**, *6*, e001016. [CrossRef]
110. Vasta, G.R. Galectins as pattern recognition receptors: Structure, function, and evolution. *Adv. Exp. Med. Biol.* **2012**, *946*, 21–36. [CrossRef]
111. Dumic, J.; Dabelic, S.; Flogel, M. Galectin-3: An open-ended story. *Biochim. Biophys. Acta* **2006**, *1760*, 616–635. [CrossRef]
112. Haudek, K.C.; Spronk, K.J.; Voss, P.G.; Patterson, R.J.; Wang, J.L.; Arnoys, E.J. Dynamics of galectin-3 in the nucleus and cytoplasm. *Biochim. Biophys. Acta* **2010**, *1800*, 181–189. [CrossRef] [PubMed]
113. Hrynchyshyn, N.; Jourdain, P.; Desnos, M.; Diebold, B.; Funck, F. Galectin-3: A new biomarker for the diagnosis, analysis and prognosis of acute and chronic heart failure. *Arch. Cardiovasc. Dis.* **2013**, *106*, 541–546. [CrossRef]
114. Diaz-Alvarez, L.; Ortega, E. The Many Roles of Galectin-3, a Multifaceted Molecule, in Innate Immune Responses against Pathogens. *Mediat. Inflamm.* **2017**, *2017*, 9247574. [CrossRef] [PubMed]
115. Henderson, N.C.; Mackinnon, A.C.; Farnworth, S.L.; Kipari, T.; Haslett, C.; Iredale, J.P.; Liu, F.T.; Hughes, J.; Sethi, T. Galectin-3 expression and secretion links macrophages to the promotion of renal fibrosis. *Am. J. Pathol.* **2008**, *172*, 288–298. [CrossRef] [PubMed]
116. Parikh, R.H.; Seliger, S.L.; Christenson, R.; Gottdiener, J.S.; Psaty, B.M.; deFilippi, C.R. Soluble ST2 for Prediction of Heart Failure and Cardiovascular Death in an Elderly, Community-Dwelling Population. *J. Am. Heart Assoc.* **2016**, *5*. [CrossRef]
117. de Boer, R.A.; van Veldhuisen, D.J.; Gansevoort, R.T.; Muller Kobold, A.C.; van Gilst, W.H.; Hillege, H.L.; Bakker, S.J.; van der Harst, P. The fibrosis marker galectin-3 and outcome in the general population. *J. Intern. Med.* **2012**, *272*, 55–64. [CrossRef]
118. Gehlken, C.; Suthahar, N.; Meijers, W.C.; de Boer, R.A. Galectin-3 in Heart Failure: An Update of the Last 3 Years. *Heart Fail. Clin.* **2018**, *14*, 75–92. [CrossRef]
119. Glatz, J.F.; van Bilsen, M.; Paulussen, R.J.; Veerkamp, J.H.; van der Vusse, G.J.; Reneman, R.S. Release of fatty acid-binding protein from isolated rat heart subjected to ischemia and reperfusion or to the calcium paradox. *Biochim. Biophys. Acta* **1988**, *961*, 148–152. [CrossRef]
120. Kleine, A.H.; Glatz, J.F.; Van Nieuwenhoven, F.A.; Van der Vusse, G.J. Release of heart fatty acid-binding protein into plasma after acute myocardial infarction in man. *Mol. Cell. Biochem.* **1992**, *116*, 155–162. [CrossRef]
121. Otaki, Y.; Watanabe, T.; Takahashi, H.; Hirayama, A.; Narumi, T.; Kadowaki, S.; Honda, Y.; Arimoto, T.; Shishido, T.; Miyamoto, T.; et al. Association of heart-type fatty acid-binding protein with cardiovascular risk factors and all-cause mortality in the general population: The Takahata study. *PLoS ONE* **2014**, *9*, e94834. [CrossRef]
122. Sieira, J.; Brugada, P. The definition of the Brugada syndrome. *Eur. Heart J.* **2017**, *38*, 3029–3034. [CrossRef] [PubMed]
123. Lindsey, M.L.; Iyer, R.P.; Jung, M.; DeLeon-Pennell, K.Y.; Ma, Y. Matrix metalloproteinases as input and output signals for post-myocardial infarction remodeling. *J. Mol. Cell. Cardiol.* **2016**, *91*, 134–140. [CrossRef] [PubMed]
124. Wilson, E.M.; Gunasinghe, H.R.; Coker, M.L.; Sprunger, P.; Lee-Jackson, D.; Bozkurt, B.; Deswal, A.; Mann, D.L.; Spinale, F.G. Plasma matrix metalloproteinase and inhibitor profiles in patients with heart failure. *J. Card. Fail.* **2002**, *8*, 390–398. [CrossRef] [PubMed]
125. Cicoira, M.; Rossi, A.; Bonapace, S.; Zanolla, L.; Golia, G.; Franceschini, L.; Caruso, B.; Marino, P.N.; Zardini, P. Independent and additional prognostic value of aminoterminal propeptide of type III procollagen circulating levels in patients with chronic heart failure. *J. Card. Fail.* **2004**, *10*, 403–411. [CrossRef] [PubMed]
126. Yanagisawa, M.; Kurihara, H.; Kimura, S.; Tomobe, Y.; Kobayashi, M.; Mitsui, Y.; Yazaki, Y.; Goto, K.; Masaki, T. A novel potent vasoconstrictor peptide produced by vascular endothelial cells. *Nature* **1988**, *332*, 411–415. [CrossRef] [PubMed]

127. Barton, M.; Luscher, T.F. Endothelin antagonists for hypertension and renal disease. *Curr. Opin. Nephrol. Hypertens.* **1999**, *8*, 549–556. [CrossRef]
128. Marasciulo, F.L.; Montagnani, M.; Potenza, M.A. Endothelin-1: The yin and yang on vascular function. *Curr. Med. Chem.* **2006**, *13*, 1655–1665. [CrossRef]
129. Abebe, W.; Agrawal, D.K. Role of tyrosine kinases in norepinephrine-induced contraction of vascular smooth muscle. *J. Cardiovasc. Pharm.* **1995**, *26*, 153–159. [CrossRef]
130. Szokodi, I.; Horkay, F.; Merkely, B.; Solti, F.; Geller, L.; Kiss, P.; Selmeci, L.; Kekesi, V.; Vuolteenaho, O.; Ruskoaho, H.; et al. Intrapericardial infusion of endothelin-1 induces ventricular arrhythmias in dogs. *Cardiovasc. Res.* **1998**, *38*, 356–364. [CrossRef]
131. Salvati, P.; Chierchia, S.; Dho, L.; Ferrario, R.G.; Parenti, P.; Vicedomini, G.; Patrono, C. Proarrhythmic activity of intracoronary endothelin in dogs: Relation to the site of administration and to changes in regional flow. *J. Cardiovasc. Pharm.* **1991**, *17*, 1007–1014. [CrossRef]
132. Yorikane, R.; Shiga, H.; Miyake, S.; Koike, H. Evidence for direct arrhythmogenic action of endothelin. *Biochem. Biophys. Res. Commun.* **1990**, *173*, 457–462. [CrossRef]
133. Yorikane, R.; Koike, H.; Miyake, S. Electrophysiological effects of endothelin-1 on canine myocardial cells. *J. Cardiovasc. Pharm.* **1991**, *17*, S159–S162. [CrossRef]
134. Wang, Z.; Li, S.; Lai, H.; Zhou, L.; Meng, G.; Wang, M.; Lai, Y.; Wang, Z.; Chen, H.; Zhou, X.; et al. Interaction between Endothelin-1 and Left Stellate Ganglion Activation: A Potential Mechanism of Malignant Ventricular Arrhythmia during Myocardial Ischemia. *Oxid. Med. Cell. Longev.* **2019**, *2019*, 6508328. [CrossRef]
135. Kiesecker, C.; Zitron, E.; Scherer, D.; Lueck, S.; Bloehs, R.; Scholz, E.P.; Pirot, M.; Kathofer, S.; Thomas, D.; Kreye, V.A.; et al. Regulation of cardiac inwardly rectifying potassium current IK1 and Kir2.x channels by endothelin-1. *J. Mol. Med.* **2006**, *84*, 46–56. [CrossRef] [PubMed]
136. Aronson, D.; Burger, A.J. Neurohumoral activation and ventricular arrhythmias in patients with decompensated congestive heart failure: Role of endothelin. *Pacing Clin. Electrophysiol.* **2003**, *26*, 703–710. [CrossRef] [PubMed]
137. Szucs, A.; Keltai, K.; Zima, E.; Vago, H.; Soos, P.; Roka, A.; Szabolcs, Z.; Geller, L.; Merkely, B. Effects of implantable cardioverter defibrillator implantation and shock application on serum endothelin-1 and big-endothelin levels. *Clin. Sci.* **2002**, *103*, 233S–236S. [CrossRef] [PubMed]
138. Muiesan, M.L.; Agabiti-Rosei, C.; Paini, A.; Salvetti, M. Uric Acid and Cardiovascular Disease: An Update. *Eur. Cardiol.* **2016**, *11*, 54–59. [CrossRef]
139. Anker, S.D.; Doehner, W.; Rauchhaus, M.; Sharma, R.; Francis, D.; Knosalla, C.; Davos, C.H.; Cicoira, M.; Shamim, W.; Kemp, M.; et al. Uric acid and survival in chronic heart failure: Validation and application in metabolic, functional, and hemodynamic staging. *Circulation* **2003**, *107*, 1991–1997. [CrossRef]
140. Yamada, S.; Suzuki, H.; Kamioka, M.; Kamiyama, Y.; Saitoh, S.; Takeishi, Y. Uric acid increases the incidence of ventricular arrhythmia in patients with left ventricular hypertrophy. *Fukushima J. Med. Sci.* **2012**, *58*, 101–106. [CrossRef]
141. Pieters, M.; Wolberg, A.S. Fibrinogen and fibrin: An illustrated review. *Res. Pr. Thromb. Haemost.* **2019**, *3*, 161–172. [CrossRef]
142. Stec, J.J.; Silbershatz, H.; Tofler, G.H.; Matheney, T.H.; Sutherland, P.; Lipinska, I.; Massaro, J.M.; Wilson, P.F.; Muller, J.E.; D'Agostino, R.B., Sr. Association of fibrinogen with cardiovascular risk factors and cardiovascular disease in the Framingham Offspring Population. *Circulation* **2000**, *102*, 1634–1638. [CrossRef] [PubMed]
143. Collins, A.J.; Kasiske, B.; Herzog, C.; Chen, S.C.; Everson, S.; Constantini, E.; Grimm, R.; McBean, M.; Xue, J.; Chavers, B.; et al. Excerpts from the United States Renal Data System 2003 Annual Data Report: Atlas of end-stage renal disease in the United States. *Am. J. Kidney Dis.* **2003**, *42*, S1–230.
144. Levin, A.; Lan, J.H. Cystatin C and Cardiovascular Disease: Causality, Association, and Clinical Implications of Knowing the Difference. *J. Am. Coll. Cardiol.* **2016**, *68*, 946–948. [CrossRef] [PubMed]
145. Choi, S.T.; Kim, J.H.; Kang, E.J.; Lee, S.W.; Park, M.C.; Park, Y.B.; Lee, S.K. Osteopontin might be involved in bone remodeling rather than in inflammation in ankylosing spondylitis. *Rheumatology* **2008**, *47*, 1775–1779. [CrossRef]
146. Wang, K.X.; Denhardt, D.T. Osteopontin: Role in immune regulation and stress responses. *Cytokine Growth Factor Rev.* **2008**, *19*, 333–345. [CrossRef]

147. Dinh, W.; Futh, R.; Lankisch, M.; Hess, G.; Zdunek, D.; Scheffold, T.; Kramer, F.; Klein, R.M.; Barroso, M.C.; Nickl, W. Growth-differentiation factor-15: A novel biomarker in patients with diastolic dysfunction? *Arq Bras. Cardiol.* **2011**, *97*, 65–75. [CrossRef]
148. Rueda, F.; Lupon, J.; Garcia-Garcia, C.; Cediel, G.; Aranda Nevado, M.C.; Serra Gregori, J.; Labata, C.; Oliveras, T.; Ferrer, M.; de Diego, O.; et al. Acute-phase dynamics and prognostic value of growth differentiation factor-15 in ST-elevation myocardial infarction. *Clin. Chem. Lab. Med.* **2019**, *57*, 1093–1101. [CrossRef]
149. Garcia-Garcia, C.; Rueda, F.; Lupon, J.; Oliveras, T.; Labata, C.; Ferrer, M.; Cediel, G.; De Diego, O.; Rodriguez-Leor, O.; Carrillo, X.; et al. Growth differentiation factor-15 is a predictive biomarker in primary ventricular fibrillation: The RUTI-STEMI-PVF study. *Eur. Heart J. Acute Cardiovasc. Care* **2018**. [CrossRef]

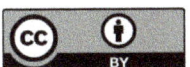

© 2020 by the authors. Licensee MDPI, Basel, Switzerland. This article is an open access article distributed under the terms and conditions of the Creative Commons Attribution (CC BY) license (http://creativecommons.org/licenses/by/4.0/).

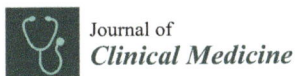 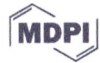

Review

Peripheral Blood Mononuclear Cells and Platelets Mitochondrial Dysfunction, Oxidative Stress, and Circulating mtDNA in Cardiovascular Diseases

Abrar Alfatni [1], Marianne Riou [1,2], Anne-Laure Charles [1], Alain Meyer [1,2], Cindy Barnig [1,2], Emmanuel Andres [3], Anne Lejay [1,2,4], Samy Talha [1,2] and Bernard Geny [1,2,*]

1. Unistra, Translational Medicine Federation of Strasbourg (FMTS), Faculty of Medicine, Team 3072 "Mitochondria, Oxidative Stress and Muscle Protection", 11 rue Humann, 67000 Strasbourg, France; aaalfatni@hotmail.com (A.A.); marianne.riou@chru-strasbourg.fr (M.R.); anne.laure.charles@unistra.fr (A.-L.C.); cindy.barnig@chru-strasbourg.fr (C.B.); alain.meyer1@chru-strasbourg.fr (A.M.); anne.lejay@chru-strasbourg.fr (A.L.); samy.talha@chru-strasbourg.fr (S.T.)
2. University Hospital of Strasbourg, Physiology and Functional Exploration Service, 1 Place de l'Hôpital, 67091 Strasbourg CEDEX, France
3. Internal Medicine, Diabete and Metabolic Diseases Service, University Hospital of Strasbourg, 1 Place de l'Hôpital, 67091 Strasbourg CEDEX, France; emmanuel.andres@chru-strasbourg.fr
4. Vascular Surgery and Kidney Transplantation Service, University Hospital of Strasbourg, 1 Place de l'Hôpital, 67091 Strasbourg CEDEX, France
* Correspondence: bernard.geny@chru-strasbourg.fr

Received: 31 December 2019; Accepted: 19 January 2020; Published: 22 January 2020

Abstract: Cardiovascular diseases (CVDs) are devastating disorders and the leading cause of mortality worldwide. The pathophysiology of cardiovascular diseases is complex and multifactorial and, in the past years, mitochondrial dysfunction and excessive production of reactive oxygen species (ROS) have gained growing attention. Indeed, CVDs can be considered as a systemic alteration, and understanding the eventual implication of circulating blood cells peripheral blood mononuclear cells (PBMCs) and or platelets, and particularly their mitochondrial function, ROS production, and mitochondrial DNA (mtDNA) releases in patients with cardiac impairments, appears worthwhile. Interestingly, reports consistently demonstrate a reduced mitochondrial respiratory chain oxidative capacity related to the degree of CVD severity and to an increased ROS production by PBMCs. Further, circulating mtDNA level was generally modified in such patients. These data are critical steps in term of cardiac disease comprehension and further studies are warranted to challenge the possible adjunct of PBMCs' and platelets' mitochondrial dysfunction, oxidative stress, and circulating mtDNA as biomarkers of CVD diagnosis and prognosis. This new approach might also allow further interesting therapeutic developments.

Keywords: cardiovascular diseases; mitochondrial dysfunction; circulating cells; PBMCS; platelets; oxidative stress; reactive oxygen species (ROS); mitochondrial DNA (mtDNA); biomarkers; herat failure

1. Introduction

Cardiovascular diseases (CVDs) rank as one of the first diseases leading to death worldwide [1,2]. The 2019 report of the American Heart Association shows that between 2013 and 2016, CVDs, including hypertension, heart failure (HF), coronary heart disease, and stroke, were present in about 48% of patients older than 20 years in the United States [3–5]. Significant progress has been made concerning CVD diagnosis and therapies, particularly considering neuro-hormonal modulation, such as natriuretic peptide (NP)-guided therapy [2,6–9], but it seems that a plateau has begun to be reached, suggesting new approaches. In this view, since CVDs are generally systemic diseases, an attempt based on circulating cells might be proposed to better understand CVD pathophysiology and to discover new biomarkers. Indeed, growing evidence suggests that the assessment of mitochondrial respiratory function of circulating peripheral blood mononuclear cells (PBMCs) and platelets might be viewed as a marker to detect the mitochondrial dysfunction in different tissues, including the heart [10–14].

The myocardium possesses one of the highest number of mitochondria in the body, allowing heart pumping activity through ATP production. Mitochondria are known contributors to the pathogenesis and outcome of several cardiovascular diseases. Indeed, regardless of cardiac disease etiology, most evidence demonstrates that mitochondrial dysfunction is widely observed in the pathological heart.

Mitochondrial dysfunction might be inferred from tissues' or cells' oxygen consumption (reflecting mitochondrial oxidative capacity) and the mitochondrial membrane potential (reflecting the ability of the electron transport system to maintain the gradient of proton driving ATP production). Thus, the failure of mitochondria to produce ATP results in an energy deficit, impairing cells, and finally, organ function [14–19].

Mitochondria have also been identified as significant sources of reactive oxygen species (ROS) [20]. Research reveals that oxidative stress, due to increased ROS and/or reduced antioxidant capacity, plays a considerable role in the development of HF and determines patient prognosis. Increased ROS accumulation and inflammation play a key role in the cardiac and vascular functional and structural damage underlying all major causes of CVDs [21]. However, the fundamental mechanism of ROS production in HF deserves to be further investigated [22]. Thus, it would be interesting to further monitor ROS levels and mitochondrial function in circulating cells in order to improve both diagnosis and follow-up of patients with CVDs.

Indeed, if tissue biopsies are relevant to the investigation of pathological changes and study of mitochondrial function in diseased organs, they are invasive and not always feasible. Alternatively, peripheral blood mononuclear cells (PBMCs) and/or platelets represent an easily available population of cells allowing mitochondrial function studies. Analysis of the energetic profile (mitochondrial function) of circulating blood cells in experimental animals and humans appears as a new research field with potential applications in the development of disease biomarkers in several settings, including respiratory and CVDs [10–14,19,23,24].

This review presents data exploring the PBMCs' and platelets' mitochondrial function, together with their ROS production and mitochondrial DNA release in order to assess whether such key parameters are modified and might be considered as biological markers of CVDs with diagnosis, prognosis, and even prognosis interests.

2. Is Mitochondrial Function Accessible in all Circulating Cells in the Blood?

2.1. Classification of Circulating Cells

There are many circulating cells in the blood, ranging from different population subtypes of white cells involved in immunity and inflammation, to platelets modulating blood aggregation and to red cells mainly transporting O_2. Several techniques might be used to separate blood cells in the blood, but gradient centrifugation is generally performed (Figure 1). Theoretically, the oxidative capacity of all circulating cells—through mitochondrial respiratory chain complexes activities assessment—might be explored, but there is a noticeable exception. Unlike in birds, for instance, human red blood cells do not present with mitochondria [25].

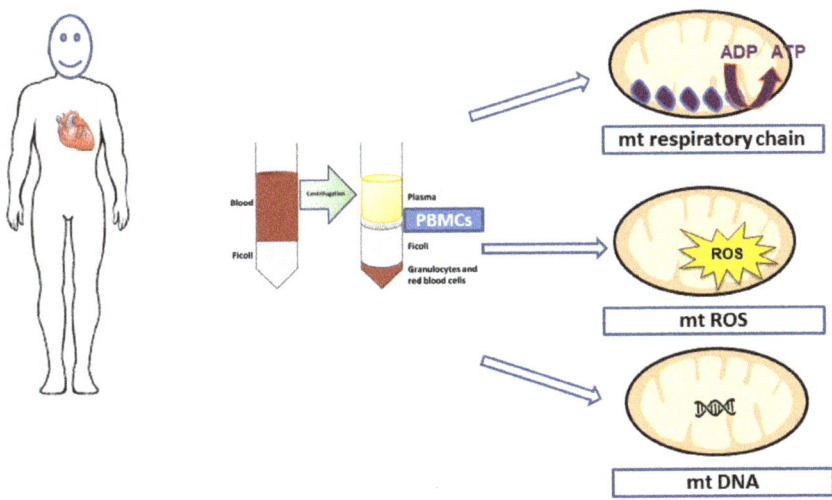

Figure 1. Density gradient centrifugation of whole blood allows peripheral blood mononuclear cells (PBMCs) isolation and then mitochondrial respiratory chain, reactive oxygen species, and DNA analysis.

The PBMC fraction consists of lymphocytes (T, B, and natural killer cells), monocytes, and dendritic cells. Circulating lymphocytes represent a mixed population of cells and ensure cellular or humoral immunity. Many types of lymphocytes can be distinguished: B cells produce antibodies, T cells support cellular immunity, and natural killer cells have their own cytolytic activity. The production of monoclonal antibodies specific for an expressed antigen can be conducted for immunophenotypic lymphocyte classification: Cluster of differentiation (CD) was created to group antibodies that recognize the same antigens. However, to date, no clear data are available on these specific cells' subtypes concerning their mitochondrial respiration. Monocytes, with a uni-lobular nucleus, have an important role in phagocytosis and the innate immune system.

Platelets are un-nucleated cells produced by cytoplasm fragmentation of megakaryocytes in the bone marrow, circulating in the peripheral blood for 7 to 10 days. They play a significant role in homeostasis and are essential for thrombus formation during the hemostatic process and are largely involved in thrombosis, myocardial infarction, stroke, and phlebitis. Platelets thus play an important role in CVDs, both in the pathogenesis of atherosclerosis and in the development of thrombotic events when presenting with qualitative and/or quantitative impairments [11,13,26,27]. Circulating platelets possess numerous mitochondria, can be obtained easily even from critically ill patients, and their isolation is performed routinely with success [28].

2.2. Isolation and Mitochondrial Respiratory Chain Activities' Determination in PBMCs and Platelets

Mitochondria are the main source of cellular energy, coupling the oxidation of fatty acids and pyruvate to the production of high amounts of ATP through the mitochondrial electron transport chain (ETC) [29]. Briefly, free electrons are transferred from complex I to complexes II, III, and IV of the ETC, thereby allowing complexes I, III, and IV to extrude protons from the matrix. The return of H+ ions from the mitochondrial membrane interspace towards the matrix allows the complex V to phosphorylate ADP into ATP.

The function of each complex is investigated by using a spectrophotometer and can be performed in cellular or tissue samples. Besides the determination of oxygen consumption, ATP synthesis and the mitochondrial membrane potential can also be investigated [30]. Specifically, Hsiao and Hoppel presented an optimal comprehensive method for analyzing the ETC activity in PBMCs [31]. There are two general techniques that have been used in vitro for the assessment of mitochondrial function and detection of delicate changes in the respiration rate of mitochondria in PBMCs and platelets isolated from peripheral blood by measuring oxygen consumption [12,13,32]. The first method is the extracellular flux analyzer. This technique provides efficient, comprehensive, and highly reproducible results and is commonly used to measure cellular bioenergetics function in intact and permeabilized cells [33]. A distinct trait of this protocol compared to others is that it does not entail mitochondrial isolation and can be operated using a minimal number of cells [33]. The second method is high-resolution respirometry (Oroboros O2K), which permits active investigation of metabolic pathways [12] and requires the availability of sufficient numbers of cells [10].

Although circulating platelets count for small numbers of functional mitochondria, they have high energy consumption levels and have been used widely to study the mitochondrial function in human disease due to their accessibility [34]. This is confirmed by a review by Kramer et al. presenting the maximal mitochondrial oxygen consumption devoted to the bioenergetic function in circulating platelets, monocytes, and lymphocytes. Interestingly, there is a distinct metabolism program between circulating platelets and leukocytes that could act as different sensors of the metabolic and inflammatory stress in many diseases [13].

3. Mitochondrial Respiratory Chain Complex Activities of PBMCs and Platelets in Patients with Cardiovascular Diseases

3.1. PBMCs Mitochondrial Respiratory Chain Activity in Cardiovascular Diseases

Interestingly, when evaluating mitochondrial respiratory chain complexes' activity in PBMCs in heart failure patients, Li et al. demonstrated that mitochondrial oxygen consumption, particularly in complex I and II, was significantly smaller as compared to the control group [29]. Such depressed PBMC mitochondrial function was observed in patients with early-stage congestive heart failure (CHF, asymptomatic patients) [29]. Possible explanations of this reduction in the electron transport chain activity in PBMCs are increased mitochondrial mitophagy and decreased biogenesis per mononuclear cell [29]. Moreover, the mitochondrial respiration was inversely related with inflammatory factors, such as high sensitivity C-reactive protein, IL6, and TNF-α. Thus, impaired mitochondrial respiratory functions of PBMCs characterize heart failure patients. Accordingly, a significant reduction of NDUFC2 expression, a subunit of mitochondrial complex I, has been detected in peripheral circulating mononuclear cells in patients with acute coronary syndrome [35]

More generally, there are several factors that might disrupt the function of the circulating leukocyte mitochondrial respiratory chain in CHF. Increased intracellular oxidants could induce mitochondrial permeability transition and inhibit respiratory coupling, which reflects mitochondrial respiratory chain disruption [36,37]. Kong et al. observed a reduction in the leukocyte, lymphocyte, and monocyte mitochondrial transmembrane potential (MTP) in congestive heart patients, in association with apoptosis and increased inflammation and ROS formation [37]. This decrease was more notable in the edematous CHF group when considering lymphocytes. Additionally, increased ROS led to mitochondrial depolarization [37]. Further, the percentage of apoptotic cells was greater in PMN than PBMCs (42.9% vs. 20%, respectively).

Song et al. found lower MTP and higher ROS levels in lymphocytes of CHF patients at low risk associated with increased serum NT-ProBNP, a diagnosis and prognosis biomarker in heart failure [36]. Furthermore, Coluccia et al., analyzing the mitochondrial membrane potential by cytofluorometric TMRM and JC-1 staining, found significant mitochondrial depolarization in PBMCs among HF patients after the administration of inflammatory stimulus lipopolysaccharide (LPS) [38]. The ultrastructural changes in mitochondria PBMCs showed a decrease in the index associated with the loss of inner mitochondrial membrane (IMM) and with an increase in the percentage of the apoptotic cells and mitophagy in HF-PBMC individuals, both at baseline and after LPS stimulation. The impairment of the inner mitochondrial membrane in PBMCs might reflect the impairment of the electron transport chain mitochondrial uncoupling [38] (Table 1). Thus, PBMCs' mitochondrial respiration can be considered as an innovative model to investigate the pathophysiology of CVDs.

3.2. Platelets' Mitochondrial Respiratory Chain Activity in Cardiovascular Diseases

Circulating platelets contain small number of functional mitochondria (averaging four mitochondria/platelet), but they are very metabolically active with a high rate of ATP turnover [39]. Platelets have higher oxygen consumption rates compared to leucocytes, since higher levels of ATP are required for the normal functioning of ion channels that maintain the intracellular ionic balance, essential for preventing platelet activation in basal conditions [13]. In platelets, mitochondrial complex III and IV are very low, underlying the severe impact of mitochondrial damage on platelet function. Electron transport chain activity in platelets is altered in many diseases [34]. However, there are few data in CVDs.

In resting platelets, mitochondrial respiration accounts for three-quarters of the energy production, with glycolysis providing the remaining [40]. The metabolic pool of ATP and ADP is located in the cytoplasm whereas non metabolic ATP and ADP are segregated into dense (δ) granules (storage pool); they are secreted during cellular stimulation and are essential for the late phase of aggregation [41]. Another important platelet trait is the fact that mitochondrial complex III and IV proteins are few, leading to increased sensitivity toward mitochondrial dysfunction [13]. Many studies have demonstrated an interest in monitoring platelet mitochondrial respiration in diabetes, Alzheimer's, or Parkinson's disease [11]. Following platelet activation, mitochondrial respiration and glycolysis enhance extra metabolic ATP production, thus sustaining shape change, aggregation, and secretion [11,39,42]. Such increased energy consumption is a main determinant of platelet function.

In cardiogenic shock (when the trigger is hypoperfusion), there is inhibition of platelet mitochondrial respiratory chain enzymes similar to that observed in sepsis. According to some authors, salicylic acid or its derivatives may interfere with platelet mitochondrial function, mainly acting as uncoupling agents. However, this issue still deserves further studies [42–44]. Petrus et al. shed light on the association between hyperpolarization of the mitochondrial membrane, ROS formation, and platelet secretion, and, for instance, diabetic patients had a lower platelet oxygen consumption rate associated with increased ROS generation [11,12]. Furthermore, circulating platelet mitochondria are not restricted to the generation of ATP, but also have an important role in initiating platelet activation through many interlinked mitochondrial processes [11,34]. Impairment of the electron transport chain leads to increased generation of ROS, which triggers platelet activation and, potentially, to a reduced mitochondrial membrane potential and mitochondrial permeability transition pore opening (Figure 2) [11].

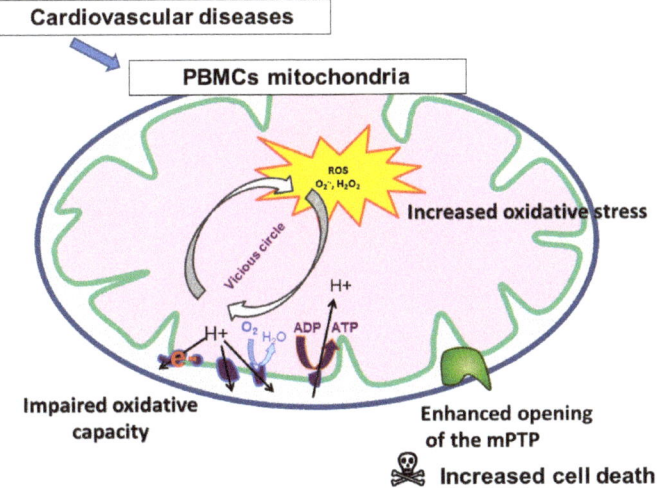

Figure 2. Mitochondrial alterations in PBMCs or platelets during cardiovascular diseases.

Table 1. Mitochondrial function, oxidative stress, and apoptosis in circulating blood cells during cardiovascular disease.

Population Characteristics	Study Design/ Cells Analyzed	Mitochondrial Function	Oxidative Stress ROS Production/ Antioxidant Level	Cell Viability/Apoptosis	Results	References
HF pediatric patients with single ventricle (SV) congenital heart disease	PBMCs	-Oxygen consumption rate (Seahorse) -Mitochondrial respiration (oroboros)	ROS (Amplex red dye)	NA	-Respiratory capacity, coupling efficiency and mitochondrial oxygen flux were reduced in SV patients. -ROS was higher in SV patients	Garcia Anastacia et al., 2019, Circulation (Abstract) [46].
-Mild Congestive Heart Failure patient (CHF) (Class I-II) n = 15, 14 male, 1 female Age: 63 ± 13 yo EF: 44.3 ± 14.5 % -Moderate-to-severe CHF (Class III) n = 16, 15 male, 1 female Age: 61 ± 14 yo EF: 26.9 ± 6%	PBMCs	-Mitochondrial respiration (oroboros) -Maximal electron transfer system capacity (ETS)	Assessment of ROS generation in permeabilized PBMCs before and after addition of mitochondrial oxidative phosphorylation uncoupler (FCCP) urinary 8-OHdG, a biomarker of oxidative DNA damage	N/A	Mitochondrial respiratory capacity of class III HF was lower than class II patients. -ETS capacity was significantly reduced in class III compared to class I-II -Mitochondrial ROS level was higher in class III CHF compared to class I-II patients, before and after FCCP.	Shirakawa et al., 2019, Scientific Report. [22]
Chronic HF patients n = 15, 12 male, 3 female Age: 56.6 ± 10.8 yo EF: 28 ± 8% Control group n = 10, 8 male, 2 female Age: 49.3 ± 8 yo EF: 65 ± 2%	PBMCs Basal and modulation by LPS	Mitochondrial membrane potential (TMRM and JC-1 staining).	-For cytoplasmic oxidative stress evaluation: PBMCs were incubate with 5 µM 2′,7′-dichlorofluorescein diacetate at 37 °C for 10 min. -For mitochondrial oxidative stress evaluation: (MitoSOX™ Red mitochondrial superoxide) -For antioxidant system (SOD GPx levels)	Assessment of overall cell damage Mitochondrial area percentage of intact cristae, and loss of inner mitochondrial membrane (IMM) -Cell damage (Annexin-v and PI staining by cytometric analysis) -Assessment of mitophagy flux (gene expression by RT-PCR quantitation).	**Baseline** -Cytoplasmic ROS: no difference between HF-PBMCs and healthy subject. -Mitochondrial ROS: increased in HF-PBMCs as compared to controls -Index associated with the loss of inner mitochondrial membrane was lower in HF patients -mitophagy flux: increased autophagy genes in HF-PBMCs **After LPS** -Mitochondrial membrane potential: depolarization in PBMCs of HF patients ($p < 0.05$). -Antioxidant system: reduced SOD ($P < 0.05$ and <0.01) and GPx ($p < 0.05$) activity in HF-PBMCs -Cytoplasmic ROS: HF-PBMCs shows marked increase cytoplasmic ROS than control group. ($p < 0.05$) -Mitochondrial ROS: increased in HF patients ($p < 0.05$). - Index associated with the loss of inner mitochondrial membrane was more deteriorated after stimulation, and reduction of mitochondrial area with intact cristae in HF-PBMCs than in healthy group ($p < 0.01$) -Cell damage: apoptotic cell percentage was increased in HF patients. ($p < 0.05$) -Mitophagy flux: the response in HF-PBMCs was increased much more after stimulation.	Colucia et al., 2018, Oncotarget. [38]

Table 1. Cont.

Population Characteristics	Study Design/ Cells Analyzed	Mitochondrial Function	Oxidative Stress ROS Production/ Antioxidant Level	Cell Viability/Apoptosis	Results	References
Congestive heart patients (CHF) n = 20, 16 male, 4 female Age: 68.9 ± 8 yo EF: 24.9 ± 5.9% -Control group n = 15, 13 male, 2 female Age:63.3 ± 9.4 yo EF: 60.0 ± 5.3%	Leukocyte were isolated by gradient centrifugation to measure cellular lipid, protein, PARP & AIF Modulation: Activation of PARP	N/A	C-reactive protein, N-terminal probrain-type natriuretic peptide, oxidative nitrative stress, plasma total peroxide level (PRX), total plasma antioxidant capacity (TAC)and Leukocyte oxidative stress index (OSI), Leukocyte lipid peroxidation, and protein tyrosine nitration (NT)were evaluated. PRX was determined by Oxystat and TAC was detected by OxiSelect™ TAC Assay kit	poly (ADP-ribose) polymerase (PARP), and apoptosis inducing factor (AIF) was measured	In CHF patients, plasma PRX level was markedly increased suggesting the increase of oxidative stress in this group. Oxidative stress of leucocytes increased in CHF group. PARP activity and AIF in circulating, mononuclear cells of CHF group was higher than in the control group. A positive correlation was demonstrated between oxidative stress (Plasma PRX level, OSI) and PARP activation in circulating leukocytes with pro-BNP levels of CHF.	Bárány et al., 2017 Oxidative Medicine and Cellular Longevity. [57]
Pulmonary hypertension patients (PH group classified as WHO Group 2) n = 20, 10 male, 10 female Age: 69 ± 7.4 Control group n = 20, 10 male, 10 female Age: 69.4 ± 17.6	Platelets	Oxygen consumption (Seahorse) Extracellular acidification rate (Seahorse)	ROS level analyzed using MitoSOX	N/A	Maximal oxygen consumption rate was significantly increased compared to controls Activity of complex II tended to increase in Group 2 PH platelets compared to controls ($p = 0.09$). Enhanced maximal capacity correlates negatively with right ventricular stroke work index No change with administration of inhaled nitrite, a modulator of pulmonary hemodynamics.	Nguyen et al., 2019, Plos one. [45]
CHFn = 54, male Age: 60 ± 10 EF% 33.3 ± 7.7 Control group n = 30, male Age: 61 ± 10 EF% 65.1 ± 7.3	PMBCs (peripheral blood Lymphocyte Serum NT-ProBNP level were assessed	Mitochondrial transmembrane potential (MTP) Analyzed by flow cytometry described as JC-1 fluorescence ratio	ROS level of PBMCs were investigated. Described as DCF fluorescence intensity.		CHF patients experienced decreased MTP, (and increase level of ROS of lymphocytes (intensity 11.12) than the control group. -CHF patients had higher Serum NT-ProBNP level -Study conclude that patients with CHF, the MTP and ROS level of PBMCs are correlated with the changes in serum NT-ProBNP level	Song et al., 2016, Heart, Lung and circulation. [58]
Early stage HF patients n = 25, 12 male, 13 female Age: 49 ± 3 years EF: 67.40 ± 0.83 Control group n = 24, 11 male, 13 female Age: 47 ± 3 yearsEF: 69.63 ± 0.99	PBMCs sample	Mitochondrial respiration (Oroboros)	Measurement of inflammatory factors: High sensitivity C-reactive protein (hs-CRP), IL6, and TNF-α -Oxidative stress biomarker: MDA Antioxidant system: SOD By using ELISA		Decreased mitochondrial oxygen consumption in HF compared to control group. -Inflammatory factors were significantly higher in patients with early stage HF. -SOD reduced, but MDA stayed unchanged in diseased patients.	Li et al. 2015 Scientific Report. [59]

Table 1. *Cont.*

Population Characteristics	Study Design/ Cells Analyzed	Mitochondrial Function	Oxidative Stress ROS Production/ Antioxidant Level	Cell Viability/Apoptosis	Results	References
HF patients with left ventricular assist device $n = 10$, 8 male, 2 female Age, median (range): 65 (57–69) EF% (median (range): 15 (10–20) Control group $n = 10$, 8 male, 2 female Age, median (range): 63 (26–74) EF%: NA	PBMCs (Circulating blood leukocyte)	N/A	-Detection of ROS in leukocyte by flow cytometry, and immunofluorescence microscopy -Antioxidant defense system; SOD activity in erythrocyte was measured by spectrophotometry. -oxidized low density (oxLDL) lipoproteins were analyzed in plasma, by ELISA. -DNA damage markers were assessed in blood lymphocyte, and measured by immunofluorescence microscopy	N/A	-In HF patients, the mean fluorescence intensity (MFI) of DCF-DA exhibited increased level of ROS in peripheral blood leukocyte than in control group. Post-operative value (1 week): Neutrophils ROS (+51%) Lymphocytes ROS (+37%) Monocytes ROS (+54%) -Quantity of ROS reach the highest 3 months later (value not specified) -SOD level decreased in HF patient than in control. And continue to decrease to reach the minimum at 3 months post-operative. -oxLDL were markedly higher in HF than in control group. These results suggested increased oxidative stress among HF patients which leads to mitochondria dysfunction. -Markers used to express DNA damage, reveals abnormal DNA repair.	Mondal et al., 2013, International Journal of Medical Sciences. [47]
Congestive heart patients (CHF) $n = 15$ 9 Male, 6 female Age: 79 ± 9 EF%=37 ± 17 Control group $n = 9$ 6 male, 3 female Age: 49 ± 22 EF% =63 ± 5	WBC and Platelets blood sampling from radial artery, brachial vein and coronary sinus	N/A	Oxidative stress (immunofluorescence microscopy analysis of nitrotyrosine) -cytoplasmic oxidative stress (incubation of resuspended buffy coat with 5-6 CM-DCF). -7 CHF and 6 health individuals were evaluated for Mitochondrial oxidative stress, (Mitotracker red CM-H2 XRos M7513 Probe). -Both cytoplasmic and mitochondrial oxidative stress (live-cells fluorescence microscopy and FACS)	N/A	CHF exhibited increased protein nitrosylation in arterial and venous WBC than control. -Cytoplasmic oxidative stress in CHF was increased in venous and arterially localized WBC and platelets. -For coronary sinus sampling, the number of ROS was higher than in venous (946 ± 475 vs. 659 ± 428 per 10,000 cells). -CHF patients had elevated mitochondrial ROS in WBC and platelets than healthy group. The number of ROS-positive venous WBC and platelets is (478 ± 261 per 10,000 cells vs. 162 ± 81 per 10,000 cells for control group). While, ROS-positive arterial WBC and platelets is 471 ± 211 per 10,000 cells vs. 85 ± 42 per 10,000 cells for healthy group. This increased number of circulating ROS suggesting increase oxidative stress in HF patients.	IJsselmuiden et al., 2008, (CardiovascularMedicine. [48]

Table 1. Cont.

Population Characteristics	Study Design/Cells Analyzed	Mitochondrial Function	Oxidative Stress ROS Production/Antioxidant Level	Cell Viability/Apoptosis	Results	References
Acute CHF Edematous $n = 15$ male 9 female 7 Age: 72.6 ± 3.7 EP% 36.2 ± 5.1 Non-edematous $n = 15$ male 10 female 5 Age: 78.5 ± 2.8 EP% 35.3 ± 2.7 Control group $n = 20$ male 18 female 2 Age: 68.5 ± 1.6	PBMCs (Peripheral blood leukocyte) 10 mL venous blood sample was collected, 5 mL was anticoagulated and assayed for fluorescence staining	Mitochondrial transmembrane potential (MTP) in leukocyte was analyzed by flow cytometry	Intracellular oxidants formation was examined by DCF for 20 min at 37°. -Fluorescence was Detected by flow cytometry -Analyzing plasma factors nitrogen metabolites. -Lipid peroxides including (MDA, HNE) -inflammatory factors: IL6, and TNF-α using ELISA.	-Cell apoptosis was measured by tunnel assay	In CHF, MTP of PBMCs was markedly decreased, with the weakening in edematous HF patients more than in non-edematous specifically in lymphocyte. -Intracellular oxidants of PBMCs were increased, with the highest was in monocytes. -Edematous CHF had higher DCF fluorescence level than the other CHF group. -Apoptotic cells percentage was higher in polymorphonuclear leukocyte (PMN) than PBMCs. -edematous leukocyte presented with higher percentage of apoptosis than another CHF group. -plasma nitrogen level, lipid peroxide, and inflammatory factors was higher in CHF than control.	Kong et al., 2001, Journal of the American College of Cardiology. [37]

Yo: years old; LPS: Lipopolysaccharide; SOD: Superoxide Dismutase; GPx: Glutathione peroxidase.

On the other hand, Nguyen et al. recently observed that the platelets of patients with pulmonary hypertension secondary to left heart diseases demonstrated an enhanced maximal respiratory capacity despite a normal basal oxygen consumption rate [45]. Increased fatty acid oxidation, together with the metabolic syndrome, likely contributed to this result. Further and interestingly, platelets' bioenergetics correlated with right ventricular dysfunction but not clearly with hemodynamic in these group 2 pulmonary hypertension (PH) patients, suggesting that non-hemodynamic parameters might play a significant role in such a setting.

4. Mitochondrial ROS Production and Antioxidant Defense of PBMCs and Platelets in Patients with Cardiovascular Diseases

4.1. Measurements of ROS in Circulating Cells

ROS include superoxide, H_2O_2, and peroxynitrite, thought to be the most common and important biological oxidants. In the cardiovascular system, different sources of ROS coexist, and NADPH oxidase, xanthine oxidase, and uncoupled eNOS, together with mitochondrial ROS, participate in endothelial dysfunction in relation to inflammation, leading to a worse prognosis. ROS production results from enzymatic reactions in different cell components, including mitochondria, and, is associated with normal basal metabolic energy generation. In the mitochondria, ROS are physiologically produced mainly across mitochondrial complex I and III of the ETC [22,49–53]. Thus, a normal balance of ROS is essential for cellular functions; however, once the level of ROS surpasses the standard concentration, cellular damage will result, leading finally to apoptosis and cellular death [54,55]. Therefore, an accurate and potent detection method of ROS is crucial for cardiovascular system studies [56], but ROS measurement with high accuracy is still challenging because of ROS' short half-life [57]. Griendling et al. listed all measurement approaches of ROS in detail [58]. In a biological system, the gold standard for measuring ROS in the form of free radicals is thought to be EPR (electron paramagnetic resonance), also recognized as electron spin resonance [55,57,58]. Other measuring techniques of ROS include chemical assays for superoxide anion radicals (O_2^-), hydrogen peroxide (H_2O_2), or peroxynitrite ($ONOO^-$) with fluorescence analysis in the presence of redox sensitive probes or direct chemiluminescent assays [58].

Another frequent method used in clinical setting to measure ROS is the measure of byproducts, such as lipid peroxidation through malondialdehyde (MDA), 4-Hydroxy-Trans-2-Nonenal (HNE), and isoprostanes F_2-IsoPs determination [57,58]. Additionally, oxidative modification of protein and nucleic acid is a classic approach in cardiovascular cells [57,58]. For example, ELISA (enzyme-linked immunosorbent assay) has been recognized as the most common measuring technique used [57]. On the other hand, flow cytometry is the most powerful technique for single cell analysis of the immune system, in particular for leukocytes and platelets [55]. Many fluorescent probes are used for ROS detection in blood cells via flow cytometry [55]. For illustration, DCFH-DA, DAF-2 DA/DAF-FM DA, DHR123, and DHE are all intercellular probes and are detected as green fluorescence except DHE, which is detected as red fluorescence for both leukocytes and platelets. However, there are multiple artifacts related to the DCFH-DA probe and its use remains discussed [59]. Thus, although progress is still to be performed for oxidative stress evaluation, PBMCs can be incubated with chemiluminescent, bioluminescent, or fluorescent redox active probes to detect cytoplasmic or mitochondrial ROS. Particularly, mitochondrial ROS evaluation is possible with specific probes that can pass through the mitochondrial membrane by the addition of a triphenylphosphonium group to a fluorescent probe, like mitosox, which is an analogue of DHE, and for selective detection of H_2O_2 within the mitochondria, MitoPY1 can be used with imaging techniques [60].

Further, the quantitation of reactive species metabolites, ROS scavengers, and antioxidant enzymes can be obtained from chromogenic and enzymatic assays from culture supernatants. Gene expression analysis of PMBCs also allows assessment of antioxidant systems and of other molecules modulating intracellular oxidative stress, such as the *OXPHOS* genes. Finally, quantitative assessment of the mitochondrial structure and function provide additional information when oxidative stress has mitochondrial genesis.

4.2. Mitochondrial ROS in PBMCs in CVDs

4.2.1. Mitochondrial ROS in PBMCs in Heart Failure

Oxidative stress plays a key role in the development and progression of CVDs and could be used as an indirect marker to predict disease severity and prognosis [61–63]. In this context, mitochondrial dysfunction appears to have increased importance [17,64]. Indeed, high levels of ROS and increased production of superoxide anion by neutrophils have been observed in the blood of HF patients, and white blood cells and platelets producing ROS can amplify oxidative stress and organ damage in HF [48,65]. A recent study showed that circulating PBMCs present structural and functional derangements of mitochondria with overproduction of ROS in HF [38]. Besides, a significant reduction of respiration was associated with a higher mitochondrial ROS production in PBMCs of patients with moderate to severe CHF compared to mild CHF [22]. Furthermore, there was a positive correlation between mitochondrial ROS formation and oxidative DNA damage and plasma BNP levels, which are related to the severity of HF. In CVDs, lymphocytes and monocytes play a key role in atherogenesis, modulating the inflammatory and immune response. Indeed, PBMCs would undergo changes similar to failing cardiomyocytes in HF [36]. Based on these data, the use of circulating leukocytes may become a relevant biomarker in cardiovascular diseases and might serve to better understand its pathogenesis [66].

The mechanisms by which mitochondrial ROS in PBMCs are increased in CVDs are multifactorial. Enhancement of myocardial ROS might stimulate ROS generation in PBMC mitochondria via the mechanism of ROS-induced ROS generation upon the passage of circulating PBMCs through the heart. Indeed, the proportion of mitochondrial ROS-loaded blood cells is higher in the coronary sinus than in the peripheral veins of CHF patients [48]. Another hypothesis is the role of inflammatory factors present in HF, such as circulating cytokines, that trigger ROS generation [29]. Further, in heart failure, tissue hypoxia may trigger an increase in the production of ROS, which is a strong stimulus of pro-inflammatory cytokines, such as IL6 and TNF-α [67]. Li et al. confirmed the involvement of mitochondrial dysfunction of PBMCs in the pathophysiology of heart failure; extreme inflammation and decreased antioxidant capacity were closely associated with heart diseases, especially in early stage heart failure patients [29].

Other markers of oxidative stress have been described, such as myeloperoxidase (MPO), oxidized low density lipoproteins (oxLDL), and F_2Isoprostane [66]. Elevated lipid peroxidation has been shown to be associated with the severity of HF, such as malondialdehyde (MDA) and 4-Hydroxy-2-nonenal (HNE) [68]. In addition, two studies showed a positive correlation between the total plasma peroxide levels (reflecting oxidative stress index) in leukocytes with serum NT-proBNP [8,36]. Mondal et al. demonstrated that HF patients with implanted left ventricular assist devices exhibit excessive production of ROS as well as DNA damage in circulating leukocytes [47]. Similarly, Garcia Anastacia et al. observed increased ROS level and deteriorated mitochondrial respiratory capacity in circulation PBMCs in pediatric HF patients who underwent cardiac transplant [46].

4.2.2. Mitochondrial ROS in Arterial Hypertension, Coronary Artery Disease, and Stroke

Yasunari et al. measured the oxidative stress of circulating leukocytes in both hypertensive and diabetic patients and concluded that the level of oxidative stress was significantly increased in arterial hypertension [69]. This study used peripheral leukocytes as a biomarker to detect hypertension-related vascular damage [51]. In fact, the role of measuring ROS in leukocytes in hypertensive patients might help monitor the effect of treatments [51].

In PBMCs, the evaluation of oxidative stress and mitochondrial function in coronary artery disease has been attempted via assessment of the gene expression profile of complex I subunit (NDUFc2). Raffa et al. found a significant reduction of complex I subunit with increased levels of ROS and decreased ATP levels [35].

Only a few works in the literature have demonstrated the role of ROS in circulating cells in the development of stroke [51]. Aizawa et al. showed that in stroke patients, the ROS levels of peripheral mononuclear cells (circulating neutrophils) are increased compared to controls [70].

4.3. Mitochondrial ROS in Circulating Platelets in CVDs

It is now clear that mitochondria modulate the pro-thrombotic function of platelets through energy generation, redox signaling, and apoptosis initiation [71–73]. Thus, studies have related increased platelet activation with mitochondrial hyperpolarization and ROS production. Yamagishi et al. demonstrated that hyperglycemia induces hyperpolarization in normal platelets, resulting in the production of mitochondrial ROS and subsequent activation [74]. Furthermore, Avila et al. observed in diabetic patients that platelets had decreased rates of oxygen consumption and hallmark signs of increased ROS production [75]. Preserving platelet mitochondrial function may therefore allow a decrease of the risk of thrombotic events in diabetic patients [76].

5. Circulating Mitochondrial DNA (mtDNA) Originating from PBMCs and Platelets in Patients with Cardiovascular Diseases

5.1. Circulating Mitochondrial DNA (mtDNA) Originating from PBMCs in Patients with Cardiovascular Diseases

Adequate numbers of mtDNA (free-cell mtDNA) or (circulating mtDNA) are important for mitochondrial as well as cellular function. mtDNA are released by cells undergoing stress or having pathological events [77]. MtDNA encodes 2 ribosomal RNAs, 22 transfer RNAs, and 13 polypeptides of the respiratory chain [78]. Mitochondria contain several copies of mtDNA. The number of mtDNA copies in cells correlates with the size and number of mitochondria, which change under different energy demands and oxidative stress and under different pathological conditions. The mtDNA copy number or content reflects the mitochondrial function through the mitochondrial enzyme activity and ATP production [79]. Quantification of the mtDNA copy number of PBMCs using real-time polymerase chain reaction (PCR) was found to produce consistent and reproducible results [80].

Unlike nuclear DNA, mtDNA is vulnerable to ROS damage because of the lack of histone protection and effective DNA repair mechanisms. When mtDNA damage occurs, it results in mitochondrial dysfunction, inflammation, and cell senescence participating in the pathogenesis of CVDs and atherosclerosis. The mtDNA copy number might reflect the level of mtDNA damage, potentially being a biomarker of mitochondrial function and a predictor of CVDs' risk and prognosis [77,79,81].

Studies have tested mtDNA for the evaluation of CVDs [81,82]. High levels of circulating mtDNA behave as a danger-associated molecular pattern molecule (DAMP), enhancing inflammation and organ damage [83]. In addition, the effective release of mtDNA requires antigen-presenting cells, such as mononuclear and lymphocytes cells, to be involved [84]. Bliksøen et al. observed a correlation between increased mtDNA content and the incidence of myocardial infarction, suggesting mtDNA as a diagnostic biomarker for acute myocardial infarction (AMI) [83]. Likewise, previous evidence emphasized that mtDNA damage might promote atherosclerosis through mitochondrial impairment [85]. As an illustration, Fetterman et al. studied mtDNA damage in PBMCs in patients presenting with diabetes mellitus, clinical atherosclerosis, and CVDs through the isolation of lymphocytes and monocytes. They found that mitochondrial DNA impairment was directly related to oxidative phosphorylation impairment, which ends up with oxidative stress and organ dysfunction [86]. However, in this study, the author found no changes in the mtDNA copy number between the three groups. Sudakov et al., indicated an increase in the circulating mtDNA content in the blood of patients with acute coronary syndrome, which could be a biomarker for the probability of death from myocardial infarction [87].

Studies support the notion that a lower level of mtDNA content indicates a high risk for CVD and sudden cardiac death [81] but others suggested that increased circulating mtDNA content was linked with reduced LV diameters and volumes and thus enhanced cardiac function [77]. By the way, at least, peripheral blood mtDNA might be a predictor of heart characteristics. Chen et al. performed a study to reveal the association between the peripheral mtDNA copy number in leukocytes and risk of CHD. A correlation between the circulating mtDNA content and the formation of atherosclerotic plaque suggested a connection among low mtDNA and a high risk of coronary heart disease [88]. Huang et al. conducted studies in heart failure and acute myocardial infarction patients with consistent results. Both patients type showed lower mtDNA content than the control group [89,90]. Discrepancies in these results might be related to the disease severity, aging, or other risk factors factor that may modify directly or indirectly the outcome. Also, the site of mtDNA extraction might be important. Indeed, in one study, the mtDNA was extracted from platelet-poor plasma while other studies have investigated mitochondria from leukocytes.

Taken together, although still needing further analysis, decreased circulating mtDNA might potentially be assumed to be a risk factor for heart failure and used as a biomarker for cardiovascular disease prognosis.

Similarly, in ischemic stroke patients, Lien et al. quantified the mtDNA content in peripheral leukocytes and found a significant reduction compared to the control individuals [91]. Furthermore, Zhang et al., in patients at risk for atherosclerosis, observed an inverse correlation between the mitochondrial copy number and the risk of sudden cardiac death [92] (Table 2).

Table 2. Mitochondrial DNA in peripheral circulating cells and cardiovascular disease.

Population Characteristics	Study Design	Mitochondrial Function/mtDNA Copy Number	Oxidative Stress	Cell Viability/Apoptosis	Results	Reference
Ischemic stroke patients Total $n = 350$ Age: 60.9 ± 9.1 Male $n = 246$ Female $n = 104$ Control group $N = 350$ Age 60.4 ± 9.1 Male $n = 246$ Female $n = 104$	mtDNA in Peripheral Blood Leukocyte	-mtDNA content (rt PCR) -The ratio of mtDNA to NuclearDNA is used to estimate the number of mtDNA per cell	-oxidized glutathione (GSSG), and reduced glutathione (GSH), (enzymatic (method) -8-hydroxy-2'-deoxyguanosine (biomarker of oxidative DNA damage, ELISA)	NA	mtDNA content in peripheral leukocyte for ischemic stroke patients was significantly lower than the control group. $P < 0.0001$ mtDNA content evaluated for 150 ischemic stroke patients $= 0.90$, while in 50 control individuals $= 1.20$ -The level of GSSG and 8-hydroxyguanosine were higher in patients with ischemic stroke than on the control group. GSSG Ischemic stroke $= 1.83$ Control $= 0.79$ 8-hydroxy-2'-deoxyguanosine ischemic stroke $= 6.33$ Control $= 4.87$ These results exhibited that oxidative stress was higher in patients with ischemic stroke than in control group	Lien et al., 2017, Journal of American Heart Association [91]
3 cohort study with a risk factor of CVD 1st Cardiovascular Health Study (CHS) $n = 4830$ Age: >65 years 2nd: Atherosclerosis Risk in Communities (ARIC) $n = 11153$ Age: Between 45 to 65 years 3rd: Multiethnic Study of Atherosclerosis (MESA) $n = 5887$ Age: 45 to 85 years Control: NA	In CHS: DNA was extracted from the buffy coat using salt precipitation following proteinase K digestion In ARIC: DNA was extracted from the buffy coat of whole blood using (Qiagen) In MESA: DNA was extracted from leukocyte using (Qiagen)	In ARIC and MESA, mtDNA copy number was measured by using probe intensities of mitochondrial single nucleotide polymorphisms (SNP) on the Affymetrix Genome-Wide Human SNP Array 6.0 In CHS: mtDNA was calculated using multiplexed TaqMan-based PCR	NA	NA	-The effect of mtDNA copy number on the incidence of coronary heart disease was higher than in stroke and in other CVDs In all 3 cohort groups, the mtDNA copy number was inversely associated with CVD events	Ashar et al., 2017, JAMA Cardiology [79]
Coronary Heart Disease (CHD) classified in 4 groups according to Gensini score 1-Gensini score: 0—22 $n = 99$, Male 72, Age: 57.3 2-Gensini score: 22—55 $n = 98$, Male 73, Age: 57.9 3-Gensini score: 55—96 $n = 102$, Male 79, Age: 58.3 4-Gensini score:96—254 $n = 101$, Male 86, Age: 58.8 -Control group $n = 110$,Age: 58.1	mtDNA of Leukocytes for CHF categorized by Gensini score	-genomic DNA was isolated from peripheral blood cells by E.Z.N.A blood DNA Midi Kit. -mtDNA quantification (Quantitative real time PCR).	NA	NA	mtDNA content of PBMCs was lower in CHD patients than in the control group. -mtDNA was reduced significantly, while Gensini score was increased suggesting the level of circulating mtDNA correlates with presence and severity of CHD.	Liu et al., 2017, Atherosclerosis [82]

Table 2. Cont.

Population Characteristics	Study Design	Mitochondrial Function/mtDNA Copy Number	Oxidative Stress	Cell Viability/Apoptosis	Results	Reference
Acute coronary syndrome (ACS) Total $n = 14$ Divided into 2 groups 1st group: (Survivor) who survive during 30 day of hospitalization $n = 11$, male 9, female 2 Age: 53 2nd group: (deceased) who died due to ACS during time of analysis $n = 3$ female Age: 67	Blood samples were collected from platelet poor plasma	-To evaluate mtDNA. Isolation performed with PROBA-NK reagent kit. -quantitation of mtDNA was performed by PCR	NA	NA	-Deceased group: the level of mtDNA level was higher (5900 copies/mL) than the survived group (36 copies/mL) $p = 0.049$ -increased level of mtDNA in plasma suggest a probability of death of 50% for ACS patients	Sudakov et al., 2017, European Journal of Medical Research [67]
Patients from the Atherosclerosis Risk in Communities (ARIC) $n = 11093$ male $n = 4971$ female $n = 6122$ Age: 57.9 ± 6.0	mtDNA in peripheral blood buffy coat	mtDNA copy number was measured by using prob intensities of mitochondrial single nucleotide polymorphisms (SNP) on the Affymetrix Genome-Wide Human SNP Array 6.0	NA	NA	-Inverse association between mtDNA copy number and sudden cardiac death	Zhang et al., 2017, Eur Heart Journal [62]
Acute myocardial infarction patient undergoing primary angioplasty $n = 55$ male $n = 47$ female $n = 8$ Age: 57.4 ± 11.4 years Control group: $n = 54$ male $n = 44$ female $n = 10$ age: 55.3 ± 7.4	Peripheral blood leukocyte	Leukocyte mitochondrial DNA copy number (MCN) was measured from venous blood using PCR -AMI patients were divided into two groups according to median baseline leukocyte mtDNA copy number = 82/cell 1st group MCN ≥ 82 2nd group MCN < 82	NA	NA	-Baseline characteristics: In AMI patients the plasma leukocyte mtDNA copy number was significantly lower than in the control group. 122.7 ± 109.3 vs. 194.9 ± 119.5/cell $p = 0.003$ -AMI patients with lower MCN, had higher left ventricle shape sphericity index (SI), at 1,3,6 months after angioplasty and higher left ventricle diastolic and systolic volume at 6 months after angioplasty.	Huang et al., 2017, Circulatiog Journal, [66]

Table 2. Cont.

Population Characteristics	Study Design	Mitochondrial Function/mtDNA Copy Number	Oxidative Stress	Cell Viability/Apoptosis	Results	Reference
Patients with diabetes mellitus and atherosclerosis cardiovascular disease Total $n = 275$ -only Atherosclerosis: $N = 55$ Female 18 Age:60 ± 10 -only DM: $N = 74$ Female 47 Age: 55 ± 10 -Atherosclerosis and DM $N = 48$ Female 31 Age: 62 ± 8 Control group $n = 98$ Female 49 Age: 55 ± 7	PBMCs	Measuring mitochondrial DNA damage in PBMCs by PCR. -Total DNA was separated using QIAmp DNA mini kit and quantification determined by using Pico-green assay kit	Oxidative stress of arterial pulsatility (increased baseline pulse amplitude $p = 0.009$)	NA	Mitochondrial DNA damage was higher in all 3 diseased group, as compared with controls, with the highest in the group combining atherosclerosis and diabetes. -mtDNA measured in DM alone (0.65 ± 1.0) -mtDNA measured in atherosclerosis alone (0.55 ± 0.65) -mtDNA measured in both atherosclerosis and DM (0.89 ± 1.32) $p < 0.05$ mtDNA damage correlated with baseline pulse amplitude	Fetterman et al., 2016, (Cardiovascular Diabetology) [66]
General population Total $n = 701$ Divided by 3 tertiles of mtDNA content -Tertile 1 mtDNA content 0.39–0.86 $N = 233$ Female 1103 Age: 51.6 ± 16.8 EP% 61.3 ± 7.0 -Tertile 2 mtDNA content 0.86–1.10 $N = 234$ Female126 Age:53.5 ± 14.7 EP%: 63.3 ± 6.56 -Tertile 3 mtDNA content 1.11–3.06 $N = 234$ Female 128 Age:54.3 ± 14.2 EP%: 62.9 ± 6.65	Peripheral blood cells	To assess the circulating mtDNA content, PCR was used. Total DNA was extracted from peripheral blood sample using QIAmp DNA Mini Kit.	NA	NA	There is a relation between peripheral blood mtDNA copy number and left ventricular function. Higher mtDNA content was associated with better systolic and diastolic left ventricular function	Knez et al. 2016, International Journal of Cardiology [77]

Table 2. Cont.

Population Characteristics	Study Design	Mitochondrial Function/mtDNA Copy Number	Oxidative Stress	Cell Viability/Apoptosis	Results	Reference
Chronic Heart Failure Total $N = 1700$ -Ischemic HF $N = 790$ Male 543 Age: 62.6 ± 10.4 EF%: 57 -Nonischemic HF $N = 910$ Male 572 Age: 53.8 ± 14.3 EF%: 40 Control group $n = 1700$ male 1115 Age: 57.7 ± 11.0 EF%: NA	Circulating; Leukocyte -Blood sample were drawn, and leukocytes were isolated in K2-EDTA tubes.	Total DNA was extracted by using QC-Mini80 workflow with a DB-S kit. And DNAs of cardiac tissues were isolated by using QIAmp DNA Mini Kit. And copy number ratio was evaluated.	ROS were quantified in heart tissues using Dihydroethidium (DHE) staining. -In lymphocyte intracellular ROS was analyzed by flow cytometry using DCFH-DA -LDL was detected		HF patients presented a low mtDNA content compared to control group. Median 0.83, IQR: 0.60–1.16 vs. median 1.00, IQR: 0.47–2.20)$P < 0.001$. Ischemic HF patients are more susceptible to lower mt DNA copy number(Median 0.77, IQR: 0.56–1.08) than non-ischemic HF median 0.91, IQR 0.63–1.22 -mtDNA content of leukocyte was not correlated with LV diameter $p = 0.988$ -in HF group, LDL was associated with the mtDNA copy number $p = 0.007$ -Lower circulating mtDNA was correlated with increased risk of HF, $p < 0.001$ -In HF patients, the level of ROS was higher than in control group in heart tissues and in lymphocytes.	Huang et al., 2016, Medicine [89]
Coronary heart Disease Patients $N = 378$ Male 279 Female 99 Age: 57.9 -Control group $n = 378$ male 279 female 99 Age: 58.9	Peripheral Blood Leukocytes -5 mL of venous blood was drawn from each individual and anticoagulated into sodium citrate tube.	-DNA was separated from peripheral blood leukocyte using E.Z.N.A blood DNA Midi Kit. -DNA content was measured using PCR	NA	NA	-mtDNA content was inversely related to increased risk of CHD -CHD group shows marked lower mtDNA content, compared to controls, $p < 0.001$. -CHF had higher neutrophils counts compared to controls (5.10 ± 1.66 vs. 4.50 ± 1.51) but no difference in WBC count $p = 0.154$	Chen et al. 2014 (Atherosclerosis) [88]
Myocardial infarction ST segment elevation MI (STEMI) $n = 20$, 5 femaleStable angina pectoris (SAP) $n = 10$, 1 female Both undergoing percutaneous coronary intervention (PCI) and categorized as transmural or non-transmural Age: between 30 and 75 years	Platelet poor plasma	Venous blood sample were gathered, and DNA was extracted from platelet poor plasma using QIAmp DNA blood Mini Kit -Quantification of mtDNA using real time PCR	NA	NA	-Baseline characteristics: Both groups were similar except SAP group which received more PCI treatment than the other group. -After PCI: 3 h later, mtDNA plasma level of NADH dehydrogenase subunit 1 (ND1) were increased in STEMI compared to SAP; $p = 0.01$ -patients with transmural: ND1 levels were greater in STEMI patients $n = 10$, than STEMI patients with non-transmural $n = 6$ -positive correlation between the severity of myocardial damage and the level of mtDNA, mtDNA being increased in myocardial infarction.	Bliksoen et al., 2012, [83]

5.2. Circulating Mitochondrial DNA (mtDNA) Originating from Platelets in Patients with Cardiovascular Diseases

Several physiological stimuli that cause platelet activation at low concentrations could induce platelet apoptosis at higher concentrations. This type of dual signaling is potentially important in the regulation of coagulation. Increased platelet apoptosis has been reported in a number of pathologies, including type 2 diabetes [93]. Activated platelets can release functional mitochondria and mtDNA. Beyond the measurement of mitochondrial function in patients with disease, and due to its lack of a nucleus, platelets provide a unique source of mtDNA [71]. An increasing number of studies support the idea that evaluation of the bioenergetic function in circulating platelets may represent a peripheral signature of mitochondrial dysfunction in metabolically active tissues (brain, heart, liver, skeletal muscle). Indeed, owing to their easy accessibility, there is interest in the use of platelets to study mitochondrial (dys) function in human disease over time. Accordingly, impairment of mitochondrial respiration in peripheral platelets might have potential clinical applicability as a diagnostic and prognostic tool as well as a potential biomarker in treatment monitoring. In sepsis, an alteration in the bioenergetics of platelet mitochondria was directly correlated with the clinical outcome [94].

In CVDs, there are few studies on circulating platelets' mitochondrial dysfunction. Baccarelli et al. suggested that platelet mDNA methylation may be implicated in the etiology of CVDs [95]. Regarding the fact that cardiovascular diseases are strongly influenced by platelet function though acute thrombotic and atherogenic mechanisms, we can expect that evaluation of the bioenergetic function in circulating platelets may represent a potential biomarker of CVD susceptibility, prognosis, or treatment.

An experimental evaluation of atherosclerosis by Yu and co-workers displayed that mtDNA damage was recognized in circulating monocytes, as well as decreased complex I and IV, which were associated with mitochondrial dysfunction [96]. However, this study showed an independent relation between atherosclerosis and reactive oxygen species, as it showed that those at high risk of atherosclerosis have extensive mtDNA damage with no increase in ROS levels [96].

6. Conclusions

In summary, this review outlines the importance of mitochondrial function in circulating blood cells and particularly, its relationship with CVDs. Impaired mitochondrial respiratory chain activity and ATP generation, changes in mitochondrial DNA content, and increased ROS formation in PBMCs and likely in platelets are often associated with several types of cardiovascular diseases. Currently, an evaluation of the mitochondrial function of circulating cells in human blood for cardiovascular disease might be considered as a new noninvasive approach that deserves further studies to improve its diagnosis and prognosis interest. Also, mitochondrial function and ROS and mtDNA involvement in CVD physiopathology support that a better knowledge of these aspects might open new therapeutic perspectives.

Author Contributions: Conceptualization, A.A., M.R., A.-L.C., A.L., and B.G.; methodology, A.A., M.R., A.-L.C., A.L., and B.G.; validation, A.A., M.R., A.-L.C., S.T., A.M., E.A., C.B., A.L., and B.G.; writing—original draft preparation, A.A., M.R., A.L.-C., and B.G. writing—review and editing, A.A., M.R.,A.L.-C., C.B., A.M., E.A., A.L., S.T. and B.G.; supervision, A.-L.C. and B.G. All authors have read and agreed to the published version of the manuscript.

Acknowledgments: The authors greatly thank Anne-Marie Kasprowicz for expert secretarial assistance. Ms Abrar Alfatni was supported by King Abdulaziz University.

Conflicts of Interest: The authors declare no conflict of interest.

References

1. Santulli, G. Epidemiology of Cardiovascular Disease in the 21st Century: Updated Numbers and Updated Facts. *J. Cardiovasc. Dis.* **2013**, *2*, 1–2.
2. Heil, B.; Tang, W.H.W. Biomarkers: Their potential in the diagnosis and treatment of heart failure. *Clevel. Clin. J. Med.* **2015**, *82*, S28–S35. [CrossRef] [PubMed]
3. Benjamin, E.J.; Muntner, P.; Alonso, A.; Bittencourt, M.S.; Callaway, C.W.; Carson, A.P.; Chamberlain, A.M.; Chang, A.R.; Cheng, S.; Das, S.R.; et al. Heart Disease and Stroke Statistics-2019 Update: A Report From the American Heart Association. *Circulation* **2019**, *139*, e56–e528. [CrossRef] [PubMed]
4. Townsend, N.; Wilson, L.; Bhatnagar, P.; Wickramasinghe, K.; Rayner, M.; Nichols, M. Cardiovascular disease in Europe: Epidemiological update 2016. *Eur. Heart. J.* **2016**, *37*, 3232–3245. [CrossRef]
5. World Health Organization. *World health statistics overview 2019: Monitoring health for the SDGs, Sustainable Development Goals*; World Health Organization: Geneva, Switzerland, 2019; Available online: https://apps.who.int/iris/handle/10665/311696 (accessed on 22 January 2020).
6. Yin, W.H.; Chen, J.W.; Lin, S.J. Prognostic value of combining echocardiography and natriuretic peptide levels in patients with heart failure. *Curr. Heart. Fail. Rep.* **2012**, *9*, 148–153. [CrossRef]
7. Taylor, C.; Hobbs, R. Diagnosing Heart Failure—Experience and 'Best Pathways'. Available online: https://www.ecrjournal.com/articles/diagnosing-hf-experience (accessed on 16 August 2019).
8. Bárány, T.; Simon, A.; Szabó, G.; Benkő, R.; Mezei, Z.; Molnár, L.; Becker, D.; Merkely, B.; Zima, E.; Horváth, E.M. Oxidative Stress-Related Parthanatos of Circulating Mononuclear Leukocytes in Heart Failure. *Oxid. Med. Cell. Longev.* **2017**, *2017*, 1249614. [CrossRef]
9. Lugnier, C.; Meyer, A.; Charloux, A.; Andrès, E.; Gény, B.; Talha, S. The Endocrine Function of the Heart: Physiology and Involvements of Natriuretic Peptides and Cyclic Nucleotide Phosphodiesterases in Heart Failure. *J. Clin. Med.* **2019**, *8*, 1746. [CrossRef]
10. Rose, S.; Carvalho, E.; Diaz, E.C.; Cotter, M.; Bennuri, S.C.; Azhar, G.; Frye, R.E.; Adams, S.H.; Børsheim, E. A comparative study of mitochondrial respiration in circulating blood cells and skeletal muscle fibers in women. *Am. J. Physiol. Endocrinol. Metab.* **2019**, *317*, E503–E512. [CrossRef]
11. Petrus, A.T.; Lighezan, D.L.; Danila, M.D.; Duicu, O.M.; Sturza, A.; Muntean, D.M.; Ionita, I. Assessment of platelet respiration as emerging biomarker of disease. *Physiol. Res.* **2019**, *68*, 347–363. [CrossRef]
12. Ost, M.; Doerrier, C.; Gama-Perez, P.; Moreno-Gomez, S. Analysis of mitochondrial respiratory function in tissue biopsies and blood cells. *Curr. Opin. Clin. Nutr. Metab. Care* **2018**, *21*, 336–342. [CrossRef]
13. Kramer, P.A.; Ravi, S.; Chacko, B.; Johnson, M.S.; Darley-Usmar, V.M. A review of the mitochondrial and glycolytic metabolism in human platelets and leukocytes: Implications for their use as bioenergetic biomarkers. *Redox Biol.* **2014**, *2*, 206–210. [CrossRef]
14. Maestraggi, Q.; Lebas, B.; Clere-Jehl, R.; Ludes, P.O.; Chamaraux-Tran, T.N.; Schneider, F.; Diemunsch, P.; Geny, B.; Pottecher, J. Skeletal Muscle and Lymphocyte Mitochondrial Dysfunctions in Septic Shock Trigger ICU-Acquired Weakness and Sepsis-Induced Immunoparalysis. *BioMed. Res. Int.* **2017**, *2017*, 7897325. [CrossRef]
15. Zhou, B.; Tian, R. Mitochondrial dysfunction in pathophysiology of heart failure. *J. Clin. Invest.* **2018**, *128*, 3716–3726. [CrossRef]
16. Pizzimenti, M.; Riou, M.; Charles, A.L.; Talha, S.; Meyer, A.; Andres, E.; Chakfé, N.; Lejay, A.; Geny, B. The Rise of Mitochondria in Peripheral Arterial Disease Physiopathology: Experimental and Clinical Data. *J. Clin. Med.* **2019**, *8*, 2125. [CrossRef]
17. Rosca, M.G.; Hoppel, C.L. Mitochondria in heart failure. *Cardiovasc. Res.* **2010**, *88*, 40–50. [CrossRef]
18. Brown, D.A.; Perry, J.B.; Allen, M.E.; Sabbah, H.N.; Stauffer, B.L.; Shaikh, S.R.; Cleland, J.G.; Colucci, W.S.; Butler, J.; Voors, A.A.; et al. Mitochondrial function as a therapeutic target in heart failure. *Nat. Rev. Cardiol.* **2017**, *14*, 238–250. [CrossRef]
19. Weiss, S.L.; Selak, M.A.; Tuluc, F.; Perales Villarroel, J.; Nadkarni, V.M.; Deutschman, C.S.; Becker, L.B. Mitochondrial Dysfunction in Peripheral Blood Mononuclear Cells in Pediatric Septic Shock. *Pediatr. Crit. Care Med.* **2015**, *16*, e4–e12. [CrossRef]

20. Muntean, D.M.; Sturza, A.; Dănilă, M.D.; Borza, C.; Duicu, O.M.; Mornoș, C. The Role of Mitochondrial Reactive Oxygen Species in Cardiovascular Injury and Protective Strategies. *Oxid. Med. Cell. Longev.* **2016**, *2016*, 8254942. [CrossRef]
21. Martin-Ventura, J.L.; Rodrigues-Diez, R.; Martinez-Lopez, D.; Salaices, M.; Blanco-Colio, L.M.; Briones, A.M. Oxidative Stress in Human Atherothrombosis: Sources, Markers and Therapeutic Targets. *Int. J. Mol. Sci.* **2017**, *18*, 2315. [CrossRef]
22. Shirakawa, R.; Yokota, T.; Nakajima, T.; Takada, S.; Yamane, M.; Furihata, T.; Maekawa, S.; Nambu, H.; Katayama, T.; Fukushima, A.; et al. Mitochondrial reactive oxygen species generation in blood cells is associated with disease severity and exercise intolerance in heart failure patients. *Sci. Rep.* **2019**, *9*, 1–8. [CrossRef]
23. Maynard, S.; Keijzers, G.; Gram, M.; Desler, C.; Bendix, L.; Budtz-Jørgensen, E.; Molbo, D.; Croteau, D.L.; Osler, M.; Stevnsner, T.; et al. Relationships between human vitality and mitochondrial respiratory parameters, reactive oxygen species production and dNTP levels in peripheral blood mononuclear cells. *Aging* **2013**, *5*, 850–864. [CrossRef] [PubMed]
24. Ederlé, C.; Charles, A.L.; Khayath, N.; Poirot, A.; Meyer, A.; Clere-Jehl, R.; Andres, E.; De Blay, F.; Geny, B. Mitochondrial Function in Peripheral Blood Mononuclear Cells (PBMC) is Enhanced, Together with Increased Reactive Oxygen Species, in Severe Asthmatic Patients in Exacerbation. *J. Clin. Med.* **2019**, *8*, 1613. [CrossRef] [PubMed]
25. Stier, A.; Bize, P.; Schull, Q.; Zoll, J.; Singh, F.; Geny, B.; Gros, F.; Royer, C.; Massemin, S.; Criscuolo, F. Avian erythrocytes have functional mitochondria, opening novel perspectives for birds as animal models in the study of ageing. *Front. Zool.* **2013**, *10*, 33. [CrossRef] [PubMed]
26. Melchinger, H.; Jain, K.; Tyagi, T.; Hwa, J. Role of Platelet Mitochondria: Life in a Nucleus-Free Zone. *Front. Cardiovasc. Med.* **2019**, *6*, 153. [CrossRef] [PubMed]
27. Gregg, D.; Goldschmidt-Clermont, P.J. Cardiology patient page. Platelets and cardiovascular disease. *Circulation* **2003**, *108*, e88–e90. [CrossRef] [PubMed]
28. Braganza, A.; Annarapu, G.K.; Shiva, S. Blood-based bioenergetics: An emerging translational and clinical tool. *Mol. Aspects Med.* **2019**, 100835. [CrossRef]
29. Li, P.; Wang, B.; Sun, F.; Li, Y.; Li, Q.; Lang, H.; Zhao, Z.; Gao, P.; Zhao, Y.; Shang, Q.; et al. Mitochondrial respiratory dysfunctions of blood mononuclear cells link with cardiac disturbance in patients with early-stage heart failure. *Sci. Rep.* **2015**, *5*, 10229. [CrossRef]
30. Spinazzi, M.; Casarin, A.; Pertegato, V.; Salviati, L.; Angelini, C. Assessment of mitochondrial respiratory chain enzymatic activities on tissues and cultured cells. *Nat. Protoc.* **2012**, *7*, 1235–1246. [CrossRef]
31. Hsiao, C.P.; Hoppel, C. Analyzing mitochondrial function in human peripheral blood mononuclear cells. *Anal. Biochem.* **2018**, *549*, 12–20. [CrossRef]
32. Horan, M.P.; Pichaud, N.; Ballard, J.W.O. Review: Quantifying mitochondrial dysfunction in complex diseases of aging. *J. Gerontol. A Biol. Sci. Med. Sci.* **2012**, *67*, 1022–1035. [CrossRef]
33. Salabei, J.K.; Gibb, A.A.; Hill, B.G. Comprehensive measurement of respiratory activity in permeabilized cells using extracellular flux analysis. *Nat. Protoc.* **2014**, *9*, 421–438. [CrossRef] [PubMed]
34. Zharikov, S.; Shiva, S. Platelet mitochondrial function: From regulation of thrombosis to biomarker of disease. *Biochem. Soc. Trans.* **2013**, *41*, 118–123. [CrossRef]
35. Raffa, S.; Chin, X.L.D.; Stanzione, R.; Forte, M.; Bianchi, F.; Cotugno, M.; Marchitti, S.; Micaloni, A.; Gallo, G.; Schirone, L.; et al. The reduction of NDUFC2 expression is associated with mitochondrial impairment in circulating mononuclear cells of patients with acute coronary syndrome. *Int. J. Cardiol.* **2019**, *286*, 127–133. [CrossRef] [PubMed]
36. Song, B.; Li, T.; Chen, S.; Yang, D.; Luo, L.; Wang, T.; Han, X.; Bai, L.; Ma, A. Correlations between MTP and ROS Levels of Peripheral Blood Lymphocytes and Readmission in Patients with Chronic Heart Failure. *Heart Lung Circ.* **2016**, *25*, 296–302. [CrossRef]
37. Kong, C.W.; Hsu, T.G.; Lu, F.J.; Chan, W.L.; Tsai, K. Leukocyte mitochondria depolarization and apoptosis in advanced heart failure: Clinical correlations and effect of therapy. *J. Am. Coll. Cardiol.* **2001**, *38*, 1693–1700. [CrossRef]

38. Coluccia, R.; Raffa, S.; Ranieri, D.; Micaloni, A.; Valente, S.; Salerno, G.; Scrofani, C.; Testa, M.; Gallo, G.; Pagannone, E.; et al. Chronic heart failure is characterized by altered mitochondrial function and structure in circulating leucocytes. *Oncotarget* **2018**, *9*, 35028–35040. [CrossRef]
39. Akkerman, J.W. Regulation of carbohydrate metabolism in platelets. A review. *Thromb. Haemost.* **1978**, *39*, 712–724.
40. Guppy, M.; Abas, L.; Neylon, C.; Whisson, M.E.; Whitham, S.; Pethick, D.W.; Niu, X. Fuel choices by human platelets in human plasma. *Eur. J. Biochem.* **1997**, *244*, 161–167. [CrossRef]
41. Daniel, J.L.; Molish, I.R.; Holmsen, H. Radioactive labeling of the adenine nucleotide pool of cells as a method to distinguish among intracellular compartments. Studies on human platelets. *Biochim. Biophys. Acta* **1980**, *632*, 444–453. [CrossRef]
42. Verhoeven, A.J.; Mommersteeg, M.E.; Akkerman, J.W. Quantification of energy consumption in platelets during thrombin-induced aggregation and secretion. Tight coupling between platelet responses and the increment in energy consumption. *Biochem. J.* **1984**, *221*, 777–787. [CrossRef]
43. Protti, A.; Fortunato, F.; Artoni, A.; Lecchi, A.; Motta, G.; Mistraletti, G.; Novembrino, C.; Comi, G.P.; Gattinoni, L. Platelet mitochondrial dysfunction in critically ill patients: Comparison between sepsis and cardiogenic shock. *Crit. Care* **2015**, *19*, 39. [CrossRef] [PubMed]
44. Penniall, R. The effects of salicylic acid on the respiratory activity of mitochondria. *Biochim. Biophys. Acta* **1958**, *30*, 247–251. [CrossRef]
45. Nguyen, Q.L.; Wang, Y.; Helbling, N.; Simon, M.A.; Shiva, S. Alterations in platelet bioenergetics in Group 2 PH-HFpEF patients. *PLoS ONE* **2019**, *14*, e0220490. [CrossRef] [PubMed]
46. Garcia, A.M.; Sparagna, G.C.; Phillips, E.K.; Miyano, C.A.; Nunley, K.; Chatfield, K.C.; Stauffer, B.L.; Sucharov, C.; Miyamoto, S.D. Reactive Oxygen Species Accumulation and Mitochondrial Dysfunction in Peripheral Blood Mononuclear Cells Are Associated With Heart Failure in Patients With Single Ventricle Congenital Heart Disease. *Circulation* **2019**, *140*, 15615.
47. Mondal, N.K.; Sorensen, E.; Hiivala, N.; Feller, E.; Griffith, B.; Wu, Z.J. Oxidative Stress, DNA Damage and Repair in Heart Failure Patients after Implantation of Continuous Flow Left Ventricular Assist Devices. *Int. J. Med. Sci.* **2013**, *10*, 883–893. [CrossRef]
48. Ijsselmuiden, A.J.; Musters, R.J.; de Ruiter, G.; van Heerebeek, L.; Alderse-Baas, F.; van Schilfgaarde, M.; Leyte, A.; Tangelder, G.J.; Laarman, G.J.; Paulus, W.J.l. Circulating white blood cells and platelets amplify oxidative stress in heart failure. *Nat. Clin. Pract. Cardiovasc. Med.* **2008**, *5*, 811–820. [CrossRef]
49. Wenzel, P.; Kossmann, S.; Münzel, T.; Daiber, A. Redox regulation of cardiovascular inflammation—Immunomodulatory function of mitochondrial and Nox-derived reactive oxygen and nitrogen species. *Free Radic. Biol. Med.* **2017**, *109*, 48–60. [CrossRef]
50. Forrester, S.J.; Kikuchi, D.S.; Hernandes, M.S.; Xu, Q.; Griendling, K.K. Reactive Oxygen Species in Metabolic and Inflammatory Signaling. *Circ. Res.* **2018**, *122*, 877–902. [CrossRef]
51. Rubattu, S.; Forte, M.; Raffa, S. Circulating Leukocytes and Oxidative Stress in Cardiovascular Diseases: A State of the Art. *Oxid. Med. Cell. Longev.* **2019**, *2019*, 2650429. [CrossRef]
52. Forte, M.; Palmerio, S.; Yee, D.; Frati, G.; Sciarretta, S. Functional Role of Nox4 in Autophagy. *Adv. Exp. Med. Biol.* **2017**, *982*, 307–326.
53. Forte, M.; Nocella, C.; De Falco, E.; Palmerio, S.; Schirone, L.; Valenti, V.; Frati, G.; Carnevale, R.; Sciarretta, S. The Pathophysiological Role of NOX2 in Hypertension and Organ Damage. *High Blood Press. Cardiovasc. Prev.* **2016**, *23*, 355–364. [CrossRef] [PubMed]
54. Senoner, T.; Dichtl, W. Oxidative Stress in Cardiovascular Diseases: Still a Therapeutic Target? *Nutrients* **2019**, *11*, 2090. [CrossRef] [PubMed]
55. Marrocco, I.; Altieri, F.; Peluso, I. Measurement and Clinical Significance of Biomarkers of Oxidative Stress in Humans. *Oxid. Med. Cell. Longev.* **2017**, *2017*, 32. [CrossRef] [PubMed]
56. Wang, Q.; Zou, M.H. Measurement of Reactive Oxygen Species (ROS) and Mitochondrial ROS in AMPK Knockout Mice Blood Vessels. *Methods Mol. Biol. Clifton. N.J.* **2018**, *1732*, 507–517.
57. Ito, F.; Sono, Y.; Ito, T. Measurement and Clinical Significance of Lipid Peroxidation as a Biomarker of Oxidative Stress: Oxidative Stress in Diabetes, Atherosclerosis, and Chronic Inflammation. *Antioxidants* **2019**, *8*, 72. [CrossRef]

58. Griendling, K.K.; Touyz, R.M.; Zweier, J.L.; Dikalov, S.; Chilian, W.; Chen, Y.R.; Harrison, D.G.; Bhatnagar, A. American Heart Association Council on Basic Cardiovascular Sciences. Measurement of Reactive Oxygen Species, Reactive Nitrogen Species, and Redox-Dependent Signaling in the Cardiovascular System: A Scientific Statement from the American Heart Association. *Circ. Res.* **2016**, *119*, e39–e75. [CrossRef]
59. Kalyanaraman, B.; Darley-Usmar, V.; Davies, K.J.; Dennery, P.A.; Forman, H.J.; Grisham, M.B.; Mann, G.E.; Moore, K.; Roberts, L.J.; Ischiropoulos, H. Measuring reactive oxygen and nitrogen species with fluorescent probes: Challenges and limitations. *Free Radic. Biol. Med.* **2012**, *52*, 1–6. [CrossRef]
60. Dikalov, S.I.; Harrison, D.G. Methods for detection of mitochondrial and cellular reactive oxygen species. *Antioxid. Redox. Signal.* **2014**, *20*, 372–382. [CrossRef]
61. Grieve, D.J.; Shah, A.M. Oxidative stress in heart failure. More than just damage. *Eur. Heart J.* **2003**, *24*, 2161–2163. [CrossRef]
62. Tang, W.H.; Tong, W.; Troughton, R.W.; Martin, M.G.; Shrestha, K.; Borowski, A.; Jasper, S.; Hazen, S.L.; Klein, A.L. Prognostic value and echocardiographic determinants of plasma myeloperoxidase levels in chronic heart failure. *J. Am. Coll. Cardiol.* **2007**, *49*, 2364–2370. [CrossRef]
63. Van der Pol, A.; van Gilst, W.H.; Voors, A.A.; van der Meer, P. Treating oxidative stress in heart failure: Past, present and future. *Eur. J. Heart Fail.* **2019**, *21*, 425–435. [CrossRef] [PubMed]
64. Rosca, M.G.; Hoppel, C.L. Mitochondrial dysfunction in heart failure. *Heart Fail. Rev.* **2013**, *18*, 607–622. [CrossRef] [PubMed]
65. White, M.; Ducharme, A.; Ibrahim, R.; Whittom, L.; Lavoie, J.; Guertin, M.C.; Racine, N.; He, Y.; Yao, G.; Rouleau, J.L.; et al. Increased systemic inflammation and oxidative stress in patients with worsening congestive heart failure: Improvement after short-term inotropic support. *Clin. Sci.* **2006**, *110*, 483–489. [CrossRef] [PubMed]
66. Tousoulis, D.; Oikonomou, E.; Siasos, G.; Chrysohoou, C.; Charakida, M.; Trikas, A.; Siasou, Z.; Limperi, M.; Papadimitriou, E.D.; Papavassiliou, A.G.; et al. Predictive value of biomarkers in patients with heart failure. *Curr. Med. Chem.* **2012**, *19*, 2534–2547. [CrossRef]
67. Ribeiro-Samora, G.A.; Rabelo, L.A.; Ferreira, A.C.C.; Favero, M.; Guedes, G.S.; Pereira, L.S.M.; Parreira, V.F.; Britto, R.R. Inflammation and oxidative stress in heart failure: Effects of exercise intensity and duration. *Braz. J. Med. Biol. Res.* **2017**, *50*, e6393. [CrossRef]
68. Dhiman, M.; Thakur, S.; Upadhyay, S.; Kaur, A.; Mantha Anil, K. Oxidative Stress and Inflammation in Cardiovascular Diseases: Two Sides of the Same Coin. In *Free Radicals in Human Health and Disease*; Rani, V., Yadav, U.C.S., Eds.; Springer: New Delhi, India, 2015; pp. 259–278.
69. Yasunari, K.; Maeda, K.; Nakamura, M.; Yoshikawa, J. Oxidative Stress in Leukocytes Is a Possible Link between Blood Pressure, Blood Glucose, and C-Reacting Protein. *Hypertension* **2002**, *39*, 777–780. [CrossRef]
70. Aizawa, H.; Makita, Y.; Sumitomo, K.; Aburakawa, Y.; Katayama, T.; Nakatani-Enomoto, S.; Suzuki, Y.; Fujiwara, K.; Enomoto, H.; Kuroda, K.; et al. Edaravone diminishes free radicals from circulating neutrophils in patients with ischemic brain attack. *Intern. Med.* **2006**, *45*, 1–4. [CrossRef]
71. Boudreau, L.H.; Duchez, A.C.; Cloutier, N.; Soulet, D.; Martin, N.; Bollinger, J.; Paré, A.; Rousseau, M.; Naika, G.S.; Lévesque, T.; et al. Platelets release mitochondria serving as substrate for bactericidal group IIA-secreted phospholipase A2 to promote inflammation. *Blood* **2014**, *124*, 2173–2183. [CrossRef]
72. Jobe, S.M.; Wilson, K.M.; Leo, L.; Raimondi, A.; Molkentin, J.D.; Lentz, S.R.; Di Paola, J. Critical role for the mitochondrial permeability transition pore and cyclophilin D in platelet activation and thrombosis. *Blood* **2008**, *111*, 1257–1265. [CrossRef]
73. Liu, F.; Gamez, G.; Myers, D.R.; Clemmons, W.; Lam, W.A.; Jobe, S.M. Mitochondrially Mediated Integrin $\alpha IIb\beta 3$ Protein Inactivation Limits Thrombus Growth. *J. Biol. Chem.* **2013**, *288*, 30672–30681. [CrossRef]
74. Yamagishi, S.I.; Edelstein, D.; Du, X.L.; Brownlee, M. Hyperglycemia potentiates collagen-induced platelet activation through mitochondrial superoxide overproduction. *Diabetes* **2001**, *50*, 1491–1494. [CrossRef] [PubMed]
75. Avila, C.; Huang, R.J.; Stevens, M.V.; Aponte, A.M.; Tripodi, D.; Kim, K.Y.; Sack, M.N. Platelet mitochondrial dysfunction is evident in type 2 diabetes in association with modifications of mitochondrial anti-oxidant stress proteins. *Exp. Clin. Endocrinol. Diabetes* **2012**, *120*, 248–251. [CrossRef]
76. Xin, G.; Wei, Z.; Ji, C.; Zheng, H.; Gu, J.; Ma, L.; Huang, W.; Morris-Natschke, S.L.; Yeh, J.L.; Zhang, R.; et al. Metformin Uniquely Prevents Thrombosis by Inhibiting Platelet Activation and mtDNA Release. *Sci. Rep.* **2016**, *6*, 36222. [CrossRef] [PubMed]

77. Knez, J.; Cauwenberghs, N.; Thijs, L.; Winckelmans, E.; Brguljan-Hitij, J.; Yang, W.Y.; Staessen, J.A.; Nawrot, T.S.; Kuznetsova, T. Association of left ventricular structure and function with peripheral blood mitochondrial DNA content in a general population. *Int. J. Cardiol.* **2016**, *214*, 180–188. [CrossRef]
78. Bayeva, M.; Gheorghiade, M.; Ardehali, H. Mitochondria as a therapeutic target in heart failure. *J. Am. Coll. Cardiol.* **2013**, *61*, 599–610. [CrossRef]
79. Ashar, F.N.; Zhang, Y.; Longchamps, R.J.; Lane, J.; Moes, A.; Grove, M.L.; Mychaleckyj, J.C.; Taylor, K.D.; Coresh, J.; Rotter, J.I.; et al. Association of Mitochondrial DNA Copy Number With Cardiovascular Disease. *JAMA Cardiol.* **2017**, *2*, 1247–1255. [CrossRef]
80. Gahan, M.E.; Miller, F.; Lewin, S.R.; Cherry, C.L.; Hoy, J.F.; Mijch, A.; Rosenfeldt, F.; Wesselingh, S.L. Quantification of mitochondrial DNA in peripheral blood mononuclear cells and subcutaneous fat using real-time polymerase chain reaction. *J. Clin. Virol.* **2001**, *22*, 241–247. [CrossRef]
81. Yue, P.; Jing, S.; Liu, L.; Ma, F.; Zhang, Y.; Wang, C.; Duan, H.; Zhou, K.; Hua, Y.; Wu, G.; et al. Association between mitochondrial DNA copy number and cardiovascular disease: Current evidence based on a systematic review and meta-analysis. *PLoS ONE* **2018**, *13*, e0206003. [CrossRef]
82. Liu, L.P.; Cheng, K.; Ning, M.A.; Li, H.H.; Wang, H.C.; Li, F.; Chen, S.Y.; Qu, F.L.; Guo, W.Y. Association between peripheral blood cells mitochondrial DNA content and severity of coronary heart disease. *Atherosclerosis* **2017**, *261*, 105–110. [CrossRef]
83. Bliksøen, M.; Mariero, L.H.; Ohm, I.K.; Haugen, F.; Yndestad, A.; Solheim, S.; Seljeflot, I.; Ranheim, T.; Andersen, G.Ø.; Aukrust, P.; et al. Increased circulating mitochondrial DNA after myocardial infarction. *Int. J. Cardiol.* **2012**, *158*, 132–134. [CrossRef]
84. Berezin, A.E. The Cell-Free Mitochondrial DNA: A Novel Biomarker of Cardiovascular Risk? *Transl. Biomed.* **2016**, *7*, 68–71. [CrossRef]
85. Yu, E.P.K.; Bennett, M.R. The role of mitochondrial DNA damage in the development of atherosclerosis. *Free Radic. Biol. Med.* **2016**, *100*, 223–230. [CrossRef]
86. Fetterman, J.L.; Holbrook, M.; Westbrook, D.G.; Brown, J.A.; Feeley, K.P.; Bretón-Romero, R.; Linder, E.A.; Berk, B.D.; Weisbrod, R.M.; Widlansky, M.E.; et al. Mitochondrial DNA damage and vascular function in patients with diabetes mellitus and atherosclerotic cardiovascular disease. *Cardiovasc. Diabetol.* **2016**, *15*, 53. [CrossRef] [PubMed]
87. Sudakov, N.; Apartsin, K.A.; Lepekhova, S.A.; Nikiforov, S.B.; Katyshev, A.I.; Lifshits, G.I.; Vybivantseva, A.V.; Konstantinov, Y.M. The level of free circulating mitochondrial DNA in blood as predictor of death in case of acute coronary syndrome. *Eur. J. Med. Res.* **2017**, *22*, 1. [CrossRef]
88. Chen, S.; Xie, X.; Wang, Y.; Gao, Y.; Xie, X.; Yang, J.; Ye, J. Association between leukocyte mitochondrial DNA content and risk of coronary heart disease: A case-control study. *Atherosclerosis* **2014**, *237*, 220–226. [CrossRef]
89. Huang, J.; Tan, L.; Shen, R.; Zhang, L.; Zuo, H.; Wang, D.W. Decreased Peripheral Mitochondrial DNA Copy Number is Associated with the Risk of Heart Failure and Long-term Outcomes. *Medicine (Baltimore)* **2016**, *95*, e3323. [CrossRef]
90. Huang, C.H.; Kuo, C.L.; Huang, C.S.; Liu, C.S.; Chang, C.C. Depleted Leukocyte Mitochondrial DNA Copy Number Correlates With Unfavorable Left Ventricular Volumetric and Spherical Shape Remodeling in Acute Myocardial Infarction After Primary Angioplasty. *Circ. J.* **2017**, *81*, 1901–1910. [CrossRef]
91. Lien, L.M.; Chiou, H.Y.; Yeh, H.L.; Chiu, S.Y.; Jeng, J.S.; Lin, H.J.; Hu, C.J.; Hsieh, F.I.; Wei, Y.H. Significant Association Between Low Mitochondrial DNA Content in Peripheral Blood Leukocytes and Ischemic Stroke. *J. Am. Heart Assoc.* **2017**, *6*, e006157. [CrossRef]
92. Zhang, Y.; Guallar, E.; Ashar, F.N.; Longchamps, R.J.; Castellani, C.A.; Lane, J.; Grove, M.L.; Coresh, J.; Sotoodehnia, N.; Ilkhanoff, L.; et al. Association between mitochondrial DNA copy number and sudden cardiac death: Findings from the Atherosclerosis Risk in Communities study (ARIC). *Eur. Heart J.* **2017**, *38*, 3443–3448. [CrossRef]
93. Cohen, Z.; Gonzales, R.F.; Davis-Gorman, G.F.; Copeland, J.G.; McDonagh, P.F. Thrombin activity and platelet microparticle formation are increased in type 2 diabetic platelets: A potential correlation with caspase activation. *Thromb. Res.* **2002**, *107*, 217–221. [CrossRef]
94. Sjövall, F.; Morota, S.; Hansson, M.J.; Friberg, H.; Gnaiger, E.; Elmér, E. Temporal increase of platelet mitochondrial respiration is negatively associated with clinical outcome in patients with sepsis. *Crit. Care* **2010**, *14*, R214. [CrossRef] [PubMed]

95. Baccarelli, A.A.; Byun, H.M. Platelet mitochondrial DNA methylation: A potential new marker of cardiovascular disease. *Clin. Epigenetics* **2015**, *7*, 44. [CrossRef] [PubMed]
96. Yu, E.; Calvert, P.A.; Mercer, J.R.; Harrison, J.; Baker, L.; Figg, N.L.; Kumar, S.; Wang, J.C.; Hurst, L.A.; Obaid, D.R.; et al. Mitochondrial DNA damage can promote atherosclerosis independently of reactive oxygen species through effects on smooth muscle cells and monocytes and correlates with higher-risk plaques in humans. *Circulation* **2013**, *128*, 702–712. [CrossRef] [PubMed]

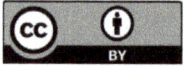

© 2020 by the authors. Licensee MDPI, Basel, Switzerland. This article is an open access article distributed under the terms and conditions of the Creative Commons Attribution (CC BY) license (http://creativecommons.org/licenses/by/4.0/).

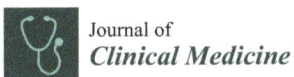 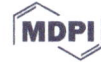

Review

Heart-Type Fatty Acid-Binding Protein (H-FABP) and Its Role as a Biomarker in Heart Failure: What Do We Know So Far?

Richard Rezar [1], Peter Jirak [1], Martha Gschwandtner [2], Rupert Derler [3], Thomas K. Felder [4], Michael Haslinger [1], Kristen Kopp [1], Clemens Seelmaier [1], Christina Granitz [1], Uta C. Hoppe [1] and Michael Lichtenauer [1,*]

1. Clinic of Internal Medicine II, Department of Cardiology, Paracelsus Medical University of Salzburg, 5020 Salzburg, Austria; r.rezar@salk.at (R.R.); p.jirak@salk.at (P.J.); mi.haslinger@salk.at (M.H.); k.kopp@salk.at (K.K.); c.seelmaier@salk.at (C.S.); c.granitz@salk.at (C.G.); u.hoppe@salk.at (U.C.H.)
2. Kennedy Institute of Rheumatology, University of Oxford, Oxford OX3 7FY, UK; martha.gschwandtner@kennedy.ox.ac.uk
3. Institute of Pharmaceutical Sciences, University of Graz, 8020 Graz, Austria; rupert.derler@hotmail.com
4. Department of Laboratory Medicine, Paracelsus Medical University of Salzburg, 5020 Salzburg, Austria; t.felder@salk.at
* Correspondence: m.lichtenauer@salk.at

Received: 10 December 2019; Accepted: 5 January 2020; Published: 7 January 2020

Abstract: Background: Heart failure (HF) remains one of the leading causes of death to date despite extensive research funding. Various studies are conducted every year in an attempt to improve diagnostic accuracy and therapy monitoring. The small cytoplasmic heart-type fatty acid-binding protein (H-FABP) has been studied in a variety of disease entities. Here, we provide a review of the available literature on H-FABP and its possible applications in HF. Methods: Literature research using PubMed Central was conducted. To select possible studies for inclusion, the authors screened all available studies by title and, if suitable, by abstract. Relevant manuscripts were read in full text. Results: In total, 23 studies regarding H-FABP in HF were included in this review. Conclusion: While, algorithms already exist in the area of risk stratification for acute pulmonary embolism, there is still no consensus for the routine use of H-FABP in daily clinical practice in HF. At present, the strongest evidence exists for risk evaluation of adverse cardiac events. Other future applications of H-FABP may include early detection of ischemia, worsening of renal failure, and long-term treatment planning.

Keywords: H-FABP; heart-type fatty acid-binding protein; FABP3; fatty acid-binding protein 3; heart failure; HF; cardiac biomarkers

1. Introduction

According to the Global Burden of Disease study, cardiovascular (CV) diseases represent the leading cause of death among non-communicable diseases, accounting for approximately 17.9 million deaths worldwide in 2015 [1]. As described in the meta-analysis by Van Riet et al., the prevalence of all-type heart failure (HF) in the older cohort of patients (>60 years) is 11.8% [2]. Additionally, health care costs, related to HF, represent a serious economic burden to healthcare systems. Heidenreich and colleagues estimated that the total medical costs of HF in the US will increase from $31 billion in 2012 to at least $70 billion in 2030 [3]. Thus, it is not only important to find new therapeutic approaches, but also to diagnose affected individuals early and monitor therapies properly. Biomarkers for HF are subject of current research and may have the potential to, not only reduce costs, but also extend symptom-free intervals through effective therapy control.

Described for the first time in 1972, a group of cytoplasmic proteins called fatty acid-binding proteins (FABPs) has been under investigation in the scientific community [4]. To date, several subtypes of FABPs, occurring in various organ systems in different concentrations, have been discovered. These low-molecular-weight proteins (about 15 kD [5]) have been widely discussed, especially given the association of H-FABP as an independent risk factor for all-cause mortality and cardiovascular (CV) death [6]. According to the HUGO Gene Nomenclature Committee, the FABP family consists of 16 members, each encoded by a distinct gene. The probably best-known members include L- (liver), I- (intestinal), H- (muscle/heart), A- (adipocyte), E- (epidermal), Il- (ileal), B- (brain), M- (myelin), and T-FABP (testis) [7]. FABPs are involved in cellular fatty acid metabolism as they reversibly bind and transport long-chain polyunsaturated fatty acids (PUFA) from cell membranes to the mitochondria. Additionally, they contribute to cellular growth and proliferation processes, and can activate peroxisome proliferator activated receptors (PPARs). Therefore, they play a functional role in lipid metabolism and energy homeostasis [8–10].

The heart-type FABP (H-FABP), also known as mammary-derived growth inhibitor, is probably the best-known member of the FABP family. H-FABP is encoded by the FABP3 gene located on the 1p33-p32 region of chromosome 1 [11], whereas, RXRa, KLF15, CREB, and Sp1 were identified as transcriptional factor binding sites for different PPARs in animal studies [12]. It is expressed in tissues with high demand of fatty-acids, such as heart, skeletal-muscle, brain, kidney, adrenal gland, and mammary gland tissues, as well as in blastocysts [8]. FABP3 was also found to be expressed in γ-aminobutyric acid (GABA)-ergic inhibitory interneurons of the male anterior cingulate cortex in mice, suggesting that it has an important role also in cerebral PUFA-homeostasis [13]. H-FABP itself is abundant in the cytoplasm of striated muscle cells and is rapidly released in response to cardiac injury [14]. H-FABP is expressed more abundantly in the heart's ventricles (0.46 mg/g wet weight) and atria (0.25 mg/g wet weight) than in skeletal muscles (e.g., the diaphragm contains 25% of the heart's H-FABP concentration) or in other organs (less than 10% of the H-FABP content of the heart) [15]. In healthy individuals, serum levels of H-FABP are in the single digit ng/ml range [16–18]. Expression of H-FABP is regulated by the microRNA miR-1, which might play a role in the progression of HF itself [19]. Upon myocardial injury, H-FABP is rapidly released from myocytes into the systemic circulation, due to its small size and free cytoplasmic localization. Also, transient increases in sarcolemmal membrane permeability are suspected to permit H-FABP leakage into the systemic circulation [20,21]. This so-called "wounding" of myocytes was observed, even after short-term ventricular stress, and it may play an important role in diverse auto- and paracrine mechanisms in the pathogenesis of HF [20]. The elimination of H-FABP takes place via the kidney, explaining a shorter diagnostic window in patients with normal renal function [22]. Kleine et al., for example, reported that H-FABP plasma levels returned to baseline within 20 hours after the onset of symptoms in patients with acute myocardial infarction [23].

Apart from its crucial role in cardiac lipid transport [24,25], several in vitro and in vivo studies investigated further functions of H-FABP. The potential role of H-FABP in cardiomyocyte differentiation was suggested by Tang et al., who observed a correlation between H-FABP expression and decreased cell proliferation in mouse cardiomyocytes [26]. A similar finding was obtained by Wang et al., using human bone marrow derived mesenchymal stem cells, by which overexpression of H-FABP inhibited proliferation [27]. Additionally, it was shown by Zhu et al., using a P19 embryonic myocardial cell line overexpressing H-FABP, that it might inhibit cell proliferation and promote apoptosis during myocardial cell development [28]. However, in a later study, H-FABP silencing instead of overexpression led to reduced proliferation and increased apoptosis in the same cell line [29]. In zebrafish, the knock-down of H-FABP resulted in impaired heart development and augmented apoptosis [30,31]. In neonatal rats, H-FABP downregulation repressed cell apoptosis and improved structural remodeling in ventricular myocytes under hypoxia. On the other hand, H-FABP upregulation enhanced phosphorylation of the MAPK signalling pathway and decreased phosphorylated protein kinase B (Akt) levels, increasing apoptosis and remodeling [32]. An anti-apoptotic role of H-FABP was also found in hypoxia/reoxygenation induced H9c2 cardiomyocytes [33]. Consistent with this,

H-FABP enhanced survival in human bone marrow derived mesenchymal stem cells in hypoxia [27]. Overexpression of H-FABP promoted growth and migration in human aortic smooth muscle cells [34]. In summary, the precise mechanism by which this protein influences cardiomyocyte proliferation and apoptosis remains elusive and further research is needed to explain its mode of action. Figure 1 provides a graphic overview of H-FABP under physiological and pathophysiological conditions.

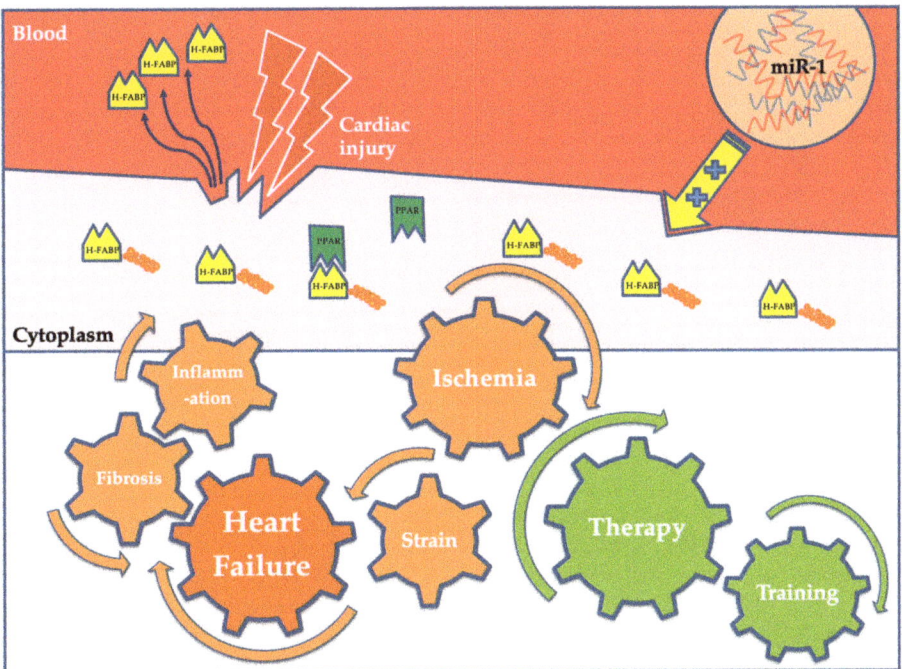

Figure 1. Under physiological conditions, H-FABP serves as a transport protein in cellular metabolism and can reversibly bind fatty acids. Furthermore, it can activate PPARs and therefore plays a role in lipid metabolism and energy homeostasis. The expression of H-FABP is regulated by the microRNA miR-1. In response to cardiac injury, H-FABP is rapidly released into the blood-stream where it can be quantified. Physical training as well as pharmacological interventions like anti-tachycardic therapy were shown to decrease plasma levels of H-FABP. Abbreviations: miR-1: microRNA 1; PPAR: peroxisome proliferator activated receptor (PPAR). H-FABP: heart-type fatty acid-binding protein.

Regarding laboratory testing, different types of assays are frequently used in research and clinical settings for the detection and quantification of H-FABP in serum, plasma, or whole blood. These assays comprise enzyme-linked immunosorbent assays (ELISA) [6,15,35–37], immunoturbidimetric assays [38,39], multiplex assays [40,41], and immunochromatographic assays [42,43]. Test times depend on the type of assay, and vary between 5 and 120 min (as reviewed in [44]). The varying characteristics of these tests allow flexibility when choosing the appropriate test for the desired readout under varying budget and time restrictions.

A number of authors have discussed the role of H-FABP in clinical routine since its discovery. The following literature review will consider H-FABP and its potential use as a biomarker in HF.

2. Methods

A structured database search regarding H-FABP and its role in HF was conducted using "PubMed Central". Three researchers (R.R., M.G. and R.D.) screened the studies independently. To select possible studies for inclusion in the definite analysis, the authors screened all available studies by title and, if suitable, by abstract. Manuscripts that appeared relevant were read in full text. References of studies included were reviewed for further reading. This review on H-FABP in HF was conducted based on the Preferred Reporting Items for Systematic Reviews and Meta-Analyses (PRISMA) guidelines [45]. The corresponding flow-chart is given in Appendix A Figure A1.

3. H-FABP as a Biomarker in Heart Failure

According to the European Society of Cardiology (ESC) guidelines, HF is a syndrome characterised by typical symptoms and clinical signs, with a "structural and/or functional cardiac abnormality" as an underlying cause, "resulting in reduced cardiac output and/or elevated intra-cardiac pressures at rest or during stress" [46]. Due to their strong negative-predictive value, the use of natriuretic peptides is well-established in standard HF algorithms [46–48]. Nevertheless, like many other biomarkers, including cardiac troponins, elevated levels of B-type natriuretic peptide (BNP) may also indicate alternative conditions and BNP release may lag in conditions with very acute onset, such as flash pulmonary edema or right-sided acute HF (AHF) [46,49]. As mentioned in the actual ESC-guidelines, their use for ruling out HF, but not for setting up the diagnosis, can be recommended [46]. These guidelines also state that, despite extensive research, no recommendation can currently be made for the use of novel cardiac biomarkers in everyday clinical practice [46]. The same holds true for the American AHA guidelines on HF [47] and even a specific sub-study of the large scale PROTECT trial failed to identify the perfect single biomarker among 48 different markers for the prognostic assessment of patients with AHF [50].

Most biomarkers are not indicative of cardio-specific events but of general pathologic processes like inflammation, ischemia, fibrosis, or general cell death. As HF is an aetiologically diversified, systemic-progressive disease, a simultaneous assessment of different pathways seems reasonable, though, a prognostic assessment based on a single factor is challenging. Possible hallmarks in the pathophysiology of HF are mechanical stress, ischemia, chronic (subclinical) inflammation, fibrosis, and angiogenesis [36]. With respect to ischemic heart disease, the potential suitability of H-FABP as an early indicator of myocardial injury has been mentioned for years in numerous publications. In contrast to cardiac troponins, which are bound to the myocyte's structural apparatus, H-FABP is present as soluble protein in the cytoplasm. Therefore, the release into systemic circulation may possibly be detected more rapidly and even after minor myocardial damage [21]. Liebetrau et al., for example, report significantly increased serum levels of H-FABP already 15 minutes after iatrogenic myocardial infarction, caused by transcoronary ablation of septal hypertrophy (TASH). in patients with hypertrophic obstructive cardiomyopathy [14]. Some authors state additional benefits of combining H-FABP with high-sensitive troponins [37,38], whereas, others do not conclude any incremental benefit of H-FABP on top of cardiac troponins for diagnosing acute myocardial infarction [42,51,52]. Regarding pulmonary embolism (PE), several publications describe the use of H-FABP for risk stratification due to its role as an early indicator of right-ventricular strain [53–55]. A strong correlation with the risk of major adverse events and mortality was demonstrated, and even the 2019 ESC Guidelines on the diagnosis and management of acute PE mention the use of H-FABP for risk stratification, despite the fact that prospective trials are still missing [56].

As mentioned before, H-FABP plays an important role in cellular signalling, lipid-transport, and myocytal homeostasis [57]. Additionally, due to the amphipathic nature of fatty acids, their accumulation and membranal storage can have noxious effects on cellular structural and functional properties [57]. Therefore, mechanical stress, as well as cellular damage, including from ischemic or inflammatory processes, may be further perpetuated by a disturbed myocytal homeostasis, reduced intracellular H-FABP content [11], and may support the (chronically) progressive character of HF. Despite its rapid, and in the case of CHF, sustained release into general circulation, H-FABP not only acted as an indicator of cellular damage, but also a marker of myocytal dyshomeostasis, and thus, functional impairment of the myocardium.

Various authors have investigated the role of H-FABP in patients suffering from HF with different methods over the last few years. Many studies postulate the independent relationship between H-FABP and outcome, as well as the risk of adverse CV events [40,58–61]. In a recent study by Ho et al., for example, high levels of H-FABP were an independent risk factor for CV death and acute HF-related hospitalization in 1071 patients with chronic coronary disease [40]. In an interesting study from 2005 with 186 patients, Niizeki et al. demonstrated superiority of the combined analysis of BNP and H-FABP for risk stratification in patients with CHF. The authors described the added benefit of H-FABP in showing persistent myocardial damage, compared to BNP, as a sole myocardial strain parameter. Interestingly, the authors only found a weak correlation between the two individual laboratory parameters, which may indicate different pathophysiological origins [58]. In a second study from 2008, involving 113 patients with CHF, the authors again associated persistently high levels of H-FABP with adverse events in patient follow-up. They suggested serial measurement of H-FABP concentrations for therapy monitoring, as they observed regredient serum levels under HF therapy in a subgroup of patients [59]. A significant decrease in H-FABP levels was also observed in a study by Jirak et al. where they investigated several biomarkers in fifty patients with CHF under therapy with the If channel inhibitor, ivabradine [62]. This was also observed in children with CHF after treatment with carvedilol [63].

Regarding AHF, Hoffmann et al. found improved specificity and positive predictive value for the diagnosis of AHF in their work including 401 patients with acute dyspnea or peripheral edema when using H-FABP in addition to BNP. H-FABP levels also correlated with adverse outcomes and AHF related rehospitalization [60]. These findings are in line with the work of Ishino et al. In their study on 134 patients with acute decompensated HF (ADHF), the authors were able to correlate high H-FABP levels with significantly higher rates of adverse cardiac events and in-hospital mortality [61]. Kazimierczyk et al. observed significantly higher rates of death and rehospitalization in patients with ADHF and both higher H-FABP concentrations at admission and discharge. Echocardiographic remodeling parameters correlated well with high initial H-FABP-levels [64]. Shirakabe et al. were able to correlate serum H-FABP levels not only with all-cause mortality in patients with ADHF, but also worsening of renal failure. The latter finding achieved a sensitivity and specificity of 94.7%, and 72.7%, respectively (AUC = 0.904) in non-chronic kidney disease patients [65].

Concerning patients with HF with reduced ejection fraction (HFrEF), Lichtenauer et al. enrolled 65 patients with dilative cardiomyopathy (DCM) and 59 patients with ischemic cardiomyopathy (ICM) in their study on novel cardiac biomarkers in CHF. H-FABP levels were significantly elevated in both patient populations, compared to controls without signs of HF or coronary artery disease. Furthermore, H-FABP levels not only correlated proportionally with NYHA functional class, but also inversely with ejection fraction [36]. Regarding, HF with preserved ejection fraction (HFpEF; left ventricular ejection fraction ≥50%), Kutsuzawa et al. observed an independent correlation of higher H-FABP-levels and the occurrence of adverse CV events in their study on 151 HFpEF-patients. Interestingly, serum levels of H-FABP did not differ between patients with HFpEF and HFrEF (left ventricular ejection fraction <50%) between each NYHA functional class [66]. Dinh et al. found markedly higher levels of Troponin T and H-FABP, even in patients with asymptomatic left ventricular diastolic dysfunction and patients with HF and normal ejection fraction, supposing ongoing myocytal damage in these patient collectives [67]. However, Jirak et al. observed significantly higher H-FABP serum levels in patients with DCM and ICM, than in patients with HFpEF. Nevertheless, significantly higher H-FABP concentrations were shown in HFpEF patients compared to the control group [68].

Considering patients with valvular heart disease, Iida et al. showed an independent association of H-FABP with clinical outcomes in hypertensive patients with aortic valve disease. Echocardiographically determined left ventricular dimensions were signs of cardiac remodelling and correlated significantly with measured levels of H-FABP, whereas Troponin T remained below cut-off levels in all patients [21]. Mirna et al. actually reported a significant reduction in H-FABP plasma concentration in 79 patients with severe aortic valve stenosis after conducting transcatheter aortic valve implantation (TAVI), indicating reduced ventricular wall stress and potential reversibility of cardiac remodeling due to valvular replacement [69].

Regarding arrhythmia as a co- and sometimes main-perpetrator in HF, Otaki et al. observed in their study with 402 patients higher levels of H-FABP in patients with CHF and atrial fibrillation (AF) than in patients with CHF and sinus rhythm (SR) [70]. Rader et al. showed that in 63 studied patients undergoing cardiac surgery that post- but not preoperative H-FABP levels correlated with onset of perioperative AF (POAF) [71]. Interestingly, Shingu et al. observed lower H-FABP gene expression in patients' atria with POAF after cardiac surgery, illustrating the complexity of cellular processes in the development of HF [72].

Mirna et al. made another interesting discovery when investigating H-FABP levels in patients with pulmonary hypertension (PH). They observed that H-FABP levels were primarily elevated in group two and three PH, namely PH related to left heart disease, pulmonary disease, and chronic hypoxia. H-FABP may, therefore, be useful as a possible indicator for post-capillary PH [73].

Application of H-FABP measurement in HF monitoring may also be found in paediatric cardiology. Zoair et al. reported a correlation of serum H-FABP levels with clinical and echocardiographic signs before, and after, HF therapy in 30 children with congestive HF compared to 20 healthy individuals. An unfavourable outcome was again associated with increased serum levels. However, the study was limited as H-FABP was investigated as a single laboratory parameter, and its superiority over biomarkers, such as BNP, was not determined [74]. Sun et al. also reported that there is a correlation between H-FABP levels with disease severity in children with CHF, but again other laboratory markers were not compared [75]. In their study on 238 children and adolescents with congenital heart disease, Hayabuchi et al. found that H-FABP did not correlate with BNP, but was affected by age, NYHA class, arterial oxygen saturation, CK-MB and creatinine, supporting a different pathophysiological pathway of the two biomarkers [76]. Table 1 gives an overview of selected studies on H-FABP and HF.

Table 1. Overview of different positive clinical studies assessing the diagnostic value of H-FABP (heart-type fatty acid-binding protein) in patients with heart failure (HF) (sorted by main topic and year of publication).

Main Findings	Study	Patient Number	Reference
High H-FABP (>4.3 ng/mL) and elevated BNP (>200 pg/mL) showed highest rates for cardiac death and cardiac events and were also independent predictors of cardiac events (H-FABP HR 5.416, $p = 0.0002$; BNP HR 2.411, $p = 0.0463$)	Prospective study for 534+/−350 days on CHF patients	186	Niizeki T. et al., 2005 [58]
Persistently high H-FABP levels at hospital discharge (>4.3 ng/mL) correlated with increased rates for CV events (HR 5.68)	Prospective study for 624+/−299 days on patients with CHF	113	Niizeki T. et al., 2008 [59]
Two-fold higher rate of primary CV events between high H-FABP (>4.143 ng/mL) vs. low H-FABP group (32% vs. 16% respectively)	Prospective multicenter study for 24 months on patients with stable coronary heart disease (SCHD)	1071	Ho S. et al., 2018 [40]
H-FABP levels of >5.7 ng/mL were correlated with significantly higher in-hospital mortality (6.7% vs. 0%, $p < 0.05$) and cardiac events	Study for 615 days on patients with ADHF	134	Ishino M. et al., 2010 [61]
Highest H-FABP level patient quartile showed increased all-cause mortality (HR: 2.1–2.5, $p = 0.04$) and AHF related rehospitalization rate (HR 2.8–8.3, $p = 0.001$); combining H-FABP & NT-proBNP improves diagnostic specificity and PPV to rule out AHF	Prospective study for up to five years on patients with acute dyspnea or peripheral edema with or without AHF	401	Hoffmann U. et al., 2015 [60]
Significant positive correlation between H-FABP with echocardiographic parameters, death and rehospitalization	Study on patients with ADHF	77	Kazimierczyk E. et al., 2018 [64]
Serum H-FABP levels were significantly higher in patients with true worsening renal failure	Retrospective study on patients with AHF	281	Shirakabe A. et al., 2019 [65]
H-FABP levels are significantly higher in patients with DCM and ICM; ejection fraction correlates inversely with H-FABP concentrations	Study on the diagnostic value of novel cardiac biomarkers in patients with HFrEF	65 patients with DCM, 59 patients with ICM, 76 controls	Lichtenauer M. et al., 2017 [36]

Table 1. Cont.

Main Findings	Study	Patient Number	Reference
Significantly higher levels of Troponin T and H-FABP in patients with asymptomatic LVDD and patients with HFnEF	Study on patients with HFnEF	49 patients with HFnEF, 51 patients with asymptomatic LVDD, 30 controls	Dinh W. et al., 2011 [67]
Higher H-FABP-levels correlated with adverse CV events; H-FABP levels did not differ between patients with HFpEF and HFrEF between each NYHA functional class	Prospective study on patients with HFpEF with a median follow-up of 694 days	151 patients with HFpEF, 162 patients with HFrEF as controls	Kutsuzawa D. et al., 2012 [66]
A greater rise in post-operative H-FABP levels is associated with AF after cardiac surgery	Prospective study on patients undergoing cardiac surgery	63	Rader F. et al., 2013 [71]
Optimal cut-off values for H-FABP as myocardial damage marker were higher in CHF patients with AF than in patients with SR (5.4 vs. 4.6 ng/mL)	Prospective study on patients with CHF and AF or CHF and SR with a median follow-up of 643/688 days	402	Otaki Y. et al., 2014 [70]
H-FABP levels correlate independently with age, NYHA-class, CK-MB, creatinine and arterial oxygen saturation	Study in children and adolescents with congenital heart disease	238	Hayabuchi Y. et al., 2011 [76]
Significant negative correlation between H-FABP levels and heart function (LVEF, CI, LVSF)	Study in pediatric patients with chronic HF	36 patients and 30 healthy controls	Sun Y.P. et al., 2013 [75]
Significant positive correlation between increased H-FABP levels and severity of HF and adverse outcome	Prospective cohort study for 3 months on pediatric patients with HF	30 patients and 20 healthy controls	Zoair A. et al., 2015 [74]

Abbreviations: ADHF: acute decompensated heart failure; AF: atrial fibrillation; AHF: acute heart failure; BNP: brain natriuretic peptide; CHF: chronic heart failure; CK-MB: muscle-brain type creatine kinase; CI: cardiac index; CV: cardiovascular; DCM: dilative cardiomyopathy; HF: heart failure; HFnEF: heart failure with normal ejection fraction; HFpEF: heart failure with preserved ejection fraction; HFrEF: heart failure with reduced ejection fraction; HR: hazard ratio; ICM: ischemic cardiomyopathy; LVDD: left ventricular diastolic dysfunction; LVEF: left ventricular ejection fraction; LVSF: left ventricular shortening fraction; NYHA: New York Heart Association; PPV: positive predictive value; SR: sinus rhythm.

4. Discussion and Conclusion(s)

In CV research, H-FABP represents a much-studied protein that is well-known for its role in lipid transport and influence on myocyte metabolism. Different assays and methods exist for measurement, allowing flexibility for the researcher and clinician. However, little is known about its precise function in cardiac development and remodelling. In vitro and animal studies suggest both, promoting and inhibitory roles in myocyte proliferation and apoptosis, but a mechanistic explanation is missing. If, and how, H-FABP that is released from damaged myocytes impacts the progression of HF and other CV diseases, in detail, remains unknown to date. Although, dyshomeostasis of cellular metabolism due to reduced intracellular H-FABP content, and hence, impaired fatty acid supply seems one reasonable consideration.

Individual investigators come to different conclusions about H-FABPs possible application in clinical routine. With BNP, a biomarker with high negative predictive value in differential diagnosis of HF and its long-term therapy surveillance already exists. The use of H-FABP in clinical settings has only been experimental in the past and large-scale studies are still lacking. Nevertheless, the different pathophysiological origins of H-FABP and BNP give hope for a more differentiated diagnostic approach in the future.

To date one possible application of H-FABP seems to be the detection of early and/or subclinical cardiac ischemia and inflammation. H-FABP could be used as a screening tool, for example, in routine health check-ups, since laboratory tests are inexpensive, and samples can be obtained in remote locations and analyzed in central laboratories. Takahashi et al. demonstrated a strong positive correlation between increased pulse pressure with BNP and H-FABP as signs of increased silent myocardial damage in 3504 participants at their annual health check [77]. On the other hand, the rapid detection of ischemia may pave the way for identifying patients with acute ischemia as an underlying cause of AHF at an early phase. As serum H-FABP levels were shown to correlate well with infarct size in patients with ST-elevation myocardial infarction [78], the measurement of H-FABP may enable the timely admission of revascularization procedures, and therefore, may even prevent the development of HF in the long run. As H-FABP and cardiac troponins show different release kinetics [14], a H-FABP-troponin ratio may be useful for distinguishing acute ischemia from chronic myocardial damage in patients with decompensated HF.

Furthermore, interactions of the various organ systems in decompensated HF are highlighted by several authors and international guidelines [46,65,79]. As the coexistence of HF and chronic kidney disease is frequently observed, the terms "cardiorenal syndromes" as well as "renocardiac syndromes" have gained attention in the last few years. A peculiarity of H-FABP compared to markers, such as BNP and troponins, could lie in detecting true worsening of renal function [65]. The exact mechanism that causes this correlation has not yet been clarified. High levels of H-FABP in patients with ADHF may be due to severely decompensated HF itself, but also due to damage of the distal tubules or due to accumulation in glomerular podocytes. Nevertheless, as Shirakabe et al. note, this correlation has not previously been shown for BNP or troponins, which may give H-FABP a unique position as a biomarker in HF diagnostics [65].

Another application of H-FABP as a biomarker might be in highly specialized areas. Dalos et al. observed an exponential increase of H-FABP levels, with decreasing left ventricular ejection fraction in patients with coronary artery disease, reflecting chronic myocardial ischemia [80]. As a strong and independent correlation of H-FABP with individual prognosis was shown in several studies, it may, therefore, be used in mid- to long-term treatment planning. This may be especially helpful when dealing with invasive and expensive approaches, like implantable cardiac resynchronization devices, valve replacement, or mechanical circulatory devices. For example, Cabiati et al. demonstrate an association between high H-FABP levels and poor prognosis in patients after LVAD implantation [81].

The clinical picture of HF comprises a group of heterogenous disease entities as an underlying cause. Novel biomarkers extend our understanding both of CV physiology and pathophysiologic processes, leading to cardiac remodelling and the development of HF. By defining an appropriate patient population in the right clinical context, the additional diagnostic value of H-FABP as a biomarker in HF may well be obtained in the future. Furthermore, an optimal point in time for sample recovery, as well as different thresholds for diagnostic, prognostic, and therapeutic consequences need to be determined.

We currently assume that H-FABP is, not only a rapid indicator of myocardial ischemia, but that its loss from the cardiomyocytes' cytoplasm may cause an intracellular metabolic dyshomeostasis, and is therefore, conducive to the progressive nature of heart failure. H-FABP's present and future in HF diagnostics may also not lie in its use as a single laboratory value, but in a combination of clinical assessment, imaging, and a multi-biomarker approach.

Author Contributions: Conceptualization: R.R., M.G. and R.D.; Writing-Original Draft Preparation: R.R., M.G., and R.D.; Writing-Review and Editing: R.R., M.G., R.D., P.J., T.K.F., M.H. and K.K.; Visualization: R.R., M.H. and C.S.; Supervision: C.S., C.G., U.C.H., and M.L.; Project administration: C.G. and M.L. All authors have read and agreed to the published version of the manuscript.

Funding: This research received no external funding.

Conflicts of Interest: The authors declare no conflict of interest.

Appendix A Flow Diagram

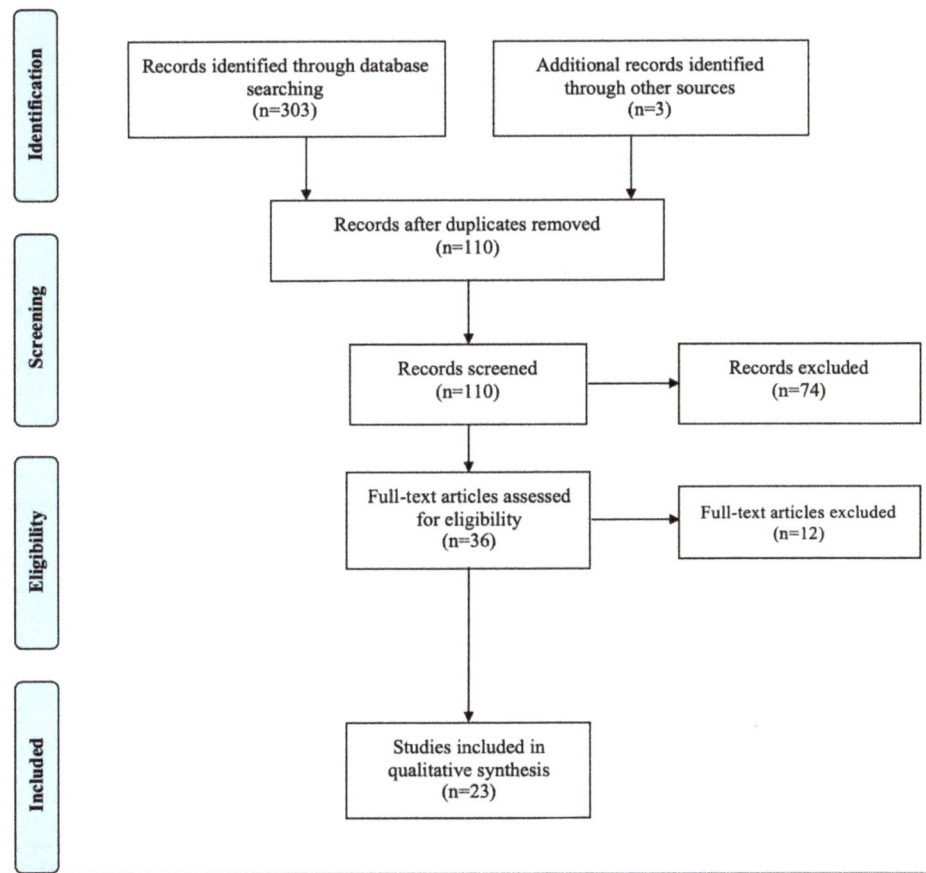

Figure A1. Flow diagram of the database search, screening and inclusion of the studies (modified after the PRISMA guidelines [45].

References

1. Wang, H.; Naghavi, M.; Allen, C.; Barber, R.M.; Bhutta, Z.A.; Carter, A.; Casey, D.C.; Charlson, F.J.; Chen, A.Z.; Coates, M.M.; et al. Global, Regional, and national life expectancy, all-cause mortality, and cause-specific mortality for 249 causes of death, 1980–2015: A systematic analysis for the Global Burden of Disease Study 2015. *Lancet* **2016**, *388*, 1459–1544. [CrossRef]
2. van Riet, E.E.S.; Hoes, A.W.; Wagenaar, K.P.; Limburg, A.; Landman, M.A.J.; Rutten, F.H. Epidemiology of heart failure: The prevalence of heart failure and ventricular dysfunction in older adults over time. A systematic review. *Eur. J. Heart Fail.* **2016**, *18*, 242–252. [CrossRef] [PubMed]
3. Heidenreich, P.A.; Albert, N.M.; Allen, L.A.; Bluemke, D.A.; Butler, J.; Fonarow, G.C.; Ikonomidis, J.S.; Khavjou, O.; Konstam, M.A.; Maddox, T.M.; et al. Forecasting the impact of heart failure in the United States: A policy statement from the American Heart Association. *Circ. Heart Fail.* **2013**, *6*, 606–619. [CrossRef] [PubMed]
4. Bass, N.M. The Cellular Fatty Acid Binding Proteins: Aspects of Structure, Regulation, and Function. In *International Review of Cytology*; Elsevier: Amsterdam, The Netherlands, 1988; Volume 111, pp. 143–184. ISBN 978-0-12-364511-1.

5. Veerkamp, J.H.; Peeters, R.A.; Maatman, R.G. Structural and functional features of different types of cytoplasmic fatty acid-binding proteins. *Biochim. Biophys. Acta* **1991**, *1081*, 1–24. [CrossRef]
6. Otaki, Y.; Watanabe, T.; Takahashi, H.; Hirayama, A.; Narumi, T.; Kadowaki, S.; Honda, Y.; Arimoto, T.; Shishido, T.; Miyamoto, T.; et al. Association of Heart-Type Fatty Acid-Binding Protein with Cardiovascular Risk Factors and All-Cause Mortality in the General Population: The Takahata Study. *PLoS ONE* **2014**, *9*, e94834. [CrossRef]
7. Fatty Acid Binding Protein Family|HUGO GENE Nomenclature Committee. Available online: https://www.genenames.org/data/genegroup/#!/group/550 (accessed on 2 January 2019).
8. Chmurzyńska, A. The multigene family of fatty acid-binding proteins (FABPs): Function, structure and polymorphism. *J. Appl. Genet.* **2006**, *47*, 39–48. [CrossRef]
9. Hostetler, H.A.; McIntosh, A.L.; Atshaves, B.P.; Storey, S.M.; Payne, H.R.; Kier, A.B.; Schroeder, F. L-FABP directly interacts with PPARalpha in cultured primary hepatocytes. *J. Lipid Res.* **2009**, *50*, 1663–1675. [CrossRef]
10. Tan, N.-S.; Shaw, N.S.; Vinckenbosch, N.; Liu, P.; Yasmin, R.; Desvergne, B.; Wahli, W.; Noy, N. Selective cooperation between fatty acid binding proteins and peroxisome proliferator-activated receptors in regulating transcription. *Mol. Cell. Biol.* **2002**, *22*, 5114–5127. [CrossRef]
11. Das, U.N. Heart-type fatty acid-binding protein (H-FABP) and coronary heart disease. *Indian Heart J.* **2016**, *68*, 16–18. [CrossRef]
12. Li, A.; Wu, L.; Wang, X.; Xin, Y.; Zan, L. Tissue expression analysis, cloning and characterization of the 5′-regulatory region of the bovine FABP3 gene. *Mol. Biol. Rep.* **2016**, *43*, 991–998. [CrossRef]
13. Yamamoto, Y.; Kida, H.; Kagawa, Y.; Yasumoto, Y.; Miyazaki, H.; Islam, A.; Ogata, M.; Yanagawa, Y.; Mitsushima, D.; Fukunaga, K.; et al. FABP3 in the Anterior Cingulate Cortex Modulates the Methylation Status of the Glutamic Acid Decarboxylase67 Promoter Region. *J. Neurosci.* **2018**, *38*, 10411–10423. [CrossRef] [PubMed]
14. Liebetrau, C.; Nef, H.M.; Dörr, O.; Gaede, L.; Hoffmann, J.; Hahnel, A.; Rolf, A.; Troidl, C.; Lackner, K.J.; Keller, T.; et al. Release kinetics of early ischaemic biomarkers in a clinical model of acute myocardial infarction. *Heart* **2014**, *100*, 652–657. [CrossRef] [PubMed]
15. Yoshimoto, K.; Tanaka, T.; Somiya, K.; Tsuji, R.; Okamoto, F.; Kawamura, K.; Ohkaru, Y.; Asayama, K.; Ishii, H. Human heart-type cytoplasmic fatty acid-binding protein as an indicator of acute myocardial infarction. *Heart Vessel.* **1995**, *10*, 304–309. [CrossRef] [PubMed]
16. Ishimura, S.; Furuhashi, M.; Watanabe, Y.; Hoshina, K.; Fuseya, T.; Mita, T.; Okazaki, Y.; Koyama, M.; Tanaka, M.; Akasaka, H.; et al. Circulating Levels of Fatty Acid-Binding Protein Family and Metabolic Phenotype in the General Population. *PLoS ONE* **2013**, *8*, e81318. [CrossRef] [PubMed]
17. Burch, P.M.; Pogoryelova, O.; Goldstein, R.; Bennett, D.; Guglieri, M.; Straub, V.; Bushby, K.; Lochmüller, H.; Morris, C. Muscle-Derived Proteins as Serum Biomarkers for Monitoring Disease Progression in Three Forms of Muscular Dystrophy. *J. Neuromuscul. Dis.* **2015**, *2*, 241–255. [CrossRef] [PubMed]
18. Gunes, F.; Asik, M.; Temiz, A.; Vural, A.; Sen, H.; Binnetoglu, E.; Bozkurt, N.; Tekeli, Z.; Erbag, G.; Ukinc, K.; et al. Serum H-FABP levels in patients with hypothyroidism. *Wien. Klin. Wochenschr.* **2014**, *126*, 727–733. [CrossRef]
19. Varrone, F.; Gargano, B.; Carullo, P.; Di Silvestre, D.; De Palma, A.; Grasso, L.; Di Somma, C.; Mauri, P.; Benazzi, L.; Franzone, A.; et al. The circulating level of FABP3 is an indirect biomarker of microRNA-1. *J. Am. Coll. Cardiol.* **2013**, *61*, 88–95. [CrossRef]
20. Fischer, T.A.; McNeil, P.L.; Khakee, R.; Finn, P.; Kelly, R.A.; Pfeffer, M.A.; Pfeffer, J.M. Cardiac Myocyte Membrane Wounding in the Abruptly Pressure-Overloaded Rat Heart Under High Wall Stress. *Hypertension* **1997**, *30*, 1041–1046. [CrossRef]
21. Iida, M.; Yamazaki, M.; Honjo, H.; Kodama, I.; Kamiya, K. Predictive value of heart-type fatty acid-binding protein for left ventricular remodelling and clinical outcome of hypertensive patients with mild-to-moderate aortic valve diseases. *J. Hum. Hypertens.* **2007**, *21*, 551–557. [CrossRef]
22. Ye, X.; He, Y.; Wang, S.; Wong, G.T.; Irwin, M.G.; Xia, Z. Heart-type fatty acid binding protein (H-FABP) as a biomarker for acute myocardial injury and long-term post-ischemic prognosis. *Acta Pharmacol. Sin.* **2018**, *39*, 1155. [CrossRef]
23. Kleine, A.H.; Glatz, J.F.C.; Van Nieuwenhoven, F.A.; Van der Vusse, G.J. Release of heart fatty acid-binding protein into plasma after acute myocardial infarction in man. In *Lipid Metabolism in the Healthy and Disease Heart*; van der Vusse, G.J., Stam, H., Eds.; Developments in Molecular and Cellular Biochemistry; Springer US: Boston, MA, USA, 1992; pp. 155–162. ISBN 978-1-4615-3514-0.

24. Binas, B.; Danneberg, H.; McWhir, J.; Mullins, L.; Clark, A.J. Requirement for the heart-type fatty acid binding protein in cardiac fatty acid utilization. *FASEB J.* **1999**, *13*, 805–812. [CrossRef] [PubMed]
25. Binas, B.; Erol, E. FABPs as determinants of myocellular and hepatic fuel metabolism. *Mol. Cell. Biochem.* **2007**, *299*, 75–84. [CrossRef] [PubMed]
26. Tang, M.K.; Kindler, P.M.; Cai, D.Q.; Chow, P.H.; Li, M.; Lee, K.K.H. Heart-type fatty acid binding proteins are upregulated during terminal differentiation of mouse cardiomyocytes, as revealed by proteomic analysis. *Cell Tissue Res.* **2004**, *316*, 339–347. [CrossRef] [PubMed]
27. Wang, S.; Zhou, Y.; Andreyev, O.; Hoyt, R.F.; Singh, A.; Hunt, T.; Horvath, K.A. Overexpression of FABP3 inhibits human bone marrow derived mesenchymal stem cell proliferation but enhances their survival in hypoxia. *Exp. Cell Res.* **2014**, *323*, 56–65. [CrossRef]
28. Zhu, C.; Hu, D.L.; Liu, Y.Q.; Zhang, Q.J.; Chen, F.K.; Kong, X.Q.; Cao, K.J.; Zhang, J.S.; Qian, L.M. Fabp3 inhibits proliferation and promotes apoptosis of embryonic myocardial cells. *Cell Biochem. Biophys.* **2011**, *60*, 259–266. [CrossRef]
29. Shen, Y.; Song, G.; Liu, Y.; Zhou, L.; Liu, H.; Kong, X.; Sheng, Y.; Cao, K.; Qian, L. Silencing of FABP3 inhibits proliferation and promotes apoptosis in embryonic carcinoma cells. *Cell Biochem. Biophys.* **2013**, *66*, 139–146. [CrossRef]
30. Liu, Y.-Q.; Song, G.-X.; Liu, H.-L.; Wang, X.-J.; Shen, Y.-H.; Zhou, L.-J.; Jin, J.; Liu, M.; Shi, C.-M.; Qian, L.-M. Silencing of FABP3 leads to apoptosis-induced mitochondrial dysfunction and stimulates Wnt signaling in zebrafish. *Mol. Med. Rep.* **2013**, *8*, 806–812. [CrossRef]
31. Wang, X.; Zhou, L.; Jin, J.; Yang, Y.; Song, G.; Shen, Y.; Liu, H.; Liu, M.; Shi, C.; Qian, L. Knockdown of FABP3 impairs cardiac development in Zebrafish through the retinoic acid signaling pathway. *Int. J. Mol. Sci.* **2013**, *14*, 13826–13841. [CrossRef]
32. Zhuang, L.; Li, C.; Chen, Q.; Jin, Q.; Wu, L.; Lu, L.; Yan, X.; Chen, K. Fatty acid-binding protein 3 contributes to ischemic heart injury by regulating cardiac myocyte apoptosis and MAPK pathways. *Am. J. Physiol. Heart Circ. Physiol.* **2019**, *316*, H971–H984. [CrossRef]
33. Zhang, Y.; Huang, R.; Zhou, W.; Zhao, Q.; Lü, Z. miR-192-5p mediates hypoxia/reoxygenation-induced apoptosis in H9c2 cardiomyocytes via targeting of FABP3. *J. Biochem. Mol. Toxicol.* **2017**, *31*, e21873. [CrossRef]
34. Chen, K.; Chen, Q.J.; Wang, L.J.; Liu, Z.H.; Zhang, Q.; Yang, K.; Wang, H.B.; Yan, X.X.; Zhu, Z.B.; Du, R.; et al. Increment of HFABP Level in Coronary Artery In-Stent Restenosis Segments in Diabetic and Nondiabetic Minipigs: HFABP Overexpression Promotes Multiple Pathway-Related Inflammation, Growth and Migration in Human Vascular Smooth Muscle Cells. *J. Vasc. Res.* **2016**, *53*, 27–38. [CrossRef] [PubMed]
35. Arı, H.; Tokaç, M.; Alihanoğlu, Y.; Kıyıcı, A.; Kayrak, M.; Arı, M.; Sönmez, O.; Gök, H. Relationship between heart-type fatty acid-binding protein levels and coronary artery disease in exercise stress testing: An observational study. *Anadolu Kardiyol. Derg.* **2011**, *11*, 685–691. [PubMed]
36. Lichtenauer, M.; Jirak, P.; Wernly, B.; Paar, V.; Rohm, I.; Jung, C.; Schernthaner, C.; Kraus, J.; Motloch, L.J.; Yilmaz, A.; et al. A comparative analysis of novel cardiovascular biomarkers in patients with chronic heart failure. *Eur. J. Intern. Med.* **2017**, *44*, 31–38. [CrossRef] [PubMed]
37. Okamoto, F.; Sohmiya, K.; Ohkaru, Y.; Kawamura, K.; Asayama, K.; Kimura, H.; Nishimura, S.; Ishii, H.; Sunahara, N.; Tanaka, T. Human heart-type cytoplasmic fatty acid-binding protein (H-FABP) for the diagnosis of acute myocardial infarction. Clinical evaluation of H-FABP in comparison with myoglobin and creatine kinase isoenzyme MB. *Clin. Chem. Lab. Med.* **2000**, *38*, 231–238. [CrossRef]
38. Dupuy, A.M.; Cristol, J.P.; Kuster, N.; Reynier, R.; Lefebvre, S.; Badiou, S.; Jreige, R.; Sebbane, M. Performances of the heart fatty acid protein assay for the rapid diagnosis of acute myocardial infarction in ED patients. *Am. J. Emerg. Med.* **2015**, *33*, 326–330. [CrossRef]
39. Ruff, C.T.; Bonaca, M.P.; Kosowsky, J.M.; Conrad, M.J.; Murphy, S.A.; Jarolim, P.; Donahoe, S.M.; O'Donoghue, M.L.; Morrow, D.A. Evaluation of the diagnostic performance of heart-type fatty acid binding protein in the BWH-TIMI ED chest pain study. *J. Thromb. Thrombolysis* **2013**, *36*, 361–367. [CrossRef]
40. Ho, S.-K.; Wu, Y.-W.; Tseng, W.-K.; Leu, H.-B.; Yin, W.-H.; Lin, T.-H.; Chang, K.-C.; Wang, J.-H.; Yeh, H.-I.; Wu, C.-C.; et al. The prognostic significance of heart-type fatty acid binding protein in patients with stable coronary heart disease. *Sci. Rep.* **2018**, *8*, 14410. [CrossRef]
41. Body, R.; Burrows, G.; Carley, S.; Lewis, P.S. The Manchester Acute Coronary Syndromes (MACS) decision rule: Validation with a new automated assay for heart-type fatty acid binding protein. *Emerg. Med. J.* **2015**, *32*, 769–774. [CrossRef]

42. Schoenenberger, A.W.; Stallone, F.; Walz, B.; Bergner, M.; Twerenbold, R.; Reichlin, T.; Zogg, B.; Jaeger, C.; Erne, P.; Mueller, C. Incremental value of heart-type fatty acid-binding protein in suspected acute myocardial infarction early after symptom onset. *Eur. Heart J. Acute Cardiovasc. Care* **2016**, *5*, 185–192. [CrossRef]
43. Bruins Slot, M.H.E.; Rutten, F.H.; van der Heijden, G.J.M.G.; Doevendans, P.A.; Mast, E.G.; Bredero, A.C.; van der Spoel, O.P.; Glatz, J.F.C.; Hoes, A.W. Diagnostic value of a heart-type fatty acid-binding protein (H-FABP) bedside test in suspected acute coronary syndrome in primary care. *Int. J. Cardiol.* **2013**, *168*, 1485–1489. [CrossRef]
44. Glatz, J.F.; Renneberg, R. Added value of H-FABP as a plasma biomarker for the early evaluation of suspected acute coronary syndrome. *Clin. Lipidol.* **2014**, *9*, 205–220. [CrossRef]
45. Moher, D.; Liberati, A.; Tetzlaff, J.; Altman, D.G.; PRISMA Group. Preferred reporting items for systematic reviews and meta-analyses: The PRISMA statement. *PLoS Med.* **2009**, *6*, e1000097. [CrossRef]
46. Ponikowski, P.; Voors, A.A.; Anker, S.D.; Bueno, H.; Cleland, J.G.F.; Coats, A.J.S.; Falk, V.; González-Juanatey, J.R.; Harjola, V.-P.; Jankowska, E.A.; et al. 2016 ESC Guidelines for the diagnosis and treatment of acute and chronic heart failure: The Task Force for the diagnosis and treatment of acute and chronic heart failure of the European Society of Cardiology (ESC)Developed with the special contribution of the Heart Failure Association (HFA) of the ESC. *Eur. Heart J.* **2016**, *37*, 2129–2200. [PubMed]
47. Yancy, C.W.; Jessup, M.; Bozkurt, B.; Butler, J.; Casey, D.E.; Colvin, M.M.; Drazner, M.H.; Filippatos, G.S.; Fonarow, G.C.; Givertz, M.M.; et al. 2017 ACC/AHA/HFSA Focused Update of the 2013 ACCF/AHA Guideline for the Management of Heart Failure: A Report of the American College of Cardiology/American Heart Association Task Force on Clinical Practice Guidelines and the Heart Failure Society of America. *J. Am. Coll. Cardiol.* **2017**, *70*, 776–803. [PubMed]
48. Pufulete, M.; Maishman, R.; Dabner, L.; Higgins, J.P.T.; Rogers, C.A.; Dayer, M.; MacLeod, J.; Purdy, S.; Hollingworth, W.; Schou, M.; et al. B-type natriuretic peptide-guided therapy for heart failure (HF): A systematic review and meta-analysis of individual participant data (IPD) and aggregate data. *Syst. Rev.* **2018**, *7*, 112. [CrossRef] [PubMed]
49. Maisel, A.; Mueller, C.; Adams, K.; Anker, S.D.; Aspromonte, N.; Cleland, J.G.F.; Cohen-Solal, A.; Dahlstrom, U.; DeMaria, A.; Di Somma, S.; et al. State of the art: Using natriuretic peptide levels in clinical practice. *Eur. J. Heart Fail.* **2008**, *10*, 824–839. [CrossRef]
50. Demissei, B.G.; Valente, M.A.E.; Cleland, J.G.; O'Connor, C.M.; Metra, M.; Ponikowski, P.; Teerlink, J.R.; Cotter, G.; Davison, B.; Givertz, M.M.; et al. Optimizing clinical use of biomarkers in high-risk acute heart failure patients. *Eur. J. Heart Fail.* **2016**, *18*, 269–280. [CrossRef]
51. Bivona, G.; Agnello, L.; Bellia, C.; Lo Sasso, B.; Ciaccio, M. Diagnostic and prognostic value of H-FABP in acute coronary syndrome: Still evidence to bring. *Clin. Biochem.* **2018**, *58*, 1–4. [CrossRef]
52. Xu, L.-Q.; Yang, Y.-M.; Tong, H.; Xu, C.-F. Early Diagnostic Performance of Heart-Type Fatty Acid Binding Protein in Suspected Acute Myocardial Infarction: Evidence from a Meta-Analysis of Contemporary Studies. *Heart Lung Circ.* **2018**, *27*, 503–512. [CrossRef]
53. Bajaj, A.; Rathor, P.; Sehgal, V.; Shetty, A.; Kabak, B.; Hosur, S. Risk stratification in acute pulmonary embolism with heart-type fatty acid-binding protein: A meta-analysis. *J. Crit. Care* **2015**, *30*, 1151-e1. [CrossRef]
54. Qian, H.-Y.; Huang, J.; Yang, Y.-J.; Yang, Y.-M.; Li, Z.-Z.; Zhang, J.-M. Heart-type Fatty Acid Binding Protein in the Assessment of Acute Pulmonary Embolism. *Am. J. Med. Sci.* **2016**, *352*, 557–562. [CrossRef]
55. Dellas, C.; Lobo, J.L.; Rivas, A.; Ballaz, A.; Portillo, A.K.; Nieto, R.; del Rey, J.M.; Zamorano, J.L.; Lankeit, M.; Jiménez, D. Risk stratification of acute pulmonary embolism based on clinical parameters, H-FABP and multidetector CT. *Int. J. Cardiol.* **2018**, *265*, 223–228. [CrossRef] [PubMed]
56. Konstantinides, S.V.; Meyer, G.; Becattini, C.; Bueno, H.; Geersing, G.-J.; Harjola, V.-P.; Huisman, M.V.; Humbert, M.; Jennings, C.S.; Jiménez, D.; et al. 2019 ESC Guidelines for the diagnosis and management of acute pulmonary embolism developed in collaboration with the European Respiratory Society (ERS). *Eur. Heart J.* **2019**, 1–61. [CrossRef]
57. van der Vusse, G.J.; Glatz, J.F.; Stam, H.C.; Reneman, R.S. Fatty acid homeostasis in the normoxic and ischemic heart. *Physiol. Rev.* **1992**, *72*, 881–940. [CrossRef]
58. Niizeki, T.; Takeishi, Y.; Arimoto, T.; Takahashi, T.; Okuyama, H.; Takabatake, N.; Nozaki, N.; Hirono, O.; Tsunoda, Y.; Shishido, T.; et al. Combination of heart-type fatty acid binding protein and brain natriuretic peptide can reliably risk stratify patients hospitalized for chronic heart failure. *Circ. J.* **2005**, *69*, 922–927. [CrossRef]

59. Niizeki, T.; Takeishi, Y.; Arimoto, T.; Nozaki, N.; Hirono, O.; Watanabe, T.; Nitobe, J.; Miyashita, T.; Miyamoto, T.; Koyama, Y.; et al. Persistently increased serum concentration of heart-type fatty acid-binding protein predicts adverse clinical outcomes in patients with chronic heart failure. *Circ. J.* **2008**, *72*, 109–114. [CrossRef] [PubMed]
60. Hoffmann, U.; Espeter, F.; Weiß, C.; Ahmad-Nejad, P.; Lang, S.; Brueckmann, M.; Akin, I.; Neumaier, M.; Borggrefe, M.; Behnes, M. Ischemic biomarker heart-type fatty acid binding protein (hFABP) in acute heart failure-diagnostic and prognostic insights compared to NT-proBNP and troponin I. *BMC Cardiovasc. Disord.* **2015**, *15*, 50. [CrossRef] [PubMed]
61. Ishino, M.; Shishido, T.; Arimoto, T.; Takahashi, H.; Miyashita, T.; Miyamoto, T.; Nitobe, J.; Watanabe, T.; Kubota, I. Heart-Type Fatty Acid Binding Protein (H-FABP) in Acute Decompensated Heart Failure. *J. Card. Fail.* **2010**, *16*, S166. [CrossRef]
62. Jirak, P.; Fejzic, D.; Paar, V.; Wernly, B.; Pistulli, R.; Rohm, I.; Jung, C.; Hoppe, U.C.; Schulze, P.C.; Lichtenauer, M.; et al. Influences of Ivabradine treatment on serum levels of cardiac biomarkers sST2, GDF-15, suPAR and H-FABP in patients with chronic heart failure. *Acta Pharmacol. Sin.* **2018**, *39*, 1189. [CrossRef] [PubMed]
63. Sun, Y.-P.; Wei, C.-P.; Ma, S.-C.; Zhang, Y.-F.; Qiao, L.-Y.; Li, D.-H.; Shan, R.-B. Effect of Carvedilol on Serum Heart-type Fatty Acid-binding Protein, Brain Natriuretic Peptide, and Cardiac Function in Patients with Chronic Heart Failure. *J. Cardiovasc. Pharmacol.* **2015**, *65*, 480–484. [CrossRef]
64. Kazimierczyk, E.; Kazimierczyk, R.; Harasim-Symbor, E.; Kaminski, K.; Sobkowicz, B.; Chabowski, A.; Tycinska, A. Persistently elevated plasma heart-type fatty acid binding protein concentration is related with poor outcome in acute decompensated heart failure patients. *Clin. Chim. Acta* **2018**, *487*, 48–53. [CrossRef] [PubMed]
65. Shirakabe, A.; Hata, N.; Kobayashi, N.; Okazaki, H.; Matsushita, M.; Shibata, Y.; Uchiyama, S.; Sawatani, T.; Asai, K.; Shimizu, W. Worsening renal failure in patients with acute heart failure: The importance of cardiac biomarkers. *ESC Heart Fail.* **2019**, *6*, 416–427. [CrossRef] [PubMed]
66. Kutsuzawa, D.; Arimoto, T.; Watanabe, T.; Shishido, T.; Miyamoto, T.; Miyashita, T.; Takahashi, H.; Niizeki, T.; Takeishi, Y.; Kubota, I. Ongoing myocardial damage in patients with heart failure and preserved ejection fraction. *J. Cardiol.* **2012**, *60*, 454–461. [CrossRef] [PubMed]
67. Dinh, W.; Nickl, W.; Füth, R.; Lankisch, M.; Hess, G.; Zdunek, D.; Scheffold, T.; Barroso, M.C.; Tiroch, K.; Ziegler, D.; et al. High sensitive troponin T and heart fatty acid binding protein: Novel biomarker in heart failure with normal ejection fraction? A cross-sectional study. *BMC Cardiovasc. Disord.* **2011**, *11*, 41. [CrossRef]
68. Abstracts Programme. *Eur. J. Heart Fail.* **2019**, *21*, 5–592. [CrossRef]
69. Mirna, M.; Wernly, B.; Paar, V.; Jung, C.; Jirak, P.; Figulla, H.-R.; Kretzschmar, D.; Franz, M.; Hoppe, U.C.; Lichtenauer, M.; et al. Multi-biomarker analysis in patients after transcatheter aortic valve implantation (TAVI). *Biomarkers* **2018**, *23*, 773–780. [CrossRef]
70. Otaki, Y.; Arimoto, T.; Takahashi, H.; Kadowaki, S.; Ishigaki, D.; Narumi, T.; Honda, Y.; Iwayama, T.; Nishiyama, S.; Shishido, T.; et al. Prognostic value of myocardial damage markers in patients with chronic heart failure with atrial fibrillation. *Intern. Med.* **2014**, *53*, 661–668. [CrossRef]
71. Rader, F.; Pujara, A.C.; Pattakos, G.; Rajeswaran, J.; Li, L.; Castel, L.; Chung, M.K.; Gillinov, A.M.; Costantini, O.; Van Wagoner, D.R.; et al. Perioperative heart-type fatty acid binding protein levels in atrial fibrillation after cardiac surgery. *Heart Rhythm* **2013**, *10*, 153–157. [CrossRef]
72. Shingu, Y.; Yokota, T.; Takada, S.; Niwano, H.; Ooka, T.; Katoh, H.; Tachibana, T.; Kubota, S.; Matsui, Y. Decreased gene expression of fatty acid binding protein 3 in the atrium of patients with new onset of atrial fibrillation in cardiac perioperative phase. *J. Cardiol.* **2018**, *71*, 65–70. [CrossRef]
73. Mirna, M.; Rohm, I.; Jirak, P.; Wernly, B.; Bäz, L.; Paar, V.; Kretzschmar, D.; Hoppe, U.C.; Schulze, P.C.; Lichtenauer, M.; et al. Analysis of Novel Cardiovascular Biomarkers in Patients With Pulmonary Hypertension (PH). *Heart Lung Circ.* **2019**. [CrossRef]
74. Zoair, A.; Mawlana, W.; Abo-Elenin, A.; Korrat, M. Serum Level of Heart-Type Fatty Acid Binding Protein (H-FABP) Before and After Treatment of Congestive Heart Failure in Children. *Pediatr. Cardiol.* **2015**, *36*, 1722–1727. [CrossRef] [PubMed]
75. Sun, Y.-P.; Wang, W.-D.; Ma, S.-C.; Wang, L.-Y.; Qiao, L.-Y.; Zhang, L.-P. Changes of heart-type fatty acid-binding protein in children with chronic heart failure and its significance. *Chin. J. Contemp. Pediatr.* **2013**, *15*, 99–101.

76. Hayabuchi, Y.; Inoue, M.; Watanabe, N.; Sakata, M.; Ohnishi, T.; Kagami, S. Serum concentration of heart-type fatty acid-binding protein in children and adolescents with congenital heart disease. *Circ. J.* **2011**, *75*, 1992–1997. [CrossRef]
77. Takahashi, T.; Shishido, T.; Watanabe, K.; Sugai, T.; Toshima, T.; Kinoshita, D.; Yokoyama, M.; Tamura, H.; Nishiyama, S.; Takahashi, H.; et al. Ventricular wall stress and silent myocardial damage are associated with pulse pressure in the general population. *J. Clin. Hypertens.* **2018**, *20*, 1319–1326. [CrossRef] [PubMed]
78. Uitterdijk, A.; Sneep, S.; van Duin, R.W.B.; Krabbendam-Peters, I.; Gorsse-Bakker, C.; Duncker, D.J.; van der Giessen, W.J.; van Beusekom, H.M.M. Serial measurement of hFABP and high-sensitivity troponin I post-PCI in STEMI: How fast and accurate can myocardial infarct size and no-reflow be predicted? *Am. J. Physiol. Heart Circ. Physiol.* **2013**, *305*, H1104–H1110. [CrossRef] [PubMed]
79. Yancy, C.W.; Jessup, M.; Bozkurt, B.; Butler, J.; Casey, D.E.; Drazner, M.H.; Fonarow, G.C.; Geraci, S.A.; Horwich, T.; Januzzi, J.L.; et al. 2013 ACCF/AHA Guideline for the Management of Heart Failure: A Report of the American College of Cardiology Foundation/American Heart Association Task Force on Practice Guidelines. *J. Am. Coll. Cardiol.* **2013**, *62*, e147–e239. [CrossRef] [PubMed]
80. Dalos, D.; Spinka, G.; Schneider, M.; Wernly, B.; Paar, V.; Hoppe, U.; Litschauer, B.; Strametz-Juranek, J.; Sponder, M. New Cardiovascular Biomarkers in Ischemic Heart Disease—GDF-15, A Probable Predictor for Ejection Fraction. *J. Clin. Med.* **2019**, *8*, 924. [CrossRef]
81. Cabiati, M.; Caselli, C.; Caruso, R.; Prescimone, T.; Verde, A.; Botta, L.; Parodi, O.; Ry, S.D.; Giannessi, D. High peripheral levels of h-FABP are associated with poor prognosis in end-stage heart failure patients with mechanical circulatory support. *Biomark. Med.* **2013**, *7*, 481–492. [CrossRef]

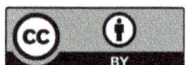

© 2020 by the authors. Licensee MDPI, Basel, Switzerland. This article is an open access article distributed under the terms and conditions of the Creative Commons Attribution (CC BY) license (http://creativecommons.org/licenses/by/4.0/).

MDPI
St. Alban-Anlage 66
4052 Basel
Switzerland
Tel. +41 61 683 77 34
Fax +41 61 302 89 18
www.mdpi.com

Journal of Clinical Medicine Editorial Office
E-mail: jcm@mdpi.com
www.mdpi.com/journal/jcm

www.ingramcontent.com/pod-product-compliance
Lightning Source LLC
LaVergne TN
LVHW070252100526
838202LV00015B/2212